Medicine: The Bare Bones

Medicine: The Bare Bones

A Comprehensive Systematic Approach

E. H. I. Friedman, M.Sc. (Community Med) MB. ChB.
Specialist in Community Medicine, South Manchester Health Authority, UK
Tutor in Community Medicine University of Manchester, UK

R. E. Moshy, FRCR
Consultant Radiologist, Peterborough District Hospital, UK.
Clinical Teacher (Radiodiagnosis) Universities of Cambridge & Leicester, UK

A Wiley Medical Publication

JOHN WILEY & SONS

Chichester · New York · Brisbane · Toronto · Singapore

Library of Congress Cataloging-in-Publication Data:

Friedman, E. H. I.

Medicine, the bare bones.

(A Wiley medical publication)
Bibliography: p.
Includes index.
1. Medicine—Outlines, syllabi, etc. I. Moshy, R. E. II. Title. III. Series. [DNLM: 1. Curriculum—outlines. 2. Medicine—outlines. W 18 F9115m]
R130.3.F74 1986 610'.02'02 85-26619
ISBN 0 471 90823 1 (pbk.)

British Library Cataloguing in Publication Data:

Friedman, E. H. I.
Medicine: the bare bones: a comprehensive systematic approach.
1. Medicine
I. Title II. Moshy, R. E.
610 R130

ISBN 0 471 90823 1

Printed and bound in Great Britain.

To Sandra Friedman

without whose help and perseverence,
this book could not have been written.

Greengages are sweet, lamb chops
exhilarating g.w.s!

Acknowledgements

Many individuals have contributed to the writing of this book and it would not be possible to thank them all. However special thanks are due to the following.

Dr. D. Ralston, Clinical Dean at University of Manchester Medical School, who kindly agreed to write a foreword.

The chapter reviewers who provided us with valuable feedback information:

Obstetrics & Gynaecology
Mr. B. Hackman Consultant Obstetrician & Gynaecologist, Peterborough District Hospital, UK

Paediatrics
Dr. A. Bradbury Consultant Paediatrician, University Hospital of South Manchester, UK

Psychiatry
Drs. R. Williams & D. Wozencroft Consultant Psychiatrists, Peterborough District Hospital, UK

Neurology
Sir John Walton, Warden Green College, Radcliffe Observatory, UK

Ophthalmology
Mr. E. Rosen Consultant Ophthalmologist, Manchester Royal Eye Hospital, UK

Ear, Nose & Throat
Mr. R. Cawood Consultant ENT Surgeon, Peterborough District Hospital, UK

Respiratory System
Dr. A. Hilton Consultant Respiratory Physician, Wythenshawe Hospital, Manchester, UK

Cardiovascular System
Dr. R. Smith Consultant Physician, North Tees General Hospital, UK

Gastroenterology
Dr. P. Miller Consultant Gastroenterologist, University Hospital of South Manchester, UK & *Mr. D. Jones*, Senior Surgical Registrar, Peterborough District Hospital, UK

Haematology
Dr. S. Fairham Consultant Haematologist, Peterborough District Hospital, UK

Endocrinology, Metabolic Disorders & the Breast
Dr. C. Beardwell Consultant Physician, University Hospital of South Manchester, UK

Infectious Diseases
Dr. E. Wilson Consultant Microbiologist, Public Health Laboratory Service, Lincoln, UK

Dermatology
Dr. P. Hudson Consultant Dermatologist, Peterborough District Hospital, UK

Rheumatology
Dr. N. Williams Consultant Rheumatologist, Peterborough District Hospital, UK

Orthopaedics
Mr. D. Markham Consultant Orthopaedic Surgeon, Manchester Royal Infirmary, UK

Genito-urinary System

Dr. D. Ralston Consultant Physician, University Hospital of South Manchester, UK & *Mr. A. Turner* Consultant Urologist, Peterborough District Hospital, UK

Community Medicine

Dr. A. St Leger Specialist in Community Medicine, South Manchester Health Authority, UK

Dr. C. Scott General Practitioner, Whittlesey Cambridgeshire, UK, for proof reading assistance.

Dr. J. Moshy, St Mary's Hospital Waterbury, CT USA for the American Appendum to the Glossary

Miss J. B. Miller–Lawson for early secretarial help, before the authors decided to write the whole book on a word processor.

Our thanks also to a number of librarians esp *Mrs. M. Rushford* & *Mrs. S. Tee* (PGMS, Peterborough District Hospital, UK)

The publishers, **John Wiley & Sons Ltd**, have given us full assistance & encouragement throughout. Special thanks are due to *Mrs. M. Granger* & *Miss V. Waite*. Last but not least *Dr. J. Jarvis* UK Medical Editor, who took a special interest in bringing this book to the bookshelf.

Contents

Preface

This book is a concise yet comprehensive review of the undergraduate medical curriculum. Although primarily intended as a means of consolidation and revision for medical students approaching their final examinations, it is also eminently suitable for many other groups in the health care professions as a quick reference source and rapid checklist of the essentials of all the major clinical specialities.

During the course of preparing this book, we have consulted many different sources, including textbooks, journals and lectures. To the junior doctor it will be of value because it summarises investigations, differential diagnoses and management; for nurses and those in the paramedical professions the book will provide some insight into the diseases of patients which they help to care for; specialists and consultants will use parts of the book to brush up on subjects with which they may have become out of touch; lecturers and teachers will use it as a convenient summary of the student curriculum. The information included in the book is much greater than is required for success in the final medical undergraduate exam, and its format may prove to be a useful revision aid for those studying for higher medical qualifications.

Each system of the body is considered in turn with respect to medical and surgical aspects so that the reader can obtain a holistic view of each topic.

The form of each chapter is such that the reader can refer to lists for quick revision and the text for a more comprehensive survey of the subject matter. In order to reduce costs and make the most economical use of space there are many abbreviations. Most of these are in everyday use, e.g. Hb—haemoglobin; FBC—full blood count; we have provided a full glossary but we are confident that as you become familiar with the style, your need to refer to it will be minimal. In fact, as it stands, the glossary probably constitutes a comprehensive list of common medical abbreviations which on its own will act as a most useful tool to unravel the mysteries of "notes" and "request forms".

We have endeavoured to ensure that there are no errors in the book and to that end we have submitted each chapter to a practising specialist in the subject for checking. We are greatly indebted to these people for their advice and guidance.

Finally, although we hope to demonstrate that this book is more than just another superficial revision aid, we should stress that it has never been our intention to provide an "easy way out" of studying detailed medical textbooks and journals. What we have tried to produce here is a workbook to which students and doctors will add their own notes to the framework we have provided—the "bare bones" of medicine to which the reader will add the flesh.

DR. E. H. I. FRIEDMAN
DR. R. E. MOSHY 1985

Foreword

Medical students in the last phase of their course face a formidable task in revising the knowledge they have acquired over the years preceeding their final degree examinations.

Like so many undergraduates the authors made extensive notes throughout their clinical course and have used these as the initial basis for this book. Its rather novel format encompasses a large body of information in a compact fashion and will I am sure facilitate revision at a time of great pressure for most students.

A. J. RALSTON
Dean of Clinical Studies
University of Manchester, UK.

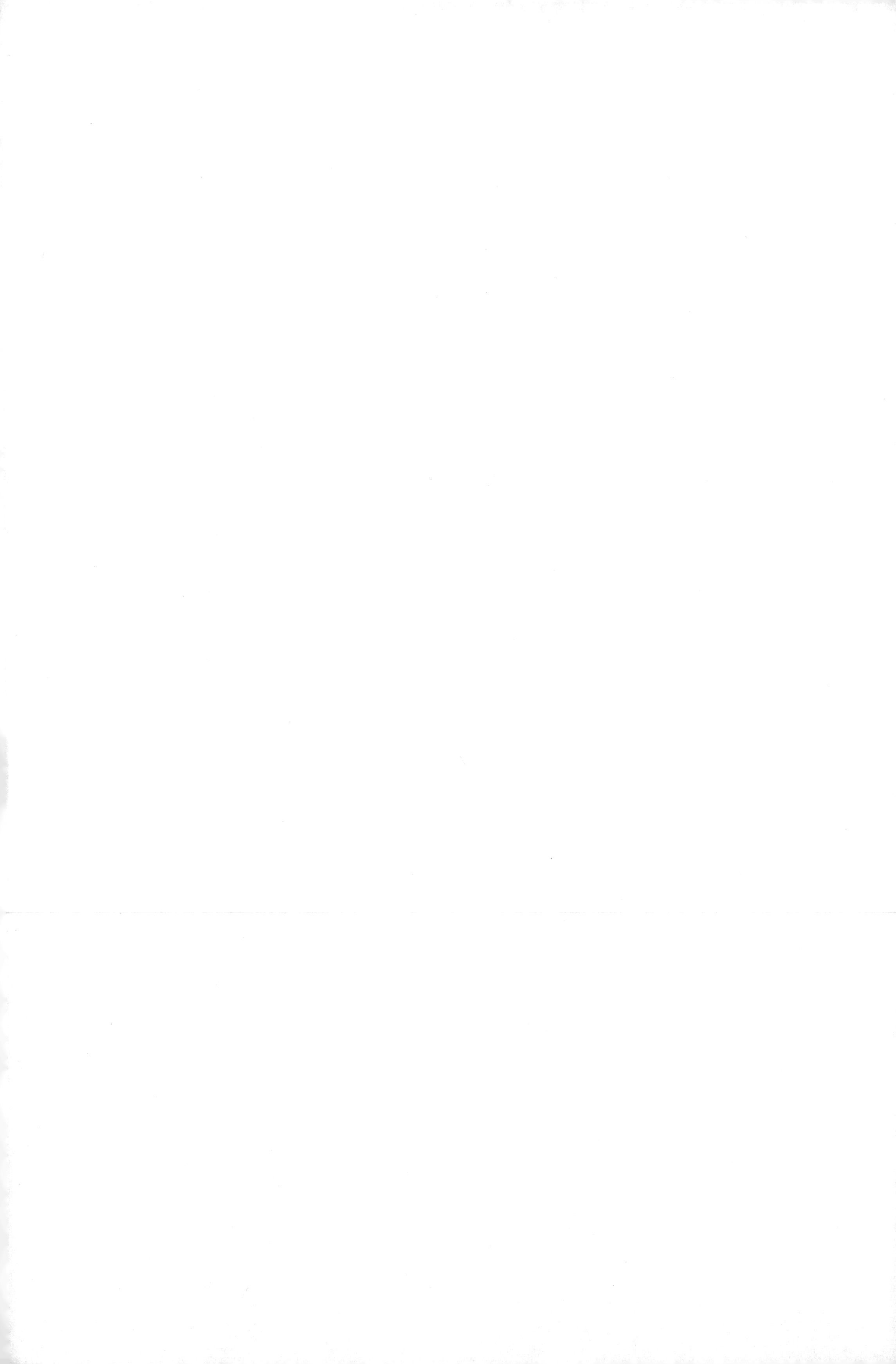

List of Lists

CHAPTER 3: PSYCHIATRY

CHAPTER 4: NEUROLOGY

CHAPTER 5: OPHTHALMOLOGY

CHAPTER 6: EAR, NOSE & THROAT

CHAPTER 7: RESPIRATORY SYSTEM

CHAPTER 11: ENDOCRINOLOGY, METABOLIC DISORDERS & THE BREAST

CHAPTER 12: INFECTIOUS DISEASES

CHAPTER 13: DERMATOLOGY

CHAPTER 14: RHEUMATOLOGY

CHAPTER 15: ORTHOPAEDICS

CHAPTER 16: GENITO-URINARY SYSTEM

CHAPTER 17: COMMUNITY MEDICINE

Glossary of Abbreviations

(*) Indicates an alternative abbreviation to be found in American Appendum to Glossary

Misc.

α	Alpha
β	Beta
γ	Gamma
&	And
?	Query(*)
#	Fracture
±	With or without
↓	Decrease or Decreasing, may refer to decrease in organ size
↑	Increase or Increasing, may refer to increase in organ size
−ve	Negative
+ve	Positive
++	To a great degree
1°	Primary
2°	Secondary
3°	Tertiary
4°	Quaternary
<	Less than
>	Greater than
⩾	Greater than or equal to
>>	Much greater than
=	Equal to
→	Leads to
μ	Micro
ˆI,II,IIIˆ	Limb ECG leads
ˆaVL,aVR,aVFˆ	Limb ECG leads
ˆV1–6ˆ	Precordial ECG leads
ˆPRˆ, ˆQRSˆ	Examples of ECG notation
[ ]	Concentration
△	Triangle
"	Inches
°	Degrees (angles)
°C	Degrees Celsius (temperature)
↑↑	Very high or very enlarged
↓↓	Very low or very diminished
£	Pound sterling
/	Per (in context)
/7	Days eg 3/7 = 3 days
/12	Months
/52	Weeks

A.

a	Artery (in context)
"a" waves	"a" venous waves
Ab	Antibody
Abd	Abduct
Abdo	Abdomen
ABO	A, B, O, blood group systems
Ac	Acute
a.c	Alternating current
ACh	Acetylcholine
ACMD	Advisory Committee on Misuse of Drugs
ACTH	Adrenocorticotrophic hormone
AdenoCa	Adenocarcinoma
ADH	Antidiuretic hormone
ADL	Activities of Daily Living
Admin	Administration
A&E	Accident & emergency(*)
AF	Atrial fibrillation
AFB	Acid fast bacillus
Afr	Africa
Ag	Antigen
AHA	Area Health Authority (now defunct)

AI	Aortic incompetence (Aortic Insufficiency)
AID	Artificial Insemination by Donor
AIDS	Acquired immune deficiency syndrome
AIH	Artificial Insemination by Husband
AIHA	Autoimmune haemolytic anaemia
AIMS	Association for Improvement in Maternity Services
Al^{3+}	Aluminium
ALA	Aminolaevulinic acid
Alc	Alcohol(*)
ALF	Acute liver failure
Alk phos	Alkaline phosphatase
ALL	Acute lymphatic leukaemia
ALT	Alanine transaminase
am	Morning
AMAb	Antimitochondrial antibodies
AML	Acute myeloid leukaemia
ANA	Antinuclear antibody
ANC	Antenatal Clinic(*)
Ank Sp	Ankylosing spondylitis
Ant	Anterior
Anticoags	Anticoagulants
AntiHBe	Hepatitis B e antibody
AntiHBc	Hepatitis B core antibody
AntiHBs	Hepatitis B surface antibody
A–P	Antero–posterior
APH	Antepartum haemorrhage
Approx	Approximately
APTT	Activated partial thromboplastin time
APUD	Amine Precursor Uptake & Decarboxylation
ARDS	Adult respiratory distress syndrome
ARF	Acute renal failure
ARM	Artificial Rupture of Membranes
As	Arsenic (in context)
AS	Aortic stenosis
Asc	Ascending
ASD	Atrial septal defect
ASOT	Anti-streptolysin "O" Titre(*)
Ass	Associated
AST	Aspartate transaminase
ATG	Anti-thymocytic globulin
ATN	Acute tubular necrosis
Aut Dom	Autosomal dominant
Aut Rec	Autosomal recessive
AV	Atrio–ventricular
A–V	Arterio–venous
Ave	Average(*)
AWR	Airways resistance
AXR	Abdominal X-Ray
B.	
Ba	Barium
BCG	Bacille–Calmette–Guerin (immunisation against TB)
bd	Twice daily(*)
b.o	Bowel open(*)
BG	Blood glucose(*)
Bi	Bismuth
Biochem	Biochemical
BMT	Bone marrow transplant
BP	Blood pressure
BPD	Biparietal Diameter
br	Branch
BS	Bowel sounds or Breath Sounds (in context)
C.	
c̄	With
C1	C1 component of complement
C3	C3 component of complement
Ca	General term for cancer
Ca^{2+}	Calcium or calcification (depends on context)
CABG	Coronary artery bypass graft
$CaCl_2$	Calcium chloride
CAH	Chronic active hepatitis
cal	Calories
C&S	Culture & sensitivity
CAPD	Continuous ambulatory peritoneal dialysis
CARD	Cardiology
CAT	Computed axial tomography (CT)(*)
$CaxPO_4$	Calcium phosphate product
CBD	Common bile duct
CCF	Congestive cardiac failure(*)
CCK-PZ	Cholecystokinin-pancreazymin
CCl_4	Carbon tetrachloride
CCNU	Chloroethylcyclohexylnitrosurea
CCU	Coronary care unit
CD	Conductive deafness
CDCA	Chenodeoxycholic acid
CDH	Congenital dislocaton of hip
CDSC	Communicable Diseases Surveillance Centre(*)
CEA	Carcino–embryonic antigen
CF	Cystic fibrosis
cf	Compare with
CFT	Complement fixation test
CGL	Chronic granulocytic leukaemia(*)
CHC	Community Health Councils
CHD	Congenital heart disease
chd	Carbohydrate(*)
Chr	Chronic
c/i	Contra-indication
Cigs	Cigarettes
CIN	Cervical Intraepithelial Neoplasia
Cl^-	Chloride
Cl.	Clostridium
Clin	Clinical(ly)
CLL	Chronic lymphatic leukaemia
CM	Community Medicine
cm	Centimetre
CMC	Carpometacarpal joint
CML	Chronic myeloid leukaemia

CMV	Cytomegalovirus
CNS	Central nervous system
CO	Cardiac output (in context)
CO	Carbon monoxide (in context)
C–O	Cardio–oesophageal(*)
CO_3	Carbonate
CoA	Coenzyme A
COAD	Chronic obstructive airways disease(*)
COCM	Congestive Obstructive Cardiomyopathy
Col Alk	Alkaline nasal wash
conc	Concentration
(C)cong	Congenital
CP	Cerebral palsy
CPAP	Continuous positive airway pressure
CPH	Chronic persistent hepatitis
CPK	Creatine phosphokinase
CPK-MB	Creatine phosphokinase isoenzyme
CPN	Community Psychiatric Nurse
Cr	Chromium
CRF	Chronic renal failure
Creps	Crepitations
CS_2	Carbon disulphide
CSOM	Chronic suppurative otitis media
Cu	Copper
Cv	Cervical
CVA	Cerebrovasular accident
CVP	Central venous pressure
CXR	Chest X-ray
Cyt.T	Cytotoxic drugs

D.

DAT	Differential agglutination test
D&C	Dilatation & Curettage
D&V	Diarrhoea & Vomiting
DD	Differential diagnosis(*)
DDAVP	Desmopressin
DDT	Chlorophenothane insecticide
Def	Deficiency
deHase	Dehydrogenase
Dept	Department
DERM	Dermatology
Desc	Descending
DGH	District General Hospital
DHAS	Dihydroisoandrosterone sulphate
1,25DHCC	1,25 Dihydroxycholecalciferol
DHSS	Department of Health & Social Security(*)
DI	Diabetes insipidus
DIC	Disseminated intravascular coagulation
Diff	Differential
Dig	Digoxin
DIP	Distal interphalangeal jt
Dip/Tet/Pert	Diphtheria/Tetanus/Pertussis triple vaccine(*)
Dir Ing	Direct inguinal hernia
Div	Division
DLE	Discoid lupus erythematosis
DMO	District Medical Officer
DMSA	Dimercaptosuccinic acid
DNA	Deoxyribosenucleic acid
DOCA	Deoxycorticosterone trimethylacetate
DOE	Department of the Environment(*)
2,3DPG	2,3 diphosphoglutinate
Dr	Doctor
DSS	Dioctyl sodium sulphosuccinate
DRO	Disablement Rehabilitation Officer
DTPA	Diethylenetriaminepentaacetic Acid
DU	Duodenal ulcer
DVT	Deep venous thrombosis

E.

E	East
E&W	England & Wales
E.coli	*Escherichia coli*
E Tube	Eustachian tube
E–B virus	Ebstein–Barr virus
EACA	Epsilon amino caproic acid
EAM	External auditory meatus
ECF	Extra cellular fluid
ECG	Electrocardiogram(*)
ECT	Electroconvulsive Therapy
ECV	External Cephalic Version
EDD	Estimated Date of Delivery(*)
Ed Psych	Educational Psychologist
EDTA	Ethylenediaminetetraacytic acid
EEG	Electroencephalogram
EFE	Endocardial fibroelastosis
eg	For example
EjSM	Ejection Systolic Murmur(*)
ELISA	Enzyme-linked Immunosorbent Assay
EMAS	Employment Medical Advisory Service
EMF	Endomyocardial fibrosis
EMG	Electromyography
EMU	Early morning urine
ENDO	Endocrinology
ENT	Ear, nose & throat
Ep	Epilepsy
EPH	Elderly Person's Home
EPS	Exophthalmos producing substance
ERCP	Endoscopic retrograde cholangiopancreatography
esp	Especially
ESR	Erythrocyte sedimentation rate
ESRF	End stage renal failure(*)
ESWL	Extra-corporeal shock wave lithotryptor
etc	Etcetera
EUA	Examination under anaesthesia
Exp	Expiration
Ext	External

F.	
F	Female
Fail	Failure (in context)
FBC	Full blood count(*)
FDP	Fibrin degradation product(*)
Fe	Iron
FEM	Full eye movements(*)
FEV_1	Forced expiratory volume in one second
FFP	Fresh frozen plasma
FH	Family history
FIGLU	Formiminoglutamic acid
F-O	Faecal-oral
FOB	Faecal occult blood(*)
αFP	Alpha fetoprotein
FPC	Family Practitioner Committee
Freq	Frequency
FSH	Follicle stimulating hormone
FTA	Fluorescent treponemal antibody
FTI	Free Thyroxine Index
5-FU	5-Fluorouracil
FVC	Forced vital capacity
G.	
g	gram (weight)
G-1-PUT	Glucose-1-phosphate uridyl transferase
G6PD Def	Glucose-6-phosphate dehydrogenase deficiency
G6phosphate	Glucose-6-phosphate
GAGS	Glycosaminoglycans
GC	Neisseria gonorrhoeae
G-cell	Gastrin cell
G-D	Gastro-duodenal
GE	Gastroenteritis
GFR	Glomerulofiltration rate
GGT	Gamma-gluteryl transferase
GH	Growth hormone
GHrH	Growth Hormone Releasing Hormone
GHRIH	Growth Hormone Releasing Inhibitory Hormone
GI	Gastrointestinal
GIP	Gastrin inhibitory polypeptide
GIT	Gastrointestinal tract
GJ	Gastrojejunostomy
GLC	Gas Liquid Chromatography
Gm	Gram stain
GMC	General Medical Council
GN	Glomerulonephritis
GNP	Gross National Product
GnRH	Gonadotrophin releasing hormone
G–O	Gastro-oesophageal(*)
Govt	Government
GP	General Practitioner(*)
Gp	Group
GPI	General paralysis of the insane
GRF	Growth Hormone Releasing Factor
GTN	Glyceryl trinitrate(*)
GTT	Glucose tolerance test
GU	Gastric ulcer (in context)
GUS	Genitourinary system
GVHD	Graft versus host disease
Gy	Grey
H.	
H_2	Hydrogen
H_1 & H_2	Histamine receptors
HAA	Hospital Activity Analysis
HAEM	Haematology
Haem	Haemorrhage
HAI	Haemagglutination inhibition
HAS	Health Advisory Service
Hb	Haemoglobin
HbA	Adult Haemoglobin
HbF	Fetal Haemoglobin
HBcAg	Hepatitis B core antigen
HBeAg	Hepatitis B e antigen
HBsAg	Hepatitis B surface antigen
Hburia	Haemoglobinuria
HCG	Human chorionic gonadotrophin
HCl	Hydrochloric acid
HCO_3	Bicarbonate
HDL	High Density Lipoprotein
He	Helium
HEO	Health Education Officer
Hep	Hepatitis
Hep A	Hepatitis A
Hep B	Hepatitis B
HepB Ag	General term for hepatitis B antigen
HFA2000	Health for All for the Year 2000
Hg	Mercury
Hgh	Height (ht)(*)
HGV	Heavy Goods Vehicle(*)
HH	Hiatus hernia
5HIAA	5-Hydroxyindole acetic acid
HIDA	Derivative of iminodiacetic acid
HIPE	Hospital In-patient Enquiry
HMG	Human Menopausal Gonadotrophin
HMSO	Her Majesty's Stationary Office
HPOA	Hypertrophic pulmonary osteoarthropathy
HPL	Human Placental Lactogen
HPT	Hyperparathyroidism
h/o	History of
HOCM	Hypertrophic obstructive cardiomyopathy(*)
hr	Hour
Hrly	Hourly
HSE	Health & Safety Executive
HSV-1	*Herpes simplex* virus type 1
HSV-2	*Herpes simplex* virus type 2
Ht or ht	Heart(*)
5-HT	5-Hydroxytryptamine
HTIG	Human Anti-tetanus Immunoglobulin(*)
HtR	Heart rate
HV	Health Visitor
HVS	High Vaginal Swab

$HyperCa^{2+}$	Hypercalcaemia
$HypoCa^{2+}$	Hypocalcaemia
$HypoMg^{2+}$	Hypomagnesaemia
HypoPT	Hypoparathyroidism
hz	Hertz ie cycles per second

I.

I_2	Iodine
IBD	Inflammatory bowel disease
IBS	Irritable bowel syndrome
IC	Intermittent claudication
ICD	International Classification of Disease
ICP	Intracranial pressure
ICRP	International Commission on Radiological Protection
ICU	Intensive care unit
IDA	Iron deficiency anaemia
IDDM	Insulin dependent diabetes mellitus
ie	That is
IF	Intrinsic factor
IFA	Immunofluorescent antibody test
Ig	Immunoglobulin
IgA	Immunoglobulin A
IgE	Immunoglobulin E
IgG	Immunoglobulin G
IgM	Immunoglobulin M
IHA	Indirect haemagglutination test
IHD	Ischaemic heart disease(*)
IM	Intra-muscular
IMF	Immunofluorescence
Immunodef	Immunodeficiency
In^{3+}	Indium (in context)
Inc	Include
Incub Pd	Incubation period
Ind Ing	Indirect inguinal hernia
Inf	Inferior
INFD	Infectious Diseases
Infect Pd	Infective period
Inflam	Inflammation
Ing H	Inguinal Hernia
Inj	Injury
Insp	Inspiratory
Insuf	Insufficiency or Insufficient
Int	Internal
Intravent	Intraventricular
In.v disc	Intervertebral disc
IOP	Intraocular pressure
IP	Interphalangeal joint
IPPV	Intermittent positive pressure ventilation(*)
IQ	Intelligence quotient
Irreg	Irregular
ISADH	Inappropriate secretion of antidiuretic hormone(*)
ITP	Idiopathic thrombocytopenic purpura
ITT	Insulin Tolerance Test
IU	International unit
IUCD	Intrauterine Contraceptive Device(*)
IUD	Intrauterine Death
IUGR	Intrauterine Growth Retardation
IV	Intravenous
IVC	Inferior vena cava
IVU	Intravenous urogram (IVP)(*)

J.

J	Jaundice
JCPT	Joint Care Planning Teams
jt	Joint(*)

K.

K^+	Potassium
KCl	Potassium chloride
kg	Kilogram
kPa	Kilopascals
KUB	"Kidney ureter bladder" abdominal X-ray

L.

L	Left
l	Litre
LA	Local anaesthetic(*)
L.A Soc	Local Authority Social
Lat	Lateral
Lab	Laboratory
L.Auths	Local Authorities
lb	Pound weight
LBBB	Left bundle branch block
LBW	Low birth weight
LDH	Lactic dehydrogenase
LDL	Low density lipoprotein
LE cells	Lupus erythematosis cells
LGV	*Lymphogranuloma venereum*
LH	Luteinising hormone
Li	Lithium
$LiCO_3$	Lithium carbonate
Lig	Ligament
LMN	Lower motor neurone
LMP	Last Menstrual Period
LN	Lymph node
LOAF	A group of small muscles of the hand supplied by the median nerve comprising: Lateral 2 lumbricals, Opponens pollicis, Abductor pollicis brevis, Flexor pollicis brevis
LOC	Loss of consciousness
LO-P	Left Occipito-posterior
LP	Lumbar puncture
LPX	Liver specific protein
LRT	Lower respiratory tract
LRTI	Lower respiratory tract infection
L:S	Lecithin/Sphingomyelin ratio
LSCS	Lower segment caesarian section
LSD	Lysergic acid diethylamide
LSE	Left sternal edge(*)
LVent	Left ventricular(*)
LVF	Left Ventricular Failure

M.

M	Male
m	Muscle
MAFF	Ministry of Agriculture, Fisheries & Foods
Maj	Majority
Mane	Morning
MAOI	Monoamine oxidase inhibitor(*)
Max	Maximum
MBC	Minimum Bactericidal Level
MCP	Metacarpo phalangeal joint
MCT	Medium chain triglycerides
MCTD	Mixed connective tissue disease
MCV	Mean cell volume(*)
MEA	Multiple endocrine adenomatosis(*)
Mech.I	Mechanical ileus
Med	Medial
Mets	Metastases
Mg	Magnesium
mg	Milligram
MHAct	Mental Health Act
MHRT	Mental Health Review Tribunal
MI	Myocardial infarct
MIC	Minimum Inhibitory Concentration
min	Minor or minutes (in context)
MInc	Mitral Incompetence(*)
MIND	MIND (Association for Mental Health)
ml	Millilitre
mm	Millimetre
mmHg	Millimetres of mercury
MND	Motor neurone disease
mod	Moderate
mol	Mole
Mort	Mortality
MRC	Medical Research Council
MS	Multiple sclerosis
msec	Milliseconds
MSt	Mitral stenosis(*)
MSU	Mid-stream specimen of urine
Mth	Month(*)
MTP	Metatarso-phalangeal joint(*)
MUA	Manipulation under anaesthesia
Multip	Multiparous
MVPP	Mustine vincristine procarbazine prednisolone
mvt	Movement

N.

N	Nausea (in context)
N	North (in context)
N/2	Half-normal saline(*)
Na^+	Sodium
NAD	Nicotinamide adenosine dinucleotide
NADP	Nicotinamide adenosine dinucleotide phosphate
$NaHCO_3$	Sodium bicarbonate
NAI	Non-Accidental Injury
NAP	Neutrophil alkaline phosphatase
NaOH	Sodium hydroxide
N&V	Nausea & vomiting
N.B	Note well
NEO	Neonatal
NEURO	Neurology
NG	Nasogastric tube
ng	Nanogram
NH_3	Ammonium
NHS	National Health Service
Ni	Nickel
NIDDM	Non-insulin Dependent Diabetes Mellitus
nm	Nanometre
NO_2	Nitrogen dioxide
Nocte	At night(*)
Norm	Normal
nos	Numbers
nr	Near
NRPB	National Radiological Protection Board
NSAID	Non-steroidal anti-inflammatory drug
NSPCC	National Society for the Prevention of Cruelty to Children
NSU	Non-specific urethritis
NTD	Neural Tube Defect

O.

O_2	Oxygen
OA	Osteoarthritis
O-A	Occipito-anterior
O&G	Obstetrics & Gynaecology
obl	Oblique
Obst	Obstruction
Obst J	Obstructive jaundice
Occ	Occasionally
o/d	Overdose
OH	Hydroxy
11OHCS	11-hydroxycorticosteroids
25(OH)D	25-hydroxy Vitamin D
OHlase	Hydroxylase
OHS	Occupational Health Service
OM	Otitis media
Op	Operation
O-P	Occipito-posterior
OPCS	Office of Population, Censuses & Surveys
OPD	Out-Patient's Department
OPHTH	Ophthalmology
ORTH	Orthopaedics
OT	Occupational therapy

P.

P	Pressure
P2	2nd pulmonary heart sound
p.a	Per annum
PA	Pernicious Anaemia
PABA/C14	Para-aminobenzoic acid/Carbon 14 test

PAED	Paediatrics(*)
Palps	Palpitations
PAN	Polyarteritis nodosa
PaO_2, $PaCO_2$	Arterial partial pressure of appropriate gas
Path	Pathological
PAS	Periodic acid schiff
PAS acid	Para-amino salicylic acid
Pb	Lead
PBC	Primary biliary cirrhosis
PBG	Protein Bound Globulin
PCV	Packed cell volume(*)
PD	Perceptive deafness
pd	Period
PDA	Patent ductus arteriosus
PE	Pulmonary embolus
pect.m	Pectoralis muscle
PEF	Peak expiratory flow
PEEP	Positive end expiratory pressure
Perf	Perforation
PET	Pre-eclamptic toxaemia(*)
Periph	Peripheral
PG	Prostaglandins
PGE2	Prostaglandin E2
PGF2α	Prostaglandin F2α
pH	Hydrogen ion concentration, a measure of acidity & alkalinity
PHC	Primary Health Care
Phenobarb	Phenobarbitone
PHLS	Public Health Laboratory Service
Physio	Physiotherapy(*)
PI	Paralytic ileus
PIF	Prolactin Inhibitory Factor
PInc	Pulmonary incompetence (Pulmonary Insufficiency)
PIP	Proximal interphalangeal joint
PKU	Phenylketonuria
PMF	Progressive massive fibrosis
PN	Percussion note
PND	Paroxysmal nocturnal dyspnoea
PNH	Paroxysmal nocturnal haemoglobinuria
PNMR	Perinatal Mortality Rate
PNS	Post-nasal space
PO_4	Phosphate
Polymorph	Polymorphonuclear leucocyte(*)
PoP	Plaster of Paris
pop	Population
Post	Posterior or after (depends on context)(*)
PPE	Plasma protein electrophoresis
PPH	Post-partum haemorrhage
ppm	Parts per million
ppt	Precipitated
PR	Pulse rate
p.r	Per rectum
Preg	Pregnancy
Prep	Preparation
Prev	Previous
Prod	Production
Prodromal Pd	Prodromal Period
Prog	Prognosis
PRV	Polycythaemia Rubra Vera
PSt	Pulmonary stenosis(*)
PSY	Psychiatry
Psych	Psychiatric
PT time	Prothrombin time(*)
PTA	Post traumatic amnesia
PTC	Percutaneous transhepatic cholangiogram
PTH	Parathormone
pts	Points
p/u	Pass urine
PUJ	Pelviureteric junction(*)
PUO	Pyrexia of Unknown Origin(*)
PUVA	Psoralen Ultraviolet Light
pv	Per Vagina
PVD	Peripheral vascular disease(*)
PVNS	Pigmented Villonodular Synovitis
PVR	Peripheral vascular resistence
Py.S	Pyloric stenosis(*)
Q.	
Q	Perfusion (as in isotope scans)
q.v.	See elsewhere
R.	
R	Right
R-a	Radioactive
Radio I_2	Radioactive Iodine(*)
RAST	Radioallergosorbent test
RAWP	Resource Allocation Working Party
RBBB	Right bundle branch block
RBC	Red blood cell
RCGP	Royal College of General Practitioners
RCT	Randomised Controlled Trial
RDS	Respiratory distress syndrome
re	Regarding, in regard to
Rehab	Rehabilitation
RES	Reticuloendothelial system
RESP (Resp)	Respiratory or Respiratory system
resus	Resuscitate
RF	Renal failure
RGM	Regional General Manager
RHA	Regional Health Authority
Rh Arth	Rheumatoid arthritis
RHEUM	Rheumatology
Rh F	Rheumatoid factor(*)
Rh fever	Rheumatic fever
Rh Ht	Rheumatic heart
RIF	Right iliac fossa(*)
RO-P	Right Occipito-posterior
Rot	Rotation
RPCFT	Reiter Protein Complement Fixation Test
RPR	Rapid Plasma Reagin
RSV	Respiratory Syncytial Virus
RTA	Road traffic accident(*)
RTbA	Renal tubular acidosis(*)
RUA	Reduction under anaesthesia(*)

RV	Residual volume
RVent	Right ventricular
RVF	Right ventricular failure
RVH	Right ventricular hypertrophy
Rx	Treatment
S.	
S	South
S1	First heart sound
S2	Second heart sound
S3	Third heart sound
S4	Fourth heart sound
SA node	Sino-atrial node
SABE	Bacterial endocarditis(*)
SACD	Subacute combined degeneration of cord
SAH	Subarachnoid Haemorrhage
S.Am	South America
Sat	Saturation, Saturated
sc	Subcutaneous(*)
SB	Still birth
SCAT	Sheep cell agglutination test
SCBU	Special care baby unit(*)
SCI	Social Class I
SCII	Social Class II
SCIIINM	Social Class III (Non-manual)
SCIIIM	Social Class III (Manual)
SCIV	Social Class IV
SCV	Social Class V
SD	Standard Deviation
SE	Side effect
secs	Seconds
SEG	Socio-Economic Group
SEN	State Enrolled Nurse
SFD	Small for dates
SGA	Small for gestational age
SH3	SH3 form
SIDS	Sudden Infant Death Syndrome
Signf	Significant(*)
SIJ	Sacroiliac joint
Sl	Slight
SLE	Systemic lupus erythematosis
SLR	Straight leg raising
Sm	Small
SMR	Submucous resection (in context)
SMR	Standardised Mortality Rate (in context)
SO_2	Sulphur Dioxide
SO_4	Sulphate
SOB	Short of breath
Soc W	Social Worker
SOL	Space occupying lesion
Sq	Squamous
SRS-A	Slow reacting substance of anaphylaxis
SSPE	Subacute sclerosing panencephalitis
Staph	Staphylococcus
STD	Sexually Transmitted Disease
Sten	Stenosis
Strep	Streptococcus
Sup	Superior
Supf	Superficial
Supps	Suppository
SVC	Superior vena cava
SVT	Supraventricular tachycardia
Sy	Syphilis
Sympath	Sympathetic
SXR	Skull X-ray(*)
T.	
T1/2	Half-life
T3	Tri-iodothyronine
T4	Thyroxine
TATT	"Tired all the time"
TAPVD	Total Anomalous Pulmonary Venous Drainage
TB	Tuberculosis
TBG	Thyroid Binding Globulin
T-cell	T-cell lymphocytes
TCAD	Tricyclic antidepressant(*)
TCCa	Transitional cell carcinoma
Tco	Transfer factor for carbon monoxide
temp	Temporary
TFT	Thyroid function tests
TGV	Transposition of Great Vessels
Thromb	Thrombosis
TI	Tricuspid incompetence
TIA	Transient ischaemic attack
TIBC	Total iron binding capacity
TLC	Total lung capacity
TLE	Temporal lobe epilepsy
TOCP	Triorthocresyl phosphate
TOF	Tracheo–oesophageal fistula(*)
TPHA	*Treponema pallidum* Haemagglutination
TPI	*Treponema pallidum* Immobilisation
TRH	Thyrotrophin Releasing Hormone
TRIC	Trachoma Inclusion Conjunctivitis
TSH	Thyroid Stimulating Hormone
TSt	Tricuspid stenosis
TTN	Transient tachypnoea of newborn
TUR	Transurethral resection
TV	Television
U.	
UA	Under anaesthesia
U&E	Urea & electrolytes(*)
UDCA	Ursodeoxycholic acid
UGS	Urogenital System
UK	United Kingdom
Ulc	Ulcerative
UMN	Upper motor neurone
Undiff	Undifferentiated
URT	Upper respiratory tract
URTI	Upper respiratory tract infection(*)
US	United States
USA	United States of America
UTI	Urinary tract infection

UVA	Ultraviolet light of waveband 280–315nm
UVB	Ultraviolet light of waveband 315–400nm
UVR	Ultraviolet Radiation

V.

v	Vein
$\dot{V}$	Ventilation
V&I	Vaccination & Immunisation
V&P	Vagotomy & pyloroplasty
Vag	Vagotomy
Vasc	Vascular
VascR	Vascular Resistence
VBI	Vertebrobasilar ischaemia
VC	Vital capacity
VDRL	Venereal disease reference laboratory
VE	Vaginal Examination(*)
Vent	Ventricular
VEs	Ventricular ectopics(*)
VF	Ventricular fibrillation
VIP	Vasoactive intestinal polypeptide
Vit	Vitamin
Vit A	Vitamin A
Vit B1	Thiamine
Vit B2	Riboflavin
Vit B3	Nicotinamide
Vit B6	Pyridoxine
Vit B12	Cyanocobalamin
Vit C	Ascorbic Acid
Vit D	Calciferol
Vit E	α-tocopherol
Vit K	Vitamin K
VLBW	Very Low Birth Weight
VLDL	Very low density lipoproteins
VMA	Vanillyl mandelic acid
vol	Volume
Vom	Vomiting
$\dot{V}/\dot{Q}$	Ventilation/perfusion
vR	Against resistance
VSD	Ventricular septal defect
VT	Ventricular tachycardia
VVs	Varicose veins

W.

W	West
WC	Water closet ie toilet
WDHA	Watery diarrhoea hypokalaemia achlorhydria syndrome
WHO	World Health Organisation
wk	Week
wkly	Weekly
WPW	Wolff–Parkinson–White syndrome
WR	Wassermann reaction
wt(s)	Weight(s)

X.

x	Times as in "$\times 3$" meaning three times
XM	Cross match blood
X-R	X-ray
X-Rad	X-irradiation therapy
XTT	Xylose Tolerance Test

Y.

yr	Year
yrly	Yearly

Z.

ZE	Zollinger–Ellison syndrome
Zn	Zinc
ZN	Ziehl–Neelsen stain
ZnO	Zinc oxide

Standard Abbreviation	American Abbreviation	
Hgh	ht	Height
HGV		Heavy Goods Vehicle (Truck)
HOCM	IHSS	Hypertrophic Obstructive Cardiomyopathy
Ht or ht	Cor	Heart
HTIG	Hypertet	Human Anti-tetanus Immunoglobulin
IHD	ASHD	Ischaemic Heart Disease
IPPV	IPPD	Intermittent Positive Pressure Ventilation
ISADH	SIADH	Inappropriate Secretion of Antidiuretic Hormone
IUCD	IUD	Intrauterine Contraceptive Device
IVU	IVP	Intravenous Urogram
jt	j	Joint
LA	Local	Local Anaesthetic
LSE	LSB	Left Sternal Edge
LVent	LV	Left Ventricular
MAOI	MAO inhibitor	Monoamine Oxidase Inhibitor
MCV		Mean Cell Volume (Mean Corpuscular Volume)
MEA	MEN-Neoplasia	Multiple Endocrine Adenomatosis
MInc	MR, MI	Mitral Incompetence or Insufficiency
MSt	MS	Mitral Stenosis
Mth	Mo	Month
MTP	MP	Metatarso–phalangeal joint
N/2	$\frac{1}{2}$NS	Half Normal Saline
Nocte	hs	At night
PAED	PED	Paediatrics (Pediatrics)
PCV	HCT	Packed Cell Volume
PET		Pre-eclampsia
Physio		Physiotherapy (Physical therapy)
Polymorph	Poly	Polymorphonuclear leucocyte
Post	p	Posterior
PSt	PS	Pulmonary Stenosis
PT time	PT	Prothrombin Time
PUJ	UPJ	Pelviureteric Junction
PUO	FUO	Pyrexia of Unknown Origin
PVD	SVR	Peripheral Vascular Disease
Py.S	P.S	Pyloric Stenosis
Radio I	RAI	Radioactive Iodine
Rh F	RF	Rheumatoid Factor
RIF	RLQ	Right Iliac Fossa (Right Lower Quadrant)
RTA	MVA	Road Traffic Accident
RTbA	RTA	Renal Tubular Acidosis
RUA		Reduction Under Anaesthesia (Closed Reduction)
SABE	SBE	Bacterial Endocarditis
sc	Subcut	Subcutaneous
SCBU	PICU	Special Care Baby Unit
Signf	sig	Significant
SXR		Skull X-Ray (Skull Series)
TCAD	TCA	Tricyclic Antidepressant
TOF	TE	Tracheo–oesophageal Fistula
U&E	BUN Lytes	Urea & Electrolytes
URTI	URI	Upper Respiratory Tract Infection
VE		Vaginal Examination (Pelvic Exam)
VEs	PVC	Ventricular Ectopics

American Appendix to Glossary

Standard Abbreviation	American Abbreviation	
?	R/O	Query
A&E	E.R	Accident & Emergency (Emergency Room)
Alc	EtOH	Alcohol
ANC		Well Baby Clinic
ASOT	ASLO	Anti-streptolysin "O" titre
Ave	Avg	Average
bd	bid	Twice daily
b.o	B.M	Bowel open
BG	BS	Blood Glucose
CAT	CT	Computed Axial Tomography
CCF	CHF	Congestive Cardiac Failure
CDSC	CDC	Communicable Diseases Centre
CGL	CML	Chronic Granulocytic Leukaemia
chd	Cho	Carbohydrate
C–O	G.E	Cardio–oesophageal
COAD	COPD	Chronic Obstructive Airways Disease
DD	DDx	Differential Diagnosis
DHSS	DHHS	Department of Health & Social Security (Department of Health & Human Services)
Dip/Tet/Pert	DPT	Diphtheria/Tetanus/Pertussis triple vaccine
DOE	DOI	Department of the Environment (Department of the Interior)
ECG	EKG	Electrocardiogram
EDD	EDC	Estimated Date of Delivery
EjSM	S.E.M	Ejection Systolic Murmur
ESRF	ESRD	End Stage Renal Failure
FBC	CBC	Full Blood Count
FDP	FSP	Fibrin Degradation Products
FEM	EOM	Full Eye Movements
FOB	Guiac test	Faecal Occult Blood
G–O	G–E	Gastro–oesophageal
GP	PMD	General Practitioner
GTN	NTG	Glyceryl Trinitrate

Reader's Guide

The following notes are intended to guide the reader in the use of this book.

1. Page structure

Each page is divided into two vertical columns which should be read in a downwards direction, starting with the left hand column.

2. Chapter structure

Within each chapter, the sequence of topics follows a logical pattern. However it is to be expected that the ordering of topics may not completely please all readers. Most conditions are dealt with in a standard manner, i.e.:

Title
General comments including epidemiology
Clinical features
Investigations
Treatment
Prognosis
Differential diagnosis

CLINICAL FEATURES: it should be recognised that the use of such words as 'rare' and 'often' are to an extent subjective and must be read as such.

INVESTIGATIONS: the order in which these are listed has no significance, nor is every investigation suggested mandatory.

TREATMENT: generic drug names have been used throughout. Not all of the drugs mentioned are universally available.

3. Subject sequence

See contents list. There is no obvious correct sequence of chapters but where possible chapters of related content have been juxtaposed.

4. Cross-referencing

The main topics covered in each chapter are shown in the contents list. Some topics are covered in more than one place; other topics might not be found in the chapter where the reader might expect them (e.g. family planning is covered in Community Medicine, not Obstetrics). In some cases cross-references are provided, but if in doubt the reader should consult the index.

5. Index

The index is largely organised on an anatomical basis (e.g. Lung, tumours of). Syndromes and diseases are listed by their specific name.

6. Glossary

Most abbreviations found in the book are in common use. Some, however, are the creation of the authors but in general will be easily understood. A full glossary of abbreviations is provided, plus an American appendum for cases where usage differs between the UK and the USA.

7. Lists

Within each chapter a number of lists are included. List titles are given in chapter order at the beginning of the book and in alphabetical order of subject at the end of the book. Within each chapter they are easily identified by their grey-tinted background.

9. Style

In the interests of stylistic uniformity, some grammatical and literary rules are occasionally broken (e.g. italicising of name of micro-organisms, the use of semicolons).

10. Readership

In general the content of the book is universally applicable, however inevitably some chapters are most relevant to UK practice (e.g. some parts of the Community Medicine chapter).

11. Sources of information

The book collects together information from many different sources (some of which do not agree with each other about exactly the same condition!) and modified according to the advice of a practising expert in the field. It is therefore to be expected that some clinicians will disagree with the authors' summaries of conditions. In cases where there is controversy about, for example, the preferred treatment for a condition, the authors have attempted to follow the more traditional medical viewpoint.

Obstetrics & Gynaecology

Obstetrics

NORMAL FETAL DEVELOPMENT

Fertilisation occurs in the distal third of fallopian tube. The fertilised egg passes along the tube entering the uterus as a morula on the 4th day. Implantation occurs on the 6th–7th day & requires the preparation of the endometrium by progesterone produced by the corpus luteum. Full implantation is achieved by the 9th day. It is conventional to time pregnancy from the date of the first day of the LMP. In the first 14 days of biological life the ectoderm, mesoderm & endoderm are formed. By 6wks from LMP a cylinder c̄ head & tail ends are formed & the heart develops. By about 8wks the limbs are formed, ossification centres are present & sex glands are differentiated. By 12wks from LMP, 1° development of all organ systems has occured. Thereafter development is mostly by growth. Organogenesis is complete by 16wks. Most cong defects develop in the first trimester
Fetal circulation is characterised by umbilical circulation & vascular shunts (Ductus venosus, Foramen ovale, Ductus arteriosus). Oxygenation is enhanced by pO_2 gradient between maternal & fetal blood, high fetal Hb, favourable O_2 dissociation curve of fetal Hb, & high fetal CO
Thoracic mvts occur in utero. Surfactant produced from 18–20wks but surge in production from about 34wks. Urine excreted from about 15wks. Swallowing & peristalsis occur by mid-pregnancy

The Placenta

The placenta is formed from the chorion & decidua basalis & covered by amniotic membrane. The chorionic plate develops buds (villi) which are made of cytotrophoblastic tissue & central mesodermal tissue from which a blood supply forms
The placenta has the following functions: Nutrition & oxygenation of fetus; Excretion of fetal waste products; Endocrine organ producing 4 hormones: 1. HCG, which prolongs the corpus luteum, is mainly produced by cytotrophoblast (Langhans' layer); 2. Oestrogen, which stimulates uterine growth & development, depends on a functioning fetal adrenal gland & liver for production; 3. Progesterone, inhibits myometrial activity; & 4. HPL is produced by syncytiotrophoblast; Immunological

protection esp as a barrier between two antigenically distinct organisms; Barrier to the passage of most large molecules

NORMAL MATERNAL CHANGES IN PREGNANCY

The Uterus & Cervix

The uterus progressively softens in early pregnancy starting at the isthmus. The uterus elongates & hypertrophies. The lower uterine segment, situated between the uterine body & cervix, chiefly develops in the last trimester from the isthmus c̄ muscle fibres mostly in a circular arrangement. The cervix effaces & dilates late in pregnancy, a process accelerated during labour

Breasts

↑ fat, connective tissue & vascularity. Pigmented areola & hypertrophied sebaceous glands (Montgomery's tubercles). Glandular proliferation. Later colostrum production
Plasma vol ↑ by approx 50% (greater in multiple pregnancy). Red cell mass ↑ by 20%. CO ↑ by 30–40%. Renal, skin & uterine bloodflow increase. Haemodilution → Hb ↓. Usually ESR ↑, WCC ↑ (esp Neutrophils), Plasma cholesterol ↑, Alk Phos ↑, Fibrinogen ↑, Plasma proteins ↓

GIT

↑ progesterone → ↓ gastric motility, ↓ colonic tone, ↓ cardiac sphincter tone

UGS

Progesterone → dilatation. elongation & kinking of ureter → urinary stasis. GFR ↑, serum urea ↓. ↓ renal threshold for glucose

Endocrine & Metabolic

↑ basal metabolic rate. +ve nitrogen balance. Na^+ & Ca^{2+} retention. Ave wt gain = 13kg (ie 5kg water retention, 3.5kg fetus, 2kg fat, 1kg amniotic fluid, 1kg uterus, 0.5kg placenta). ↑ pituitary hormone output. ↑ output of steroids & aldosterone. ↑ TBG

SYMPTOMS & DIAGNOSIS OF PREGNANCY

CLIN: Amenorrhoea. Often N&V esp mane; Breast enlargement & tenderness; Montgomery's tubercles; Darkened breast areola; Frequency; ↑ Vaginal discharge. Occ False period ie small vaginal bleed at expected date of first post fertilisation period. Increased uterine size & Hegar's sign are usually detectable at 6–12wks by int examination. Later Abdo distension; Fetal mvts. Occ Heartburn; Constipation; VVs; Headaches; Palps; Fainting; Drowsiness; Backache; Leg cramps; Oedema. Rarely Carpal tunnel syndrome; Osteitis pubis

INVESTIGATIONS:
- Urine pregnancy test: Detect high levels of HCG & most become +ve at about 6wks
- Ultrasound: Can often detect pregnancy by 6wks
- Occ β chain HCG monoclonal test, become +ve at about 1wk

ROUTINE ANTENATAL CARE

The aim of ANC is to achieve complete physical, mental & emotional well being of the mother & fetus. Pregnancy is not an illness & the desires of the mother for the management of the pregnancy are therefore an important factor in achieving these aims

The aim is to prevent illness in mother & fetus, promote healthy lifestyle during pregnancy, prepare for childbirth & child rearing, & treat illness. ANC should usually be a partnership between the mother & the health care professions. ANC is primarily concerned c̄ sequential screening to forestall problems in pregnancy

First Antenatal Visit

As the first wks of preganancy are a critical period in organogenesis the idea of preconceptual advice eg on diet & smoking has been proposed. Most F have pregnancy confirmed & have made initial antenatal visit by 12wks. Late first visit for antenatal care is ass c̄ high risk pregnancy. The function of the first visit can be divided into four categories:

HISTORY: Previous medical history; FH; Menstrual history; Previous obstetric history; Dietary, smoking, drugs, alcohol & social histories

EXAMINATION: General inc BP, Resp system, CVS, legs, spine; VE; Abdo examination; Breast examination

INVESTIGATIONS:
- MSU
- Urinalysis
- FBC
- Blood Gp
- Rhesus gp & Abs
- Rubella Abs
- Sy serology
- αFP
- Cervical smear
- Occ Sickle cell screen; CXR

ADVICE: Dietary advice; Dental advice; Anti-smoking; Parentcraft; Welfare benefits. Occ Genetic counselling. Discuss options for further care c̄ mother eg shared care c̄ GP, Home delivery

Further Visits

Most women are seen monthly to 28wks, then fortnightly till 36wks & weekly thereafter. At each visit Examine size of uterus & estimate amount of liquor; Record wt; Urinalysis; BP; Presence of any oedema; Lie, position, presentation & station of fetus; Check number of foetuses; Fetal ht. Note date of first fetal mvts. Compare expected gestational age from date of LMP c̄ clin & investigatory findings

Special Examinations & Investigations

1. ULTRASOUND

   Carried out at approx 16 & 24wks, to assess Maturity; Rate of growth; Number of fetuses; Placental site; Morphology, can detect many fetal abnormalities eg Anencephaly, Hydrocephaly, Spina bifida, Absent kidneys; Viability esp suspected fetal death

2. AMNIOCENTESIS

   Carried out in some high risk pregnancies eg Suspected spina bifida, some inherited metabolic diseases, Mothers over 35yrs. Can determine fetal sex

3. ESTIMATION OF ADEQUACY OF BIRTH CANAL

   May be by manual examination $\pm$ X-R Pelvimetry. Usually carried out at about 36wks

4. PLACENTAL FUNCTION TESTS

   Sequential measurements of HPL or Oestriol give an indication of fetal well being

5. LECITHIN/SPHINGOMYELIN RATIO

   To test lung maturity in pregnancies where early delivery is considered

6. KICK CHART
7. FETOSCOPY

ABNORMAL CONDITIONS & DISEASES IN PREGNANCY

Prenatal Diagnosis

Often high risk couples can be identified before pregnancies begin & counselling can start pre-conceptually. Most of the tests required for pre-natal diagnosis carry small but significant risk to the fetus & parents should be aware, before the test is performed, of the risks & their decision should a test prove +ve

Amniocentesis at about 16wks followed by culture of amniotic fluid cells & chromosomal analysis yields a result at 18–19wks c̄ good sensitivity & specificity. Amniocentesis in experienced hands → 1% ↑ in complications eg miscarriage.

Indications for amniocentesis inc: Raised maternal age eg >35yrs (ass c̄ ↑ risk of Down's syndrome); Previous child c̄ chromosomal abnormality; Fetal sexing to identify M in sex-linked condition eg Duchenne muscular dystrophy, when mother is a known carrier; Parent c̄ balanced chromosome rearrangement (ass c̄ h/o recurrent abortions)

NEURAL TUBE DEFECTS

Maternal αFP screening identifies F who may be carrying an affected fetus

Causes of Raised Serum αFP (LIST 1 O&G)

1. Neural tube defect
2. Multiple pregnancy
3. Fetal abdominal wall defects
4. Fetal renal disease
5. Threatened abortion
6. Hepatoma

Confirmation of NTD is made by a second elevated serum αFP sample & ultrasonography. Occ confirmation by elevated amniotic αFP level or acetylcholinesterase gel electrophoresis is required

INBORN ERRORS OF METABOLISM

A number of metabolic disorders can be identified by amniocentesis & amniotic fluid cell culture. Fetoscopy allows the acquisition of fetal blood, skin & liver which may allow diagnosis of metabolic disorders eg Hbopathies

STRUCTURAL DEFECTS

Ultrasonography can detect many structural abnormalities eg CHD; NTD; Abdo wall defects; Cysts; Hydronephrosis. Detection may allow for abortion or occ for early corrective surgery. Fetoscopy allows direct observation of the fetus

Vomiting in Pregnancy

Usually due to pregnancy itself but occ due to HH, PU, Pyelonephritis. About 50% of F complain of symptoms. Usually Vom begins by 6wks & ends by 12–14wks. The cause is unknown. ? due to oestrogens or HCG

Late Vom in pregnancy is usually due to abdo mass pushing up stomach &/or a HH. Vom in labour is common

CLIN: Vom esp mane; N. Most cases are mild but about 1 in 1000 have severe form (Hyperemesis gravidarum) c̄ Vom++ → dehydration, hypovolaemia, acidosis, Vit def. Rarely → liver failure, encephalopathy, polyneuritis

INVESTIGATIONS (in severe cases):
- FBC
- U&E
- Urinalysis
- Exclude other diseases

RX: In mild cases frequent small non-spicy meals; Reassure; Drugs occ helpful eg Phenergan. In severe cases admit to hospital, correct fluid & electrolyte balance c̄ IV regime; Vit supplements. When Vom abates give oral antiemetics eg Mecloxine HCl (Ancoloxin) ± mild sedative. Hypnotherapy may benefit. Very rarely therapeutic abortion required

Ectopic Pregnancy

A pregnancy implanted outside the

cavity of the uterus. In UK about 1 in 300 mature pregnancies; In W.Indians about 1 in 30 mature pregnancies. 95% occur in the fallopian tube. Rarer sites are the cornu of uterus, ovary, cervix & abdomen. Predispositions inc "Luteal phase defects"; Previous pelvic inflamm disease eg TB, GC; Endometriosis; Previous pelvic surgery; Infertility; IUCDs; Developmental tubal abnormalities. Ass c̄ high maternal age

CLIN: If implantation in isthmial med 2/3 of tube, early rupture at 4–8wks is usual c̄ sudden acute lower abdo pain, tender rigid abdo, shock & fainting. Occ develop pleuritic pain
If implantation occurs in ampullary lat 1/3 of tube presentation usually occurs at 8–12wks following short period of amenorrhoea c̄ mild lower abdo pain. Occ Vaginal bleeding (prune juice); Dyspareunia; Dyschezia; Tender uterus & pouch of Douglas; Adnexal mass. May develop acute episode c̄ severe pain & fainting (indicating tubal rupture or incomplete abortion) or further episodes of vaginal bleeding & pain may gradually abate (indicating complete abortion ± haematocoele)

INVESTIGATIONS:
- Pregnancy test: +ve in about 75%
- WCC sl ↑
- FBC: Occ Hb ↓
- Ultrasound
- Laparoscopy

SEQUELAE: **1. Tubal Rupture:** If rupture occurs on anti-mesenteric side usually → intraperitoneal haem & pelvic haematocoele. If rupture occurs on mesenteric side of tube a broad ligament haematoma forms

2. Tubal Abortion: The ovum is either completely absorbed, aborted into the peritoneal cavity, incompletely aborted (the conceptus distends the tubal ostium), or a tubal blood mole is formed

3. 2° Abdominal Pregnancy: Very rarely the ovum is expelled into the abdo & continues to grow

RX: Analgesia. If tubal pregnancy suspected transfer to hospital without VE. Treat any shock c̄ blood transfusion. When diagnosis is made immediate laparotomy, operative procedure depends on state of other tube & whether patient desires further children. Salpingectomy or salpingostomy

PROG: About 60% become pregnant again. The risk of a second ectopic is about 10%. A term baby occurs in about 50% of subsequent pregnancies

DD:
1. Uterine abortion
2. Pelvic infection
3. Torsion of ovarian cyst
4. Acute appendicitis

Abortion

An abortion is the expulsion or attempted expulsion of a fetus before 28wks of pregnancy (as medical technology → more viable fetuses <28wks, definitions may require alteration). All abortions whether spontaneous or therapeutic may be ass c̄ social & psychological sequelae eg guilt

SPONTANEOUS ABORTIONS

Very common, occuring in 10–25% of all pregnancies. Most occur between 6–12wks. The cause of many abortions is not known. 25–50% show anatomical malformations & >25% have chromosomal abnormalities. There is ↑ risk c̄ Defective implantation eg ectopic pregnancy; Local disorders of the genital tract eg bicornute uterus, myomata distorting uterine cavity; Cervical incompetence. Abortion is the commonest cause of bleeding in early pregnancy

Causes of Bleeding in Early Pregnancy (LIST 2 O&G)

1. Abortion
2. Ectopic Pregnancy
3. Hydatidiform mole
4. Cervical erosions
5. Cervical polyps
6. Vaginitis
7. Cervical Ca
8. Bleeding from adjacent organs: Eg Haemorrhoids
9. Implantation bleed

The varieties of spontaneous abortions are classified as Threatened, Inevitable, Incomplete, Complete & Missed

THREATENED: Vaginal bleeding during the first 28wks of pregnancy. The cervical int os is closed

Clin: Sl bleeding; No or sl uterine contractions & pain

Investigations: • Pregnancy test

• Ultrasound

Rx: Bed rest. Avoid speculum & bimanual examination

Prog: About 75% continue pregnancy to term

INEVITABLE:

Clin: Vaginal bleeding; Pain; Uterine contractions; Dilated os. Occ Shock. May be preceded by signs of threatened abortion. Later incomplete or complete abortion occurs

INCOMPLETE: Following abortion some products of conception remain in the uterine cavity. Commoner than complete abortion

Investigation: • Ultrasound

Rx: Syntometrine. Analgesia. Occ blood transfusion. EUA & surgical evacuation of products

COMPLETE: All products of conception are passed following abortion

Investigation: • Ultrasound

Rx: Syntometrine. Analgesia. EUA, D&C

MISSED: All products of conception are retained following fetal death. If occurs in early wks a carneous mole develops containing layers of blood clot. Later fetal death → mummification or absorption

Clin: Often h/o threatened abortion, then bleeding stops & signs of pregnancy disappear. Later Brown discharge. May result in later spontaneous abortion

Investigation: • Ultrasound

Rx: If uterus is <12wks in size, EUA & vaginal evacuation of products of conception preceded by Oxytocin infusion. If uterus is >12wks in size use high dose Oxytocin to stimulate uterine contractions. Occ Prostaglandin IV or pessaries

SEPTIC ABORTION

May occur c̄ any abortion. Commonest after incomplete & criminal abortions. Esp Strep, Staph, *E.coli*

CLIN: Fever; PR ↑; Vaginal discharge. Occ Boggy tender uterus. Rarely Peritonitis

INVESTIGATIONS: • WCC ↑

• High vaginal or Cervical swab

• Blood culture

• Occ: U&Es; Urinalysis

SEQUELAE: In a minority of cases infection spreads to involve myometrium & tubes. Rarely generalised peritonitis. These sequelae are both ass c̄ *Cl.welchii* infection & septic shock

RX: Antibiotics; Bed rest. Occ blood transfusion. EUA & evacuation 12hrs after starting chemotherapy. If Clostridial infection suspected give anti-gas gangrene serum & steroids. Rarely if no response to Rx, hysterectomy

HABITUAL ABORTION

A women who has had 3 or more successive abortions is termed a habitual aborter & has about a 30% chance of aborting again. History & examination may indicate a uterine abnormality eg bicornute uterus or an incompetent cervix. In many no cause can be found

RX: If no specific cause identified, traditional to suggest early cessation of work, avoidance of exertion, good diet

THERAPEUTIC ABORTION

In the UK the Abortion Act of 1967 permits therapeutic abortion. 2 doctors must certify that one of the 4 indications for legal abortion is present ie Continuation of pregnancy involves risk to the life of the pregnant woman or to the physical or mental health of the mother or risk of injury to the physical or mental health of any existing children of the pregnant woman's family or substantial risk that the child if born, would suffer severe physical or mental handicap. The termination must be carried out in approved premises before 28wks. Abortions after 24wks are rare

Septic Shock

A rare complication of septic abortion, pyelonephritis, puerperal endomyometritis & chorioamnionitis. Incidence has been falling in UK. Usually due to Gm-ve bacteria eg *E.coli.* Partly mediated by effects of endotoxins

CLIN: Symptoms & signs of underlying cause. PR ↑; BP ↓; Warm peripheries; Pyrexia. Later Pale clammy peripheries; Temperature ↑ or ↓. May develop DIC; ARF; CCF; ARDS; Coma

INVESTIGATIONS: • MSU
- Blood cultures
- HVS
- FBC
- WCC
- Platelets
- U&Es
- Astrup
- Urinalysis
- Coagulation profile
- CXR
- AXR: To exclude foreign body

RX: Antibiotics eg Ampicillin, Gentamicin, Metronidazole. Remove septic focus, usually by D&C or Oxytocin but occ laparotomy ± hysterectomy. Correct fluid & electrolyte balance under CVP control. $NaHCO_3$ for metabolic acidosis. Occ O_2 ± mechanical ventilation required. Steroids may benefit. Digoxin if CCF. Vasoactive drugs may aid eg Dopamine, Naloxone

Causes of DIC in Pregnancy (LIST 3 O&G)

1. Septic abortion
2. Missed abortion
3. Intrauterine death
4. Abruptio placentae
5. Amniotic fluid embolism
6. Eclampsia
7. Ruptured uterus
8. Trophoblastic disease
9. Other sepsis:
   Eg Gm-ve septicaemia,
   Disseminated herpes simplex infection
10. Saline abortion

Cervical Incompetence

About 20% of habitual aborters have cervical incompetence. Incompetence of int os allows membranes to bulge into cervical canal

CLIN: h/o abortions usually occuring at 14–16wks c̄ painless dilatation of os. May be h/o pre-term labour

INVESTIGATIONS: • Ultrasound
- HSG: May show shelving of lower uterus into upper cervical canal

RX: If cervical incompetence suspected a purse string suture (Shirodkar stitch) is inserted at the level of the int os at about 14wks pregnancy. If abortion becomes inevitable cut suture. Surgery c/i if infection or if membranes have ruptured. Remove suture about 1wk before term. If severe incompetence, proceed to ARM & delivery

Incarcerated Retroverted Gravid Uterus

Rare. Occurs at 12–14wks. Often idiopathic occ due to adhesions

CLIN: Frequency; Dysuria. Later UTI; Retention. Occ Palpable bladder; Abortion. If sacculation → palpable abdo mass

INVESTIGATIONS: • MSU
- Ultrasound

RX: Pass catheter & if uterus does not antevert spontaneously try vaginal pessary. Occ MUA

Malformations of Uterus & Vagina

Cong malformations may occur if only one Mullerian duct is present, fusion of the two ducts is abnormal or if embryonic septum persists. Commonest abnormalities are the bicornute, arcuate & subseptate uterus. Ass c̄ ↑ incidence of Infertility; Abortion; Premature labour; Malpresentation; Inco-ordinate uterine action; PPH; Obstructed labour; Retained placenta

RX: Corrective surgery for persistent septa. Caesarian section for some malpresentations

Trophoblastic Disease

HYDATIDIFORM MOLE

In UK about 1 per 1000 pregnancies. Commoner in Afr, Latin Am., Far E.

PATHOGENESIS: Abnormal development of placenta. Young chorionic villi undergo a cystic dilatation. The cysts are covered c̄ trophoblastic tissue which obtains food from the decidua. Paucity of blood supply in villous → death of embryo. Partial moles are rare & often ass c̄ chromosomal abnormalities

CLIN: Early uterine bleeding, often heavy. Discrepancy between actual size & expected size of uterus (usually larger than expected). Occ N&V; Malaise;

Passage of vesicles; PET; Ovarian luteal cysts; Anaemia. Rarely Convulsions; ↑ risk of sepsis; Hyperthyroidism

INVESTIGATIONS: • Pregnancy test: HCG ↑↑
- CXR
- Ultrasound: No fetal parts, Multiple cysts. Rarely a live fetus from a twin pregnancy is present
- Histology

RX: Admit to hospital. If bleeding heavy transfuse. IV Oxytocin to induce contractions & control bleeding. EUA & remove vesicles by vacuum extraction. About 5 days after tumour expulsion perform D&C. If woman has completed her family, hysterectomy. All women require follow-up for at least 2yrs c̄ CXR, Urinary HCG & regular VE

PROG: Good in benign form. 10% develop choriocarcinoma. Risk of mole in subsequent pregnancy is 1–4%

MALIGNANT TROPHOBLASTIC DISEASE

Metastatic disease usually occurs in the presence of choriocarcinoma. Lung mets >Vaginal >Liver, Brain. Divided into low & high risk gps

CLIN: Lung mets often → Acute chest pain; SOB; PR ↑; Resp rate ↑. Occ Cough; Haemoptysis. Rarely Pulm BP ↑

INVESTIGATIONS: • Serial HCG levels
- CXR
- Ultrasound
- U&Es
- LFTs
- CAT Scan
- Liver scan
- IVU

RX: For low risk, Methotrexate. Hysterectomy for older women. For high risk, combination chemotherapy ± hysterectomy. X-Rad for CNS mets. Careful follow-up

PROG: Very good. Fertility often preserved after Methotrexate Rx

Hypertension in Pregnancy

Common. BP usually falls during first half of normal pregnancy. Pre-eclampsia (PET) refers to pregnancy induced BP ↑ occurring in 2nd half of pregnancy & resolving after delivery. Chr BP ↑ is less common than PET & usually presents before 20wks

PET

Cause unknown, ? immunological

Factors Predisposing to PET (LIST 4 O&G)

1. FH of PET
2. Primigravidity
3. Hypertensive renal disease
4. Diabetes
5. Chr BP ↑
6. Multiple pregnancy
7. Hydatidiform mole
8. Hydrops fetalis
9. Mothers aged <20yrs & >35yrs

PATHOPHYSIOLOGY: Not well understood. GFR ↓. Proximal tubular dysfunction → non-selective proteinuria. Widespread vasospasm

CLIN: BP ↑. In more severe cases Proteinuria; Oedema. Occ Migraine. Usually BP ↑ increases in later pregnancy. Occ BP ↑ worse nocte. Rarely → Eclampsia. Occ Fetal growth retardation; Premature labour; LBW child. PET rapidly settles following delivery

INVESTIGATIONS: • Serial serum urates: Gradually ↑
- Placental function tests
- Urinalysis
- Platelets: Occ ↓

RX: Bed rest. Regular monitoring eg weekly clinic vists. If BP>160/100mmHg probably best to admit to hospital & if BP level does not fall start anti-BP ↑ drug Rx eg Methyldopa, Hydrallazine, Labetolol. Higher BP require more urgent anti-BP ↑ drugs Rx. Diuretics are not indicated (they affect urate levels & are relatively ineffective as plasma volume is ↓ in PET). Occ fetal cardiotachographic monitoring. If signs of maternal or fetal problems develop early delivery should be considered. Indications for early delivery inc: RF, Hepatic dysfunction, Eclampsia, DIC, Signs of poor fetal growth

ECLAMPSIA

Rare in Western countries. Postpartum >Antepartum, Intrapartum

CLIN: Antepatum eclampsia is preceded by worsening PET c̄ oedema & proteinuria. Vom, oliguria, epigastric pain & J often immediately precede development of convulsions. Confusion;

Muscular clonus; Headaches. Ass c̄ fetal distress, abruptio placentae, fetal death. Ass c̄ ↑ risk of maternal death

RX: Prompt Rx of PET should prevent development of eclampsia. Eclampsia is a medical emergency. Maintain airway. Nurse in dimly lit quiet room. IV Diazepam to control seizures, then maintenance infusion. Anti-BP ↑ drugs. Immediate delivery of baby. Occ use $MgSO_4$. Regular monitoring of reflexes, Resp rate, urine output, BP, fetal parameters

CHRONIC HYPERTENSION

Usually antedates pregnancy. May coexist c̄ PET. Usually due to essential BP ↑ but occ 2° to Coarctation of aorta, SLE, Phaeochromocytoma

CLIN: BP ↑, usually apparent in first trimester. Occ Ht ↑; Retinal haem & exudates

INVESTIGATIONS:
- U&Es
- Urate
- Urinalysis
- Placental function tests
- Urinary VMA

RX: Anti-BP ↑ drugs

Heart Disease In Pregnancy

Esp Afr, India (ass c̄ Rh Ht disease). In developed countries usually due to CHD. Pregnancy should usually be avoided in cases of COCM, 1° Pulm BP ↑, Inoperable cyanotic CHD eg Eisenmenger's syndrome, Marfan's syndrome

GENERAL CLIN: Common symptoms are Oedema; SOB; PR ↑. Acute LVF, Cough & 2° infection are not uncommon in Rh Ht disease. In coarctation risk of rupture of aorta in late pregnancy

GENERAL INVESTIGATIONS:
- ECG
- CXR
- Placental function tests
- Ultrasound
- Occ Echocardiography, Dig levels

RX: Preconceptual counselling may prevent inadvisable pregnancy or allow corrective surgery pre-pregnancy. Known cardiac disease requires regular monitoring & delivery in specialist centres. Cover surgery & dentistry by antibiotics as risk of SABE

Often require bed rest. Advise stop smoking, dental care. Admit if ↑ SOB, 2° infection, cough, acute LVF, tachyarrhythmias. Prophylactic Iron & Folate to avoid anaemia. Anticoags may be teratogenic & Heparin should be substituted esp in early pregnancy. Occ Dig for arrhythmia, PR ↑
If ↑ SOB or Haemoptysis occur c̄ Rheumatic mitral valve disease, closed mitral valvotomy is indicated. This carries the normal small operative risk (but ? ↑ risk of teratogenesis due to the use of anticoags)
If pregnancy occurs in conditions c̄ high risk of maternal mort try to terminate pregnancy before 10wks
Admit to hospital before delivery. Allow spontaneous labour or induce c̄ PGE2 pessaries. Keep membranes intact. Try to avoid VE. In first stage, nurse in reverse lithotomy position. IV antibiotics eg Ampicillin & Gentamicin throughout labour; Adequate analgesia (avoid epidural as it → vasodilation). Electively shorten 2nd stage by using forceps. O_2. Avoid Ergometrine in 3rd stage. Give Oxytocin ± Frusemide c̄ birth of ant shoulder. Monitor closely in puerperium. Mobilise early. Encourage breast feeding

PROG: Major cause of maternal death. Slight ↑ risk to fetus

DD: Cardiac features of normal pregnancy inc: SOB; Periph oedema; Syncope; Collapsing pulse; Displaced apex beat; Loud split S1; S3; EjSM LSE. ECG features inc ^L axis deviation^; ^ST^ depression; Ectopics

PERIPARTUM CARDIOMYOPATHY

Esp Blacks. Rare

CLIN: Present late in pregnancy or in puerperium. Symptoms & signs resemble COCM

RX: Diuretics, Hydrallazine. Occ antiarrhythmics

PROG: About 50% fully recover

DVT

Ass c̄ ↑ maternal age; Obesity; LSCS; ↓ mobility. Common in pregnancy as woman is in a "hypercoagulable" state

INVESTIGATIONS:
- Venography (Shield fetus by Pb apron)

- Doppler studies

RX: Warfarin c/i in first trimester. Use Heparin. Monitor by APTT estimations. Can use Heparin throughout pregnancy or use Warfarin in 2nd trimester & up to 4wks pre-term when Heparin is again substituted. Firm bandage, early ambulation

COMPLICATION: PE

Renal & Urinary Tract Disease in Pregnancy

BACTERIURIA

Common, about 2–7% have significant bacteriuria on booking. Ass c̄ multiparity. Partly due to increased progesterone levels → ureteric dilatation → urinary stasis. Untreated about 30–40% develop acute pyelonephritis esp if structural abnormalities of urinary tract

CLIN: Bacteriuria is usually initially asymptomatic. May develop acute pyelonephritis, esp 2nd or 3rd trimester, c̄ Backache; Loin pain esp R; Headache; Vom; Frequency; Dysuria. Slight ↑ risk of PET; BP ↑; Megaloblastic anaemia; Prematurity

INVESTIGATIONS:
- MSU
- WCC
- Creatinine clearance
- IVU: >4mths after delivery, if persistent bacteriuria or pyelonephritis

RX: Bed rest. Plentiful fluids. Alkalinise urine c̄ $NaHCO_3$. Antibiotics if significant bacteriuria or if symptomatic

PROG: Prompt Rx of bacteriuria c̄ appropriate antibiotic can virtually eradicate acute pyelonephritis during pregnancy. If pyelonephritis, 6mths after pregnancy about 25% have abnormal X-Ray &/or persistent bacteriuria

Causes of Abdo Pain in Pregnancy (LIST 5 O&G)

1. Acute pyelonephritis
2. Acute appendicitis
3. Concealed APH
4. Acute cholecystitis
5. Red degeneration of fibroid
6. Perf PU
7. Torsion, rupture or haem of ovarian tumour
8. Round ligament tenderness
9. Ectopic pregnancy
10. Labour pains: Inc Abortion, Premature labour
11. Incarcerated gravid uterus
12. Broad ligament haematoma
13. Acute polyhydramnios
14. Urinary calculi
15. Ruptured splenic artery aneurysm
16. Severe PET
17. Uterine rupture
18. Rectus haematoma
19. Acute fatty liver of pregnancy

CHRONIC PYELONEPHRITIS

CLIN: May be past h/o renal disease. Occ Early BP ↑ c̄ later superadded PET; Proteinuria; Oedema; Acute episode of pyelonephritis; Fetal growth retardation, placental malfunction

SERIAL INVESTIGATIONS:
- Urinalysis
- U&Es
- MSU
- Placental function tests
- Ultrasound

RX: Monitor regularly. Bed rest, Anti-BP ↑ drugs. Treat infections early. May require early delivery, occ LSCS

RENAL FAILURE

Obstetric Causes of ARF (LIST 6 O&G)

1. Due to Hypovolaemia:
   a) Abortion
   b) Abruptio placentae
   c) Eclampsia
   d) PPH
   e) Adrenal failure
2. Infection:
   a) Septic abortion
   b) Pyelonephritis
   c) UTI
   d) Puerperal genital tract infection
3. Haemolysis:
   a) Trauma
   b) Abruptio placentae
   c) Haemolytic crisis
4. Chemicals:
   Eg Hg, Phenol
5. Incompatible blood transfusion

RX: If due to hypovolaemia restore blood volume eg packed cell transfusion. Close monitoring. Normal Rx of ARF. Often require dialysis

PROG: Good prog c̄ ATN. Renal cortical necrosis is rarer & has worse prog

URINARY CALCULI

Symptomatic in approx 1 in 1000 pregnancies

CLIN: Variable presentation. Occ Ureteric colic; Loin pain; Haematuria; Frequency; Dysuria. May → Acute pyelonephritis; Recurrent UTIs

INVESTIGATIONS:
- MSU: Occ microscopic haematuria
- Ultrasound
- Occ IVU

RX: Good hydration, analgesia. Strain urine (analyse any calculi passed). If continued obst, surgical removal usually by cystoscopy & basket extraction. Often extensive evaluation of urinary tract is delayed until puerperium

Anaemia in Pregnancy

Common. IDA >Megaloblastic anaemia >Other anaemias

IDA

AETIOLOGY: Fe is required for the approximate 35% ↑ in maternal red cell mass. Full term infant has a total body Fe content of about 300mg. Each pregnancy requires a net gain of about 500–600mg of Fe. Without Fe supplements F are Fe depleted by the end of pregnancy. Contributory factors to IDA can inc poor diet, lack of Vit C, Vom, multiple pregnancy, PU, haemorrhoids, infections, drug induced gastritis & low pre-pregnancy Fe stores eg pregnancies close together, 2° to menorrhagia

CLIN: May be asymptomatic. Occ Tiredness; Oedema; Pallor

INVESTIGATIONS:
- FBC: MCV ↓, MCH ↓
- Serum Fe ↓
- Reticulocytes: ↑ in response to Rx
- Transferrin sat ↓
- TIBC ↑

RX: Prophylactic dietary Fe supplements. Use oral Fe preparation for mild anaemia. Vit C aids absorption. If early severe anaemia exclude other anaemia, give IM or IV Fe & monitor regularly. If late severe anaemia require blood transfusions or rarely exchange transfusion

FOLIC ACID DEF ANAEMIA

Due to Poor intake eg poor diet, vom; Poor absorption eg malabsorptive states; or ↑ utilisation esp multiple pregnancy, infection, fetal haemolysis, drugs (esp anticonvulsants)

AETIOLOGY: Pregnancy increases the requirement for folate & B12 due to the rapid growth of fetal placental & uterine tissues. As stores of folate are small compared to demands of pregnancy folate def is not uncommon

CLIN: May be asymptomatic. Occ Tiredness; SOB; Oedema. Ass c̄ slight ↑ risk of abortion, fetal malformation, abruptio placentae, prematurity

INVESTIGATIONS:
- FBC: MCV ↑, MCH ↑
- Red cell folate ↓ (more accurate than serum folate & FIGLU test)
- Serum Fe
- Occ Bone marrow

RX: Prophylactic Folic acid supplements (risk of masking PA & SACD is very small). Oral Folic acid for mild anaemia, severe cases may require IM Folate ± oral Fe, blood transfusion

HAEMOLYTIC ANAEMIA

Women c̄ chr haemolytic anaemias eg Spherocytosis, Thalassaemia, Hbopathies can react to fall in Hb level c̄ an acute haemolytic crisis

THALASSAEMIA: Esp Mediterranean littoral, Afr, Orient

Investigations:
- FBC
- Serum Fe ↑
- RBC fragility ↑

Rx: Folate. Prompt Rx of potential stresses eg infection, hypoxia. Treat crisis c̄ careful transfusion

SICKLE CELL DISEASE: Esp Blacks

Clin: Complications are common in pregnancy c̄ ↑ risk of Sickling crisis c̄ bone necrosis; Emboli; Pulm infarct; CCF; Cerebral haem; PET; Recurrent infections; Abortion; Prematurity; IUGR

Investigations:
- FBC
- Hb electrophoresis

Rx: Folic acid. Avoid hypoxia. Monitor

closely. If severe anaemia, slow transfusion of packed RBCs under diuretic cover. If crisis, correct any ppt factor (eg fever, infection, hypoxia), rehydrate, rest, O_2. Occ sterilisation advised

HAEMOGLOBINOPATHIES:

Investigations: • Hb electrophoresis (screen at risk populations)
• FBC
• Blood film

Rx: Folate. Prevent or early Rx of Hypoxia, Dehydration, Trauma. In crisis transfuse c̄ packed cells covered by diuretic. Deliver if BP ↑↑

MICROANGIOPATHIC HAEMOLYTIC ANAEMIA: Rare. Ass c̄ severe PET & Eclampsia. May → DIC

Vaginal Infections During Pregnancy

During pregnancy ↑ oestrogens → ↑ vaginal acidity but cervical epithelial discharge of alkaline mucus largely counteracts this effect. An exaggeration of the normal vaginal secretion is common in pregnancy

TRICHOMONAS

Common

CLIN: Red tender vagina; Thin irritant odourous discharge

INVESTIGATION: • Microscopy of discharge: Flagellate protozoan

RX: Saline bath or douches. Metronidazole (c/i first trimester) to F & her partner

PROG: Usually no effect on fetus

CANDIDA

Common. Esp Diabetics

CLIN: Thick creamy irritant odourous discharge (thrush). Occ vaginal tenderness

INVESTIGATION: • HVS

RX: Saline baths or douches. Antifungal pessaries or creams

PROG: Usually no effect on fetus

GONORRHOEA

Increasing incidence. In pregnant, affects vulva & vagina as well as cervix & urethra, cf GC in non-pregnant which affects tubes, uterus & cervix

CLIN: Vaginal discharge; Frequency. Occ asymptomatic

INVESTIGATION: • Urethral Swab
• HVS

RX: Antibiotics—often sensitive to Penicillin

PROG: If untreated, GC spreads in mother following delivery & may → neonatal ophthalmia in the fetus

HERPES

↑ in incidence

CLIN: Irritant vesicles on lower & upper vagina. Occ Thin vaginal discharge

INVESTIGATION: • Vesicle scrapings for virology

RX: Acyclovir. If active herpes in vagina deliver baby by LSCS

LGV

Rare. Esp W.Indies

CLIN: Bilat inguinal LN ↑. Occ Inguinal abscesses (buboes); Vaginal strictures; Vulval lymphoedema; Proctitis

INVESTIGATION: • Skin test

RX: Antibiotics eg Tetracycline. If extensive fibrosis or strictures, elective LSCS may be indicated

Disease of Resp System

PULM TB

Esp Indian sub-continent. Exacerbation in puerperium is common

RX: Anti-TB Rx as in non-pregnant. If mother has +ve sputum separate baby from mother at birth & give BCG to baby at 7 days & return baby to mother at 6wks. Bottle feeding usually advised

ASTHMA

Not usually affected by pregnancy. Rarely acute attack ppt premature labour

RX: Continue pre-pregnancy Rx. ↑ Dosage of any steroid Rx during labour

CHR BRONCHITIS & EMPHYSEMA

Uncommon in pregnancy

CLIN: SOB may ↑ in late pregnancy. ↑ risk of LRTI

RX: Normal Rx. May shorten 2nd stage to ↓ resp embarassment

Neurological Conditions

CHOREA GRAVIDARUM

Rare. Approx 1 in 3000 pregnancies. Ass c̄ Rheumatic carditis. Often recurs in later pregnancies

CLIN: Chorea. Occ Carditis; Pericarditis; Acute Psychosis

RX: Sedatives

MYASTHENIA GRAVIS

Pregnancy has no consistent effect. Puerperal exacerbations are common. Ass c̄ slight ↑ in SGA babies, perinatal death & maternal mort. About 20% of infants have neonatal myasthenia gravis c̄ hypotonia, poor feeding, facial weakness, feeble cry

RX: Neostigmine ± Atropine ± Steroids. Occ Thymectomy required during pregnancy. Occ shorten 2nd stage by forceps. Neonates respond to anticholinesterases

GIT Conditions

ACUTE CHOLECYSTITIS

Commoner in pregnant due to altered gall bladder function inc ↓ gall bladder emptying & ↑ biliary excretion of cholesterol

ACUTE APPENDICITIS

Incidence is about 1 in 1500 pregnancies. Diagnosis can be difficult partly due to reluctance to procede to laparotomy. Late diagnosis is ass c̄ the development of peritonitis

CLIN: Anorexia; N&V; Abdo pain. Occ Frequency; Fever. Site of pain differs in the pregnant as appendix is higher & more lat in late pregnancy

PROG: 30–40% fetal death if peritonitis

HEARTBURN

Common. ↑ progesterone → relaxation of cardiac sphincter → ↑ incidence of reflux

RX: Frequent small meals. Sleep propped up. Antacids may benefit

CONSTIPATION

Common. Due to ↓ gut muscle tone & affect of P by enlarged uterus in later pregnancy. May → development of haemorrhoids. Occ prevents engagement of head

RX: ↑ fluid intake. High fibre diet. Occ require laxatives

ACUTE INFECTIVE HEPATITIS

Not uncommon in pregnancy. Clinical picture similar to non-pregnant. Occ → premature labour. Slight ↑ in fetal death. Rarely → acute fulminant hepatitis

CHOLESTASIS OF PREGNANCY

Cause unknown. Similar condition occurs c̄ the "Pill"

CLIN: Pruritus; Malaise; N&V; Upper abdo pain; Liver ↑. Later J. Pruritis & J clear within 10 days of delivery. Does not → chr liver disease. Ass c̄ ↑ prematurity, ↑ perinatal mort. Recurrence in subsequent pregnancies is common

INVESTIGATIONS:
- Alk phos ↑
- ALT, AST ↑
- Bilirubin
- Hep B Ag –ve

RX: Cholestyramine. Vit K supplements

ACUTE FATTY LIVER OF PREGNANCY

May be idiopathic or due to drugs esp Tetracycline. Rare. Esp primagravida

CLIN: Sudden severe ALF in late pregnancy. N&V; Abdo pain; J; No fever. Occ Oliguria, DIC

INVESTIGATIONS:
- Bilirubin ↑↑
- Alk Phos ↑↑
- WCC ↑↑

RX: Correct dehydration, electrolyte imbalance. Give Vit K. Normal Rx of ALF. Emergency LSCS

PROG: High maternal & fetal mort. Rarely recurrence in subsequent pregnancy

Diabetes & Endocrine Conditions

DIABETES

Pregnancy is ass c̄ hormonal changes affecting the body's insulin requirements. An ↑ insulin requirement is needed to offset the

↑ in progesterone, oestrogens, HPL & free cortisol. Diabetes is ass c̄ at least 2–3× ↑ perinatal mort partly due to ↑ cong malformations. Complications are commoner if control is poor

Increased Risks of Diabetic Pregnancies (LIST 7 O&G)

1. Premature labour
2. PET
3. Cong malformations
4. Perinatal mort
5. Obstructed labour (large baby)
6. Hydramnios
7. Late IUD
8. Macrosomia
9. Shoulder dystocia
10. Essential BP ↑
11. Fetal growth retardation
12. Candidiasis

CLIN OF INFANT OF DIABETIC MOTHER: Poorly controlled diabetes → ↑ birth wt; ↑ length; Normal head circumference; Visceromegaly esp Liver, Ht which may → obst labour, shoulder dystocia, birth inj, asphyxia. Long standing diabetes may → placental insuf which may → SGA baby. ↑ Cong malformations eg TGV, VSD, PDA, NTD, Hydrocephalus esp in severe diabetes. RDS is common in diabetes (even when compared c̄ matched controls for gestational age, sex, Apgar score & mode of delivery) Maternal BG ↑ is ass c̄ neonatal BG ↓. Neonatal BG ↓ may → Sweating, Irritability, Hypotonia, Resp rate ↑, Fits. Less commonly HypoCa^{2+} &/or HypoMg^{2+} are seen which may → Irritability, Tremor, Fits. Rarely Renal vein thromb; Hypoplastic colon
Later ↑ incidence of CP, Ep. 1–5% develop diabetes

SERIAL INVESTIGATIONS:
- BG
- Urinalysis
- Ultrasound
- HPL
- Occ Unconjugated oestrogens, Glycosated Hb

RX: Encourage early antenatal attendance. Monitor regularly eg 2wkly until 32wks & wkly thereafter at the ANC. High fibre diet. Insulin Rx required if preprandial BG >5.8mmol/l. N.B Oral hypoglycaemics are c/i in pregnancy. Usually can control c̄ b.d human Insulins. Most diabetics can perform pre-prandial home BG monitoring. Early assessment by ophthalmologist c̄ follow up & Rx as necessary. Usually vaginal delivery near term is possible. If early delivery considered measure L:S ratio to assess maturity. During labour control BG level by infusion of 10% dextrose & insulin pump monitored by hrly BG estimations. Continuous fetal HtR monitoring. Fetal scalp blood for pH & blood gasses
Premature labour treated c̄ β sympathomimetics requires ↑ Insulin dosage to prevent hyperglycaemia
Post delivery insulin requirements fall rapidly. Encourage breast feeding. Diabetic control can be difficult to achieve & requires close monitoring

HYPERTHYROIDISM

About 1 in 1000 pregnancies. Ass c̄ slight ↑ risk of abortion, prematurity, SB, early neonatal mort. In fetus approx 1% develop neonatal hypothyroidism or thrombocytopenia

RX: Continue anti-thyroid drugs. If control difficult consider thyroidectomy. Carbimazole can → goitre &/or hypothyroidism in child. Avoid use of Radio I_2

ADDISON'S DISEASE

Require careful monitoring in pregnancy & puerperium. If vom in early pregnancy, care to ensure adequate cortisol dosage. Cortisol requirements usually ↑ during labour

SLE in Pregnancy

SLE may present as infertility or recurrent abortions. The severity of SLE is usually unchanged during pregnancy but often ↑ in puerperium. In fetus there is an ↑ risk of abortion, IUD, poor fetal growth, prematurity, hydrops, cong Ht block & skin rashes. Rarely neonatal SLE

INVESTIGATIONS:
- FBC
- ANA
- Urinalysis
- U&Es
- Platelets
- WCC
- Placental function tests
- Ultrasound

RX: Monitor closely. Often require steroids ± Azathioprine. ↑ steroids required during labour & puerperium. May require anti-BP ↑ drug Rx

Rh Arth in Pregnancy

Rh Arth may present as infertility. About 75% remit during pregnancy. Post-partum deterioration common

The Skin & Pregnancy

↑ pigmentation occurs on areolae, nipples, linea nigra, genitalia & face (Melasma), fading after delivery. Striae (stretch marks) are common—they are probably due to ↑ steroid production. The ↑ oestrogen production → ↑ incidence of spider naevi & palmar erythema. Hair growth usually ↑ in pregnancy & may be followed by excess hair loss in the puerperium (telogen effluvium). An itchy erythematous papular rash occ occurs in the 3rd trimester. Pruritus is also ass c̄ cholestatic J

Antepartum Haemorrhage

APH is genital tract bleeding between 28wks & delivery. Antepartum bleeding occurs in about 2% of pregnancies. About 50% are due to placenta praevia or abruptio placentae, 45% are unclassified

Causes of Bleeding in Late Pregnancy (LIST 8 O&G)

1. Abruptio placentae
2. Placenta praevia
3. Idiopathic
4. Cervical polyp or erosion
5. Vaginitis
6. Vaginal varicosities
7. Rarely:
   Ca Cervix, ITP, Leukaemia
8. Vasa praevia

DD: 1. Haematuria
2. Rectal bleeding

PLACENTA PRAEVIA

A placental encroachment onto the lower uterine segment. Esp seen in multiple pregnancy & multiparous. About 1 in 200 deliveries. Classified into 4 Stages of increasing severity: Stage 1—placenta encroaches on lower segment but does not reach int os; Stage II—placenta reaches but does not cover int os; Stage III—placenta covers int os before dilation occurs but would not cover fully dilated int os; Stage IV—placenta covers int os & would do so even when os fully dilated

CLIN: Painless fresh vaginal bleeding which often recurs. Uterus soft & non-tender. More severe forms may → persistent malpresentations esp transverse lie. Abnormalities of placenta are common eg battledore & velamentous cord insertions, membranacea & bipartite placenta

INVESTIGATION: • Ultrasound

RX: If bleed, admit to hospital, confirm diagnosis (not by VE) & XM blood. If confirmed stage II–IV placenta praevia, elective LSCS at 38wks. If unconfirmed or stage I do EUA at 38wks & if stage I rupture membranes & allow vaginal delivery. Syntometrine to ↓ risk of PPH. Occ vaginal delivery is tried c̄ type II placenta praevia on ant uterine wall

PROG: Good. ↑ risk to fetus if early delivery necessary

ABRUPTIO PLACENTAE

Bleeding from a normally sited placental bed after the 28th wk of pregnancy until birth. About 1 in 150 deliveries. Esp low social class, multiparous. Ass c̄ PET, Previous abruptio, Folate def, Trauma eg ECV, Circumvallate placenta, Sudden decompression of overdistended uterus eg post rupture of membranes c̄ polyhydramnios & Post delivery of a first twin

CLIN: May be bleeding p.v (revealed abruptio) or int bleed (concealed abruptio), usually mixture of both. Abdo pain; Shock. Often Uterus tender & woody hard. Foetal Ht may be absent. In more severe cases often → premature labour. Occ ARF; Clotting defects which may → DIC

INVESTIGATIONS:
- FBC
- XM
- Ultrasound
- Fibrinogen
- FDPs

RX: Analgesia; Urgent hospital admission. Monitor urine output. Often require transfusion c̄ FFP, fresh blood. If fetus alive & norm fetal Ht, LSCS when mother stable. If IUD or fetus compromised, ARM & Oxytocin when mother stable. Standard Rx of DIC, ARF

UNCLASSIFIED APH

Probably due to minor degrees of placenta praevia or abruptio placentae

RX: Manage expectantly. Ultrasound excludes placenta praevia. When bleeding settles may be allowed home. Closely monitor fetal growth

PROG: ↑ risk of perinatal mort

VASA PRAEVIA

In about 1 in 5000 pregnancies there is a velamentous insertion of the cord which passes across the lower cervical segment in front of the presenting part (vasa praevia). During labour the vessels may be compressed → asphyxia or the vessels may be traumatised eg at ARM → bleeding

CLIN: Bleeding p.v after spontaneous or ARM. Then fetal distress

INVESTIGATIONS:
- Kliehauer test: Detects fetal RBCs
- Abt test: HbF is resistant to alkalinisation

RX: Immediate delivery

Polyhydramnios

A ↑ vol of amniotic fluid

Causes of Polyhydramnios (LIST 9 O&G)

1. Multiple pregnancy
2. Maternal diabetes
3. Anencephaly
4. Hydrocephalus
5. Duodenal atresia
6. Oesophageal aresia
7. Chorioangioma
8. Rhesus incompatibility

CLIN: Large tense abdo. Abdo discomfort. Often SOB; Heartburn; Haemorrhoids; VVs. Rarely acute presentation c̄ Sudden rapid abdo distension; Tense tender uterus; & occ Oedema; N&V; SOB. Ass c̄ premature labour

INVESTIGATION: • Ultrasound

RX: Bed rest. In acute case may drain off some amniotic fluid if patient uncomfortable by slow release following amniocentesis. Often require early delivery

DD:
1. Ovarian cyst
2. Fibroids
3. Incorrect dates
4. Hydatidiform mole (early preg)
5. Large baby

Oligohyramnios

A ↓ vol of amniotic fluid. Rare

Causes of Oligohydramnios (LIST 10 O&G)

1. Renal agenesis
2. Intrauterine growth retardation
3. Retained dead fetus
4. Prolonged pregnancy
5. Severe PET

CLIN: Uterus small for dates (early). Later uterus feels full of fetus. Often premature labour. Fetus is often born relatively dehydrated. Common malformations are talipes & excessive lordosis. Ass c̄ abnormal placenta (Amnion nodosum)

INVESTIGATION: • Ultrasound

Fibroids & Ovarian Cysts Complicating Pregnancy

FIBROIDS

Fibromyomata are benign uterine tumours. Esp Blacks. Often ↑ in size during pregnancy & may become symptomatic. Can complicate pregnancy in a number of ways: Abortion; Red degeneration; Pressure effects → oedema, SOB, constipation, frequency; Obst labour (very rare); Uterine dysfunction. Most fibroids do not affect pregnancy

RED DEGENERATION:

Pathogenesis: In pregnancy ↑ in uterine growth & vascularity → enlarged vascular uterine fibroid. Oedematous fibroid may block venous supply → ischaemia & infarction (red degeneration)

Clin: Acute local pain & tenderness. Occ Mild fever; Vom; Anorexia. Pain abates in a few days

Investigations: • Ultrasound
• WCC: Occ ↑

Rx: Rest; Analgesia. Rarely laparotomy required to make diagnosis

OVARIAN CYSTS

May cause acute pain if they undergo torsion, rupture or bleed. Torsion is commonest in early pregnancy or the puerperium. Rarely obst labour

CLIN: Acute unilat pain. Occ Tenderness ± rebound on affected side. In early pregnancy, tumour often palpable

INVESTIGATIONS: • Ultrasound
• Tumour histology

RX: Laparotomy. Remove tumour & any infarcted tissue

Intrauterine Growth Retardation

IUGR is an imprecise definition concerning intrauterine growth factors → SGA babies (often defined as birth wt <10th centile for gestational age). About 30% of LBW babies suffer from IUGR. IUGR may be asymmetric c̄ relative sparing of head size or symmetric c̄ reductions in head & body size. Asymmetric IUGR is ass c̄ uteroplacental vascular insuf

Aetiology of IUGR (LIST 11 O&G)

1. Infections:
   Eg CMV, Rubella, Herpes, Toxoplasmosis
2. Chromosomal abnormalities
3. Cong anomalies inc dysmorphic syndromes
4. Genetic
5. Irradiation
6. Multiple pregnancy
7. Cyt.T drugs
8. Idiopathic
9. Maternal factors affecting placental perfusion:
   a) PET
   b) Recurrent APH
   c) Chr BP ↑
   d) Renovascular disease
   e) Diabetes
   f) Cyanotic Ht disease
   g) Sickle cell disease
   h) Malnutrition
   i) Smoking
   j) Heavy alcohol consumption

CLIN: Occ h/o low wt before pregnancy, alcoholism, smoking &/or poor diet. Occ Detectable low wt gain during pregnancy. Ass c̄ prematurity, perinatal asphyxia, ↑ perinatal mort

INVESTIGATIONS: • Serial ultrasounds: Measure BPD (good predictor of IUGR), head circumference, fetal abdo circumference
• Serial symphysis–fundus height measurement
• Serial measurements of Oestriol, HPL (less accurate than ultrasound)
• L:S ratio: Ratio of <2:1 is ass c̄ pulm immaturity
• Phosphatidylglycerol: Presence indicates pulm maturity

RX: Control of maternal complications eg BP ↑. Bed rest, β sympathomimetics may help. Balance risk of early delivery eg RDS against risks of further IUGR. Assess by biophysical profile ie ultrasonic assessment of fetal mvts, tone, reactive HtR (eg using non-stress or contraction stress test) & breathing mvts, alongside assessment of amniotic fluid vol. Often deliver at 35–37wks The biophysical profile score has been successfully used to determine high risk pregnancies requiring immediate delivery & reduce perinatal mort compared to a control gp

PROG: Some fetal & neonatal death unavoidable due to severe malformations. Prog depends on severity of perinatal asphyxia & extent of prematurity. Worse prog c̄ symmetric IUGR

PHYSIOLOGY, MECHANISMS & MANAGEMENT OF NORMAL LABOUR

Normal labour is the expulsion of the conceptus through the lower uterine segment. The child is born by the vertex, spontaneously within 24hrs, without injury to mother or baby
Labour is divided into 3 stages. The first stage is from the onset of labour until full dilation of the cervix. During this stage contractions increase in frequency & intensity. 2nd stage is from full dilation of the cervix until the birth of the baby. Strong regular contractions occur every 2–3mins. The 3rd stage is concerned c̄ the separation, descent & expulsion of the placenta & membranes
Prior to labour the lower uterine segment thins out & the cervix ripens ie softens & shortens. In late pregnancy episodes of unco-ordinated uterine contractions (Braxton–Hicks) are common
Mechanism of onset of labour not completely known. PGE2 & PGF2α are released by myometrium → ↑ cytosol free Ca^{2+} → contractions. Maternal ACTH may stimulate fetal adrenal DHAS release → ↑ oxytocin release. Mechanical factors eg uterine distension may also influence onset of labour
Uterine muscle can contract & retract. During first stage there is a heaping up & thickening of upper uterine segment. The lower segment is pulled up over the presenting part of the fetus. Cervix effaces & dilates. Onset of pain is variable. The first stage lasts about 12hrs in the primigravid & about 6hrs in the multiparous. In the 2nd stage the regular uterine contractions are enhanced by voluntary expulsive efforts by mother
At onset of labour the fetus is well flexed lying longitudinally & presenting by the vertex. As the fetal head descends to the pelvic floor, flexion is increased & the fetal head becomes moulded. Resistance of the pelvic floor → int rot of the fetal head. The head extends as it passes through the pelvic outlet. Once born the head rotates back to its normal relationship c̄ the shoulders (restitution). Further ext rotation of the head occurs as the ant shoulder reaches the pelvic floor & is rotated anteriorly. Expulsion of the fetal trunk occurs by lat flexion
In the third stage, the uterine muscle contracts constricting blood vessels & preventing excessive bleeding. The uterus becomes hard & globular & seems to rise up the abdo. The umbilical cord lengthens at the vulva

Management of Normal Labour

In UK most F are delivered in hospital but in many countries eg Holland, home delivery is common
Check BP, Temperature, PR, Urine. Clean vaginal area. VE to assess degree of cervical dilatation. Determine presentation of fetus. Occ catheterise &/or enema. Record frequency, duration & strength of uterine contractions. Record fetal HtR & rhythm in relation to contractions (phonocardiography). Progress of first stage is also monitored by vaginal assessment of descent in relation to ischial spines & dilation of cervix, & abdo assessment of descent in relation to pelvic brim. Plot labour on partogram. Food is not encouraged in first stage in case LSCS is required. Analgesia eg Pethidine, Entonox or epidural analgesia
Baseline fetal HtR is usually between 120–160 beats/min. There is a norm baseline variability of between 5–15 beats/min. During stronger contractions HtR may decelerate. Occ meconium is passed but this is commoner if fetal hypoxia. Occ fetal scalp capillary blood pH is measured, norm is >7.25
In the 2nd stage, woman is encouraged to bear down during uterine contractions. Analgesia. As head descends onto perineum inject LA into perivaginal tissues in preparation for an episiotomy if tearing of tissues appears likely. Avoid too rapid a delivery to help prevent tearing. When ant shoulder is born give IM Oxytocic eg Syntometrine. Following birth cord is clamped twice & divided. Suck out baby's nose & mouth
Oxytocic drugs eg Syntometrine to

expedite placental separation & descent. Placenta is delivered by controlled cord traction ie gentle traction on umbilical cord & upward counter pressure on uterus. Check placenta & membrane for completeness. Estimate blood loss (usually 100–200ml). Repair any tear or episiotomy. Close observation for at least 2hrs. Examine baby. Keep baby warm. Give baby to mother. Encourage early breast feeding

The benefits of invasive techniques for intrapartum monitoring eg scalp electrodes are not proven in low risk labour

Analgesia During Labour

The experience of pain during labour is variable. Many factors contribute inc psychological. Fear of labour pains may be ameliorated by ante-natal relaxation classes. Supportive, sympathetic staff & other attendants eg husband may help relieve apprehension

Entonox is a mixture of 50% nitrous oxide & 50% O_2. It should be used by inhalation as contraction is felt, taking 15–20secs to work

Pethidine is an effective analgesic given IM or slowly IV. Can → depression of fetal respiration. Best avoided within 2hrs of expected delivery

General anaesthesia should be performed c̄ empty stomach & c̄ precautions to avoid aspiration

Epidural anaesthesia (Rare SE: Infection, Inadvertent spinal anaesthesia, Injection of wrong drug, BP ↓) gives rapid pain relief by the introduction of anaesthetic eg Xylocaine into peridural fat numbing T11–S4 nerve roots. Repeat doses can be given through indwelling catheter → loss of sensation from the uterus & in 2nd stage patient requires help to recognise & bear down c̄ contractions

Indications for Epidural Analgesia (LIST 12 O&G)

1. Elective pain relief
2. Pain relief for potentially prolonged labour
3. Pain relief when other analgesics have failed
4. To help control BP in cases of BP ↑
5. Prevention of premature bearing down:
   Eg Breech presentation, Multiple pregnancy
6. Prevention of forceful 2nd stage contractions:
   Eg Cardiac disease, Severe resp disease
7. If risk of shoulder dystocia
8. For operative deliveries:
   Inc LSCS

Local nerve blocks involve infiltration of vulva & labia & injection of pudendal nerve c̄ Xylocaine. Indicated for pelvic manipulations in 2nd stage eg forceps & prior to episiotomy or repair of tear

MANAGEMENT OF ABNORMAL LABOUR

Planned Induction of Labour

Inductions for social reasons are generally disliked. These inductions may → LSCS or premature delivery. Induction to suit the operational policy of maternity units is often to the detriment of the mother's experience of giving birth

Gestational maturity of infant must be determined before any induction is considered

Induction is usually achieved by

Indications for Induction of Labour (LIST 13 O&G)

A. MATERNAL
   1. Postmaturity
   2. Severe BP ↑ (inc PET)
   3. Persistent APH
   4. Social
   5. Diabetes

B. FETAL
   1. IUGR
   2. Intrauterine death
   3. Some cong abnormalities
   4. Rhesus haemolytic disease

ARM (amniotomy) & infusion c̄ Oxytocin or by use of a vaginal pessary of PGE2. Monitor carefully (if uterus overstimulated → prolonged contractions → fetal hypoxia & occ uterine rupture). If amniotomy is carried out when the presenting part is not in the pelvis, cord prolapse may occur. If induction fails proceed to LSCS

Effectiveness of all methods of induction increases as the uterus nears term. If the cervix is soft, canal taken up & os dilated, high chance of early delivery post induction

Premature Rupture of the Membranes

Rupture of the membranes before the onset of regular uterine contractions. Occurs in 10% of pregnancies. Ass c̄ pre-term deliveries

CLIN: Sudden feeling of vaginal loss of fluid or wetness. Occ Smelly vaginal discharge (anaerobic infection). Occ Pelvic infection is asymptomatic. Rarely Uterine pain & tenderness

INVESTIGATIONS:
- Nitrazine swab
- Ferning
- Liquour C&S
- L:S ratio
- WCC
- MSU

RX: Confirm diagnosis by sterile speculum examination. Risk of preterm delivery must be weighed against risk of infection. Admit to hospital. Regular monitoring of pulse, temperature & uterine activity

If >34wks gestational age usually deliver. 85% go into spontaneous labour within 24hrs; induce before 24hrs to ↓ risk of puerperal fever

If <34wks give steroids every 7 days. Steroids ↓ risk of RDS. Transfer to centre c̄ neonatal intensive care unit. If confirmed pelvic sepsis, give Ampicillin & Metronidazole & deliver. If LSCS indicated, give single IV dose of antibiotic to ↓ risk of puerperal sepsis even if no proven infection. If fluid leak continues may → oligohydramnios & fetal crush syndrome, therefore deliver within 2wks of development of any oligohydramnios. Avoid tocolytic drugs

Pre-term Labour

Pre-term labour is labour before 37 completed wks of gestation. In UK about 7% of deliveries are pre-term. Pre-term delivery is ass c̄ LBW & fetal immaturity & hence most cases of perinatal death. RDS is common in children born before 34wks gestation

Factors Ass c̄ Pre-term Labour (LIST 14 O&G)

1. Previous spontaneous 2nd trimester abortion
2. Previous pre-term labour
3. Young maternal age
4. Smoking
5. Single F
6. Low social class
7. High alcohol intake
8. Grand multiparity
9. Low maternal wt pre-pregnancy (<50Kg)
10. Cong uterine abnormalities
11. Cervical incompetence
12. Polyhydramnios: Inc Multiple pregnancy
13. Premature rupture of membranes
14. Pyelonephritis
15. Fetal abnormality or death
16. ARM: Inc Wrongly timed induction, Rhesus haemolytic disease
17. Severe PET
18. APH
19. IUGR

The best predictor of pre-term delivery is previous pre-term labour. About 50% of multiple pregnancies → pre-term delivery. Generally the factors ass c̄ pre-term delivery are not specific enough to describe an at risk gp of practical value

INVESTIGATIONS:
- Serial ultrasound
- L:S ratio
- HVS

PREVENTION: Advice re smoking, diet & alcohol. Suture for any cervical incompetence (qv). Early Rx of UTIs. In F c̄ h/o repeated pre-term delivery, strict bed rest between 26–32wks is often advised on empirical grounds

RX: Bed rest. Inhibition of pre-term labour c̄ tocolytic drugs eg sympathomimetics, antiprostaglandins, $MgSO_4$, Ethanol.

Sympathomimetics eg Ritodrine, Salbutamol usually used (SE: Cardiac arrhythmias; BP ↓; Pulm oedema; Maternal BG ↑; ?neonatal BG ↓. c/i: Maternal cardiac disease; Thyrotoxicosis; When fetus is deemed safer delivered than remain in utero). Slowly ↑ dose of infusion until contractions stop or maximum dose is reached or unacceptable SE occur. If proven infection, antibiotics. Monitor c̄ continuous cardiotocography: prolonged, profound or recurrent decelerations are the result of fetal hypoxia, & deceleration in ass c̄ uterine contractions is abnormal

If F is in inevitable pre-term labour Rx depends on condition, maturity & presentation of fetus & place of confinement. Try to arrange for confinement in special centre (c̄ tocolytic Rx cover if necessary). Epidural analgesia is often preferred pain relief as it does not affect fetal respiration

Deliver if >34wks, though if membranes ruptured may deliver even slightly earlier. Give steroids if 27–33wks to hasten lung maturity. Give tocolytic drugs for contractions occuring before 33wks. If membranes ruptured but no contractions avoid tocolytic drugs. If evidence of infection & gestation >28wks, deliver early. LSCS is usually indicated if breech presentation (commoner in early pregnancy), intrauterine infection, signs of fetal hypoxia, placenta praevia, severe PET, IUGR, poor obstetric history. If vaginal delivery permissible a large episiotomy is essential c̄ good control of fetal head at crowning to ↓ risk of intracranial haem

Indications for Episiotomy (LIST 15 O&G)

1. Pre-term labour
2. Previous 3rd degree tear
3. Forceps
4. Ventouse
5. Fetal distress
6. Breech
7. Multiple pregnancy
8. Shoulder dystocia
9. Cord prolapse
10. Large fetal head
11. Face presentation
12. Rigid perineum

Non-Progressive Labour

Labour not progressing over time in a norm fashion. Often expressed as abnormal increase in one of the three phases of the Friedman labour curve. Friedman's curve compares duration of labour against cervical dilatation. The curve differs for primigravid & multiparous patients. In the first (latent) phase the cervix dilates slowly, in the 2nd acceleration phase the cervix dilates at maximal rate & in the 3rd deceleration phase cervical dilatation slows as ↑ fetal descent. It is practical to monitor progress of labour by assessing cervical dilatation & fetal descent against time. Non-progression of labour should always → a search for underlying cause & thus rational Rx

Causes of Non-progression of Labour (LIST 16 O&G)

A. THE POWERS
   Dysfunctional uterine action
B. THE PASSAGES
   1. Soft tissue obst:
      Eg Fibroid
   2. Bony obst:
      Eg Contracted pelvis
C. THE PASSENGER
   1. Large baby
   2. Malposition
   3. Malpresentation
   4. Fetal anomaly

GENERAL RX: Establish cause. If necessary transfer to specialist unit. ARM, if not already ruptured. Correct inefficient uterine action. Closely monitor fetal condition eg continuous fetal HtR monitoring, uterine activity, maternal condition eg BP. Give psychological support to F & relatives ie explanation, reassurance. Ensure adequate pain relief. Empty bladder & rectum. Avoid dehydration. Assess pelvis by clinical pelvimetry & occ X-Ray

Most cases result in cephalopelvic disproportion requiring LSCS or descent allowing spontaneous or low forceps delivery. Cases of mid-pelvic arrest require immediate LSCS or trial of forceps or vacuum c̄ theatre prepared for LSCS if trial fails

DYSFUNCTIONAL UTERINE ACTION

The inability to produce cervical

effacement & dilatation due to inefficient uterine action. Contractions may be too weak or too infrequent. Occ the problem is frequent strong or irregular inco-ordinate contractions. It may be difficult to distinguish between early labour & forced labour in those patients who present c̄ a partially effaced dilated cervix, but a "show" or rupture of membranes usually indicates true early labour

RX: Nurse in lat position. Amniotomy often improves uterine action. Usually possible to wait 1–2hrs to assess effect & possibly avoid other interventions
In the nulliparous, early non-progression is quite common & Oxytocin can be safely used to stimulate contractions. Monitor closely, avoid uterine overstimulation
Non-progression in the multiparous is rarely due to dysfunctional uterine action. Oxytocin must be used c̄ care as serious risk of tonic contraction & fetal distress which may → uterine rupture, if underlying cause is disproportion. If contractions too strong, analgesia esp epidural is often helpful

OBSTRUCTED LABOUR

Disproportion occurs when a fetal part is too big to pass through the maternal pelvis. There are 4 basic types of pelvis (although many pelvices are of mixed type): Gynaecoid; Anthropoid; Android; Platypelloid. The android pelvis has a narrowed outlet & may cause disproportion as the head descends. The platypelloid (flat pelvis) often does not allow passage of head through brim
The fetal part involved in disproportion is usually the head as this is the largest & least compressible part of the fetus. Disproportion may be caused by the angle of approach of the fetal part to the pelvis

INVESTIGATIONS: • Ultrasound: Eg to measure fetal head size
• X-Ray pelvimetry
• Head fitting test

GENERAL RX: If cephalopelvic disproportion is obvious eg head will not engage in late pregnancy c̄ overlap of pubic symphasis, elective LSCS in 39th wk or earlier if labour supervenes. If cephalopelvic disproportion borderline, if spontaneous labour has not occured, induce at 39wks & proceed to trial of labour. Prepare for shoulder dystocia

CONTRACTED PELVIS: Usually defined as a pelvic brim c̄ either AP or transverse diameter of reduced by 2cm. In UK usually due to general pelvic contraction preventing engagement of head. In underdeveloped countries abnormal shaped pelvis are common & engagement is no guarantee that fetal head can pass through pelvis. Ass c̄ maternal Hgh <5ft

Rx: If assessment of bony pelvis indicates disproportion LSCS indicated. If diagnosis of disproportion questionable do trial of labour if head presenting & facilities for immediate LSCS. In trial of labour allow spontaneous onset of labour unless baby at term when induction may be indicated. Monitor descent of head abdominally & vaginally, continuous fetal Ht monitoring, periodic assessment of cervix. Avoid oral food & fluids. Trial of labour failed if: No ↑ in cervical dilatation despite good contractions; Non-engagement of head c̄ fully dilated cervix; No cervical dilatation for 4hrs following rupture of membranes; Labour of >24hrs; Serious

Causes of Disproportion (LIST 17 O&G)

1. Large fetus:
   a) Genetic
   b) Diabetes
   c) Occ young multiparous F
   d) Rarely: Abnormalities of aorta & left Ht; Fetal ascites; Brain, thyroid or kidney tumours
2. Abnormal fetal head:
   Eg Hydrocephaly, Anencephaly (shoulders too wide)
3. Malpositions & malpresentations:
   Eg Brow, Transverse lie
4. Bony obst:
   a) Small normally shaped pelvis
   b) Abnormally shaped pelvis
      eg Naegele's pelvis, Rickets, Osteomalacia, Fracture, Trauma
5. Soft tissue obst:
   Eg Fibroids esp post cervical; Ovarian tumours; Pelvic kidney

deterioration in fetal or maternal condition. If trial of labour succeeds, often require forceps delivery. Give IV Syntometrine c̄ delivery of head, & be prepared for PPH

Prog: About 80% entered into trial of labour deliver vaginally. Approx 20% of F c̄ h/o LSCS for disproportion subsequently deliver a child vaginally

SHOULDER DYSTOCIA: Shoulder dystocia occurs when the head of the baby is born but the shoulders cannot be delivered by normal means. Approx incidence is 1 in 400 deliveries. Ass c̄ Large babies; Diabetes; Postmaturity

Pathogenesis: If shoulders enter pelvis in AP diameter the ant shoulder will impact behind pubic symphesis compressing fetal chest

Clin: Often prolonged 2nd stage & assisted mid-pelvic delivery. Normal amount of traction on head fails to deliver shoulders. Ext rot of head does not occur. ↑ risk of Fetal hypoxia; Upper body #; Erb's palsy; Genital tract trauma; PPH

Rx: Obstetric emergency. Put in lithotomy position. Try & rotate fetal shoulders to oblique diameter of pelvic brim by inserting hand between symphesis & fetal neck. If successful apply head traction c̄ backward flexion. If fails, enlarge episiotomy & prepare to bring down post arm. Following delivery of whole arm norm head traction will usually deliver ant shoulder. If not, rotate the body 180° & bring down 2nd arm

Prog: Prompt action can usually prevent morbidity & death

MALPRESENTATIONS & MALPOSITIONS

A malpresentation occurs when some part of the fetus other than the head is the presenting part. A malposition occurs when the head presents, but the lower pole is not the vertex region. The vertex is an area bounded by the two parietal eminences, the post border of the ant fontanelle & the ant border of the post fontanelle. The commonest malpresentations are breech & shoulder. The commonest malposition is O-P. All are ass c̄ non-progressive labour, ↑ risk of prolapsed cord & early rupture of membranes

Breech

About 1 in 40 of all deliveries. Commoner if Pre-term labour; Fetal malformations eg Hydrocephalus; Hydramnios; Abnormal pelvic brim or uterus; Placenta praevia; Multiple pregnancy. Occ May be due to splinting by extended legs of the fetus

Types: 4 Types. Complete flexed breech; Frank breech ie both legs extended; Incomplete breech ie one leg extended, one flexed; Footling breech ie both legs to hips extended

Clin: Head felt at upper end of uterus. No head palpable on VE. Occ Early rupture of membranes ± prolapsed cord. ↑ risk of PPH

Investigations:
- Ultrasound
- Assessment of pelvic size

Rx: If breech present after 33wks attempt ECV (c/i: Multiple pregnancy, BP ↑, previous uterine scar, ruptured membranes, bleeding in late pregnancy, Rhesus – ve). Review wkly, ECV may be repeated if previously unsuccessful or fetus has turned back. If version has not occured by 36–38wks prepare for breech delivery

Vaginal delivery is ass c̄ ↑ risks inc fetal hypoxia, intracranial haem, #, intra-abdominal organ damage, prolapsed cord, cervical spine inj & Erb's palsy & therefore often safer to deliver by LSCS. LSCS is usually indicated if large baby or other signf risk of disproportion, any complication of late pregnancy eg PET, previous LSCS, multiple pregnancy, non-progression of attempted vaginal delivery & fetus <32wks gestation. If no spontaneous labour by term proceed to induction or LSCS as appropriate

If vaginal delivery attempted: Bed rest to ↓ risk of early rupture membranes; Immediate VE after rupture of membranes to assess for prolapsed cord; Restrict oral intake in case of op delivery. Epidural analgesia is good method of pain relief. Be prepared for urgent LSCS. With knee & footling presentations, & c̄ premature breech, presenting part may be visible at introitus before full dilatation & it is important to ensure full dilation of cervix before proceeding c̄ delivery. When buttocks are on point of crowning perform episiotomy. Assist birth of legs. Relieve tension on cord by bringing down loop. Ensure that baby does not rotate into a sacro–posterior position. If arms are extended, manipulate eg by rotation & traction (Lovset's manoeuvre). Deliver body & apply gentle traction to legs until suboccipital region is below maternal pubis. Deliver head by forceps c̄ the body held horizontal by an assistant. As face is delivered clear nose & mouth of mucus allowing baby to breathe. Deliver rest of head slowly to prevent sudden decompression. Alternative method if forceps are not available is the Mauriceau–Smellie–Veit manoeuvre when a finger is placed in the fetal mouth (which gently flexes the head) whilst the other fingers lie on the shoulders & the other hand is placed on the fetal back. As head is delivered give Syntometrine. Deliver placenta in norm manner

Accelerated delivery is indicated if fetal or maternal distress or lack of progress in 2nd stage

Prog: Breech delivery is ass c̄ ↑ PNMR, prematurity, hypoxia & intracranial haem. Asphyxia is commonest c̄ a footling breech

Shoulder Presentation

Approx 1 in 250–300 pregnancies. Esp if: Polyhydramnios; Contracted pelvis; Placenta praevia; Pelvic obst eg fibroid; Abnormal uterus eg arcuate, subseptate; Fetal abnormalities; Prematurity; Multiple pregnancy; Lax uterus of grand multip

Clin: Fetus in transverse lie

Investigation: • Ultrasound: Eg To confirm diagnosis & to look for multiple pregnancy &/or fetal abnormality

Rx: Between 33–35wks, attempt ECV weekly if no c/i. If longitudinal lie not achieved admit to hospital & attempt ECV daily if >36wks in multiparous or >38wks in nulliparous. If patient goes to term c̄ fetus in transverse position may do elective LSCS or attempt ECV in labour ward followed by hind water rupture c̄ Drew–Smythe catheter. If F admitted in labour c̄ transverse lie & ruptured membranes, impacted shoulder presentation ± prolapse of arm will have occured c̄ risk of uterine rupture & requires Caesarean section often of the classical type

Occipito–posterior Position

About 5% of cephalic presentations rotate into an O–P position. A further 10% undergo long 270° int rot through the O–P position to become O–A. RO–P is commoner than LO–P. Esp if: Android pelvis; Inco-ordinate uterine action; Poor flexion of head; Epidural analgesia

Clin: Occ Palpation reveals fetal limbs in front; Non-palpable back & high head. P of head on sacrum & rectum often → early desire to push. Usually prolonged labour. Occ constriction ring occurs round baby's neck. ↑ risk of PPH, maternal & fetal distress, sepsis. May extend into face/brow presentation

Rx: Observe closely. Many cases will rotate spontaneously. Expect long labour. Check for cord prolapse immediately after rupture of membrane. Ensure that F does not push before cervix is fully dilated. Adequate analgesia eg epidural. Restrict oral intake. If head stays O–P delivery face to pubis may occur spontaneously & large episiotomy will be needed. If head stays in occipito–transverse position it will not deliver spontaneously & requires rotation under anaesthesia by Kielland's straight forceps, manual rotation to O–A position or vacuum extraction. With crowning of head give IV Syntometrine. Deliver placenta promptly. Suture episiotomy. LSCS may be indicated if failure to progress, fetal or maternal distress

Causes of High Head at Term (LIST 18 O&G)

1. O–P position
2. Full bladder or rectum
3. Wrong dates
4. Steep inclination of pelvic brim
5. Twins
6. Hydramnios
7. Cephalopelvic disproportion
8. Some fetal abnormalities: Eg Hydrocephalus
9. Non-bony obst to passages: Eg Placenta praevia, Fibroids, Ovarian tumours

Face Presentation

The face is the area from chin to nasion. Occurs in 1 in 300 deliveries. Ass c̄: Lax uterus; Multiple pregnancy; Prematurity; Fetal malformations esp anencephaly & thyroid tumours; Dolichocephalic skull (long head); Spasm of fetal neck muscles; Platypelloid pelvis

Clin: Usually diagnosed in labour. 85% engage in the mento–transverse. Most rotate to mento–anterior & can deliver spontaneously. A rotation to mento–posterior → obst labour

Rx: After rupture of membranes exclude prolapsed cord. If ant rotation expect longer 2nd stage. Occ low forceps required. If mento–transverse arrest, Keilland's forceps or manual rotation to mento–anterior & extraction. With birth of head give Syntometrine. If rotation to mento–posterior, fetal chin is in the curve of the mother's sacrum & head cannot extend further. Hence proceed to LSCS

Prog: ↑ risk of fetal hypoxia

Brow Presentation

Brow is area bounded by nasion, biparietal eminences & ant fontanelle. Approx 1 in 1000 deliveries

Clin: High head. Abdominally, head felt on both sides of fetus. Often membranes rupture early ± prolapse of cord

Rx: In labour may convert to face or vertex. If presentation persists perform LSCS

Cord Presentation

The presence of the umbilical cord below the presenting part c̄ intact membrane. Esp seen in incomplete breech presentation. If discovered at time of inducing labour, defer induction & nurse in bed for 24hrs. Often cord will now be placed above presenting part. If not, LSCS

Prolapse of Cord

Approx 1 in 400 deliveries. Occurs when part of umbilical cord falls in front of presenting part following rupture of membranes

Predispositions to Cord Prolapse (LIST 19 O&G)

1. Malpresentations:
   Esp Transverse lie, Breech, O-P, Face, Brow
2. Abnormal fetus
3. Pre-term fetus
4. Multiple pregnancy
5. Premature rupture of membranes
6. Polyhydramnios
7. Placenta praevia
8. Pelvic tumours
9. Obstetric procedures:
   Eg ECV

CLIN: Occ sudden appearance of cord loop at introitus following rupture of membranes. Usually diagnosis made on VE. If baby alive cord pulsates. Fetal distress

INVESTIGATIONS: • Ultrasound
• Fetal Ht monitoring

RX: If baby dead deliver vaginally. If baby alive immediate relief of cord compression. Gently replace cord in vagina (to ↓ risk of umbilical artery spasm from cooling). With whole hand in vagina & cord cradled in palm of hand, elevate presenting part c̄ tips of fingers. Place mother in knee–chest or Sims lat position. If cervix fully dilated & presenting part low perform immediate assisted vaginal delivery, otherwise immediate LSCS

PROG: ↑ fetal death esp if prolapse occurs outside hospital

Postmaturity

Labour occuring after 42wks of pregnancy. Incidence in UK is low as intervention prevents most F going to 42wks. Important to assess maturity accurately

CLIN: Uterus feels "full of baby". Occ Oligohydramnios. Postmaturity is ass c̄ long labour, inefficient uterine action, disproportion, malpositions. ↑ risk of fetal hypoxia (due to ↓ placental efficiency); PPH

INVESTIGATION: • Assessment of maturity inc: LMP, Serial ultrasounds, Serial clin assessments, X-R (occ)

RX: If postmaturity confirmed intervene to induce labour. If cervix ripe: ARM & IV Oxytocic. If cervix unripe: PGE2 pessary to ripen, then ARM. If disproportion or failure of induction: LSCS

PROG: ↑ risk of perinatal mort which is reduced by early intervention

Interventional Procedures to Assist Delivery

FORCEPS

Forceps are devices to apply to fetal head. Usually used to hasten delivery by application of gentle traction. Other value may be in controlling speed of descent eg breech delivery & protecting fetal head eg in very premature. Many types of forceps eg Wrigley's,

Kielland's. Frequency of usage variable, approx 5–15% of deliveries

Indications for Forceps (LIST 20 O&G)

1. Delay in 2nd stage of labour:
   a) Poor maternal effort
      eg Exhaustion, Non-cooperation, Inability to push adequately following epidural
   b) Malrotation eg Transverse arrest, O–P position
2. Previous pelvic surgery
3. To expedite delivery when there is fetal distress
4. To reduce maternal effort:
   Eg Maternal BP ↑, PET, Cardiac disease, Resp disease
5. To prevent rapid delivery & protect fetal brain:
   Eg Aftercoming head in breech delivery, Very premature

Three basic types of forceps:

1. Long curved forceps: Used when fetal head is in a direct A–P position no higher than the level of ischial spines. They all have a pelvic curve & crossover handles forming a fixed lock. Eg Neville–Barne's
2. Short curved forceps: Similar to long curved forceps but shorter handles limits amount of traction. Used for lift out when head is on perineum. Eg Wrigley's
3. Long straight forceps: Used to aid rotation of fetal head. Have no pelvic curve. Have a sliding lock to allow correction of any asynclitism. Eg Kielland's

All forceps procedures are possible causes of trauma to mother &/or fetus esp in inexperienced hands. Certain conditions must be fulfilled before application: Cervix must be fully dilated; Membranes must be ruptured; Bladder should be empty; Head must be at level of ischial spines or below; Position must be accurately determined; Adequate analgesia; Adequate uterine contractions; Aseptic technique; Episiotomy; Intervention must have reasonable chance of success. A LSCS is preferable to a difficult forceps delivery

VACUUM EXTRACTION (VENTOUSE)

A metal cup connected to a chain for traction & via a rubber tube to a suction pump to produce a vacuum. Cup is applied over post fontanelle & traction applied during contractions. Advantages over forceps inc: ↓ risk of trauma to mother; No necessity for episiotomy & catheterisation; Can be used without full dilation of cervix; ↓ risk of trauma to fetus as strong traction detaches cap. If used for >20mins may → scalp trauma. If delivery not achieved or imminent in 3 pulls, discontinue. Indications for use similar to forceps but c/i in disproportion, prematurity, malpresentation. In fetal distress forceps are quicker to apply

CAESAREAN SECTION

The surgical delivery of the fetus through the abdominal wall. Approx 5–15% of deliveries in UK

Indications for Caesarean Section (LIST 21 O&G)

1. 2 or more previous Caesarean sections
2. Previous classical Caesarean section
3. Major cephalopelvic disproportion
4. Previous section complicated by post-op infection
5. Placenta praevia (more than Stage I)
6. Fetal distress in first stage of labour
7. Failed trial of labour
8. Some breech presentations: Esp Premature, In elderly primagravida, Disproportion
9. Previous major uterine surgery
10. Failed forceps
11. Maternal distress: Eg Severe PET
12. Obst labour: Eg Malpresentation, Constriction ring
13. Genital herpes
14. Prolapsed cord
15. Death of mother in late pregnancy

Occ elective op can be planned. Often obstetric procedures eg trial of labour are carried out in knowledge that Caesarean section facility may be required & should be available c̄ patient prepared eg restricted oral intake. Some cases are true emergency ops. Vast majority of ops are of the LSCS type as this has fewer post-op complications, better scar healing & lower risk of uterine rupture than classical op. Classical op indicated if transverse lie or unapproachable lower segment eg Adhesions, Contracted pelvis, Fibroids

COMPLICATIONS: 1. Haem
2. Thromboemboli inc Pelvic vein thrombosis, DVT & PE
3. Wound infections
4. Other general op complications eg PI, Adhesions, LRTI

Uterine Rupture

May be complete involving full thickness of uterine wall or incomplete. Rare in developed countries (approx 1 in 3000 deliveries) but not uncommon in underdeveloped nations

Causes of Uterine Rupture (LIST 22 O&G)

1. Previous Caesarian section:
   Esp Classical type
2. Previous hysterotomy
3. Other major uterine surgery:
   Eg Myomectomy, Uteroplasty
4. Excessive Oxytocic drugs
5. Neglected obst labour:
   Esp In multiparous
6. Trauma:
   Eg Forceps, Shoulder dystocia

Uterine rupture is ass c̄ Uterine anomalies, Cornual pregnancy, Placenta increta & percreta, & Trophoblastic disease

CLIN: Variable presentation. Symptoms & signs may be severe or mild. Occ Severe abdo pain; Vaginal bleeding; Abatement of contractions; Shock; Fetal Distress. Rarely Haematuria; Swelling & crepitus over lower uterine segment

RX: Treat shock. Laparotomy to remove fetus & placenta, & secure haemostasis. If major rupture, total or subtotal hysterectomy. If simple rupture c̄ no infection, laceration repair ± tubal ligation

PROG: High risk of fetal death. Risk of maternal death

Fetal Distress During Labour

During uterine contractions intervillous blood flow is transiently halted → ↓ O_2 supply to fetus. If fetus unable to withstand this stress → fetal distress ie hypoxia & acidosis

Causes of Fetal Distress During Labour (LIST 23 O&G)

1. ↓ Maternal oxygenation:
   Eg Cyanotic Ht disease, Severe anaemia, COAD, Eclampsia
2. Fetal anaemia:
   Eg Rhesus haemolytic disease, Vasa praevia, Twin to twin transfusion
3. Cord compression:
   Eg Cord prolapse, P on cord from presenting part
4. ↓ Intervillous blood flow & placental transfer:
   a) BP ↓ eg APH, Drugs, Epidural
   b) Vasoconstriction 2° to BP ↑
   c) Excessive uterine action
      eg Excess Oxytocics, Abruptio placentae
   d) Idiopathic placental insufficiency

Three main methods of assessing fetal distress in labour: Meconium staining, Fetal HtR monitoring, Fetal blood acid–base determination

FETAL HtR MONITORING: Normal rate is 120–160 beats/min. Patterns suggesting fetal hypoxia are:
1. Late decelerations: Start after contraction peaks c̄ return to baseline well after contractions have ceased
2. Variable decelerations: Shape, duration & timing of decelerations are variable. Often abrupt fall & rise of HtR. Usually due to cord compression. Severest types last >60secs
3. Prolonged decelerations: Any decelerations lasting >2mins
4. Mixed deceleration patterns: Defy precise classification eg variable deceleration c̄ gradual return of HtR
5. Fetal tachycardia >160 beats/min
6. Reduction in beat to beat variability
7. Fetal Bradycardia: Marked bradycardia ie <90 beats/min may be ass c̄ cong Ht block

Early decelerations ie those starting early in contraction c̄ uniform shape & returning to norm rate by end of contraction, are benign. Accelerations & mild bradycardia are usually benign. Fetal hypoxia rarely exists in presence of normal baseline variability

Rx: Look for correctable cause eg Drugs. Correct any BP ↓. Exclude cord prolapse. O_2 to mother. Consider early delivery esp if supporting evidence eg Fetal acidosis, passage of fresh thick meconium

FETAL BLOOD ACID–BASE DETERMINATION: Normal pH is >7.25. If pH <7.20, expedite delivery. If pH 7.20–7.25, recheck pH after 10–15 mins

PPH

PRIMARY PPH

Bleeding from the genital tract in excess of 500mls within 24hrs of delivery. If active management of 3rd stage practised, incidence approx 2–5% of deliveries

Predisposing Factors to 1° PPH (LIST 24 O&G)

1. Atonic uterus:
   Ass c Multiple pregnancy, Multiparity, Prolonged or ppt labour, Polyhydramnios, APH, Deep anaesthesia
2. Mechanical prevention of retraction:
   a) Retained placenta
   b) Retained clots
   c) Uterine fibroids
   d) Uterine anomalies
      eg Cornual implantation, Previous scar on uterus
3. Trauma:
   Eg Lacerations of vagina, episiotomy
4. Coagulation defects
5. Uterine inversion

INVESTIGATIONS: • Ultrasound
• FBC
• XM
• Clotting screen

PREVENTION: Give Oxytocic c̄ delivery of ant shoulder. After delivery of placenta, massage uterus firmly to help expel clot. Close surveillance for 2–3hrs post delivery. In high risk eg Grand multip c̄ h/o PPH may give IV infusion of Oxytocin for 2hrs post-partum

RX: Contract uterus by fundal massage & IV Oxytocin or Ergometrine. Deliver placenta by controlled cord traction or if this fails, manually under a GA. Suture any lower genital tract laceration. Treat any shock c̄ IV fluids & blood. Rarely laparotomy required ± hysterectomy. If not in hospital, emergency technique such as bimanual compression of uterus may be required during transit

COMPLICATIONS: 1. ARF
2. Sheehan's syndrome
3. Post partum anaemia
4. Maternal death (rare)

SECONDARY PPH

Abnormal bleeding from the genital tract between 24hrs & 6wks post partum. Occurs in approx 1% of deliveries

Causes of 2° PPH (LIST 25 O&G)

1. Retained placental fragments ± infection
2. Lacerations
3. Retained old clots
4. Trophoblastic disease (rare)
5. Submucous fibroid
6. Chr uterine inversion

CLIN: Fresh vaginal bleeding. Occ Pyrexia; Offensive discharge; Large uterus; Open cervix

INVESTIGATIONS: • Ultrasound
• FBC
• XM
• HVS

RX: If slight bleed, Syntometrine. Treat any infection c̄ appropriate antibiotic
If heavy bleed, gently explore uterus under anaesthesia using finger & sponge forceps. Loosen & remove any placental tissue & then cautious curettage. Risk of Uterine perf; Inducing severe haem eg by tearing adherent strip of myometrium

COMPLICATIONS: 1. Anaemia
2. Infection → infertility
3. Subinvolution of myometrium

PERINEAL & VAGINAL TEARS

Tears are ass c̄ ppt delivery, large head, cephalopelvic disproportion, O–P position, breech delivery, use of forceps. Three degrees of perineal laceration. In first degree, damage to skin. In 2nd degree, tearing of post vaginal wall & perineal muscles. In 3rd degree, tearing of anal canal

RX: Adequate analgesia. Repair in lithotomy position. Check genital tract systematically for tears. Repair tears

RETAINED PLACENTA

About 2% of deliveries. The longer the placenta is retained the greater the risk of PPH. Retention of separated placenta may be due to uterine atony or a constriction ring. Retention of adherent placenta is more likely if uterus is subjected to previous surgery, trauma or infection

Placenta accreta indicates adherence to myometrium. Placenta increta invades myometrium. Placenta percreta penetrates serosal layer

RX: If retained separated placenta, treat as for 1° PPH. Try controlled cord traction. If retained placenta is unresponsive to Oxytocics, manual removal under GA indicated c̄ infusion of Oxytocics. Any trapping of placenta in cornual pockets must be identified & relieved by careful exploration c̄ fingers. In rare case of pathological adherence, piecemeal manual removal may be indicated

ACUTE UTERINE INVERSION

Rare. Approx 1 in 20,000 deliveries. May be incomplete or complete depending on degree to which uterine fundus turns itself inside out

CLIN: Often follows 3rd stage. Complete inversion usually → Sudden shock; Heavy PPH; Lower abdo pain

RX: Treat shock. Transfuse. Early attempt to replace uterus without removing placenta by manual replacement. If fails try inserting douche of warm antiseptic raised above vagina into the post fornix. If fails, surgical correction at laparotomy

Abnormal Placentas

PLACENTA EXTRACHORIALIS

The area of the chorionic plate is reduced & deep irregular invasion by trophoblast occurs in lat direction. Types inc: Placenta marginata ie superficial decidua appears as a ring on surface of placenta; Placenta circumvallata where membranes enfold decidua

Occur in 1 in 6 pregnancies. Ass c̄ mild APH

PLACENTA MEMBRANACEA

Implantation deeply into decidua. Entire fetal membranes covered by thin functioning placenta

PLACENTA SUCCENTURIATA

Main placenta is connected to an accessory small placenta by vessels passing through membranes. Risk of retained small placenta → PPH; Infection

PLACENTA ACCRETA, INCRETA, PERCRETA

Danger of retained placenta (qv)

PLACENTA HAEMANGIOMATA

May be small & asymptomatic. Occ large → APH, premature labour

MULTIPLE PREGNANCY

Twins occur in approx 1 in 100 pregnancies. Other multiple deliveries are much rarer, approx 1 in 5–10,000 deliveries. Rates are commoner in some families, if previous multiple pregnancy & if "fertility" drugs used. Binovular twins are commoner than monovular. Binovular twins are commoner if maternal FH of non-identical twins, mother aged >35yrs, high parity

PATHOGENESIS: Monovular twins are produced by one ovum fertilised by one sperm which at the two cell stage divides into two separate cell bodies c̄ common chromosomal material &

hence later identical twins. Binovular twins occur when two separate ova are fertilised by different sperms, non-identical twins develop

CLIN: May be FH or past obstetric h/o twins. Often Hyperemesis gravidarum; VVs; Heartburn; Breathlessness. Uterus larger than dates. Later "lot of limbs" can be felt & >2 poles determined. ↑ risk of: Polyhydramnios; Abortion; Pre-term labour; PET; Anaemia; Placenta praevia; APH. In 80%, first twin has cephalic presentation. Frequency of presentations in twin birth are Vertex–Vertex >Vertex–Breech >Breech–Vertex >Breech–Breech >Others. In labour ↑ risk of: Early rupture membranes; Prolapsed cord; PPH; Retained placenta. Ass c̄ ↑ PNMR esp for 2nd twin. After delivery of 2nd twin examine abdo for 3rd baby. In puerperium ↑ risk of: Infection; Anaemia; Feeding problems eg insuf milk for both babies

INVESTIGATIONS: • Ultrasound
• FBC
N.B A significant minority (3–20%) of twin pregnancies are not diagnosed until labour

RX: Extra Fe & Folate supplements. Treat any PET. Book for hospital delivery. If first twin is transverse lie do LSCS. Check for cord prolapse after rupture of membranes. Monitor both fetal hearts. Be prepared for LSCS, fetal resus & therefore anaesthetist & paediatrician should be available. Often episiotomy indicated. Do not give Syntometrine c̄ delivery of first twin. Clamp cord securely (occ vascular connection between twins)
Following delivery of first twin, check lie of 2nd twin. If lie not longitudinal, convert preferably by ext version but if unsuccessful by int version & breech extraction. Important to deliver 2nd twin without delay ie within 15mins of first twin. Rupture membranes of 2nd sac. Check for cord prolapse. Occ require Oxytocin drip to enhance contractions. Give Syntometrine on delivery of 2nd twin. Deliver placenta as soon as uterus is contracted. Continue Oxytocin drip for 3–4hrs post delivery to ↓ risk of PPH

COMPLICATION: Rarely shunting of blood between the fetuses → J; Anaemia; Disparity of fetal size. If one twin dies, esp in early pregnancy, a small squashed dehydrated fetus may be found in the placental membranes (fetus papyraceas)

PROG: ↑ PNMR due mainly to Hypoxia; Immaturity; Operative delivery risks. 2nd twin at ↑ risk due to Trauma eg 2° to malpresentation & intrauterine manipulation; Partial placental separation → asphyxia; Haemodynamic changes after delivery of first twin → asphyxia

DRUGS IN PREGNANCY

Experience has taught doctors to be very cautious in the use of drugs during pregnancy. All non-essential drugs should be avoided in the first trimester when the risk of teratogenicity is highest. If a drug is required, favour well established remedies. Some drugs are well known to be teratogenic eg Thalidomide, whilst many others are suspected either on experimental grounds or suggestive case histories

SE of Some Drugs During Pregnancy (LIST 27 O&G)

A. ANTIBIOTICS
1. Chloramphenicol → Grey Syndrome
2. Tetracycline → Teeth staining, Bone deformities

B. HORMONES
1. Diethylstilboesterol → Genital tract abnormalities, Vaginal AdenoCa in young adult
2. Oral Hypoglycaemics → Neonatal hypoglycaemia
3. Anti-thyroid drugs → Neonatal hypothyroidism
4. R-a I_2 → Hypothyroidism
5. Oestrogen/Progestogen pill → ↑ fetal abnormalities
6. Progestogens → F virilisation

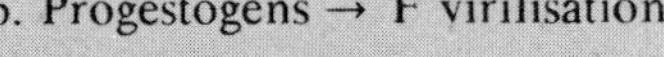

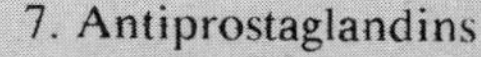

7. Antiprostaglandins
   → Premature closure of Ductus Arteriosus

C. CYTOTOXIC DRUGS
Most known or presumed to be teratogenic

D. NARCOTICS
1. Heroin → IUD, Resp depression, Neonatal withdrawal syndrome
2. Methadone → neonatal withdrawal syndrome

E. ANTICONVULSANTS
1. Phenytoin → Cleft lip & palate, CHD, Craniofacial & limb abnormalities
2. Phenobarbitone → Haemorrhagic disease of newborn

F. ANTI-BP ↑
1. Propranolol → Preterm labour, Neonatal BG ↓ & PR ↓
2. Diazoxide → Fetal BG ↑
3. Hydrallazine → ?cleft palate

G. ANTICOAGS
Warfarin → IUD, Neontal haem, Limb & facial defects

F. MISC
1. Lithium → BG ↓, Neonatal lethargy
2. Aspirin → Bleeding

Alcohol Abuse In Preganacy

Alcohol abuse in pregnancy is ass c̄ the fetal alcohol syndrome. Moderate alcohol intake in pregnancy may also → morbidity

FETAL ALCOHOL SYNDROME

A syndrome ass c̄ chr large alcohol consumption ie >80g alcohol/day before & during pregnancy

CLIN: Often Mental retardation; Microcephaly; Hypotonia; IUGR; SGA; Failure to thrive; Cleft palate; Hypoplastic maxilla; Short palpebral fissures; Short upper lip; Hypoplastic philtrum. Occ Cong malformations; Hyperactivity

PREVENTION: Advise no alcohol during pregnancy
N.B Most cases are diagnosed retrospectively

MODERATE ALCOHOL INTAKE

The effects of moderate alcohol intake are a cause of debate. It is difficult to accurately estimate the alcohol intake of pregnant women. There is evidence linking moderate drinking c̄ ↑ risk of cong malformations, spontaneous 2nd trimester abortions & lower birth wt. Heavy drinkers who also smoke appear at particular risk of delivering a small baby

Narcotic Abuse in Pregnancy

Ass c̄ ↑ in: IUGR; PNMR; Prematurity; Neonatal withdrawal syndrome ie hypertonia, tremor, resp rate ↑, irritability, fits, high pitched cry

RX: Slowly withdraw drug during pregnancy (sudden withdrawal may → IUD or fetal distress). Methadone substitution early in pregnancy is beneficial

NEURAL TUBE DEFECTS

Esp low social class. Esp Ireland, S.Wales. Probably due to poor periconceptual maternal diet.
↑ recurrence risk if previous NTD

GENERAL INVESTIGATIONS:
- Ultrasound
- Serum αFP
- Amniocentesis & αFP

PREVENTION: Periconceptual vit supplements probably beneficial. Advise good diet

ANENCEPHALY

Bony vault of the skull & scalp are absent. F>M. Approx 1 in 400 births in UK. Ass c̄ other fetal malformations eg CHD

CLIN: Often Hydramnios; Premature labour; Face presentation; Prolonged labour. Occ Shoulder dystocia; PPH. All die before or shortly after birth

RX: If diagnosed, terminate pregnancy

SPINA BIFIDA

A bony defect in the encasement of the spinal cord which may involve cord or meninges. Often ass c̄ hydrocephaly

CLIN: Born c̄ variable degree of disability. Spina bifida occulta may be ass c̄ a hairy patch or dimple over bony defect but is asymptomatic. Meningocoeles are usually small, occ ass c̄ hydrocephalus. Meningomyelocoeles are ass c̄ sphincter paralysis, hydrocephalus, CDH, talipes, kyphoscoliosis, CHD, Imperforate anus, paraplegia

RX: Occ corrective op for defect is indicated. A meningocoele is usually closed at 3–6mths. A meningomyelocoele should be covered c̄ a sterile dressing whilst assessment for op is carried out

HYDROCEPHALY

An excess of CSF within the ventricles → large head. Approx 1 in 1500 births. Ass c̄ other cong malformations eg spina bifida

CLIN: Often hydramnios. Head may be palpably large in utero. Occ h/o cong infection. Usually vaginal delivery impossible due to non-engagement or cephalopelvic disproportion. Often malpresentation eg brow. In breech delivery (approx 30%) aftercoming head will not deliver

INVESTIGATION: • Ultrasound

RX: Occ elective LSCS. If diagnosed in labour & cephalic presentation, collapse skull by needle withdrawal of CSF. If breech presentation, decompress head via meningocoele, if present, or by direct puncture of foramen magnum

NORMAL PUERPERIUM

The period following delivery in which the mother returns to her normal physiological state. Usually defined as the 6wk post delivery period, as most pregnancy-induced changes have returned to norm by this time

The uterus rapidly involutes. By 10–12 days the uterus has returned to normal size (sl larger than nulliparous state). The endometrium regenerates in 2–6wks

Lochia is initially red but gradually becomes yellow/white over 2wks. Diuresis starts on first day & lasts till day 4. Often mild constipation

Management of Puerperium

Check uterine size daily for first wk; BP, PR, Temperature periodically for 2 days. Analgesia for after-pains &/or episiotomy. Check Hb on day 4, may need Fe. High fibre diet. Mobilise early. Exercise to restore muscle tone. Encourage breast feeding. Encourage bonding eg allow baby to stay c̄ mother, arrange early physical contact c̄ baby at birth. Psychological support to mother; Reassurance & instruction in infant care esp important after birth of first child. If medical & social factors allow, early discharge is advantageous. Check that episiotomy is well healed. Discuss contraception. Examine mother & child at 6wks. If necessary give anti-D Ig &/or rubella vaccine

ABNORMAL PUERPERIUM

Genital Tract Infection

Major cause of maternal morbidity. Esp anaerobic Strep, *E.coli*, Klebsiella, Proteus & Bacteroides. Predispositions inc LSCS; Prolonged labour; Traumatic delivery c̄ tissue necrosis. Ass c̄ low social class

PATHOGENESIS: The initial infection is usually an endomyometritis. The source of infection is usually endogenous ie from the floor of the lower genital tract. Spread may occur to surrounding organs directly or via lymphatics

CLIN: Variable symptoms. Mild cases → sl pyrexia, sl uterine tenderness & pain. More severe cases → Malaise; Anorexia; Pyrexia; Abdo pain & tenderness; Foul lochia. Infection may spread → salpingitis, parametritis, pelvic or generalised peritonitis, pelvic abscess, septicaemia

INVESTIGATIONS:
- Vaginal & cervical cultures
- MSU
- Blood cultures
- Swab of any incision site
- Intrauterine aerobic & anaerobic cultures at time of LSCS (in high risk cases)

PREVENTION: Limit number of VEs during labour. Minimise tissue trauma during op delivery. Aseptic technique. Prophylactic antibiotics for LSCS probably helpful

RX: Bed rest, analgesia. Mild cases post vaginal delivery usually respond to Ampicillin. Mild cases following LSCS usually require IV Ampicillin & Gentamicin. In severe cases often use three antibiotics eg Ampicillin, Gentamicin & Metronidazole (SE in mother: Necrotising enterocolitis). Treat rare septic shock in usual manner. Drain any pelvic abscess—if in pouch of Douglas drain via post colpostomy. Septic pelvic thrombophlebitis requires an IV Heparin infusion. Occ removal of episiotomy sutures to allow drainage. The very rare necrotising fasciitis requires early extensive surgical debridement & high dose antibiotic Rx

PROG: Early Rx → good prognosis. Chr endometritis may → menorrhagia. Chr salpingitis may → infertility

UTI

Common. Predisposed to by Urinary stasis; ↓ bladder sensation; Catheterisation in labour. Esp asc *E.coli* infection

CLIN: Frequency; Dysuria; Loin pain; Pyrexia. Rarely → Pyelonephritis; Chr cystitis

INVESTIGATIONS:
- FBC
- WCC
- MSU
- HVS

RX: Bed rest; Analgesia; Antibiotics

Breast Infection

Occ mastitis occurs as epidemic on ward. Esp *Staph aureus* >Strep, *E.coli.* Predispositions inc Nipple fissures; Milk stasis; Poor hygiene

CLIN: Local tenderness, redness, swelling of breast esp upper outer quadrant; Pyrexia; Pain. Esp 1–3wks post partum. May → brawny swelling ± fluctuance (breast abscess)

INVESTIGATIONS:
- Culture of expressed milk from affected side
- Look for infection in baby, mother & other contacts eg staff

RX: Antibiotics eg Cloxacillin (often organism is Penicillin resistant) for 7–10 days. Do not discontinue breast feeding. The breast should be emptied by feeding & manual expression. Local poultice may comfort. If abscess, drain by radial incision under GA

PROG: Early Rx should prevent abscess formation

Puerperal Psychiatric Problems

Post partum mental illness is quite common. Three main types can be recognised ie post partum "blues", post partum depression, post partum psychosis

POST PARTUM "BLUES"

Affects approx 50% of F

CLIN: Usually present between 3–5th day post partum. Weeping; Anxiety; Irritability; Lack of confidence; Lethargy

RX: Reassurance; Explanation; Support from staff & family

PROG: Usually full spontaneous recovery in <1wk

POST PARTUM DEPRESSION

Approx 10% of F. Occ previous h/o neurotic illness

CLIN: Degree of depression is variable, usually mild. Often Weeping; Lethargy; Inability to cope; Lack of confidence; Sleep disturbance. May neglect child. Occ present c̄ Infant feeding problems;

Lack of libido; Dyspareunia

RX: Antenatal & post natal classes to discuss implications of having a child. Reassurance & support from staff & family. Occ explanation to & support of husband is required. If possible arrange assistance so that mother can get out of house & has some respite from looking after child. Occ short term course of tranquilisers or TCAD are indicated

POST PARTUM PSYCHOSIS

Approx 1 in 500 births. Esp if h/o affective disorder, psychosis. Esp primiparous

CLIN: Usually presents after 5th day post partum. May be acute or insidious onset. Often early clin picture of delirium developing into functional psychosis in next few days. Depressive psychosis >Schizophrenia >Mania

RX: Exclude organic cause. Admit to hospital. Require appropriate psychiatric care eg ECT, TCAD, Phenothiazines

PROG: About 15–20% have recurrence in subsequent pregnancies

DD: Toxic confusional states

DVT

↑ risk in pregnancy & post partum. About 66% of pregnancy related cases occur post partum. Esp following LSCS

CLIN: Often clin signs imprecise. Classically Oedema; Pain; Tenderness; +ve Homan's sign. Risk of PE

INVESTIGATIONS:
- Venography
- Isotope venography
- Doppler ultrasound

PROPHYLAXIS: Early ambulation. In high risk cases eg obese, >35yrs old, CVS disease, LSCS, previous thromboembolism related to pregnancy give low dose sc Heparin from onset of labour until 1wk post partum. Avoid exogenous oestrogens. Pressure stockings during pregnancy for high risk F

RX: Raise end of bed. Bandage leg from toes to groin. Mobilise early. Support stockings when ambulant. Exercise leg in pain free range. Heparin by constant IV infusion for 7–14 days. Warfarin for 12wks

Amniotic Fluid Embolism

Very rare. 1 in 50,000 births. Ass c̄ Polyhydramnios; Abruptio placentae; Multiparity; Operative delivery

PATHOGENESIS: The entry of amniotic fluid into the maternal circulation eg via a uterine op wound → amniotic fluid in pulm circulation → acute pulm vascular obst

CLIN: Sudden shock; BP ↓; Hypoxia; Cyanosis; Acute pulm BP ↑. Often Pulm oedema; Ep; Coma; DIC; Death

RX: IPPV; IV Dopamine infusion; IV $NaHCO_3$; IV Steroids. Treat any haem & DIC c̄ FFP, blood

PROG: Poor. Approx 85% die, many within 1hr of onset. Often diagnosis made at post mortem

PERINATAL MORTALITY

PNMR is the number of SB plus deaths in first wk per 1000 live plus SB in a defined population. Rates have been falling in western countries due to improved social & medical factors. Risk in M sl>F. PNMR is a reflection of the standard of perinatal health services. The rate in the UK is now about 9 per 1000 total births. Identification of high risk pregnancies should allow greater attention to be given to these mothers & their babies during & after their pregnancy

Factors Ass c̄ ↑ PNMR (LIST 28 O&G)

A. SOCIAL FACTORS
1. Low social class
2. Immigrants
3. Mothers aged <20 & >35yrs
4. Cigarette smoking
5. Moderate to high alcohol intake
6. Poor maternal diet
7. Short stature <5ft
8. Late booking at ANC
9. Illegitimacy

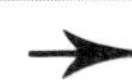

B. OBSTETRIC FACTORS
1. PET
2. Malpresentations & malpositions
3. Cong malformations
4. LBW
5. IUGR
6. Primiparity
7. Grand multiparity
8. Rhesus haemolytic disease
9. Postmaturity
10. Prematurity
11. Cord prolapse
12. Abruptio placentae
13. BP ↑
14. Diabetes
15. Prolonged labour
16. Birth injury
17. PROM
18. APH
19. Multiple pregnancy
20. Previous poor obstetric history:
    Eg Previous still birth, neonatal death, LBW baby

Definitions of other mort rates relevant to this period are:
SB rate: Number of SB per 1000 live plus SB
Early neonatal mort rate: Number of deaths in 1st wk/1000 live births
Late neonatal mort rate: Number of deaths in 1st to 4th wk/1000 live births
Neonatal mort rate: Number of deaths in first 4wks/1000 live births
Infant mort rate: Number of deaths in first yr/1000 live births

MATERNAL MORTALITY

A maternal death is a death occuring during pregnancy or within 6wks of its termination. In UK Confidential Enquiry into Maternal Deaths covers all maternal deaths within 1yr of termination of pregnancy. In industrialised countries rate has been falling & is now very low ie approx 1 in 15,000 births
The commonest causes of maternal death are: PE; BP ↑; Abortion; Ectopic pregnancy; Haem; Anaesthetic death; Amniotic fluid embolism; Sepsis; Ruptured uterus

TEENAGE PREGNANCY

In many countries the rate of teenage pregnancy is increasing. The greater acceptance of intimate sexual relations → many unplanned pregnancies in this age gp as they are less likely to use contraception
Teenage pregnancy is ass c̄ LBW babies; SGA; ↑ risk of child abuse & neglect; Poor compliance c̄ antenatal care; Anaemia; Cong malformations; Disproportion due to small pelvis. The normal psychosocial development of the girl is disrupted. Often the mother is not supported by a partner

RX: If pregnancy diagnosed early, discussion re therapeutic abortion can be undertaken. Need support & reassurrance from staff & if possible partner & family during & after pregnancy. If possible arrange to allow schooling to continue

GRAND MULTIPARITY

A woman having her 5th or subsequent child is termed a grand multip. Grand multiparity is ass c̄ ↑ risk of Cong malformations eg Down's syndrome; BP ↑; Multiple pregnancy; Anaemia; Preterm labour; APH; PROM; Cephalopelvic disproportion; Unstable lie; Precipitate labour; Uterine rupture; Malpresentations; PPH

PHANTOM PREGNANCY (PSEUDOCYESIS)

A condition in which a non-pregnant women believes herself pregnant & develops objective signs of pregnancy. Esp African Blacks. F usually naive about medical matters

CLIN: Usually amenorrhoea or oligomenorrhoea; Abdo swelling; Tender swollen breasts; Areolar pigmentation; Secretion of milk or colostrum; Sensation of fetal mvts reported. Occ Morning sickness; Wt ↑

RX: Confront patient c̄ diagnosis. Usually symptoms disappear but recurrence is common. Occ Psychotherapy needed

Gynaecology

THE MENSTRUAL CYCLE

Menstruation is the discharge of blood from uterus at regular approx 4wkly intervals in F during their reproductive period. Menstruation starts at menarche when aged approx 12yrs & continues until the menopause at approx 50yrs. The menstrual cycle describes the regular pattern of events occuring in the approx 28 day period between menstruations

The cycle is controlled by hormonal interactions between the hypothalamus, ant pituitary & ovaries. GnRH is released by the hypothalamus & stimulates the production of FSH & LH in the ant pituitary. FSH stimulates the growth & maturation of 1° ovarian follicles. LH stimulates the follicles to secrete Androstenedione which is converted into Oestradiol in the presence of FSH. As Oestradiol levels rise a −ve feedback loop ↓ release of FSH, but a further rise of Oestradiol near midcycle → a +ve feedback both to the hypothalamus c̄ ↑ GnRH release & to the pituitary → ↑ sensitivity to GnRH. This surge of LH in mid cycle is ass c̄ release of an ovum from its follicle

After ovulation, LH causes transformation of theca granulosa cells of collapsed follicle into lutein cells. The corpus luteum produces Oestrogen & Progesterone which inhibit FSH release. In the absence of pregnancy, levels fall after 8–10 days allowing FSH levels to rise, thereby initiating a new cycle

The endometrium follows a cyclical pattern under this hormonal influence. In the post menstrual "resting" phase (days 6–7), the endometrium is thin & non-vascular. During the follicular "proliferative" phase (days 7–14) the endometrial glands grow & become more tortuous. Ovulation occurs at about day 15 & thereafter the endometrium enters the luteal phase, becoming thick & glandular. If the ovum is fertilised the endometrium develops into the decidua. If no fertilisation occurs menstruation occurs about 14 days post ovulation c̄ arteriolar spasm, haem & shedding of endometrial cells

The cervix is also influenced cyclically by the F sex hormones. In the follicular phase, the cells of the cervical canal proliferate secreting a thin watery mucous. Mucous production reaches a peak at ovulation. In the luteal phase, progesterone causes the cervical mucous to become more viscous & less easily penetrable by sperm

In the vagina, supf large cells are common in the follicular phase. During the luteal phase the supf cells are replaced by white cells & intermediate cells c̄ folded edges which tend to clump

The normal cycle lasts 28 days c̄ bleeding lasting about 6 days. However cycles between 21–35 days are probably within norm limits & bleeding may last from 2–7 days. The menstrual flow is initially heavy & bloody but later becomes a scanty brown discharge. The norm blood loss during the cycle is approx 50mls

The basal body temperature has a typical pattern during the cycle. Following menstruation the temperature falls during the follicular phase. At ovulation there is a further temperature drop followed by a rise the next day which is maintained until 2 days before menstruation. The temperature rise is due to ↑ progesterone levels

↑ progesterone levels

In the luteal phase there may be fluid retention, wt gain & breast tenderness. Abdominal or pelvic pain ass c̄ ovulation (Mittelschmerz) is quite common

For a few yrs following menarche some cycles are often anovular & therefore painless. As the menopause approaches, periods usually become less heavy & less frequent

Disorders of Menstrual Cycle

PREMENSTRUAL TENSION

Esp F>35yrs. Approx 10% of F. ?due to relative def of progesterone

CLIN: Symptoms vary in severity even in same F. Symptoms start 2–12 days before menstruation & are relieved by its onset. Often Lower abdo swelling; Anxiety; Irritability; Depression; Lassitude; Emotional lability; Constipation; Oedema; Wt ↑; Mastalgia; Headaches

RX: Reassurance; Explanation of symptoms. If severe fluid retention, diuretics. Occ tranquiliser of benefit. Ergotamine for migraine. Progestogens given daily from day 12–26 may help. Severe mastalgia may be relieved by Bromocriptine

AMENORRHOEA

Amenorrhoea may be 1° ie menstruation has never occured or 2°. About 5% of cases are 1°; 30% are due to Wt ↓; 30% to prolactin ↑; 25% to post pill amenorrhoea; 5% to ovarian failure; 5% to systemic disease, endocrine disease, polycystic ovary syndrome or others

Causes of Amenorrhoea (LIST 29 O&G)

1. Physiological:
   a) Prepubertal
   b) Post menopausal
   c) Pregnancy
   d) Lactation
   e) In 2–3yr period post menarche
2. Ovarian:
   a) Agenesis
   b) Dysgenesis eg Turner's syndrome
   c) Ablation
   d) Polycystic ovary syndrome
   e) Granulosa theca cell Ca
3. Hypothalamic/Pituitary:
   a) Prolactin secreting tumours
   b) Severe wt ↓ eg Anorexia nervosa, Crash dieting
   c) Ablation eg Infarcts, Tumours, Surgery
4. Psychogenic
5. Post oral contraception
6. Severe chr disease:
   Eg CRF, Hypothyroidism, Thyrotoxicosis
7. False amenorrhoea (cryptomenorrhoea):
   Eg Vaginal atresia, Imperforate hymen → haematocolpos
8. Uterine:
   a) Surgical removal
   b) Radiation
   c) Trauma → adhesions (Asherman's syndrome)
   d) Endometrial TB
9. Adrenal:
   a) Cushing's disease
   b) Adrenogenital syndrome
   c) Mild post pubertal adrenal hyperplasia
10. Testicular feminisation syndrome

INVESTIGATIONS: • Hgh & Wt
- Pregnancy test
- Presence or absence of 2° sexual characteristics
- Buccal smear
- X-R pituitary fossa
- FSH
- LH
- Prolactin
- Oestrodiol
- Urinary 17-oxosteroids
- TSH
- T4
- Progestogen stimulation test
- Chromosomes

DYSMENORRHOEA

Pain in ass c̄ menstruation. 2 forms: Spasmodic or 1°; Congestive or 2°

SPASMODIC DYSMENORRHOEA: Common. Severe pain of uterine origin related to the onset of menstruation. ?due to uterine muscle ischaemia. Esp 15–25yrs. Esp F who have not had child by vaginal route

Clin: Pain starts a few hrs before menstruation & usually persists for <12hrs. Lower abdo pain which may be colicky or continuous

Rx: Hot bath during menstruation may help. Analgesics esp Aspirin, Mefenamic acid. Occ hormone Rx to inhibit ovulation

Special Cases of Spasmodic Dysmenorrhoea:

a) MEMBRANOUS DYSMENORRHOEA: Rare. Occ FH. Due to shedding of endometrium in very large pieces

Clin: Severe pain at start of menstruation. Passage of endometrial casts

Rx: Resistant to Rx. Can try D&C; Oral contraceptive

Prog: Does not affect conception or pregnancy. Not cured by childbirth

b) DYSMENORRHOEA ASS c̄ PASSAGE OF CLOTS

c) DYSMENORRHOEA ASS c̄ UTERINE MALFORMATIONS: Eg Rudimentary horn; Bicornuate uterus

SECONDARY DYSMENORRHOEA: Esp >30yrs. Usually due to endometriosis or chr pelvic infection eg Salpingo-oophoritis

Clin: Pain starts 2–7 days before menstruation reaching a peak at onset of bleeding & abating after about 2 days. Pain esp pelvis & back. Symptoms & signs of underlying condition

Rx: Rx of underlying condition

Abnormal Uterine Bleeding

Menorrhagia is excessive blood loss in a cycle of norm duration
Polymenorrhagia is excessive blood loss in a cycle of ↓ length
Epimenorrhoea is abnormally frequent bleeding
Metrorrhagia is irregular bleeding often of ↑ duration
Breakthrough bleeding is the result of oestrogen levels being in a middle range ass c̄ haem in mid-cycle

Causes of Abnormal Uterine Bleeding (LIST 30 O&G)

1. Lesions of Uterine Body:
   a) Endometritis
   b) Fibroids
   c) Polyps
   d) TB
   e) Endometriosis
   f) Myohyperplasia
   g) Malignancy eg Ca, Sarcoma
2. Lesions of Cervix:
   a) Erosion
   b) Polyp
   c) Chr cervicitis
   d) Ca
3. Lesions of Ovary:
   a) Endometriosis
   b) Chr infection
   c) Oestrogen secreting tumours
4. Complications of pregnancy:
   a) Abortion
   b) Ectopic pregnancy
   c) Hydatidiform mole
   d) Malignant trophoblastic Ca
5. Trauma
6. Foreign bodies:
   Eg IUCD
7. Drugs:
   Eg Gonadotrophins; Synthetic progestogens → breakthrough bleeding; Excess oestrogens endogenous or exogenous
8. Dysfunctional (idiopathic):
   Inc Psychosomatic eg Anxiety, Sexual problems
9. Endocrine:
   a) Hypothyroidism
   b) Hyperthyroidism
   c) Pituitary disease → ↑ gonadotrophins
10. Haematological:
    Eg ITP, Chr liver disease

Commonest causes are: Dysfunctional uterine bleeding, if aged >20yrs; Organic cause or complication of pregnancy, if aged 20–40yrs; Ca if aged >40yrs

GENERAL INVESTIGATIONS: • FBC
- Ultrasound
- D&C
- Rarely: Eg Hormone assay, Clotting screen

DYSFUNCTIONAL UTERINE BLEEDING

Abnormal haem without identifiable cause. Important to distinguish between anovular & ovular cases

ANOVULAR CAUSES:

Metropathia Haemorrhagica: Esp Premenopausal; Postpubertal adolescents. Characterised by absent luteal tissue, ovarian follicular cysts, hypertrophy of endometrium ("Swiss cheese" endometrium). Bleeding due to failure of uterine spiral retraction

Breakthrough Bleeding: Less than 1% of all F. May also occur if on "pill". Endometrium may be atrophic

OVULAR CAUSES: Usually due to irregular shedding of endometrium (?resulting from slow involution of corpus luteum), or irregular endometrial ripening (?resulting from slow formation of corpus luteum). Esp >40yrs

GENERAL RX: Exclude organic cause. Diagnostic D&C cures some cases. Synthetic Progestogens between days 15–25 of cycle controls bleeding. Anovular bleeding may respond to Clomiphene in those wishing to conceive. In F >40 consider hysterectomy

POSTMENOPAUSAL BLEEDING

Bleeding from the genital tract >1yr after completion of menopause. Usually due to Ca

Causes of Post Menopausal Bleeding (LIST 31 O&G)

1. Malignancy:
   a) Cervix
   b) Vagina
   c) Vulva
   d) Uterine body
   e) Ovary
   f) Rarely eg Urethral, Fallopian tube
2. Benign tumours:
   a) Uterine or cervical polyps
   b) Fibroids
3. Vaginitis:
   Esp Senile atrophic
4. Urethral caruncle
5. Trauma
6. Foreign bodies
7. Hormone Rx:
   Esp Following withdrawal of oestrogens
8. Senile endometritis
9. Spurious:
   ie Rectal bleeding, Haematuria

INFERTILITY

About 90% of couples produce a pregnancy within a year of normal coitus. In UK about 8% of couples fail to achieve a pregnancy despite wishing to start a family. In about 30% of cases the M partner is at fault, in 30% the F & in 40% there are factors affecting both M & F. Esp middle aged & elderly

Causes of Infertility (LIST 32 O&G)

Any cause of failure to ovulate → infertility (See LIST 29 O&G Causes of Amenorrhoea)

A. FEMALE
1. Uterine anomalies:
   a) Cong malformations
   b) Fibroids
   c) Polyps
   d) TB
   e) Retroverted uterus
2. Fallopian tube:
   Infection esp TB, GC, Post abortal

3. Ovarian:
   Eg Endometriosis, Streak ovaries, Resistant ovary syndrome
4. Lower genital tract:
   Eg Cong malformations, Intact hymen, Cervical hostility to spermatozoa
5. Systemic disorder:
   a) Hypothyroidism
   b) Diabetes
   c) CRF
6. Pelvic adhesions
7. Idiopathic
8. Vaginismus

B. MALE
1. Cong malformations:
   Eg Hypospadias
2. Azoospermia, Oligospermia:
   Eg 2° to Maldescent of testes, Previous orchitis, Exposure of testes to heat
3. Impotence
4. Premature ejaculation
5. Bilat obst of Epididymis, Vas or Ejaculatory ducts:
   Eg Cong malformation, Surgery
6. Endocrine:
   Eg Hypopituitarism

PATHOGENESIS IN F: Various factors inc Failure to ovulate; Mechanical obst interfering c̄ passage of ovum from ovary to tube; Uterine hostility to sperm or newly fertilised ovum eg malformation, TB endometritis; Cervical hostility to sperm ?due to pH ↓, infection, malformation; Coital errors eg infrequent coitus, apareunia, dyspareunia

CLIN: May be h/o 1° or 2° amenorrhoea. Occ h/o infection

INVESTIGATIONS IN F: • Basal temperature chart
- Post coital test c̄ examination of cervical mucous
- D&C c̄ examination of endometrium inc guinea pig inoculation for TB
- Ultrasound
- Laparoscopy
- Hysterosalpingography
- CO_2 insufflation
- Hormone levels

INVESTIGATIONS IN M: • Seminal fluid analysis: Total count, vol, motility, % of abnormal forms
- Sperm antibodies
- Bacterial culture of semen

RX: Determine from history if full investigations are required. Advise on frequency & timing of coitus. Treat any active infection. Remove any intact hymen or vaginal septum

In anovulatory cases hormone levels may indicate cause. Often require laparoscopy ± ovarian biopsy. Standard Rx of atrophic ovaries, polycystic ovaries. If endometriosis, cautery of endometriotic nodules may benefit. If hyperprolactinaemia, exclude a pituitary tumour, may require Bromocriptine Rx. If low FSH, LH & Oestrogen, may respond to HMG & HCG injections, under close monitoring.

If low FSH & LH c norm Oestrogen levels use Clomiphene to induce ovulation, c̄ close monitoring as risk of hyperstimulation of ovaries (N&V; Abdo pain; Hypovolaemic shock; Ovary ↑. Multiple pregnancy). If 1° or 2° ovarian failure, ovulation usually not possible, Oestrogen replacement Rx may be indicated to combat SE of low endogenous Oestrogen levels

If tubal blockage, op to restore patency eg salpingolysis to free adhesions, salpingostomy, reimplantation of tubes when the isthmus is blocked. If failure, may consider extracorporeal in-vitro fertilisation ("test tube" baby)

Uterine lesions may respond to D&C. Occ myomectomy for fibroids. Rarely correct retroversion by ventrosuspension

Occ when cervical hostility is suspected, give subovulatory suppressant dose of Oestrogen in first half of cycle. Cautery or cryosurgery for erosions

In M, defective spermatogenesis may respond to Wt ↓, avoidance of tight warm underpants. Treat any UTI or prostatic infection. Surgery for varicocoele. Gonadotrophin Rx rarely effective. Standard Rx for impotence or premature ejaculation

AIH may be used in cases of impotence, premature ejaculation or oligospermia

If the F is fertile & partner infertile, AID & adoption can be considered. Counselling by experienced staff is necessary

PROG: In UK about 25% of F seeking advice for infertility subsequently become pregnant. Following tubal surgery, best results if minor adhesions & worst if salpingostomy. Pregnancy rate following tubal surgery is approx

5–40%. However having achieved pregnancy, ↑ abortion rate, ectopic pregnancy rate & PNMR compared to norm pop

DYSPAREUNIA

Causes of Dyspareunia (LIST 33 O&G)

1. Lower genital tract:
   - a) Unruptured rigid hymen
   - b) Vaginal septum
   - c) Infection or inflam
   - d) Post-op → scarring, narrowing &/or shortening of vagina
   - e) Episiotomy scarring
   - f) Post X-Rad Rx
   - g) Postmenopausal atrophic changes
2. Upper genital tract:
   - a) Infection/Inflam eg Chr salpingitis, Pelvic endometriosis, Cervicitis
   - b) Malignancy eg Ca cervix, Ca ovary
   - c) Retroverted uterus
   - d) Ovarian cyst
   - e) Degenerating fibroid
3. Psychogenic: Inc Frigidity
4. Vaginismus

CLIN: Pain on sexual intercourse. May be slight or severe, supf or deep

RX: Treat any infection. In deep dyspareunia exclude pelvic disease. Dilate &/or excise rigid hymen. Vaginismus may respond to psychotherapy & course of graduated vaginal dilators or Fenton's op. A tight perineum may require perineotomy. Occ enlargement of vagina by plastic op is indicated. Oestrogens for post menopausal atrophy

INFECTIONS OF THE GENITAL TRACT

Infections of the genital tract are usually generalised rather than confined to individual organs. Infections of upper tract are therefore often diagnosed as pelvic inflam disease rather than related to a specific organ. The genital tract is protected from infection by vaginal acidity → ↓ bacterial growth, mthly shedding of endometrium, & the fact that vagina is only a potential tube & is thus normally closed. Infections are mainly 2° to coitus, childbirth & abortion esp illegal. Infection is uncommon in children & virgins

Vulval Infections

HAIR FOLLICLE INFECTION

Esp if poor personal hygiene, debilitated. Esp Staph. *Ducrey bacillus* infection → chancroid

CLIN: Boils or carbuncles. Tender painful vulva. Occ Supf ulcers c̄ sl discharge

INVESTIGATIONS: • Swab of ulcer • Urinalysis

RX: Topical Chlorhexidine or K^+ permanganate. Oral antibiotics

CANDIDIASIS

Common. Esp diabetics

CLIN: Red, wrinkled, oedematous vulva. Occ 2° infection

RX: Advise cotton underwear as nylon prone to encourage hot, moist climate favoured by candida. Clean & dry vulva after p/u & apply topical anti-fungal cream. If 2° infection apply anti-fungal cream in high vagina, occ antibiotics.

Avoid douching as risk of allergic reaction

BARTHOLINITIS

Quite common. *E.coli*, Staph >GC

CLIN: Acute onset c̄ red swollen painful posterior labia. If untreated may resolve or → abscess or chr retention cyst

RX: Bed rest. Analgesia. Antibiotics. If abscess or cyst, marsupialisation

GENITAL HERPES

Usually due to HSV 2. ↑ in prevalence worldwide

SYPHYLIS

Vulva is common site of chancre

CONDYLOMATA ACUMINATA (VIRAL WARTS)

Common. Due to viral infection

CLIN: Usually multiple & grouped in clusters. Esp vulva, vagina & around anus. Often enlarge & multiply in pregnancy

RX: Remove vulval hair. Apply topical Podophyllin. Occ Diathermy or laser excision

LYMPHOGRANULOMA VENEREUM

Due to a virus of the psittacosis gp. Usually a STD. Esp Blacks

GRANULOMA INGUINALE

Due to *Donovania Granulomatis*. Esp Blacks

Vaginal Infections

In the prepubertal, the vagina does not produce acid secretions & different organisms infect vagina compared c̄ the adult. Inc GC, Strep, Pneumococcus. Vaginal infection in children is rare. Occ occurs 2° to foreign body or as part of systemic infection
In the adult the main causes of vaginitis are 1° infection esp Trichomonas, Candida, Chlamydia; Infection 2° to cervicitis; Foreign bodies; Chemicals eg douches, deodorants

TRICHOMONAL VAGINITIS

Common. 2–20% of married F (although many asymptomatic). Usually spread by intercourse. Due to the protozoan, *Trichomonas vaginalis*

CLIN: Often asymptomatic. Irritating yellow-green frothy vaginal discharge; Tender vagina. Occ Dysuria; Frequency; Dyspareunia; Urethritis. Attacks often ppt post coitally, post menstruation or if intercurrent illness. May recur. May coexist c̄ GC infection. M partner usually asymptomatic but occ urethritis c̄ discharge

INVESTIGATIONS:
- Microscopic examination of vaginal discharge mixed c̄ saline
- Incubate vaginal discharge on Kupferberg's medium
- Gm stain smear

RX: Metronidazole to F & her M partner. In first trimester pregnancy use Natamycin pessaries

CANDIDAL VAGINITIS

Esp diabetics, pregnant, 2° to systemic antibiotic Rx

CLIN: Pruritus; Thick white cheesy vaginal discharge. M partner may have post coital irritation of sex organs

INVESTIGATIONS:
- Microscopic examination of discharge
- Place swab in Nickerson's medium: Colonies obvious after 2 days

RX: Various effective drugs eg Nystatin pessaries, Miconazole. If recurrence, give 2nd course. If further recurrences suspect intestinal infective reservoir, Rx oral Nystatin

NON-SPECIFIC VAGINITIS

May be due to Chlamydia

CLIN: In M, NSU. In F, Vaginal discharge occ malodorous

RX: Tetracycline

Cervical Infections

ACUTE CERVICITIS

Due to GC or in puerperal infection esp Staph, Strep, 2° to trauma of childbirth

CHR CERVICITIS

Chr non-specific infection of cervical crypts. Often ass c̄ cervical ectropion

CLIN: Non-specific symptoms. Often mucopurulent vaginal discharge. Occ Deep dyspareunia; Dull pelvic pain; Backache. ?ass c̄ infertility

RX: Cautery or cryosurgery of cervix

Uterine Infections

ACUTE ENDOMETRITIS

Rare. Usually due to GC, Puerperal infection or post abortal infection. Often ass c̄ infection of ovaries & fallopian tubes

CLIN: Blood stained uterine discharge

CHR ENDOMETRITIS

Rare. Usually due to GC or 2° spread from other pelvic organs

CLIN: Menorrhagia. Symptoms & signs of underlying condition

RX: Treat underlying condition

Fallopian Tube Infections

Fallopian tubes may be infected by 3 routes: Blood esp TB; Via pelvic peritoneum; Ascending infection from lower genital tract. Salpingitis may be acute, subacute or chr

ACUTE SALPINGITIS

Usually due to GC, Puerperal infection, Post abortion, Post op, Foreign bodies, or 2° to Ca cervix

CLIN: Classical form due to GC infection. Bilat lower abdo tenderness & pain; Pyrexia; PR ↑; Frequency. Occ Bloodstained purulent vaginal discharge; Vom; Tender bilat swellings in pouch of Douglas; Abdo rigidity. Later may → Pyosalpinx c̄ abdo distension; Pelvic abscess which may point in vagina or rectum; Tubo–ovarian abscess; Salpingo–oophoritis. If pyosalpinx or pelvic abscess ruptures → shock, peritonitis. Rarely, usually 2° to illegal abortion, present c̄ shock & ARF. If inadequate Rx, chr salpingitis may develop. ↑ risk of susequent infertility or tubal pregnancy

INVESTIGATIONS:
- WCC: ↑↑, Polymorphs ↑↑
- FBC
- Cultures from cervix & urethra: Occ GC isolated
- Laparoscopy

RX: Admit to hospital. Bed rest. Analgesia. High doses of appropriate antibiotic(s) usually for 14 days but longer if symptoms & signs persist. Drain pelvic abscess by posterior colpotomy. Laparotomy indicated if Failure of medical Rx; Rupture of pyosalpinx; Intestinal obst; Doubt about diagnosis

DD:
1. Ectopic pregnancy
2. Acute appendicitis
3. Infection, torsion or rupture of ovarian cyst
4. Acute pyelonephritis

SUBACUTE SALPINGITIS

Similar but less severe symptoms than acute salpingitis. Recurrences common

CHRONIC SALPINGITIS

Usually h/o acute or subacute salpingitis

PATHOGENESIS: Variable path: May be chr oviductal inflam, adhesions, hydrosalpinx, pyosalpinx, tubo–ovarian abscesses. A hydrosalpinx is the end result of low virulence high irritation infection → retention of large vol of exudate within closed tube. A pyosalpinx is due to acute blockage at the fimbrial end & at one or more points along the tube which → accumulation of infected exudate in blocked section & inflam thickening of tubal wall. Often ovary is involved → chr tubo–ovarian abscess formation

CLIN: Variable symptoms. Occ General malaise; Lower abdominal ache esp premenstrual; Sterility; Menstrual irregularity esp polymenorrhoea, dysmenorrhoea; Deep dysparuenia; Mittelschmerz; Mucopurulent vaginal discharge

INVESTIGATIONS:
- FBC
- WCC
- Laparoscopy
- Cervical & urethral cultures

RX: Full course of appropriate antibiotics. Analgesia. Short wave diathermy may help. Occ surgery to restore tubal patency including removal of adhesions & plastic implants. Usually surgery indicated if failure of medical Rx—Remove uterus & fallopian tubes ± ovaries. Menorrhagia may respond to 6mths Rx c̄ Norethisterone or Danazol

PROG: Ops to restore tubal patency are usually

unsuccessful

DD:
1. Pelvic endometriosis
2. Pelvic TB
3. Ovarian tumours esp bilat
4. Impacted fibroid
5. Bowel disease eg Diverticulitis, Appendix abscess

Pelvic Cellulitis

Usually due to cervical laceration 2° to childbirth, pelvic ops, abortion. Often ass c̄ infection of cervix, fallopian tubes & ovaries. May spread to utero–sacral ligaments & bladder. May be acute, subacute or chr; Unilat or bilat

CLIN: Acute infection → lower abdo pain, fever, fixed uterus. Occ abscess pointing in vagina or rectum. In chr infection, symptoms & signs too difficult to distinguish from underlying condition eg Chr salpingitis

RX: Analgesia, antibiotics. Short wave diathermy may be useful. Occ hysterectomy required

Female Genital TB

Esp low social class. Esp 20–40yrs. Always a 2° infection. Usual 1° site is lung; Occ abdo, kidneys, bones. Spread to genital tract occurs in 5–10% of pulm TB cases. Commonest sites of infection are the fallopian tubes & endometrium. Rarely affects vulva or vagina

CLIN: Symptoms depend on disease severity. May be asymptomatic. Often infertility. Occ in severe disease, chr pelvic pain, irregular uterine bleeding, amenorrhoea. Rarely Constitutional symptoms eg fever, night sweats, malaise, wt ↓; Pelvic mass (due to TB pyosalpinx); Fistulae

INVESTIGATIONS:
- CXR
- Curettage c̄ histology, ZN stain, culture
- Hysterosalpingography (risk of reactivation of disease)
- FBC
- AXR
- EMUs

RX: Standard triple anti-TB therapy. Surgery occ required if large caseous pelvic masses, pyosalpinx, fistulae. Delay surgery until medical Rx has been given for at least 12wks

PROG: Very good cure rate c̄ Rx. Moderately high risk of infertility. ↑ risk of abortion & ectopic pregnancy

Ovarian Infections

Usually part of a generalised pelvic inflam disease process. Acute oophoritis is an uncommon sequelae of mumps

NON-INFECTIVE CONDITIONS OF THE VULVA

Pruritus Vulvae

Irritation of the vulva → scratching. Common

Causes of Pruritus Vulvae (LIST 34 O&G)

1. Psychogenic
2. Irritating vaginal discharges:
   Esp Trichomonas, Candida
3. Systemic disease:
   Esp Diabetes, Cholestatic J, IDA
4. Skin diseases:
   Eg Scabies, Intertrigo, Lichen planus, Psoriasis, Threadworms, Fungal infections
5. Allergy:
   Esp to Disinfectants, Soaps, Underwear material, Topical drugs
6. Vulval neoplasm
7. Chr epithelial dystrophies:
   a) Leukoplakia
   b) Lichen sclerosus et atrophicus

GENERAL INVESTIGATIONS: • BG, GTT
• FBC
• Swab for infection
• Occ vulval skin biopsy

Chr Epithelial Dystrophy

Esp postmenopausal. Degenerative conditions

LEUKOPLAKIA OF VULVA

Uncommon. Premalignant

PATH: Thick hypertrophied vulva. White patches. Occ fissures. May spread to anus, groins

INVESTIGATION: • Vulval biopsy

RX: Steroid cream. Careful follow-up. Surgical removal if evidence of progression

PROG: Vulval dysplasia is a pre-malignant vulval dystrophy. About 5% develop Ca in 15yrs

Vulval Atrophy

Common in very elderly due to withdrawal of ovarian hormones. Rarely occurs in younger F

CLIN: Usually asymptomatic. Occ dyspareunia

RX: If symptomatic, Oestrogen containing cream. Occ weak steroid cream or Testosterone ointment of benefit

Vulval Cysts

Inc sebaceous cysts, Bartholin cyst, implantation cyst, Skene's duct cyst, Cyst of canal of Nuck

VULVAL TUMOURS

Benign Vulval Tumours

Inc Squamous papilloma, Naevus, Hidradenoma, Lipoma, Fibroma

Malignant Vulval Tumours

Causes about 4% of all F genital tract Ca. Esp postmenopausal. Probable pre-malignant conditions inc Leukoplakia, Lichen sclerosus et atrophicus, X-Rad, TB, LGV, Sy, Granuloma inguinale

SQUAMOUS CELL CARCINOMA

Commonest malignant tumour. Esp elderly postmenopausal. ?ass c̄ early menopause. ?? due to HSV or papilloma wart virus

CLIN: Usually affects ant half of vulva. Presents as ulcer c̄ raised everted edge or as nodule which increases in size. Later develops into fungating mass or ulcerated infiltrating lesion. Occ multiple primaries (may give rise to "kissing ulcers"). Rarely arises from clitoris. Often coexisting leukoplakia. Bleeding; Discharge; Soreness; Dyspareunia. Usually inguinal LN ↑. Spread by lymph

INVESTIGATION: • Vulval biopsy

RX: Radical vulvectomy inc groin node dissection. Skin grafts may aid healing. Palliative surgery if mets. High dose X-Rad for vulval recurrences ± Bleomycin

PROG: If no mets at presentation, about 70% 5yr survival

MALIGNANT MELANOMA

2nd commonest vulval tumour. Cause of 5% of vulval malignancy

RX: Radical vulvectomy

PROG: Poor

BASAL CELL CARCINOMA (RODENT ULCER)

Rare. Presents as ulcer

RX: Wide excision of ulcer or X-Rad

PROG: Good

BARTHOLIN'S GLAND TUMOUR

An adenoCa. Rare. Solid tumour

RX: Radical vulvectomy c̄ gland dissection

CA-IN-SITU

3 main gps: Ca-in-situ simplex; Bowen's disease; Paget's disease

RX: Wide local excision

PROG: Good

URETHRAL CONDITIONS

Urethral Caruncle

Esp postmenopausal

CLIN: Bright red tender swelling at post-meatal margin; Dysparuenia; Dysuria. Occ Bleeding

RX: Oestrogen cream. If fails, diathermy excision of caruncle

Urethral Diverticulum

CLIN: Occ Dysuria; Dribbling; Vulval swelling

RX: Excision

Urethral Prolapse

May be acute or chr, partial or total

CLIN: Red tender meatal swelling; Dyspareunia; Dysuria. Occ Bleeding

RX: Excise prolapse & repair

Urethral Ca

Rare. May be squamous or AdenoCa

CLIN: Occ Dysuria; Bleeding; Pain; Dyspareunia. Spread via lymph

RX: Radical surgery inc LN, bladder & urethral excision & transplantation of ureters. Occ X-Rad

NON-INFECTIVE CONDITIONS OF VAGINA

Atrophic Vaginitis

A degenerative condition due to inadequate oestrogenic stimulation. Esp postmenopausal

CLIN: Vaginal discharge occ bloodstained or purulent. Occ Mild vaginal tenderness; Dyspareunia; 2° infection

INVESTIGATIONS:
- Colposcopy
- HVS

RX: Treat any infection. Local Oestrogen replacement. Rarely if introitus narrowed, perineotomy

DD: Other causes of postmenopausal bleeding

Imperforate Hymen

CLIN: Occ cause of cryptomenorrhoea by obstructing menstrual flow c̄ bulging vulva, periodic episodes of lower abdo pain, abdo mass & occ 2° infection

RX: Excision c̄ antibiotic cover

Rigid Hymen

CLIN: Often dyspareunia

RX: Dilators or excision under GA. Occ perineotomy may be required

Vaginal Cysts

Inc Mesonephric (Gartner duct) cyst, Mucous cysts, Inclusion cysts, Endometriotic cysts

CLIN: May simulate cystocoele or rectocoele

RX: Excise or marsupialise

Vaginitis Emphysematosa

Rare. Esp pregnant. Numerous gas filled bullae. Cause unknown ?Trichomonal

RX: Usually remits spontaneously

Vaginal Prolapse

Predisposing factors inc Obstetric trauma; Postmenopausal atrophy; ↑ intra-abdominal P eg chr cough

ANT WALL PROLAPSE

A prolapse of the upper ant vaginal wall → cystocoele. Lower ant wall laxity → urethrocoele

CLIN: May be asymptomatic. Cystocoele may → UTI; Dysuria; Frequency. Urethrocoele may → Stress incontinence

POST WALL PROLAPSE

Middle wall prolapse → rectocoele ie rectal herniation. Upper post wall prolapse → prolapse of post fornix which may contain bowel loop & is termed an enterocoele

CLIN: Often asymptomatic until large. A large enterocoele may → deep dyspareunia. A large rectocoele may → difficulty in emptying rectum

GENERAL RX: Cystocoele, Rectocoele & other vaginal wall prolapse are dealt c̄ by ant &/or post colporrhaphy

Genital Tract Fistulae

Commonest are vesicovaginal & rectovaginal fistulae. Causes are Obst labour; Pelvic ops; Ca eg bladder, vagina, cervix; X-Rad; TB; Sy; Cong ectopic ureter

CLIN: Depends on size & site. Vesico-vaginal fistula → urinary incontinence

INVESTIGATIONS:
- IVU
- Cystoscopy
- Proctoscopy
- Introduction of dyes eg Methylene blue
- Colposcopy

RX: Small fistulae may heal if bladder is drained for up to 3wks. Usually operative repair eg Latzko's op, interposition ops eg of gracilis muscle

TUMOURS OF VAGINA

Benign Tumours

Rare. Inc squamous papilloma, fibroma, leiomyoma, haemangioma

Malignant Tumours

1° tumours are rare, accounting for 1–2% of F genital tract tumours. 2° tumours arise by direct spread or mets esp from cervix, uterus, bladder, vulva, rectum & sigmoid colon. Esp elderly

SQUAMOUS CELL CARCINOMA

Commonest 1° vaginal tumour. Esp 50–70yrs. Post wall upper third >ant wall lower third >other sites

CLIN: Occ Abnormal vaginal bleeding (usually postmenopausal); Vaginal discharge; Pain; Dyspareunia. May cause urinary or bowel symptoms. Spread by lymph & local invasion

INVESTIGATIONS:
- Biopsy & histology
- EUA
- Ultrasound
- CAT scan
- Contrast X-R of bowel & urinary tract

RX: Treat early stage Ca by partial vaginectomy, radical vaginectomy, or X-Rad. Treat stage II & III by ext beam X-Rad ± interstitial or intracavity X-Rad. Stage IV tumours require ant, post or total exenteration usually c̄ X-Rad. X-Rad is usually Rx of choice, surgery being used for some cases of stage I & IV disease & recurrences

PROG: Stage I 75% 5yr survival. Stage IV 20% 5yr survival

ADENOCARCINOMA

Rare. Maternal ingestion of diethyl stilboestrol during the 8th–18th wk of gestation is the usual cause → development of Ca in child about 20yrs later

RX: Radical hysterectomy ± X-Rad

MALIGNANT MELANOMA

Very rare

CLIN: Bleeding; Discharge. Often early mets but occ lies dormant for years

RX: Radical surgery ± X-Rad

SARCOMA BOITRYOIDES

Very rare. Esp young children

CLIN: Bloody vaginal discharge. Occ polypoidal tumour visible at introitus

RX: Radical surgery

PROG: Poor

NON-INFECTIVE CONDITIONS OF THE CERVIX

Cervical Erosion

The cervix is that part of the uterus lying below the int os. The cervical canal is lined c̄ columnar epithelium & extends onto the vaginal portion of the cervix to a varying degree beyond the ext os where the epithelium becomes squamous (the squamo–columnar junction). The position of the junction depends on hormonal influences & local tissue conditions

Squamous metaplasia is a process by which the norm cervical columnar epithelium is replaced by stratified squamous epithelium. Possible sites inc ectropion & cervical polyp. If a neck of an endocervical gland is closed off by this process, a retention cyst is formed (Nabothian follicle)

An area of exposed columnar epithelium visible on VE is termed an ectropion, eversion or erosion. Eversion is a norm consequence of the increasing vol of the cervix during times of maximal hormonal influence eg pregnancy, first few ovulatory periods. Cervical erosions are commoner in F taking "pill"

CLIN: Although often claimed to cause symptoms, little evidence. Occ ↑ mucorrhoea

INVESTIGATION: • Cervical smear

RX: This area of the cervix is the zone where cervical Ca develops therefore a smear should usually be taken. Cryosurgery if mucorrhoea or dysplasia

Cervical Polyp

Common. Often ass c̄ cervical ectropion. May be single or multiple. Squamous metaplasia & malignant change may occur

CLIN: Bright red polyp arising in cervical canal & usually protruding into vagina. Vaginal discharge; Irregular vaginal bleeding esp post coital. May coexist c̄ endometrial polyps or Ca

INVESTIGATIONS: • Cervical smear
- D&C
- Histology of polyp
- Occ Cervical biopsy

RX: Remove polyp

Cervical Ulcers

Rare. Types inc Traumatic; TB; Sy; Malignant; Granulomatous

TUMOURS OF CERVIX

Ca cervix is the 2nd commonest malignant tumour in F in UK. In UK accounts for 60% of F genital tract tumours. Esp 45–55yrs. Esp married F, particularly those c̄ many sexual partners who have first intercourse in their teens. ?transmission by coitus due to virus (?HSV 2, ?? human papillovirus), thus M c̄ many sexual partners may be high risk to F. Strong occupational links eg wives of fishermen, long distance lorry drivers have ↑ risks. Esp lower social class. Cervical polyps may be pre-malignant.

Use of contraceptive sheath may be protective

PATHOGENESIS: Cervical epithelium is known to pass through a series of stages which may → malignancy. The transitional stages can be described as: Norm epithelium → low degree dysplasia (CIN I) → high degree dysplasia (CIN II) → Ca-in-situ (CIN III) → invasive Ca. The early transitional stages are reversible. Indeed perhaps only about 25% of Ca-in-situ cases would normally become invasive. The period from initial abnormal epithelial change to malignancy is usually about 20yrs but a more aggressive form is also probably present → most cases of early cervical Ca. Most arise from squamous epithelium in region of squamo–columnar junction. 95% of cervical Ca is squamous cell Ca & 5% adenoCa

CLIN: Often abnormal vaginal discharge esp bloody post-coital discharge. Occ Severe bleeding; Anaemia; Frequency. Later Pain; Malaise; Wt ↓. Occ Vesico–vaginal fistula; RF

Local spread to vagina, parametrium & occ bladder, uterine body. Early spread to LN. Late mets via blood esp to lungs, bones

INVESTIGATIONS:

- Cervical cytology: Smears can be graded as norm, inflam, dyskaryotic, possibly malignant, frankly malignant. All abnormal smears require further investigation
- Cone biopsy (a biopsy of the squamo–columnar junction & most of the cervical canal)
- Curettage
- Colposcopy
- IVU
- Cystoscopy
- CXR
- CAT scan

PREVENTION: Screening by cervical cytology allows the determination of possible pre-malignant states. In UK & many other countries a screening service for the high risk gps is in operation. Screening is carried out at antenatal, postnatal, STD & family planning clinics opportunistically in those aged <35 & at 5yr intervals for those aged 35–65yrs. In suspicious smears: Colposcopy & cone biopsy or laser therapy

RX: Depends on stage of disease & general condition of F. For Stage I(a) ie cases c̄ minimal stromal invasion & confined to cervix, total hysterectomy c̄ an adequate vaginal cuff & block disection of pelvic LN. For all other stages, X-Rad (SE: Radiation sickness, Proctitis, RF, ↑ infections eg cystitis). Radical surgery is occ used for adenoCa, pelvic infection, failure to respond to X-Rad

If invasive Ca cervix in pregnancy, deliver fetus early by classical Caesarian section

PROG: Unfortunately in UK screening programme many of the high risk gp women do not attend for smears, even when invited. Incidence of cervical Ca is roughly constant in UK, but may have been higher if there had been no screening programme. Some screening programmes eg Iceland have been ass c̄ a fall in incidence

5yr survival rates approx: Stage I 80%, stage II 60%, Stage III 30%, Stage IV 5–10%. Best results in specialised centres

NON-INFECTIVE CONDITIONS OF THE UTERINE BODY

Uterine Displacements

The uterus is a mobile organ. Normally uterus is anteverted & anteflexed. Displacements may occur in several directions but are usually of no significance. Retroflexion & retroversion are occ symptomatic

UTERINE RETROFLEXION & RETROVERSION

In retroflexion the long axis of the corpus is bent backwards on the long axis of the cervix

In retroversion the long axis of the corpus & cervix are in line, & the

uterus has pivoted backwards in relation to the birth canal
Common in infancy. 20% of adult F have retroverted uterus which usually has persisted from childhood but occ is 2° to Adhesions; Tumours; Endometriosis; Pregnancy esp puerperium

CLIN: Usually asymptomatic. 2° causes more likely to cause problems. Occ complain of Pelvic pain, Heaviness. Rarely a contributor to Infertility; Abortion. May be signs of underlying condition

INVESTIGATIONS:
- Speculum examination
- Ultrasound
- Pessary test of uterine mobility

RX: A pessary to antevert uterus eg the Hodge pessary, is indicated if retroverted uterus after 12th wk of pregnancy & occ for infertility. If uterus fixed & major symptoms eg pain, dyspareunia, op may be indicated eg Gilliam's ventrosuspension op

COCHLEATE UTERUS

Rare. Uterus acutely angled forward

CLIN: Occ Pin-hole meatus; Dysmenorrhoea; Infertility

RX: Dilatation of uterus

Uterovaginal Prolapse

Descent of the uterus is always ass c̄ some descent of the vagina. Often ass c̄ cystocoele, rectocoele &/or enterocoele. Classified into 3 degrees:
1st degree: Sl uterine descent, cervix remains within vagina
2nd degree: Cervix projects through vulva on straining
3rd degree (Procidentia): Entire uterus prolapsed outside vulva

PATHOGENESIS: Due to weakness of one or more of the three uterine supports ie the round ligaments, the transverse cervical (cardinal) ligaments, the muscular vagina. Causes inc Cong weakness (rare); Stretching of supporting tissues at childbirth; Obstetric trauma; Peri- & postmenopausal tissue atrophy. May be ppt by ↑ intra-abdominal P; Pelvic tumours
When cervix prolapses through vulva, supf epithelium becomes keratinised & prone to trauma & ulceration. Cervix elongates → cervical oedema. In 3rd degree prolapse, the lower ureters may become obst → hydroureter & hydronephrosis

CLIN: Symptoms depend on degree of prolapse. Often Vaginal fullness; Sensation of "something coming down"; Difficulty in p/u &/or defaecation; Backache. Occ Frequency; Incontinence; Vaginal discharge (may be blood stained 2° to ulceration). Symptoms usually relieved by lying down. Prolapse may be observed during straining or coughing

INVESTIGATIONS:
- Sims' speculum examination in L lat position
- p.r
- MSU
- Bonney's digital elevation test: +ve if stress incontinence

PREVENTION: During pregnancy: Avoid difficult instrumental delivery; Avoid delivery before full cervical dilatation; Repair episiotomy well. Postnatal pelvic floor exercises

RX: Usually surgery. Medical Rx ie ring pessary, pelvic floor exercises & faradic stimulation may be indicated if Unfit for op; Failed op; Refusal of op; Further pregnancy planned soon; In puerperium; 3rd degree prolapse esp elderly, prior to op. Patients wearing pessaries should be seen every 4mths, when pessary is changed
All 3rd degree prolapse should be reduced & the vagina packed c̄ an Oestrogen impregnated gauze to allow ulcer healing, reduction of oedema. Op 2–3wks later
Variety of ops eg Ant colporrhaphy, Post colpoperineorrhaphy, Manchester repair (ant & post colporrhaphy, amputation of cervix, shortening of transverse cervical ligaments, & Fothergill suture ie plication of transverse cervical ligaments to cervical stump), vaginal hysterectomy & repair

DD:
1. Cervical polyp
2. Vaginal cysts
3. Vaginal tumours
4. Inversion of uterus

Endometrial Hyperplasia

Generalised endometrial overgrowth due to persistent oestrogenic stimulation. Esp perimenopausal.

Usually anovulatory. Predisposes to myohyperplasia. May be pre-malignant Two main forms, cystic & adenomatous. Cystic hyperplasia may be due to exogenous oestrogens, follicular cysts, granulosa theca cell tumours of the ovary & is part of the metropathia haemorrhagica syndrome. Adenomatous type may be ass c̄ Stein–Leventhal syndrome

CLIN: Often Bulky uterus; Dysfunctional uterine bleeding; Short periods of amenorrhoea

INVESTIGATION: • Curettage & histology: Commonest finding is cystic hyperplasia

RX: D&C may be curative. If symptoms recur, use gestogen eg Norethisterone for 3–6mths (unless pregnancy desired). If pregnancy desired, often require investigation of infertility & Rx c̄ Clomiphene. In older F, esp if histology shows atypical hyperplasia, may perform hysterectomy

Myohyperplasia

Endometrial & myometrial hyperplasia due to excess oestrogen stimulation

CLIN: Usually menorrhagia; Uterus size of 8–10wk pregnancy

INVESTIGATION: • EUA, Curettage & histology

RX: Norethisterone in 2nd half of cycle. If fails, consider hysterectomy

UTERINE TUMOURS

Polyps

Local benign tumours of endometrial glands & stroma. Esp >30yrs; Perimenopausal F. May be sessile or pedunculated. May be pre-malignant

CLIN:

May be asymptomatic. Occ abnormal uterine bleeding

INVESTIGATION: • Curettage & histology

RX: D&C. May require use of polyp forceps

Uterine Fibroids

Commonest F tumour. Benign tumour of smooth muscle (leiomyoma). Esp 35–45yrs. Esp nulliparous & para >2. Esp Blacks. Often ass c̄ Endometriosis; Endometrial hyperplasia. ?due to excess oestrogen stimulation. Fibroids usually regress after menopause

PATHOGENESIS: Minute seedlings in uterine muscle which grow very slowly. 70% remain intramural; 10% grow inward becoming submucous myoma ± pedunculation; 20% grow outwards becoming subserous ± pedunculation. If origin is cervical muscle → cervical myoma. Outward growth in lat uterine wall may → fibroid in broad ligament. Fibroids are often multiple. May undergo degenerative changes

Degenerations in Fibroids (LIST 35 O&G)

1. Hyaline degeneration
2. Cystic degeneration
3. Red degeneration
4. Lipoid degeneration
5. Myxomatous degeneration
6. Atrophy
7. Calcification
8. Ossification
9. Malignant change

CLIN: Often asymptomatic. Symptoms likelier if large fibroid close to endometrial cavity. Occ Menorrhagia (due to ↑ vascularity, ↑ bleeding area, impaired uterine contractility, ass endometrial hyperplasia); Irregular bleeding (may be due to ulceration of submucous fibroid, sarcomatous change); P effects eg frequency, constipation, VVs; Pain (may be due to torsion, spasmodic dysmenorrhoea, P on nerves, sarcomatous change, ass endometriosis); Abdo swelling. Rarely Infertility; Polycythaemia; Sarcomatous change; Intraperitoneal haem (rupture of subserous myoma); Torsion → gangrene
In pregnancy, fibroid often ↑ in size. Ass c̄ Abortion; Premature labour; Malpresentations & malpositions; Inco-ordinate uterine action; PPH; Torsion;

Infection of fibroid; PPH. Rarely Red degeneration; Obst labour (esp cervical or broad ligament myoma)

INVESTIGATIONS: • FBC
• Laparoscopy
• Ultrasound
• Hysterosalpingography
• Cervical smear
• Diagnostic curettage

RX: Depends on age, parity, size of fibroid, symptoms & complications. No treatment if small & symptomless, unless likely to complicate delivery or diagnosis in doubt. Hysterectomy in non-pregnant if Uterus larger than 14wk gestation; F has completed family; P symptoms; Menorrhagia unresponsive to hormones. Myomectomy (relative c/i during pregnancy) is op of choice in F who wish to preserve reproductive function but risk of uterine rupture in pregnancy. If fibroid is cervical or submucous & pedunculated, vaginal myomectomy or polypectomy

PROG: Generally good. About 50% conceive following myomectomy op

DD:
1. Ovarian tumour
2. Pregnant uterus
3. Uterine polyps
4. Adenomyosis
5. Constipation

Uterine Sarcoma

Rare but commonest sarcoma of genital tract. Many types eg Leiomyosarcomas, Mixed mesodermal, Endometrial stromal. Esp Blacks. Often ass c̄ fibroids

CLIN: Abnormal vaginal bleeding; Back &/or abdo pain; Mass

RX: Combination Cyt.T & X-Rad

Endometrial Carcinoma

Esp 50–70yrs. About 25% are premenopausal. Esp W.Europe, N.Am

Risk Factors for Endometrial Ca (LIST 36 O&G)

1. Obesity
2. Late menopause
3. Early menarche
4. Nulliparity
5. Diabetes mellitus
7. Exogenous oestrogens: Eg Sequential "Pill", Replacement Rx for gonadal dysgenesis
8. Endogenous oestrogens: Eg Granulosa theca cell tumours of ovary, Adrenal Ca
9. Polycystic ovary syndrome
10. ?high fat diet
11. BP ↑

PATHOGENESIS: ?due to local excess oestrogens → endometrial hyperplasia → atypical adenomatous hyperplasia → endometrial Ca. Tumour usually starts in fundus & spreads slowly & diffusely over endometrium. Usually invasion of cervix & myometrium occurs late. Usually an adenoCa but occ squamous metaplasia or anaplastic form

CLIN: Abnormal vaginal bleeding (usually postmenopausal). Later Pain; Mets. Ass c̄ ↑ risk of other 1° Ca eg breast Ca; Gall bladder disease

INVESTIGATIONS: • Fractional curettage & histology
• Endometrial biopsy

RX: 75% are confined to the body of uterus on diagnosis (Stage I) & are treated by total hysterectomy & bilat oophorectomy followed 7–10 days later by X-Rad to pelvis in low grade tumours. If spread to cervix (Stage II), Rx as if Ca cervix ie X-Rad etc. Stage III, IV & recurrences, analgesia & hormone therapy ie gestagens for palliation. Occ Cyt.T for Stage III & IV

PROG: Worse if Later Stage; Squamous or Anaplastic histology; Pyometra; Elderly. Approx 5yr survivals: Stage I 85%, Stage II 50%; Stage III 30%; Stage IV 10%

ENDOMETRIOSIS

Abnormally located functioning endometrial tissue. May be in uterine muscle, when termed adenomyosis or extrauterine. Commonest extrauterine sites are the ovaries & pelvic peritoneum. Cause is unknown, theories inc coelomic metaplasia, implantation by retrograde menstruation, lymphatic or venous spread. Esp high social class

PATHOGENESIS: Ectopic endometrium is hormonally sensitive. At menstruation, bleeding & shedding of cells → cyst distension. Between menstruation some resorption of blood & cells → "chocolate cyst". Cysts gradually enlarge. Cysts may Rupture; Infiltrate adjacent tissues → adhesions; Become non-functional due to P destroying endometrial cells

ADENOMYOSIS

Esp multiparous, >35yrs, high social class. Usually multiple foci. In 50% ass c̄ fibroids. In 15%, extrauterine endometriosis

CLIN: Occ asymptomatic. Occ Progressively increasing dysmenorrhoea; Menorrhagia or Polymenorrhagia (due to ↑ bleeding area, ↑ vascularity, & occ endometrial hyperplasia); Enlarged hard uterus (rarely >size of 12wk pregnancy)

RX: If symptomatic, usually hormone Rx or hysterectomy. Occ excision (difficult as not encapsulated like fibroids)

EXTRAUTERINE ENDOMETRIOSIS

Commoner than adenomyosis. Esp Nulliparous; High social class.Commonest sites are ovaries, pouch of Douglas, broad ligaments, uterosacral ligaments, sigmoid colon & rectum. Less common sites are rectovaginal septum, vagina, bladder, round ligament, appendix, incisions. Rarely found in umbilicus, lungs & limbs

CLIN: May be asymptomatic. Variable symptomatology. Often Menstrual irregularities eg menorrhagia, polymenorrhagia or polymenorrhoea; Progressive dysmenorrhoea usually c̄ peak in last days of menstruation; Deep dyspareunia. Occ Constant lower abdominal or pelvic pain; Backache; Pain on defaecation esp at menstruation; Infertility (but tubes usually patent); Retroverted uterus; Tender enlarged ovaries; Fixed firm tender nodules in pouch of Douglas. Rarely Painful scar; Intermittent pyrexia at menstruation

INVESTIGATIONS: • Laparoscopy ± biopsy
• Occ Ba studies, IVU, Laparotomy, Other investigations of infertility

RX: Depends on size & extent of lesions, seriousness of symptoms & desire to have children. Small lesions & minor adhesions can be treated at laparoscopy by cautery & division
Medical Rx can involve use of gestagen only "pill" (SE: Wt ↑, Amenorrhoea which may persist for mnths after drug is stopped), combined "pill" (to suppress ovulation & menstruation producing a "pseudopregnancy") or Danazol (SE: Amenorrhoea, Wt ↑, Acne). Rx is for 3–6mths for Danazol, & 9–12mths for other hormonal treatments. If later relapse occurs, further course can be given
Surgical Rx is indicated if medical Rx fails, diagnosis uncertain & when lesions are larger esp if ovaries are involved (risk of rupture of ovarian cyst). If possible, even if surgery indicated, a 3mth course of hormone Rx should be given. In younger F wanting children, conservative op avoiding oophorectomy but dissecting out cysts & releasing organs from adhesions ± ensuring uterus in anteverted position. In older F, total hysterectomy & oophorectomy. Occ bowel or urinary tract surgery required. Rarely use X-Rad

PROG: Extrauterine disease more likely to respond to hormone Rx than adenomyosis. About 80% have pain relief c̄ hormone Rx, Danazol usually relieving symptoms quickest. In those wanting children, subsequent pregnancy is uncommon following Rx

DD:
1. Pelvic inflam disease
2. Ovarian tumours
3. Diverticulitis

NON-INFECTIVE CONDITIONS OF THE OVARY

Non-Neoplastic Ovarian Cysts

Various types inc Inclusion cysts; Follicular cysts; Cysts of the corpus luteum, Theca lutein cysts, Corpus albicans cyst; Endometriosis

FOLLICULAR CYSTS

Enlarged unruptured Graffian follicles in which the ovum has degenerated but lining cells have continued to secrete fluid. May be large or small, single or multiple. May be ass c̄ endometrial cystic hyperplasia, Stein–Leventhal syndrome or sclero–cystic disease

CLIN: May have ↑ or ↓ length of menstrual cycle; Menorrhagia. Cyst is never >5cm in diameter

POLYCYSTIC OVARY SYNDROME (STEIN-LEVENTHAL SYNDROME)

Uncommon. A syndrome of multiple bilat follicular cysts c̄ Hirsutism, Infertility, Obesity, Amenorrhoea or Oligomenorrhoea

PATHOGENESIS: ↑ basal level of LH → theca interna hypertrophy → ↑ androgen secretion. ↓ FSH level → ↓ granulosa cell growth & ↓ conversion of androgens to oestrogens. Thus Low ovarian oestrogen secretion → anovulation, amenorrhoea; High androgen output → hirsutism

INVESTIGATIONS: • LH ↑
- FSH: Sl ↓
- Testosterone ↑
- Prolactin: Occ ↑
- Laparoscopy

RX: Diet. Cimetidine or Cyproterone acetate may benefit hirsutism. If prolactin ↑, Bromocriptine. If prolactin norm, Clomiphene. If pregnancy does not occur after 4–6 courses of Clomiphene may perform wedge resection of ovary or add HMG

SCLERO–CYSTIC DISEASE (SMALL CYSTIC OVARY)

Thickening of tunica albuginea prevents ovulation → development of small follicular cysts

THECA LUTEIN CYSTS

Due to excessive HCG. Seen in trophoblastic disease & occ c̄ use of fertility drugs

CORPUS LUTEAL CYSTS

Occ a corpus luteum persists instead of degenerating after failure of implantation, to form a corpus luteum cyst. Secretes oestrogen & progesterone → amenorrhoea

RX: Observe. Surgery if cyst enlarges or fails to disappear within 3mths of detection

PAROVARIAN CYST (BROAD LIGAMENT CYST)

Not a true ovarian tumour. Arises in broad ligament. Usually unilocular. Benign

CLIN: Usually presents as ovarian swelling

RX: Surgical removal

OVARIAN TUMOURS

Quite common. Esp industrialised countries. About 25% are malignant. Peak incidence 50–70yrs

Classification of Primary Ovarian Tumours (LIST 37 O&G)

1. Epithelial tumours:
   a) Benign or malignant serous tumours

b) Benign or malignant mucinous tumours
c) Endometrioid tumours
d) Clear cell (mesonephroid) tumours
e) Brenner tumours
f) Mixed epithelial tumours
g) Undifferentiated Ca
2. Sexcord stromal tumours:
a) Benign or malignant granulosa–theca cell tumours
b) Benign or malignant androblastoma (Sertoli–Leydig)
c) Gynandroblastoma
d) Gonadoblastoma
e) Unclassified
3. Lipid cell tumours
4. Germ cell tumours:
a) Dysgerminoma
b) Endodermal sinus tumour (yolk sac)
c) Embryonal Ca
d) Polyembryoma
e) Choriocarcinoma
f) Teratoma inc Immature, Mature & Monodermal eg Struma Ovarii

Commonest tumours are the benign & malignant mucinous & serous tumours, & teratomas

GENERAL CLIN OF OVARIAN TUMOURS: Excluding those which are hormonally active ovarian tumours are usually quiet & rarely give rise to symptoms other than due to the size of the mass. Thus malignant tumours often present in late stage. Often abdo swelling. Occ Cachexia; Dyspepsia; Ascites; P effects eg Vom, Frequency. Most tumours may Haem; Tort; Become infected; Rupture;Obstruct. Menstrual function is usually unaffected unless tumour is hormonally active. Occ sl postmenopausal bleeding. Pain is a late sign

GENERAL DD OF OVARIAN TUMOURS:

1. Pregnancy
2. Ascites
3. Distended bladder
4. Uterine fibroids
5. Endometriosis
6. Ectopic pregnancy
7. Abscess eg Pelvic, Appendix
8. Pyo- or hydrosalpinx
9. Hydronephrosis
10. Pelvic kidney
11. Cystic ovary
12. Tumours eg Rectum, Colon, Retroperitoneal, "Phantom"
13. Obesity
14. Hydatid cyst

Ovarian Tumours Complicating Pregnancy

About 1 in 1500 pregnancies is complicated by an ovarian tumour, usually a teratoma or serous adenoma

RX: If detected before 12wks, observe (may be a corpus luteum cyst) & remove by ovarian cystectomy at 12–18wks if cyst is same size or growing. If detected after 28wks, op may need to be delayed until puerperium

Common Epithelial Tumours

About 70% of all ovarian tumours

GENERAL CLIN OF MALIGNANT EPITHELIAL TUMOURS: Palpable mass. Occ Abdo distension; Abdo pain; Vom; Obst; P symptoms eg frequency; Resp embarassment; Ascites; Wt ↓. Spread by peritoneal seeding >LN, direct spread >Blood

GENERAL INVESTIGATIONS OF EPITHELIAL TUMOURS:
- FBC
- U&Es
- LFTs
- CXR
- Ultrasound
- Laparoscopy
- Occ CAT scan, IVU, Ba studies, Lymphangiogram

GENERAL RX OF MALIGNANT EPITHELIAL TUMOURS: Often require pre-op high calorie, high protein diet to combat cachexia. Bowel preparation inc Neomycin for 2 days pre-op, enema, prophylactic antibiotics c̄ pre-med & continuing for 1–2 days post-op. Laparotomy for staging
If surgery can clear all obvious disease or substantially reduce tumour bulk (allowing better response to further X-Rad & Cyt.T) perform total hysterectomy, bilat salpingo–oophorectomy, omentectomy, appendicectomy & resection of any involved segments of GIT or GUS. Then Cyt.T eg Melphalan or Platinum

compounds. Later 2nd look surgical reassessment to decide whether to continue or stop Rx
If deemed inoperable, biopsy & close

GENERAL PROG OF MALIGNANT EPITHELIAL TUMOURS: Most patients present in advanced stage disease. Stage I & II disease, approx 75% 5yr survival. Stage III & IV disease, median survival 2yrs

BENIGN SEROUS CYSTADENOMA

Esp 30–40yrs. Cysts lined by cuboidal epithelium resembling that of fallopian tube. About 20% of all ovarian tumours. 30% bilat. Usually unilocular. Pre-malignant

CLIN: Ovarian enlargement. Occ Haem; Torsion; Infection; Rupture; Malignant change

RX: In young, conservative surgery. In F >40yrs, total hysterectomy & bilat salpingo–oophorectomy

MALIGNANT SEROUS CYSTADENOMA

Usually 2° to a benign serous cystadenoma. Esp >50yrs. Occ malignant papilliferous cysts contain calcerious granules (psammoma bodies)

BENIGN MUCINOUS CYSTADENOMA

Cysts lined by tall columner cells resembling that of endocervix. Usually multilocular. Rarely pre-malignant. About 20% of all ovarian tumours. Esp 30–50yrs

CLIN: Ovarian enlargement, occ massive. Occ Haem; Torsion; Infection; Meig's syndrome; Rupture → pseudomyxoma peritonei. Rarely malignant change

RX: In young, conservative surgery. In F >40yrs, total hysterectomy & bilat salpingo–oophorectomy

ENDOMETRIOID TUMOURS

Presumed to arise from malignant change of ovarian endometriosis. Rare

MESONEPHROID TUMOURS

Malignant ovarian tumour. Rare. Tubular pattern resembling that of renal cortex

BRENNER TUMOUR

A fibroepitheliomatous tumour. Rarely malignant. About 2% of ovarian tumours. Usually solid but larger tumours are partially cystic

CLIN: Ovarian enlargement. Occ Meig's syndrome ie ascites & hydrothorax; Hyaline degeneration; Fatty degeneration; Calcification

RX: Surgical removal of tumour

OTHER EPITHELIAL OVARIAN CARCINOMAS

Rare. Inc mixed epithelial tumours & undifferentiated Ca

Sex-cord Stromal Tumours

Account for 1–3% of all ovarian tumours

GENERAL INVESTIGATIONS:
- CXR
- Ultrasound
- FBC
- U&E
- LFTs
- Laparoscopy
- Hormone levels eg Urinary 17ketosteroids
- Occ ovarian biopsy

GRANULOSA–THECA CELL TUMOURS

3–5% of ovarian malignancy. Esp peri- or postmenopausal F. Usually unilat. Produce oestrogen & therefore cystic or adenomatous endometrial hyperplasia. Usually slow growing

CLIN: Irregular vaginal bleeding or postmenopausal bleeding. Effects of ↑ oestrogen eg Uterus ↑; Breast ↑; Breast tenderness. In children may → precocious puberty. ↑ incidence of endometrial Ca

RX: Total hysterectomy & bilat salpingo–oophorectomy. Lifelong follow-up

PROG: 50–80% survival rate. Late recurrences are occ observed

ANDROBLASTOMA (SERTOLI–LEYDIG CELL TUMOUR)

<1% of all ovarian tumours. Esp young adults. Usually unilat. In tubular type, tubules resemble Sertoli cells of testes & may produce oestrogens. Often cells resembling the interstitial

Leydig cells of testes are present & may produce androgens

CLIN: Tumour may show effects of ↑ androgens or ↑ oestrogens eg Hirsutism; Atrophy of genital organs; Amenorrhoea. Malignant behaviour is characterised by intra–abdominal spread

RX: Surgical removal

PROG: 80% 5yr survival. Tumour removal may reverse virilism

GYNANDROBLASTOMA

Very rare. Mixed or indeterminant cell tumours

GONADOBLASTOMAS

Derived from germ cell & stromal tissue. Benign. Occ ass c̄ dysgerminomas. Seen in cases of intersex c̄ streak gonads. Patient is apparently F, often there is a sex chromosomal abnormality eg X0/XY. Call–Exner bodies may be seen histologically

RX: Surgical removal

LIPOID CELL TUMOURS

Rare. Tumour cells have high lipoid content. May cause masculinisation & hypercorticoidism eg Obesity, Striae, Diabetes, BP ↑

Ovarian Germ–Cell Tumours

Commonest type is the benign cystic teratoma (Dermoid cyst) which accounts for 25% of all ovarian tumours

DYSGERMINOMA

Rare. Histologically similar to seminomas. Usually unilat. Age at onset 15–25yrs. Often malignant

CLIN: Usually present c̄ Abdo pain; Abdo swelling. Occ Torsion → acute abdomen. Mets to LN & distant sites

INVESTIGATIONS:
- FBC
- U&Es
- CXR
- Ultrasound
- αFP
- β HCG
- Occ IVU, CAT scan, Lymphangiogram

RX: 70% are confined to ovary at diagnosis (Stage I). In Stage I disease, if there is no ascites, washings are cytologically –ve, & the tumour is non-adherent & < 10cm in diameter, do a unilat salpingo–oophorectomy. Follow-up carefully. If relapse detected early, X-Rad or Cyt.T are likely to be curative In more advanced stages more radical surgery c̄ X-Rad &/or Cyt.T is performed. The tumour is very radiosensitive but chemotherapy is potentially preferable as it may preserve fertility

PROG: Very good

ENDODERMAL SINUS TUMOUR

May occur in combination c̄ teratoma or dysgerminoma. Rare

CLIN: Often Ascites; Transperitoneal spread; Distant mets

RX: Unilat salpingo–oophorectomy & Cisplatin based combination Cyt.T. Monitor tumour response by serial αP & β HCG levels

PROG: Majority remit on Cyt.T. Long term survival not yet known

Embryonal Ca

May occur in combination c̄ dysgerminoma or teratoma. Rare. May spread by transcoelomic route

RX: Unilat salpingo–oophorectomy & Cisplatin based combination Cyt.T

TERATOMAS

Most are mature & cystic. Significant minority are solid & may contain mature &/or immature elements. Benign tumours are usually cystic & malignancy is commonest in immature solid tissues. Teratomas may be composed of one tissue (monophyletic) eg Struma ovarii is composed of thyroid tissue

CYSTIC TERATOMAS: About 15% of all ovarian tumours. Occur throughout age range. Occ bilat. Usually unilocular & benign. May contain many tissues eg Hair, Teeth, Bone, Nervous tissue

Clin: May present as abdo mass; Interfere c̄ pregnancy. Occ Infection; Rupture; Torsion → acute abdo (quite common as teratoma often has a long pedicle);

Malignant change

Rx: In younger F, ovarian cystectomy. In elderly, oophorectomy

SOLID TERATOMAS: Usually malignant. Usually have elements of all 3 germinal layers. May present in childhood

Rx: Excise tumour & combination Cyt.T

Prog: Related to stage & grade. Very good prog if histologically grade 0 or 1

Special cases of Solid Teratomas:

a) CARCINOID TUMOURS: May develop in solid teratoma or mucinous cysts. Usually unilat & confined to ovary. Can produce typical carcinoid syndrome

Rx: Surgery

b) STRUMA OVARII: May develop in solid or cystic teratoma. May occur along c̄ carcinoid like tumours. May be malignant

Rx: Surgery or occ Radio I_2

Secondary Ovarian Tumours

About 20% of all ovarian malignancies. Ovarian mets from extragenital tumours are quite common esp from breast, stomach & large intestine. Occ mets may reach large size & cause symptoms whilst 1° growth is still small. Tumours often bilat. If unilat, R>L. Spread from extragenital sites is usually transcoelomic but occ spread by lymph or blood. Histologically the tumours are usually either adenoCa or Krukenberg tumours. Extragenital deposits occur esp in F aged 30–50yrs. Direct spread of cancer from genital tract sites is also quite common

PROG: Poor

THE MENOPAUSE

In UK average age of menopause is 51yrs. There is usually a gradual transition from ovulatory cycles to ovarian quiescence. The climacteric is the period usually lasting yrs of waning ovarian function

PATHOGENESIS: At about 35–40yrs, FSH levels start to rise → disturbance of ovarian follicular function, which is increasingly likely over time to → irregular or infrequent ovulation. In the climacteric the ovary's responsiveness to gonadotrophins diminishes. Although FSH & LH levels rise, few follicles are stimulated & hence oestrogen secretion falls → oligomenorrhoea & eventually amenorrhoea

CLIN: Various menstrual patterns may occur during climacteric eg Oligomenorrhoea; Episodes of menorrhagia alternating c̄ oligomenorrhoea; Sudden cessation of menses. Often vasomotor disturbances occur in climacteric eg Hot flushes; Sweating; Palps; Fainting. Psychological adjustment to the menopause can cause psychiatric morbidity eg Irritability; Depression; ↓ sexual responsiveness Postmenopausally Vagina becomes thin & atrophic occ → dyspareunia; Breasts ↓ in size; Fibroids, if present, atrophy. ↑ incidence of prolapse; Osteoporosis

RX: Reassurance. Oestrogen Rx for atrophic vaginitis or occ for vasomotor symptoms

Neonatology & Paediatrics

Neonatology

PERINATAL INFECTIONS

Uncommon. Ass c̄ maternal low social class, multiple pregnancy, polyhydramnios, maternal UTIs, prolonged rupture of membranes, preterm birth, LBW. M>F

PATHOGENESIS: Amniotic fluid has anti-infective properties. Placenta acts as a barrier to many infections but Toxoplasma, CMV, Rubella are exceptions. Foetal defence mechanisms develop steadily in utero. Maternal colostrum & breast milk contain protective IgA. Infection may occur just before or during labour esp if early rupture of membranes
Foetal infections eg Rubella, Toxoplasma, CMV, Sy, can → severe problems. Infections from birth canal inc Herpes, GC, Candida, Chlamydia. Early neonatal infections are commonly due to *E.coli*, Gp B Strep, Staph; Breast feeding is protective

GENERAL CLIN: Commonest presentations of bacterial infection are pneumonia, septicaemia. Occ Meningitis. Symptoms often non-specific. Early foetal viral infection may → SB, cong abnormalities, LBW

GENERAL INVESTIGATIONS:
- Blood cultures
- LP: CSF, C&S
- Swabs
- MSU
- CXR
- WCC inc Neutrophil count

GENERAL RX OF BACTERIAL INFECTION: Early Rx is important for good prog. Antibiotics; O_2; IV fluids. Occ require ventilation. Rarely granulocyte transfusion

Neonatal Pneumonia

PATHOGENESIS: 1. Intrauterine inhalation
2. Aspiration pneumonia
3. Droplet spread esp Staph, *H.influenza*, *E.coli*, Strep, Pneumococci

CLIN: Temperature ↑, ↓ or norm; Fine creps. Occ SOB; Cyanosis; Expiratory grunt; Tachypnoea; Indrawing of ribcage; Poor feeding; Poor wt gain

INVESTIGATIONS:
- CXR
- WCC inc neutrophil count

RX: O_2, Antibiotics

Neonatal Septicaemia

Esp due to *E.coli*; Staph; Strep. May be 2° to infected placenta or umbilical vein sepsis

CLIN: Variable picture. Occ Vom; Poor feeding; Temperature ↑ or ↓; J; Haem

INVESTIGATION: • Blood cultures

RX: Rehydrate. Treat any shock. O_2; Antibiotics

Neonatal Meningitis

Esp LBW. Causes *E.coli* >Strep, Listeria, Staph, Proteus. Usually ass bacteraemia. Transplacental infection can occur c̄ Listeria

CLIN: Non-specific. Occ Lethargy; Vom; Irritability; Poor sucking. Fontanelle ↑, Opisthotonos, stiff neck & fits are uncommon. May have resp distress, diarrhoea or J

INVESTIGATIONS: • LP: Cells ↑, Protein ↑
• WCC & diff
• Blood cultures

RX: Antibiotics eg Ampicillin & Gentamicin c̄ monitoring of antibiotic levels. May need intrathecal or intraventricular antibiotics. Restrict fluids. Prophylactic anticonvulsants

COMPLICATIONS: 1. Hydrocephalus
2. Subdural haematoma
3. Blindness
4. Ep
5. IQ ↓

PROG: 30% mort. About 30% of survivors have sequelae

Conjunctivitis

In UK common causes are Staph & Strep. GC ophthalmia neonatorum, contracted from birth canal, is common in developing countries. Occ viral, chlamydial

CLIN: Usually present at 2–3 days old. Acute swelling & oedema of eyelids; Sticky eyes

INVESTIGATION: • Eye swab

RX: Wipe eyes after birth prophylactically. Repeated irrigation c̄ antibiotic & saline

Neonatal Candidiasis

CLIN: Usually affects mouth. Occ napkin area. Rarely causes problems c̄ feeding. Esp bottle feeders

RX: Cleanliness, Nystatin

E.Coli

A common neonatal pathogen. May → septicaemia, meningitis, pneumonia, UTI, GE

Skin Infections

Usually Staph. Many varieties eg pustules, impetigo, furuncles, umbilical infections, epidermal necrolysis

RX: Good staff hygiene. Hexachlorophane to stump & 1% chlorhexidine to bath prophylactically. Cover infected skin. Antibiotics

DD: Benign Urticaria Neonatorum

Neonatal GE

May occur as epidemic in SCBU. Often due to *E.coli*

CLIN: Poor feeding; Poor wt gain; Apathy; Watery diarrhoea. Occ Vom; Dehydration; Fever

RX: Rehydrate. Occ require IV therapy. Antibiotics if suspected septicaemia

Neonatal UTI

Usually 2° to cong abnormality

CLIN: Occ Poor feeding; Fever; J; Pallor

INVESTIGATIONS: • Urine C&S
• Ultrasound
• Later IVU, Micturating cystogram

RX: Antibiotic. Later surgery to correct cong abnormality

Neonatal Tetanus

Esp E.Europe, China. Due to use of contaminated dressings on umbilicus

CLIN: Usually present at 3–10 days age. Spasms; Opisthotonos; Ep. Occ Resp distress, Death

RX: Tetanus antitoxin, Penicillin; IPPV if resp distress

Toxoplasmosis

A rare transplacental infection. Esp 2nd trimester

CLIN: Hydrocephalus or Microcephaly; Ep; J; Liver ↑; Spleen ↑; Maculopapular rash; Microphthalmos; Chorioretinitis; Encephalitis

INVESTIGATIONS:
- Toxoplasma Ab
- LP
- SXR: Ca^{2+} esp basal ganglia

RX: Pyrimethamine & Sulphadiazine

CMV

Causes approx 400 cases of mental retardation in E&W per yr. A transplacental infection. Mother usually asymptomatic

CLIN: Variable picture. LBW; J; Liver ↑; Spleen ↑; Purpura; Haem. Occ Microcephaly; Hydrocephalus; IQ ↓; Microphthalmos; Haemolytic anaemia; Chorioretinitis; Ep

INVESTIGATIONS:
- CMV Ab
- SXR: Occ Ca^{2+}

RX: Steroids. (Vaccine being developed)

PROG: Poor

Rubella

In non-epidemic yrs seriously affects about 200 live births per yr in E&W

CLIN: Mother has overt infection. Variable presentations depending on time of infection. Can → SB. In seriously affected → SFD; PDA; Septal defects; Myocarditis; Cataract; Retinopathy; Glaucoma; Microphthalmos; Deafness; Microcephaly; Liver ↑; LN ↑; J; Spleen ↑; Purpura; Rash; Metaphyseal changes; Pneumonitis. Follow up studies show that more mildly affected at birth often later develop deafness, IQ ↓ & behavioural disorders

INVESTIGATION: • Rubella HAI test

PREVENTION: In UK immunise F at 10–14yrs. Check immunity in pregnancies

Congenital Syphilis

Rare. Should be prevented by serological screening of pregnant women & Rx of those found to be +ve

CLIN: Variable severity. SB; SFD; Failure to thrive; Maculopapular rash; Pemphigus bullae & desquamation esp palms & soles; Rhagades (scars); Condylomata; Bloody rhinitis; Depressed nasal bridge; Liver ↑; Spleen ↑; Cirrhosis; Pneumonia alba; Periostitis; Skull bossing; Osteochondritis → pseudoparalysis; Dactylitis; Blindness; Deafness; Hydrocephalus; Anaemia

INVESTIGATION: • Syphilis serology

RX: Penicillin

DD OF PERIOSTITIS:
1. Scurvy
2. Leukaemia
3. Osteomyelitis
4. Fracture
5. Physiological
6. Infantile Cortical Hyperostosis

Other Viral Congenital Infections

1° HERPES SIMPLEX INFECTION

Can → Abortion or cong malformations esp of CNS. Infection can be transmitted from birth canal

RX: If genital herpes, LSCS

VARICELLA

Rarely → CNS malformations

HEPATITIS B

Transmission to child esp likely if HBeAg +ve. Esp China. Risk of transmission esp c̄ 3rd trimester infection

RX: Specific HBsAg Ig after birth & at 1mth

COXSACKIE B

Can → SB, Acute myocarditis

MUMPS, INFLUENZA, POLIO, MEASLES & ENTEROVIRUSES

Increased risk of miscarriage

PERINATAL ASPHYXIA

Risk Factors for Perinatal Asphyxia (LIST 1 NEO)

1. Intrauterine growth retardation
2. Pre-term delivery
3. PET or severe BP ↑
4. LSCS
5. Low or ↓ urinary Oestriol
6. Multiple delivery
7. Abruptio placentae or APH
8. Meconium stained liquor
9. Breech presentation
10. Forceps delivery
11. Polyhydramnios
12. Foetal malformation
13. Maternal diabetes
14. Recent maternal drugs: Eg Pethidine
15. Rhesus haemolytic disease
16. Cerebral haem
17. Prolapse of cord or strangulation by cord
18. Trauma
19. Post-maturity
20. Resp tract obst: Eg By Meconium, Blood, Mucus
21. Maternal anaemia or BP ↓

PATHOGENESIS: Chr hypoxia → initial vasodilation → cerebral oedema → irreversible injury. Brain esp affected as perinatal asphyxia → BP ↓ → failure of perfusion. In pre-term, BP ↓ may be ass c̄ intraventricular haem. In full term, BP ↓ may be ass c̄ periventricular leucomalacia

CLIN: Most babies are born in 1° apnoea ie HtR >100, blue colour, some flexion of extremities, reflex response to manipulation. An asphyxiated baby makes a few gasps then enters stage of terminal apnoea c̄ HtR ↓; Weak resp effort; BP ↓; Poor reflex irritability; Cyanosis; White trunk; Flaccidity. Occ an asphyxiated baby is born in terminal apnoea

INVESTIGATIONS:
- Foetal scalp pH ↓
- Apgar score: Low
- Cord blood pH

RX: Careful monitoring of at risk foetus. Prompt Rx. Maintain body temperature, clear airway, O_2, Aspirate, if required IPPV c̄ humidifier, cardiac massage if HtR <60/min despite IPPV. Naloxone if mother had been given pre-delivery opiates. Occ Mannitol. Later reduce fluids (anticipating ISADH). Monitor & Rx any BG ↓, Ca^{2+} ↓; Na^+ ↓; K^+ ↑.
If fits give Phenobarbitone

COMPLICATIONS:
1. Cerebral Haem
2. SAH
3. Cerebral oedema
4. ADH secretion & oliguria
5. BG ↓
6. HypoCa
7. $HyperK^+$
8. Ep
9. Necrotising enterocolitis

PROG: Depends on degree of hypoxia. Causes of failed resus inc Cong abnormalities esp cardiac or resp; Severe meconium aspiration; Pneumothorax & equipment failure. Poor prog if fail to establish spontaneous resp within 20mins; If severe Ep

BIRTH INJURY

Esp pre-term infant & large for dates

Caput Succedaneum

Oedematous swelling & ecchymosis over presenting portion of foetus in prolonged labour. Maximal at birth, usually subsides in 2–3 days

Cephalhaematoma

Subperiosteal haem → fluctuant swelling limited by suture lines. Maximal 2nd day. Resolves spontaneously

of Skull

Small undisplaced #s are not uncommon

Subaponeurotic Haem

Rare serious disorder. Esp if clotting defect. Haem over skull can → death. Rarely due to vacuum extraction

RX: Rapid transfusion. Correct any clotting defect

Forceps Injuries

May → trivial ecchymoses or deep lacerations

Nerve Palsies

Difficulty in delivering infant's shoulders may → Erb's or Klumpke's palsy. Facial palsy may be due to forceps injury

Intracranial Injuries

Important cause of neonatal morbidity or mort. May cause or be caused by hypoxia

INJURIES WITHOUT HAEM

Common. Normally recover

CLIN: Variable presentation eg flaccid c̄ asphyxia or restless & irritable c̄ fits

INVESTIGATION: • Ultrasound

DD: Hypoglycaemia & other metabolic fits

INJURIES WITH HAEM

Commonest cause is SAH. May be fatal esp 2° to Subdural

RISK FACTORS:
1. Breech
2. Forceps
3. Disproportion
4. Precipitate labour
5. Low prothrombin eg LBW
6. Hypoxia

CLIN: Usually present at birth. Shock; Apnoea; Cyanosis. Fails to suck & cry. Occ Twitching, Fits

INVESTIGATION: • Ultrasound

RX: Careful monitoring. Maintain body temperature; O_2; Vit K; Phenobarbitone for fits

COMPLICATIONS:
1. Hydrocephalus
2. Chr subdural haematoma
3. CP
4. Ep

LOW BIRTH WEIGHT BABIES

LBW is defined as a live born baby c̄ wt <2.5kg at birth. % of LBW is related to socioeconomic conditions. Low rate in Sweden. Causes of LBW are pre-term delivery & intrauterine growth retardation. Pre-term = <37wks gestation. Pre-term children who are growth retarded are termed small for gestational age (SGA)

SGA infants are identified using a wt percentile chart c̄ a known or estimated gestational age. Gestational age is based on morphology, CNS signs, menstrual dates & obstetric test observations eg ultrasound. SGA infant at term appears underweight, scraggy yet mature. Pre-term infants have a large head/body ratio, low subcutaneous fat & a wrinkled appearance. In very

Causes of LBW (LIST 2 NEO)

A. CAUSES OF PRE-TERM DELIVERY
1. Idiopathic
2. Maternal infections
3. Foetal abnormality
4. BP ↑ disease of Pregnancy
5. Amnionitis
6. Uterine abnormalities
7. Multiple pregnancy
8. Cervical incompetence

B. CAUSES OF GROWTH RETARDATION
1. Severe maternal malnutrition
2. Chr maternal infection: Eg Malaria
3. BP ↑ disease of pregnancy
4. Maternal smoking

immature, red, thin, shiny skin

Problems of LBW Babies (LIST 3 NEO)

1. Respiratory:
   a) RDS
   b) Atelectasis
   c) Persistent pulm BP ↑
   d) Aspiration → pneumonitis
   e) Apnoeic attacks
2. Perinatal asphyxia
3. Metabolic:
   a) BG ↓
   b) $HypoCa^{2+}$
   c) Hypothermia
   d) Dehydration
   e) J
   f) Def diseases eg Rickets
   g) Acidosis
4. Wt loss
5. Oedema
6. Anaemia
7. Bleeding:
   Esp Intraventricular Haem, Periventricular haem
8. Neurological problems:
   Eg Ep
9. Infections ↑
   Eg Necrotising enterocolitis, Pneumonia
10. ↑ incidence of cong malformations
11. Complications of Rx:
   a) O_2 → retrolental fibroplasia, pulm damage
   b) Iatrogenic infection eg via umbilical catheter
   c) Prolonged ventilation → chr lung disease

Particular problems of SGA are: BG ↓; Hypothermia; Meconium aspiration; Perinatal asphyxia & pulm BP ↑

GENERAL CLIN: Cold; J; Somnolent; Irreg shallow resp

INVESTIGATIONS: • BG
- If problems: FBC, WCC, CXR, AXR, Ca^{2+}, Astrup, Ultrasound

GENERAL RX: Often require admission to SCBU. Regular monitoring of HtR, Resp, Temperature, pre-prandial BG. NG feeding usually required if <34 wks, resp or CNS problems. Use breast milk 3–4hrly. Check for gastric retention. Correct dehydration. Maintain body heat by wrapping infant in warm dry towel post delivery & transfer infant, covered by heat shield, to incubator. Add vitamin supplements after 2–4wks. If BG ↓, IV 10% dextrose. Rx bilirubin ↑ if high or increasing bilirubin level, acidotic, severe asphyxia by phototherapy or exchange transfusion. O_2, limited handling, Vit K, Fe. Phenobarbitone for fits

GENERAL PROG: In West, improved mort & morbidity in recent yrs. Poor prog factors are birth wt <1kg, fits, symptomatic BG ↓, prolonged mechanical ventilation, large cerebral haem. Long term follow up shows > expected problems of learning, reading, behaviour, parent bonding

Severe Hypothermia

PATHOGENESIS: ↓ brown fat, ↓ subcutaneous fat, large surface area/vol ratio, poor vasoconstriction

CLIN: Failure to suck; Apathy; HtR ↓; Cyanosis; Cold skin; Oedema; Reddening; Oedematous non-fluctuant hardening of skin (sclerema)

RX: Gradual warming in incubator. Occ antibiotics, steroids, exchange transfusion for sclerema

COMPLICATIONS: Ht failure, pulm haem if rewarming too rapid

Periodic Breathing & Apnoeic Attacks

30–50% of premature babies esp in first wk have spells of periodic breathing comprising 5–10sec pauses alternating c̄ periods of ventilation at a rate of 50–60/min
In first 2wks some premature esp VLBW have apnoeic episodes lasting >15secs (apnoeic attacks). May be ass c̄ PR ↓; Cyanosis; Metabolic acidosis. Apnoeic attacks may be ass c̄ underlying conditions eg BG ↓; Intracranial haem

PREVENTION: Aminophylline. Use of 25–30% O_2 is justified if an accurate O_2 analyser is used & health staff are vigilant

RX: Monitor all babies of <34wk gestation. Apnoea monitors, either PR↓-dependent or Resp-dependent. In attack, most respond to cutaneous stimulation. If not, ventilate until spontaneous resp resumed

RDS

Ass c̄ preterm babies esp <34wks gestation. Ass c̄ intravent haem

PATHOGENESIS: Decreased Surfactant (a surface tension lowering phospholipid) in pre-term. Surfactant also destroyed by hypoxia, acidosis & hypothermia → atelectasis → increased hypoxia which may → persistent pulm hypertension & persistent foetal circulation

CLIN: Present 1–2 hrs post-birth. Rapid, laboured breathing c̄ rib retraction & expiratory grunt; Cyanosis (R to L shunt)

INVESTIGATIONS: • Astrup: Acidosis, pO_2 ↓
• CXR : Ground glass appearance, Air bronchogram

RX: Usually need resp support for 4–5days to enable lung to make sufficient surfactant. O_2; CPAP, IPPV ± PEEP; Maintain body temperature. Humidify. Occ antibiotics

COMPLICATIONS:

1. **Bronchopulmonary Dysplasia:** Rare. Persistent resp distress. Ass c̄ prolonged mechanical ventilation c̄ O_2
   Investigation: • CXR: Hyperaeration & patchy opacities
   Prog: Considerable morbidity for 1–2yrs. Many then improve
   N.B Wilson–Mikity syndrome describes premature infants that become apnoeic & cyanotic at 2–3wks of age. Cause unknown. Identical CXR findings to Bronchopulmonary dysplasia
2. **Persistent Pulm BP ↑:** R to L shunt through PDA. May also be 2° to Ht disease, Other resp disease
   Clin: Mild resp signs; Cyanosis
   Investigation: • CXR: Oligaemic lung fields
   Rx: O_2, IPPV. Occ use pulm vasodilators
3. **PDA:** Usually occurs in recovery phase of infants ventilated for RDS
   Clin: Resp distress. Systolic murmur
   Rx: Fluid restriction or diuretics. Indomethacin to close PDA, if fails surgical ligation
4. **Pneumothorax**

PROG: In good centres mort approx 5% in infants of >1250g. Poor prog if develop bronchopulmonary dysplasia, persistent pulm BP ↑

DD: 1. Transient tachypnoea (TTN)
2. Pneumonia

Causes of Neonatal SOB (LIST 4 NEO)

1. RDS
2. TTN
3. Pneumonia
4. Pneumothorax
5. Acidosis
6. CHD
7. Cerebral irritation
8. TOF
9. Diaphragmatic hernia
10. Choanal atresia
11. Bronchopulmonary dysplasia

Oedema

May be 2° to Protein ↓; Hypothermia; Fluids ↑; Renal function ↓

DD: 1. CCF
2. Turners syndrome

Retrolental Fibroplasia

Esp in <1kg babies. Usually due to prolonged high conc O_2 Rx

Necrotising Enterocolitis

Probably anaerobic infection 2° to ischaemic GIT episode

CLIN: Bile vomit; Blood & mucous in stools; Shock; Abdo distension

INVESTIGATION: • AXR: Air in bowel wall ± Portal venous tree

RX: Stop oral feed. Feed IV; Antibiotics

COMPLICATIONS: 1. Perf
2. Stricture

Periventricular Haemorrhage

Ass c̄ very LBW, breech delivery, perinatal asphyxia

CLIN: May be asymptomatic. Occ Shock; Fits. Often ass resp disease eg pneumothorax. May → CP, hydrocephalus

INVESTIGATIONS: • Ultrasound
• CAT scan
• Coagulation tests
• Astrup
• CXR

JAUNDICE

Causes of Neonatal Jaundice (LIST 5 NEO)

A. NON HAEMOLYTIC UNCONJUGATED HYPERBILIRUBINAEMIA
1. Delayed enzyme maturation:
   a) Physiological
   b) J in pre-term infant
   c) Hypothyroidism
2. Enzyme inhibition:
   Esp Breast milk J
3. Enzyme def:
   a) Crigler–Najjar
   b) Gilbert's disease

B. HAEMOLYTIC UNCONJUGATED HYPERBILIRUBINAEMIA
1. Congenital:
   Eg Spherocytosis, G6PD def, Pyruvate Kinase def, Thalassemia
2. Acquired:
   a) Rhesus haemolytic disease
   b) Incompatible blood transfusion
   c) Excess Vit K
3. Sepsis:
   Eg UTI

C. INTRAHEPATIC CONJUGATED HYPERBILIRUBINAEMIA
1. Infection:
   Eg Gm -ve septicaemia, CMV, Rubella, Herpes, Toxoplasma, Sy
2. Metabolic:
   a) Galactosaemia
   b) Tyrosinaemia
   c) Fructosaemia
   d) α_1-antitrypsin def
   e) CF (Rarely)
3. Dubin Johnson syndrome
4. Rotor syndrome
5. Neonatal hepatitis syndrome

D. EXTRAHEPATIC CONJUGATED HYPERBILIRUBINAEMIA
1. Extrahepatic biliary atresia
2. Choledochal cysts
3. Total parenteral nutrition

Physiological Jaundice

Common approx 50% of babies. Esp pre-term infants

PATHOGENESIS: Large bilirubin load from RES breakdown of Hb excedes albumin binding capacity. The splenic vein may bypass liver via ductus venosus. Lack of glucuronyl transferase to conjugate bilirubin. Immature active transport mechanism & good enterohepatic circulation contribute

CLIN: J starts on 2nd day, peaks on 4th & usually disappears by 10 days. In pre-term J may be more prolonged & severe

INVESTIGATION: • Unconjugated Bilirubin ↑ (not >175umol/l)

RX: Phototherapy if bilirubin >250umol/l c̄ pads to protect eyes

DD: Pathological J: J starts in 1st 24hrs or persists >2wks in term or >3wks in pre-term

Rhesus Haemolytic Disease

Alleles at 3 loci (C, D & E) determine Rhesus constitution. D is the most common Rhesus antigen. ABO blood gp incompatibility can also cause haemolytic disease of newborn. Other blood gps rarely produce haemolytic disease

PATHOGENESIS: Typically a Rhesus D -ve woman is sensitised by Ag from D +ve foetus usually late in pregnancy due to foetal leak. In a subsequent pregnancy, a 2nd Rhesus D +ve foetus will stimulate IgG anti-D Ab which passes across placenta destroying foetal red cells. However most Rhesus D -ve mothers never produce Ab

CLIN: Variable severity. Most severe is SB (Hydrops foetalis). Predominant features may be oedema (Hydrops foetalis), severe J (Icterus gravis neonatorum), haemolysis (Haemolytic anaemia). Spleen ↑; Liver ↑. Risk of kernicterus

INVESTIGATIONS: • Maternal ABO & Rhesus typing
- Ab levels: If Rhesus D -ve
- Amniotic optical density & L:S ratio
- Maternal blood Kleihauer test: +ve if foetal leak

- Foetal ABO & Rhesus typing
- Coombs test
- Foetal Hb
- Foetal bilirubin

PREVENTION: Anti-D Ig after delivery reduces incidence of Rhesus sensitisation. Also give Anti-D Ig after abortion, amniocentesis & ectopic pregnancy

RX: If Ab levels high consider early delivery. Assess foetal maturity. If immature try intrauterine transfusion. Exchange transfusion (SE: Infection, CCF, Trauma) is indicated if: +ve Coombs' & low cord Hb; High unconjugated bilirubin

COMPLICATION: Kernicterus: Occurs if unconjugated bilirubin from any cause is >340umol/l when bilirubin is toxic to neurones

Clin: Lethargy; Opisthotonus; Ep; J. Later Athetosis

Rx: Prevent by Phototherapy; Exchange transfusion

Neonatal Jaundice Due to Infection

Common. Esp if hypoxia, acidosis or BG ↓. Esp Pre-term; Post mature. Causes inc CMV, Gm -ve septicaemia

Biliary Atresia

Rare

CLIN: Usually presents at 2wks c obst J; Liver ↑; Spleen ↑

INVESTIGATIONS:
- Bilirubin: Total & direct
- Liver biopsy
- Ultrasound
- HIDA scan
- Laparotomy

RX: Difficult. Liver transplant or Kasai procedure

PROG: Most die at 18–24mths

DD:

1. α_1-antitrypsin def
2. Intrahepatic bile duct dysplasia
3. Severe neonatal hepatitis syndrome

α_1-Antitrypsin Def

CLIN: Often present in 1st few wks of life c̄ severe cholestasis. J clears by 6mths but present c̄ cirrhosis at 5yrs. In adults ass c̄ emphysema

INVESTIGATIONS:
- Liver biopsy: PAS +ve intracellular inclusions
- Protease inhibitor typing

RX: Genetic counselling. However most c̄ def are asymptomatic

Neonatal Hepatitis Syndrome

?cause. Probably many conditions. Diagnosis of exclusion but liver biopsy usually shows giant cells

Choledochal Cyst

F>M. Rare

CLIN: May present any time in early life. Many presentations. Classically J; Palpable mass, Pain

INVESTIGATION:
- Ultrasound

NEONATAL HAEMORRHAGE

Causes of Neonatal Haemorrhage (LIST 6 NEO)

1. Birth trauma
2. Improper tying of cord
3. Infection
4. Haemorrhagic disease of the newborn
5. Thrombocytopenia: Eg Leukaemia, ITP. Haemangioma
6. Any cause of severe J

Haemorrhagic Disease of Newborn

Usually due to temp clotting factor def. Esp pre-term baby

CLIN: Usually present at 3–4 days. Occ Malaena; Haematemesis; Umbilical cord haem; Vaginal haem; Haematuria. If blood loss severe → shock

INVESTIGATION:
- PT time ↑

RX: Vit K. Occ require transfusion

DD: Swallowed maternal blood

NEONATAL CONVULSIONS

Causes of Neonatal Convulsions (LIST 7 NEO)

1. Pre-natal infection:
   Eg CMV, Toxoplasmosis
2. Cerebral malformation
3. Birth trauma
4. Perinatal asphyxia
5. Intracranial haem
6. Meningitis, Septicaemia
7. Metabolic:
   a) BG ↓
   b) HypoCa^{2+}
   c) HypoMg^{2+}
   d) HypoNa & water overload
   e) Hyperbilirubinaemia
8. Inborn errors of metabolism:
   Eg Galactosaemia, Fructosaemia, Pyridoxine def
9. Drug withdrwal in addicted mothers

M>F. 40% of fits occur in days 0–3 max 24hrs; Main causes are perinatal anoxia, cerebral trauma. 35% of fits occur in days 4–9 max 120hrs; Main causes are metabolic

CLIN: Fits may be multifocal, tonic, focal, clonic or myoclonic. Child may be irritable or apathetic

INVESTIGATIONS:
- LP
- BG
- Ca^{2+}
- Mg^{2+}
- U&E
- WCC
- Blood cultures
- Ultrasound
- EEG

RX: Dextrose IV if BG ↓. Ca^{2+} gluconate or $MgSO_4$. Diazepam followed by Phenytoin

PROG: Poor if early Ep. 20% of survivors have Ep. 40% of survivors have some handicap

DD:
1. Breath holding attacks
2. Cardiac arrhythmias
3. Jittery baby

CHROMOSOMAL ABNORMALITIES

Approx 4 in 1000 babies in the UK are born c̄ handicapping chromosomal abnormalities. Also causes many abortions. Ass c̄ SGA

Down's Syndrome

Three types: Trisomy 21 (90%); Translocation of chromosome 21 onto another chromosome (5%); Mosaic of normal & trisomy (5%). Incidence of Trisomy 21 increases c̄ maternal age. Approx 1 in 600 births

CLIN: IQ ↓; Upward slanting eyes; Prominent epicanthic skin folds; Short nose; Protuding tongue; Flat occiput; Transverse palmar crease; Incurved little finger; Delayed dentition; Short stature; Underdeveloped 2° sexual characteristics; Floppiness. Occ Brushfield spots on iris; Cataract; Nystagmus; Poor speech. 40% have CHD esp Fallots, VSD, Ostium primum defect. Ass c̄ Leukaemia; Duodenal atresia; ↑ illness susceptibility

RX: Correct any duodenal atresia

PROG: Poor if pre-term; CHD; or Leukaemia

Trisomy 18 (Edwards Syndrome)

CLIN: Micrognathia; Low set ears; Prominent occiput; Rocker bottom feet; Overlapping fingers. Occ CHD

PROG: Usually die in 1st yr

Trisomy 13–15 (Patau Syndrome)

Microcephaly; Microphthalmia; Sloping forehead; Bilat cleft lip & palate; Aplasia cutis congenita. Occ Polycystic kidneys

PROG: Most die in 1st yr

Partial Deletion Trisomy 22

Very rare

CLIN: Anal atresia; Iris colobomatas

Cri-du-chat Syndrome (Partial Deletion Chromosome 5)

Very rare. F>M

CLIN: "Mewing cry". Microcephaly; Anti-mongoloid slant to eyes; IQ ↓. Occ CHD

INFANT FEEDING

Babies usually treble birth wt in 1st year. Wt should be monitored by sequential plotting on growth chart. Babies crossing centiles & those on >97th & <3rd centile require further follow up. Main nutritional requirements in infancy are water, calories (100–120cals/kg/day), Vit C (15mg/day), Vit D (400IU/day), Ca^{2+} (600mg/day) & Fe (6mg/day). Expected wt gain in first 3mths is 170g/wk
Causes of feeding problems inc infection, prematurity, cerebral irritation, Ht failure, J, SOB, cleft palate. Now increasing evidence of benefits of breast compared to bottle feeding
Problems of breast feeding inc Breast milk J, the need to add Vit supplements & occ psychological objections. Social factors eg the concept of bottle feeding as convenient & more acceptable in public lead many mothers to soon stop breast feeding. Breast feeding in the West is commoner in higher social classes. c/i to breast feeding is rare eg maternal TB, PKU, mother on anticoags. More advanced bottle feeds closely mimic composition of breast milk but still lack maternal Ig, lactobacilli & antiviral factors which protect against infection esp *E.coli.* Breast feeding should initially be on demand. Milk flow is usually well established between 4–10 days. Introduction of solids is necessary at 4–6mths. Early introduction may ppt severe coeliac disease

Problems of Bottle Feeding
(LIST 8 NEO)

1. Problems Due to Composition of Feed:
   a) Neonatal tetany (PO_4 ↑ → HypoCa^{2+}) (Rare)
   b) Hyperosmolality
   c) ↑ sat fats ? → ↑ atheroma
2. Problems in Preparation:
   a) ↑ infections
   b) Concentrated feeds → hypernatraemia
3. Increased Infection:
   Esp GE, Resp infection, OM, Candida
4. Obesity
5. Cows milk allergy
6. Increased susceptibility to disease:
   a) Necrotising enterocolitis
   b) Dental caries
   c) ? ↑ incidence of cot death
   d) ?Asthma, ?Eczema
7. Constipation
8. ? ↓ maternal bonding

Paediatrics

GROWTH & DEVELOPMENT

Growth is best assessed by serial measurements of Wt, Height & head circumference plotted on a centile chart & estimation of growth velocity. Child assessment can be considered under 5 headings: Motor development inc posture & large mvt; Vision & fine mvt; Hearing & speech; Social behaviour; Sexual maturity. Milestones in these areas can be assessed by developmental charts; however the charts should be used c̄ caution. Some ave milestone guides in normal are:

6wks:	Smile in response to stimulus
3mths:	Lose Moro & sucking reflex; Coos when pleased
4mths:	Able to roll over; Full head control
6mths:	Palmar grasp; Localise soft sounds
7mths:	Able to sit up unaided
9mths:	Crawl; Stands c̄ support
12–15mths:	Walk; 1st words
24mths:	Run; Says own name; 50% control bladder
M Wt (kg):	3.5 (birth); 7.9 (6mths); 10.2 (1yr); 30.3 (10yrs)
F Wt (kg):	3.4 (birth); 6.9 (6mths); 9.7 (1yr); 31.1 (10yrs)
M Hgh (cm):	54 (birth); 76 (1yr); 87 (2yr); 108 (5yrs)
F Hgh (cm):	53 (birth); 74 (1yr); 86 (2yr); 107 (5yrs)

There are two growth spurts one starting in utero & ending at 2yrs; the other occuring at puberty.

Physical growth potential is genetically determined. 2 sets of genes concerned, genes to determine adult stature & genes to determine growth rate & bone development. Potential for growth is influenced by nutrition, disease or handicap & emotional factors
In early childhood non achievement of expected growth is termed failure to thrive. Most disease in childhood → failure to thrive

Causes of Failure to Thrive (LIST 1 PAED)

1. Defective intake:
   a) Feeding mismangement
   b) Kwashiorkor, Marasmus
   c) Anorexia
   d) Mechanical eg cleft palate
2. Defective absorption:
   a) Intestinal eg Coeliac disease, Giardiasis, Post-GE, Milk allergy, Immune def, Tropical sprue, Hirschprung's disease, Blind loop
   b) Pancreatic eg CF, Pancreatitis
   c) Liver eg Biliary atresia, Neonatal hepatitis
4. Increased loss by Vom: Eg Py.S, HH, Chr ICP ↑, Rumination
5. Metabolic: Eg Hypothyroidism, Diabetes, RTbA, Nephrogenic DI, PKU, Idiopathic HyperCa^{2+}, Adrenocortical hyperplasia, Hypophosphatasia, Galactosaemia
6. CNS disease: Eg Cerebral palsy, Tumours, Subdural haematoma
7. CHD
8. Recurrent UTI, CRF
9. Resp disease: Eg Bronchiectasis, Asthma, CF
10. Cirrhosis
11. Chr infections: Eg TB, Malaria, Hookworm, Cong CMV
12. Emotional deprivation
13. Severe prematurity
14. Chromosomal abnormalities

Short stature indicates Hgh below 3rd centile for age. Infantilism implies general developmental retardation

Causes of Short Stature (LIST 2 PAED)

A. DWARFISM WITHOUT INFANTILISM
1. Familial & genetic short stature
2. Cong dwarfism: Eg Trisomy syndromes, Silver's syndrome
3. Skeletal disease: Eg Achondroplasia, Mucopolysaccharidoses, Rickets, Spina bifida, Polio, HPT
4. 2° to Precocious puberty
5. Emotional deprivation

B. DWARFISM WITH INFANTILISM
1. SGA (Chr intrauterine growth retardation)
2. VLBW ie <1kg
3. Endocrine:
   a) Hypothyroidism
   b) Panhypopituitarism
   c) Diabetes
   d) Isolated GH def
   e) 1° Hypogonadism eg Turner's
   f) Prader–Willi syndrome
   g) Excess steroids inc Cushing's
   h) Pseudohypoparathyroidism
4. Infection Eg Malaria, TB, Hookworm
5. Systemic disease:
   a) Renal eg CRF, RTbA
   b) GIT eg Coeliac disease, Crohn's
   c) Cardiac eg CHD
   d) Cerebral eg Mental retardation
   e) Resp eg CF, Bronchiectasis, Asthma
6. Glycogen storage diseases
7. Down's syndrome
8. Dysmorphic Syndromes: Eg de Lange, Dubowitz, Bloom's

Most children below 3rd centile are familiarly predisposed. Other common causes are Psychosocial short stature & Intrauterine growth retardation Investigate children c̄ low growth velocity, small stature & illness, non-familial small stature & extremely small stature (ie >3 SD below mean)

GENERAL INVESTIGATIONS OF SHORT STATURE:
- Serial accurate Hgh Measurements: To assess rate of growth
- Social history
- Bone age
- SXR
- CXR
- Urinalysis
- U&E
- FBC
- BG
- Occ eg: TFT, Ca^{2+}, Sweat test, Fundoscopy & visual fields, Chromosomes (F), Jejunal biopsy, CAT scan, GH. (N.B ↑ in early sleep, exercise & c̄ insulin)

Russell Syndrome

Very rare

CLIN: Short stature; LBW; Small triangular face; Syndactyly; Hypomandibulosis

Silver Syndrome

Very rare

CLIN: Short stature; LBW; Hemihypertrophy

GH Def

Occ Aut Rec. May be 2° Craniopharyngioma; X-Rad; Emotional deprivation. Usually present at 2yrs

CLIN: Normal birth wt; Short stature; Relatively obese; Small genitalia

INVESTIGATIONS:
- Bone age ↓
- ITT: No rise in GH

RX: Human GH

Hypothyroidism

NEONATAL HYPOTHYROIDISM

1 in 5000 births. Commonest cause is thyroid dysgenesis

CLIN: Slow to cry; Somnolent; Poor feeder; Constipation; Wrinkled forehead; Developmental delay; Umbilical hernia. Occ Goitre; J. Later yellow pallor, gingery hair (β carotinaemia); Short stature; Large tongue; Obese; IQ ↓

INVESTIGATION: • TFT

RX: Prophylactic screen. Thyroxine

PROG: Very good if early Rx

JUVENILE HYPOTHYROIDISM

Commonest cause is chr lymphocytic thyroiditis

CLIN: Usually present at 8–10yrs. Short stature; Early puberty; Obese. Occ IQ ↓

INVESTIGATIONS: • TFT
• Bone age ↓

RX: Thyroxine

Hypopituitarism

Rare. May be 1° or 2° to tumour, infection, haem. May → retention of childhood habitus into adult life

Pseudohypoparathyroidism

FH. Failure of organ to respond to PTH

CLIN: Short; Obese; Long index finger; Round face; IQ ↓

INVESTIGATIONS: • Ca^{2+} ↓
• Low urinary PO_4
• PTH ↑

RX: Vit D

Steroid Excess

Usually due to prolonged drug Rx. Cushing's syndrome very rare in children. Suppress GH release → short stature

Prader–Willi Syndrome

CLIN: LBW; Feeding problems; Small stature; Undescended testes; Hypotonia. Later Obesity; Diabetes

Cerebral Gigantism (Soto's Syndrome)

Rare. ?Hypothalamic lesion

CLIN: IQ ↓; Clumsy; Large head; High arched palate; Hypertelorism; Rapid growth from infancy

Gigantism indicates large size & precocity advanced development for age

Causes of Gigantism & Precocity (LIST 3 PAED)

A. GIGANTISM WITHOUT PRECOCITY
1. Familial & genetic gigantism
2. Eunochoidism:
   Eg Klinefelter's Syndrome
3. Marfan's Syndrome
4. Cerebral Gigantism
5. Infants of diabetic mothers
6. Homocystinuria
7. Beckwith–Wiedemann syndrome

B. GIGANTISM & PRECOCITY
1. Endocrine:
   a) Hypergonadal eg Testicular or Ovarian tumours
   b) Hyperadrenalism eg Cong adrenal hyperplasia
   c) Hyperpituitary Gigantism
   d) Hyperthyroidism (rare)
2. Neurological:
   Eg Hypothalamic disorders, Hydrocephalus, Cerebral degenerations, Meningoencephalitis, Tuberous sclerosis
3. Idiopathic Familial

Beckwith–Wiedemann Syndrome

Rare. Exomphalos, Macroglossia, Gigantism

Hyperpituitary Gigantism

Rare. Due to ant pituitary adenoma

CLIN: Giants—very tall c̄ enlarged extremities eg jaw. Delayed puberty. Often diabetes. Occ Hypogonadism

INVESTIGATIONS: • GH ↑
• BG

- PO_4 ↑
- X-R of extremities

RX: Stereotactic surgery

Hyperthyroidism

Rare. F>M. Usually an autoimmune thyroiditis

CLIN: Wt ↓; Good appetite; PR ↑; Goitre. Tall. Occ Ht ↑; Irritability; Exophthalmos

INVESTIGATIONS:
- TFT
- Bone age ↑
- BG
- CXR

RX: Carbimazole or partial thyroidectomy

PUBERTY

Signs of puberty normally start to appear in M & F at about 11 yrs. Growth spurt starts earlier in F. Menarche usually occurs at 13yrs.

RX PRECOCIOUS PUBERTY: Cyproterone acetate suppresses puberty but generally adult height cannot be attained. Rx of underlying cause

Causes of Early Puberty
(LIST 4 PAED)

1. Familial
2. Hypothalamic:
   Eg ICP ↑, McCune–Albright Syndrome
3. Hypothyroidism
4. Gonadal tumours
5. Adrenal:
   a) Cong adrenal hyperplasia (21OHlase, 11 β-OHlase defs)
   b) Adrenal Ca
   c) Cushing's syndrome
6. Excess gonadotrophins:
   a) Pinealoma
   b) Hepatoblastoma
   c) Exogenous gonadotrophins
7. Other neurological conditions:
   Eg Hydrocephalus, Post encephalitis

Causes of Delayed Puberty
(LIST 5 PAED)

1. Chr systemic illness
2. Familial
3. Severe malnutrition
4. Emotional:
   Esp Anorexia nervosa
5. Prolactinoma
6. Kallman's syndrome
7. Gonadal defects:
   Eg Anorchia, Cryptorchidism, Mumps, Turner's syndrome, Klinefelter's Syndrome, Noonan–Ullrich syndrome, Tumour, Testicular feminisation syndrome
8. Cong adrenal hyperplasia (3β-OHsteroid deHase, 17α-OHlase defs)
9. Cong adrenal hypoplasia
10. GnRH def
11. Sex hormone biosynthesis disorders

Precocious puberty can be defined as puberty at <8yrs in F & <9yrs in M. Delayed puberty is at >13.5yrs in F & >14yrs in M

GENERAL INVESTIGATIONS OF PRECOCIOUS PUBERTY:
- FSH
- LH
- TFT
- SXR
- Bone age

GENERAL INVESTIGATIONS OF DELAYED PUBERTY:
- FSH
- LH
- Prolactin
- GnRH test
- HCG test in M (Testosterone should rise)
- Bone age
- SXR

RX: If M gonadotrophin def give HCG. If M gonadal failure give testosterone. In F gonadal failure give ethinyloestradiol

Congenital Adrenal Hyperplasia

Aut Rec. M=F. 4 poss enzyme def, 21 OHlase def is commonest

PATHOGENESIS: 21-OHlase def →↓ cortisol →↑ ACTH → adrenocortical hyperplasia & ↑ 17β-OH-progesterone →↑ 17 ketosteroids & therefore masculinisation. If severe def then excess salt loss in urine
11β-OHlase def → ↑11deoxycorticosterone → BP ↑ & salt retention
3β-OHsteroid deHase def →↓ cortisol →↑ 17ketosteroids
17α-OHlase def →↓ corticosterone → BP ↑. No salt loss

CLIN: In 21-OHlase def M are norm at birth but soon develop large penis, pubic hair & tall stature, yet testes are small. F at birth have masculinised genitalia. For both M & F later short stature due to premature epiphyseal fusion; Often skin pigmentation. Occ neonatal acute adrenal crisis c̄ D&V, dehydration & shock
3 β-OHsteroid deHase def → F virilisation & incomplete masculinisation of male eg cryptorchidism, bifid scrotum

INVESTIGATIONS: • Blood 17α OHprogesterone
• Urinary 17 ketosteroids, Pregnanetriol: ↑ in 21 OHlase def
• Chromosomal sex typing

RX: Long term Cortisone therapy. In salt losing crisis give IV fluids, DOCA & cortisone. "Salt losers" require maintenence Rx of salt c̄ Fludrocortisone or DOCA. Cover any injury, infection or op c̄ steroids. Surgery on virilised F eg partial cliteroidectomy at 1–4yrs

DD: Adrenal adenoma or carcinoma

Kallman's Syndrome

Anosmia, Hypogonadism. Congenital

Stages of Sexual Differentiation

Genetic (Chromosomal) sex: At conception; Gonadal sex: 8–10th intrauterine wk; Genital sex: 12th intrauterine wk; Psychological sex: 18–30 mnth; Hormonal sex: Puberty
At 6wks a bipotential gonad appears. If Y chromosome present → testes development, if no Y → ovary development. 2 X chromosomes needed for full ovary development. In presence of testosterone Wolffian duct forms epididymis, vas & seminal vesicles. In F, Mullerian duct forms fallopian tube, uterus & vagina. Ext M sex structures depend on presence of testosterone

Abnormal Gonadal Differentiation

KLINEFELTER'S SYNDROME

47,XXY syndrome. 1 in 500 births. Rarely mosaic XY/XXY

CLIN: Small testes; Azoospermia. Occ ↓ body hair, IQ ↓, Gynaecomastia. Not usually impotent

INVESTIGATIONS: • Chromosomes
• FSH ↑ (Post puberty)
• Testosterone ↓

RX: Androgens

TURNER'S SYNDROME

45,XO syndrome. 1 in 5000 births. Occ mosaic 46,XX/45,X. Ass c̄ diabetes & Hashimoto's thyroiditis

CLIN: Growth ↓; Dwarfism. Streak gonads; Amenorrhoea; High arched palate; Infantilism. Occ Naevi; Webbed neck; Lymphoedema; L sided CHD eg coarctation; Widely spaced nipples; Short 4th metacarpals; GUS malformations eg Horseshoe kidney; ↑ carrying angle. Rarely IQ ↓

INVESTIGATIONS: • Chromosomes
• FSH, LH ↑
• Oestradiol ↓

RX: Oestrogens

NOONAN–ULLRICH SYNDROME

Affects both sexes. F (Noonan syndrome) have norm 46,XX karyotype c̄ a Turner phenotype but norm ovarian function & R sided CHD. In M (Ullrich syndrome) have norm 46,XY karyotype c̄ cryptorchidism & features of Turner's syndrome

PURE GONADAL DYSGENESIS

1 in 40,000 births. Streak gonads. May be genetic XX, XY

CLIN: 1° Amenorrhoea; No 2° sexual characteristics; Norm Hgh

ASYMMETRICAL GONADAL DYSGENESIS

Presents c̄ either unilat ovarian dysgenesis or unilat testicular dysgenesis. The latter is ass c̄ X/XY mosaicism & gonadoblastoma

TRUE HERMAPHRODITISM

1 in 50,000 births. Both ovarian & testicular tissue. Ambiguous 2° sexual characteristics. Usually best to rear as F

Abnormal External Genital Differentiation

FEMALE PSEUDOHERMAPHRODITISM

Masculinisation of external genitalia in a 46,XX karyotype c̄ 2 ovaries. Commonest cause is cong adrenal hyperplasia. Rarely due to exogenous androgens eg progestogens to pregnant F

MALE PSEUDOHERMAPHRODITISM

Feminisation of ext genitalia in a 46,XY karyotype c̄ 2 testes. Causes inc abnormal testicular differentiation, disorders of testicular function c̄ ↓ testosterone production & abnormal target organ resistance to androgen. Androgen receptor defects are the commonest cause of the testicular feminisation syndrome in which patients have F phenotype, 1° amenorrhoea, IngH (testes) & develop breasts at puberty. Occ X-linked inheritance

INVESTIGATIONS OF TESTICULAR FEMINISATION: • LH, FSH ↑
• Testosterone: High normal

RX: Remove gonads post puberty to prevent risk of Ca. Raise as F

OTHER ENDOCRINE DISORDERS

Diabetes

Most childhood cases occur at age 10–13yrs. Almost all are IDDM. Occ FH. Incidence approx 1 in 700

CLIN: Thirst; Polyuria; Wt ↓; Lethargy; Constipation; Enuresis. Later Vom; Abdo pain; Acidotic breathing; Shock; Coma; ↑ infections. Mauriac syndrome ie infantilism, liver ↑, short stature, poor diabetic control is rare esp c̄ modern insulins. Complications in adult life eg Neuropathy; Nephropathy; Retinopathy; IHD

INVESTIGATIONS: • Random BG & Urinalysis
• Fasting BG

RX: Admit to hospital for stabilisation. Generally use bd human insulin. Avoid obesity; High fibre diet. Involve family in treatment

Hypoparathyroidism

Rare. Mostly idiopathic

CLIN: Tetany; Ep; Poor dentition. Occ IQ ↓; Moniliasis; Cataract

RX: Ca^{2+} gluconate for tetany. Long term calciferol Rx

Hyperparathyroidism

1° HPT is rare & usually due to an adenoma. 2° HPT is usually due to CRF

CLIN: Bone pains; Weakness; Thirst; Polyuria; Anorexia; Vom; Constipation. Occ Spontaneous #s

INVESTIGATIONS OF 1° HPT: • Ca^{2+} ↑
• PO_4 ↓
• Alk phos ↑
• PTH ↑
• Cortisone suppression test: No ↓ of Ca^{2+}
• X-Rs inc KUB

RX: Remove parathyroid adenoma

INBORN ERRORS OF METABOLISM

A gp of inherited disorders c̄ genetically determined abnormalities of metabolic pathways. Prenatal diagnosis by amniocentesis or foetal blood sampling can identify many enzyme defects eg Lipidoses, Mucopolysaccharidoses. Neonatal screening can be used for amino acid errors of metabolism eg PKU

TYPES OF RX: 1. Restrict intake of accumulating substrate eg restrict fructose in fructose intolerance
2. Post block augmentation eg cystine in homocystinuria, tyrosine in PKU
3. Addition of missing end product eg thyroxine
4. Promote excretion of unwanted substances eg penicillamine to bind Cu^{2+} in Wilson's disease
5. Replace missing protein eg Factor VIII in Haemophilia

Classification of Inborn Errors of Metabolism (LIST 6 PAED)

1. Carbohydrate Metabolism:
   Eg Glycogen storage diseases, Galactosaemia
2. Lipid Metabolism:
   Eg Tay–Sachs, Metachromatic Leucodystrophy, Gaucher's, Niemann–Pick, Krabbe's
3. Mucopolysaccharidoses (GAGS metabolism):
   Eg Hurler's, Hunter's, Sanfilippo, Morquio, Scheie, Maroteaux–Lamy
4. Amino Acid Metabolism:
   Eg. PKU, Homocystinuria, Maple Syrup urine, Histidinaemia, Urea cycle disorders
5. Purine & Pyrimidine Metabolism:
   Eg Lesch–Nyhan syndrome
6. Metal Metabolism:
   Eg Wilson's disease
7. Hormonal Metabolism:
   Eg Cong adrenal hyperplasia

Glycogen Storage Disease

Many types have been described

HEPATORENAL GLYCOGENOSIS (VON GIERKE'S DISEASE)

Due to def of G6phosphatase. Aut Rec

CLIN: Liver ↑↑; Kidney ↑; BG ↓; Failure to thrive; Short stature; Lumbar lordosis; Genu valgum; Excess fat deposits; Xanthomata. Later Gout; Haem; Delayed puberty; ↑ infections

INVESTIGATIONS: • GTT
• Liver biopsy & G6phosphatase assay

RX: Frequent chd feeds. Occ portacaval shunt to ↓ liver glycogen

COMPLICATIONS: 1. Lactic acidosis
2. Hyperlipidaemia
3. Uric acid ↑

GLYCOGEN STORAGE DISEASE OF LIVER & MUSCLE

Aut. Rec. Debrancher enzyme def

CLIN: Liver ↑; Muscle weakness; Hypotonia. Occ BG ↓. Growth sl ↓

RX: Frequent chd feeds

GLYCOGEN STORAGE DISEASE OF THE HEART (POMPE'S DISEASE)

Aut Rec. Acid maltase def

CLIN: Present neonatally c̄ Vom; SOB; Failure to thrive; Ht ↑; Systolic murmur. Occ Hypotonia; Macroglossia. Later liver ↑

PROG: Die in 1st yr

Galactosaemia

Aut Rec. Two types. Commoner is Galactose-1-phosphate uridyl transferase def (G-1-PUT) c incidence of 1 in 70000. Galactokinase def is rarer

PATHOGENESIS: G-1-PUT def → ↑ galactose-1-PO_4 which accumulates toxically in liver, kidney, brain, Ht & lens & ↑ galactose. Galactokinase def only → ↑ galactose. ↑ galactose → ↑ galactitol & cataracts

CLIN: Neonatal presentation. Vom; Failure to thrive; Liver ↑; J; Cataracts; RTbA. Often 2° infection eg Gm -ve septicaemia. Later Cirrhosis; Mental retardation. Galactokinase def → cataracts

INVESTIGATIONS: • Tests for urine reducing sugar (Clinistix -ve; Benedict's test +ve)
- Chromatography
- Beutler's screening test
- Urine: Aminoaciduria, Glycosuria, Proteinuria

RX: Early removal of Lactose & Galactose from diet. Continue diet strictly for 2yrs & at least till puberty

PROG: Cataracts are reversible. With Rx most children have slightly ↓ IQ & Hgh

Hereditary Fructose Intolerance

Aut Rec. Def of Fructose Aldolase

CLIN: Presents when fructose introduced to diet. Failure to thrive; D&V; Liver ↑; J. Occ Ep

INVESTIGATION: • Liver biopsy & enzyme assay

RX: Remove fructose from diet

Lipidoses

GAUCHER'S DISEASE

Familial esp Jews. F>M. Due to deposition of cerebroside. 2 forms

CLIN OF INFANTILE FORM: Onset at 0–1yr. Spleen ↑↑; Liver ↑; IQ ↓. Occ Trismus; Opisthotonus; Strabismus

CLIN OF CHR FORM: Onset in childhood or early adult life. Spleen ↑↑; Liver ↑; Anaemia; Bone pains; Pigmentation

INVESTIGATIONS: • Bone marrow: Gaucher cells
- X-R Long bones: Flask shaped lower femora
- WCC ↓
- Platelets ↓

RX: Splenectomy for hypersplenism

PROG: Infantile form die by 3yrs. Chr form die early

NIEMANN–PICK DISEASE

Due to accumulation of sphingomyelin

CLIN: Present in infancy. Spleen ↑↑; Liver ↑↑; Ascites; Hypotonia; Mental retardation; Pigmentation; Anaemia. Occ Cherry-red macular spot; Resp disease; Blindness; Deafness

INVESTIGATION: • Bone marrow: Niemann–Pick cell

PROG: Die by 2yrs

TAY–SACHS DISEASE (GM2 GANGLIOSIDOSIS)

Aut Rec. Esp Jews. Due to deposition of GM2 ganglioside in brain

CLIN: Onset at 4–6mths. Developmental delay; Blindness; Deafness; Weakness; Cherry-red macular spot. Later Ep; Dementia. Resp infections

PROG: Death by 2yrs

GENERALISED GANGLIOSIDOSES GM1

Aut Rec

CLIN: Present at birth. Mental retardation; Ep; Hypotonia; Liver ↑; Spleen ↑; Gargoyle features; Cherry-red macular spot

PROG: Death by 2yrs

METACHROMATIC LEUKODYSTROPHY

Due to sulphatide defect

CLIN: Onset at 3–18mths. Hypotonia; Spasticity; Progressive mental retardation

PROG: Death by 3yrs

KRABBE'S DISEASE

Aut Rec. Due to excess hexosides in brain

CLIN: Onset in 1st yr. Irritability then apathy; Ep; Blindness; Dysphagia; Periph neuropathy

PROG: Death by 2yrs

Mucopolysaccharidoses

Rare conditions. Commonest are Hurler, Hunter & Morquio types

HURLER'S SYNDROME (TYPE 1)

Aut Rec. Deposition of dermatan- & heparitin-SO_4. Facial features termed gargoylism

CLIN: Onset 0–2yrs. Mental retardation; Hypertelorism; Thick lips; Wide nostrils; Thick purulent nasal discharge; Heavy nasolabial folds; Large square head; Low set ears; Liver ↑; Spleen ↑; Kyphosis; Flexion deformities; Claw hand; Systolic murmur. Occ Hernia; CCF; Deafness

INVESTIGATIONS: • X-R: Hooked lumbar vertebrae; Kyphosis; Bone age ↓; CXR
• Toluidine blue test

PROG: Die in early adult life

HUNTER'S SYNDROME (TYPE 2)

X-linked Rec

CLIN: Slight mental retardation; Deafness; No kyphosis; Gargoyle facies

PROG: Better than Hurler's

SANFILIPPO SYNDROME (TYPE 3)

CLIN: Severe mental retardation; Hyperactivity; Claw hand

MORQUIO'S SYNDROME (TYPE 4)

Aut Rec. Chondro–osteodystrophy

CLIN: Short neck; Dwarfism; Kyphosis; Deformities of sternum, vertebrae, jts; Genu valgum. Normal IQ

INVESTIGATIONS: • X-Rs
• Urine: Keratan sulphate ↑

PROG: Survive into adulthood

SCHEIE SYNDROME (TYPE 5)

CLIN: Stiff jts; AI; Corneal clouding; Gargoyle facies; IQ sl ↓

PROG: Survive into adulthood

MAROTEAUX-LAMY SYNDROME (TYPE 6)

CLIN: Severe skeletal changes; Corneal clouding; Liver ↑; Spleen ↑; Gargoyle facies; IQ normal

GENERAL RX: Occ BMT

Amino Acid Metabolism

PHENYLKETONURIA

Aut Rec. Due to def of phenylalanine OHlase

PATHOGENESIS: Enzyme def blocks conversion of phenylanaline to tyrosine

CLIN: Present 6–12mths unless screened. IQ ↓↓; Dwarfism; Ep; Hypotonicity; Poor dentition. Often Fair hair; Blue eyes; Eczema.

INVESTIGATIONS: • Guthrie test
• Scriver test
• Serum Phenylalinine ↑
• Urinary phenylpyruvic acid ↑

RX: Screen all children at 6–14 days. Early Rx prevents abnormalities. Low phenylalanine diet for at least 6yrs c̄ tyrosine supplementation. Also low phenylalanine diet for PKU mothers during pregnancy to protect unborn child

HOMOCYSTINURIA

Aut Rec. 1 in 90,000 live births. Cystathionine synthase def

PATHOGENESIS: Enzyme def → ↑ homocysteine & methionine & ↓ cysteine

CLIN: Kyphoscoliosis; Genu valgum; Pes planus; ↓ jt mobility; Tall; IQ ↓; Ep; Dislocated lens; Loss of hair colour. Occ A-V thromb → MI; PE; Glaucoma; Buphthalmos; Blindness; Asthma

INVESTIGATIONS: • Cyanide nitroprusside urine test
• Chromatography
• X-R: Osteoporosis

RX: 2 gps. The pyridoxine sensitive respond to pyridoxine c̄ a sl dietary protein restriction. The pyridoxine resistant gp require a high cysteine, low methionine diet c̄ added vitamins & trace metals. Early screening & Rx prevents complications

DD: Marfan's syndrome

MAPLE SYRUP URINE DISEASE

CLIN: Urine has odour of maple syrup. Feeding difficulty; Spacticity; Opisthotonus

RX: Screen by Scriver test. Diet low in Valine, Leucine & Isoleucine

PROG: Die in few months if untreated

HISTIDINAEMIA

Aut Rec. 1 in 12000. Histidase def

CLIN: Speech retardation. Occ IQ ↓

RX: Screen by Scriver test. Low histidine diet

TYROSINAEMIA

Def of enzyme to convert tyrosine to homogentisic acid

CLIN: Acute or chr course. Occ D&V; Liver ↑; Spleen ↑; Haem; Cirrhosis; J; Vit D resistant rickets; BG ↓

RX: Screen by Scriver test. Diet low in tyrosine, phenylalanine & methionine

HARTNUP DISEASE

CLIN: Pellagra-like rash; Ataxia; Nystagmus; Tremor. Slow mental deterioration

INVESTIGATION: • Chromatography: Gross aminoaciduria

RX: Nicotinamide

PROG: Poor

Idiopathic Hypercalcaemia of Infancy

?Inborn error in Vit D metabolism. Rare

CLIN: Failure to thrive; Vom; Anorexia; Constipation; Thirst; Polyuria; Hypotonia; Elf like facies. Occ Supravalvar AS; BP ↑; IQ ↓. Later RF; Dwarfism

INVESTIGATIONS: • Ca^{2+}: Usually ↑
- Urinalysis: pH ↓
- KUB: Occ nephrocalcinosis
- ECG
- CXR

RX: Low Ca^{2+} diet. Steroids to reduce hyperCa^{2+}

Hypophosphatasia

Rare. Aut Rec. Alk phos def

CLIN: Poor dentition; Kyphoscoliosis; Bowing of long bones. Occ Spontaneous #; RF

INVESTIGATIONS: • X-R: Poor mineralisation
- Alk Phos ↓
- Ca^{2+}: Occ ↑

RX: Vit D

PROG: Poor

DISORDERS OF NUTRITION

Kwashiorkor

Due to protein def diet. Esp poor tropical countries

CLIN: Usual onset when breast feeding stops. Gross oedema; Dry, coarse hair; Depigmentation; Dermatoses; Anaemia; Apathy; Mental retardation. Often 2° infections; Vit defs

INVESTIGATIONS: • Proteins ↓
- U&E: Urea, K^+ ↓
- FBC
- BG: Occ ↓

RX: Prevent by good diet. Rehydrate, high protein diet. Rx of infections

PROG: Cost of diet can be prohibitive. Severe kwashiorkor has high mort

Marasmus

Due to poor calorie intake, usually dietary but occ due to severe diseases of infancy

CLIN: Thin; Wt ↓; sc Fat ↓; Inelastic skin; Muscle wastage; Sunken eyes; Irritability. Later Oedema; 2° infections; Apathy; Purpura

INVESTIGATIONS: • Are of "failure to thrive"

RX: Gradual increase in cal intake. Treat intercurrent infections. Treat any underlying cause

Rickets

Vit D def. Due to low intake, lack of sunlight. Esp Asians

PATHOGENESIS: Vit D def → ↓ Ca^{2+} → ↑ PTH → ↓ PO_4 & ↓ $CaxPO_4$ product. Serum Ca^{2+} can only be maintained by Ca^{2+} removal from bone → Osteoporosis, Defective ossification

CLIN: Usually presents at 6/12 to 2yrs. Variable severity. Hypotonia; Walk late; Abdo distension; Alternating constipation & green stools; Kyphoscoliosis; Large ant fontanelle; Craniotabes (soft skull); Frontal bossing; Beading of ribs (rachitic rosary); Swollen wrists, ankles. Occ Bowing of long bones; Harrison's sulci; Pigeon breast; Spasmus nutans; Recurrent bronchitis; Anaemia

INVESTIGATIONS: • X-R esp wrist, long bones, pelvis: Splaying & fraying of metaphysis, Osteoporosis
- CXR, SXR
- Alk phos ↑
- Ca^{2+}
- PO_4
- Urinalysis: Glycosuria, Aminoaciduria

RX: Screen for sub clin cases &/or prophylactic low dose Vit D supplements for at risk gps. Vit D analogue replacement therapy. Ensure adequte Ca^{2+} in diet

COMPLICATION: Tetany (↓ ionizable Ca^{2+}) → Laryngeal stridor; Carpopedal spasm; Ep

PROG: Good if early Rx

Scurvy

Due to Vit C def. Esp poor countries

PATH: ↑ Permeability of capillary bed, osteoblast function ↓ → spontaneous haem esp subperiosteal

CLIN: Usually presents 6–18mths. Anaemia; Pain in lower extremities → "frog position"; Swollen bleeding gums; Haem eg Haematuria, Ecchymosis. Occ Swelling ant ends of ribs; Fever

INVESTIGATIONS: • X-R: Ground glass osteoporosis, "Signet ring" epiphysis
- White cell Vit C
- FBC

RX: Vit C

Vit A

Common in underdeveloped countries. Ass c̄ protein–cal def

CLIN: Night blindness → Xerophthalmia → Bitot's spots & photophobia → keratomalacia & blindness. Dermatoses

RX: Vit A

DISORDERS OF GIT

Hare Lip & Cleft Palate

May occur singly or together; Unilat or bilat. Occ ass c̄ chromosomal or dysmorphic syndromes. Approx 2 in 1000 births. Occ FH. 3 types pre-alveolar, alveolar, post alveolar

CLIN: Occ Speech defect; Difficulty in feeding; Nasal infections; OM

RX: Repair hare lip at 1-3mths (Le Mesurier's op). Cleft palate may require orthodontic measures prior to repair at 15–18mths (Wardeal's op). Speech therapy

Hypomandibulosis

May be ass c̄ cleft palate (Pierre–Robin anomaly). Occ ass c̄ CHD; Talipes

CLIN: Tongue can easily fall back blocking epiglottis c̄ danger of resp obst

RX: Care whilst feeding

Oesophageal Atresia

Cong. Many forms. Commonest is blind ending upper oesophagus c̄ fistula between trachea & lower segment (TOF). Ass c̄ other cong defects

CLIN: Polyhydramnios. Occ Excess mucus; Cyanosis at birth. If fluid given → Cough, Choking, Cyanosis

INVESTIGATIONS: • CXR, AXR: If TOF, air in stomach

RX: Close fistula & feed through gastrostomy. Later reconstructive op eg end to end oesophageal anastomosis

Diaphragmatic Hernia

Rare. L>R

CLIN: Acute emergency as lung expansion is prevented by abdo viscera. SOB; Cyanosis. Occ BS over chest; Ht pushed to R

INVESTIGATION: • CXR

RX: IPPV to inflate lungs. Aspirate stomach, then repair diaphragm.
N.B Do not give O_2 via face mask

Hiatus Hernia

Cong. Sliding hernia commoner than para-oesophageal. Often short oesophagus. 1 in 1000 live births. Occ ass c̄ Py.S

CLIN: Persistent vom from 1st week. Occ Constipation; Haematemesis; Reflux oesophagitis → stricture; Anaemia; Failure to thrive

INVESTIGATION: • Ba swallow

RX: Feed upright. Thickened feeds. Occ require op

Congenital Pyloric Stenosis

4M:1F. Esp 1st born. Occ FH. 1 in 300 live births

PATHOGENESIS: Pyloric circular muscle hypertrophy → obst to passage of food

CLIN: Usually present at 2–3wks. Palpable tumour; Projectile vom; Wt ↓; Infrequent stools; No loss of appetite. Occ Visible peristalsis; Dehydration; Haematemesis

INVESTIGATIONS:
- Test feed
- Ba meal or Ultrasound
- Urine Cl ↓
- Astrup: Metabolic alkalosis
- U&E

RX: Drip & suck. Pyloromyotomy (Fredet–Ramstedt op). Rarely medical Rx of atropine methyl nitrate

PROG: Good. Op mort <1%

Causes of Vomiting (LIST 7 PAED)

A. INFANCY
1. Posseting & Rumination
2. Feeding mismanagement
3. Cong abnormalities:
   Eg Oesophageal atresia, TOF, Vascular ring, HH, Duodenal atresia, Hirschprung's disease
4. Intestinal obst:
   Eg Pyloric stenosis, Meconium ileus, Intussusception
6. Infections:
   Eg Meningitis, Septicaemia, Whooping cough, Winter vom disease, GE, UTI
7. Drugs & Poisons
8. Coeliac disease
9. Appendicitis
10. Metabolic:
    Eg Diabetes, PKU
11. ↑ ICP
12. Kernicterus

B. CHILDHOOD
1. Psychogenic:
   Eg Attention seeking behaviour
2. Travel sickness
3. Intestinal obst
4. Infections:
   Eg Tonsillitis, OM, Meningitis, GE
5. Appendicitis
6. Mesenteric adenitis
7. Torsion of Testes
8. Diabetes
9. ICP ↑
10. Drugs & poisons:
    Eg Anticonvulsants, Lead poisoning

Causes of Haematemesis (LIST 8 PAED)

A. INFANCY
1. Haemorrhagic disease of newborn
2. G-O reflux
3. Py.S

B. CHILDHOOD
1. Severe Vom
2. HH
3. PU
4. Varices
5. Acute tonsillitis
6. Swallowed blood from epistaxis
7. Blood dyscrasias
8. Swallowed foreign body
9. Drugs & poisons:
   Eg Corrosives, Iron
10. Rarely:
    Eg ZE syndrome, Enterogenous cyst, DIC, Gaucher's

Duodenal Obst

May be due to duodenal atresia or rarely web. Ass c̄ Hydramnios; Down's syndrome

CLIN: Dehydration; Vom occ bile stained

INVESTIGATIONS:
- U&E: Metabolic alkalosis
- AXR: Double bubble sign

RX: Treat early. Rehydrate. Duodenojejunostomy

Infantile GE

Acute infective D&/orV. Common esp in poor socioeconomic conditions. Peak incidence 9–24mths. In temperate countries esp winter. Breast feeding is protective. Viral >bacterial cause. Esp Rotavirus, *E.coli*, Campylobacter, Giardiasis. M>F

PATHOGENESIS: Rotaviruses have Incub Pd 2–3 days & may → subtotal villous atrophy. *E.coli* enteropathic strains act by their invasiveness &/or toxin production. Intestinal damage → lactase def → unabsorbed lactose which is fermented by gut bacteria → ↑ osmotically active gut material → marked diarrhoea high in sugar

CLIN: D&V; Dehydration (3–5% loss of body Wt → loss of skin turger; 5% loss → depressed fontanelle, sl sunken eyes; 10% loss → severe dehydration, sunken eyes, weak PR ↑, cold blue extremities; 12–14% loss → limpness, acidotic breathing, moribund). Occ Venous thromb; RF; Intercurrent infection, DIC. Occ Hypernatraemia (esp bottle fed) → Doughy skin, good periph circulation, CNS signs; Acidosis

INVESTIGATIONS:
- Stools for C&S
- U&E: In hypertonic dehydration Na ↑, Osmolality ↑, Urea ↑
- Throat swab
- Urinalysis
- Blood cultures
- LP

RX: Most can be managed at home. Admit to hospital if detectable dehydration, persistent vom, diagnostic doubt, poor home conditions, intercurrent infections. Need to maintain adequate electrolyte & fluid balance. Care c̄ hygiene, most are F-O spread (Rarely barrier nurse). In many cases removal of milk & carefully monitored fluid replacement c̄ oral glucose–electrolyte solution for 24–48hrs c̄ gradual subsequent reintroduction of milk is sufficient. If severely dehydrated require IV rehydration. Hypernatraemic dehydration must be slowly corrected c̄ fluids, rapid rehydration may → cerebral oedema & Ep. Little evidence that antibiotic or antidiarrhoeal agents are useful

LATE COMPLICATION:

Post GE Syndrome: Esp in <6mths & malnourished. Due to Lactose intolerance, Cow's milk protein intolerance, Multiple food intolerances esp transient gluten intolerance

Clin: Prolonged period of Diarrhoea, Failure to thrive following episode of acute GE

Rx: Special diet eg lactose free

PROG: Still appreciable mort esp in epidemics, in LBW, severely dehydrated

DD:
1. Coeliac disease
2. Food intolerances
3. Other infections: Esp Shigella, Salmonella
4. Pyloric stenosis
5. Intussusception
6. Hirschprungs's disease
7. CF
8. Poisoning

Winter Vomiting Disease

Virus infection. Incub Pd 1–3 days

CLIN: Vom, occ recurrent, usually at night. No fever. Rarely diarrhoea

Causes of Diarrhoea (LIST 9 PAED)

1. Faulty feeding: Esp excess sugar in feed
2. Infections: Eg Viral GE, E.coli, Shigella, Salmonella, Campylobacter, Necrotising enterocolitis, Giardia
3. Hirschprung's disease
4. Malabsorption: Eg CF, Coeliac disease, chd intolerance
5. Drugs & poisons
6. IBD
7. Spurious diarrhoea
8. Rarely: Eg Appendicitis, Intussusception, Malrotation, Staph lung abscess, Immunodef, Ganglioneuroma, Thyrotoxicosis, Stress (irritable colon)

GENERAL INVESTIGATIONS: • Stool culture
- U&E
- Sigmoidoscopy: If blood or mucus

Cow's Milk Protein Intolerance

Usually strong FH & ass c̄ other allergies. Most are allergic to β lactoglobulin. M>F. Esp 3–6mths of age. May be 2° to GE

CLIN: Usually present as young infant c̄ D&V; Abdo distention Snuffles. Occ Failure to thrive; Blood in stools; Wheezing; Urticaria; Recurrent OM. Rarely Anaphylactic reactions
Occ present later at 6–18mths c̄ recurrent D&V

INVESTIGATIONS: • Response to removal & subsequent challenge c̄ cow's milk (monitoring includes jejunal biopsy)

RX: Replace cows milk c̄ protein which is tolerated eg Breast milk, Soya protein milk. Vit supplements. Reintroduce cow's milk 6–12mths later

PROG: Most children can tolerate cow's milk by 2yrs of age

Lactose Intolerance

Familial, cong & late onset forms. May be 2°, usually post GE. Familial form is rare. Other forms have similar Clin & Path signs but late onset form presents some yrs after birth esp in some races eg Black Americans. May co-exist c̄ Cow's milk protein intolerance

CLIN: Diarrhoea; Abdo distention; Abdo pain. Occ Failure to thrive; Steatorrhoea

INVESTIGATIONS: • Response to removal & subsequent challenge c̄ lactose load
- Small bowel biopsy: Def lactase activity

RX: Lactose free diet

PROG: Many appear to have partial lactase def & can tolerate some dietary lactose

Bowel Duplications

Rare. Arise from mesenteric bowel border. Usually small (enterogenous cysts). Ass c̄ Cv vertebral anomalies

CLIN: Occ PU; Malaena; Intestinal obst

INVESTIGATIONS: • AXR
- Ba studies

RX: Surgery. Occ transfuse

Abdo Pain

Causes of Abdo Pain (LIST 10 PAED)

1. Wind
2. Evening colic
3. Appendicitis
4. Pain from Vom, Coughing, Diarrhoea
5. Mesenteric adenitis
6. Acute peritonitis: Eg Ruptured appendix, Pneumococcal, TB
7. Intussusception
8. CF
9. UTI
10. Intestinal obst
11. Acute nephritis
12. Renal colic
13. Hepatitis
14. Diabetic acidosis
15. Basal pneumonia
16. Torsion of testes
17. Rh fever
18. Bowel infections
19. Henoch–Schonlein purpura
20. Periodic syndrome
21. Psychogenic
22. Trauma
23. Rare causes: Eg Pb poisoning, Sickle cell anaemia, PU, IBD, Meckel's diverticulitis, Gallstones, Renal stones

Commonest cause of acute abdo pain if >2yrs is appendicitis. Recurrent abdo pain is usually psychogenic in origin. In infancy common causes are colic, cong abnormalities, intussusception & pyelonephritis

Causes of Recurrent Abdo Pain (LIST 11 PAED)

1. Wind
2. Evening colic
3. Psychogenic
4. Constipation
5. PU
6. Lactose intolerance
7. Worms
8. Pb poisoning
9. Intermittent volvulus
10. Hydronephrosis
11. Ep
12. Sickle cell disease
13. Periodic syndrome

Evening Colic (3 mths Colic)

Esp well thriving babies. Esp 2–3mths old

CLIN: Evening abdo pain → restlessness, drawing up of legs, recurrent screaming attacks lasting 2–10mins

RX: Dicyclomine hydrochloride (SE: Apnoea)

PROG: Disappears spontaneously

Mesenteric Adenitis

Often ass c̄ URTI. Esp children

CLIN: Abdo pain in RIF; Fever. Occ Tonsillitis; Vom

RX: Observe. Occ laparotomy to exclude appendicitis

Emotional Stress & GI Symptoms

In School children, Abdo pain ± vom is quite common. In the toddler, "stress" usually presents c̄ loose stools, constipation or anorexia. In adolescents, anorexia & vom are common presentations

Intestinal Obst

Causes of Intestinal Obst (LIST 12 PAED)

1. Foreign body
2. Intussusception
3. Volvulus
4. Bands, adhesions
5. Strangulated hernia
6. Duodenal atresia
7. Imperforate anus
8. Meconium ileus
9. Meckel's
10. Malrotation
11. Cysts
12. TB
13. Crohn's
14. Ca

GENERAL CLIN: Abdo pain; Vom; Abdo distension; Constipation. Occ PR ↑; Pallor; Dehydration

INTUSSUSCEPTION

The invagination of one part of the bowel into another. Ileo-colic >Ileo-caecal. 2M:1F. Esp 3–9mths. In older children, adults usually 2° to Meckel's, Polyp or Ca

CLIN: May have preceding constipation. recurrent episodes of severe colic c̄ pallor, screaming, drawing up of legs. After 24–36hrs, Vom; Dehydration; Abdo mass eg R hypochondrium; Pyrexia; Blood & mucus pr ("Red currant jelly stool")

INVESTIGATIONS:
- AXR
- Ba Enema
- WCC: Occ ↑

RX: Drip & suck. Try to reduce by barium enema. If fails op reduction

PROG: 1–2% recurrence

DD:
1. Henoch–Schonlein purpura
2. Dysentery

Causes of Blood in the Stool (LIST 13 PAED)

1. Pharyngeal—2° to epistaxis
2. Oesophageal:
   a) HH
   b) Varices
   c) Foreign body
3. Gastric:
   a) PU
   b) Aspirin
4. Small Intestinal:
   a) Intussusception
   b) Dysentery
   c) Meckel's
   d) Enterogenous cyst
   e) Henoch–Schonlein purpura
   f) Haemolytic uraemic syndrome
   g) Tumours
   h) Hookworm
5. Large Intestinal:
   a) Constipation
   b) IBD
   c) Haemangioma
6. Rectal:
   a) Prolapse
   b) Polyp
   c) Foreign body
7. Anal fissure
8. Blood dyscrasias

FOREIGN BODY OBST

Quite common in young children. Obst usually occurs at oesophagus, pylorus, duodenum or ileo-caecal valve. The hair ball (trichobezoar) occurs in children who eat their hair

INVESTIGATION: • Serial X-Rs

RX: If asymptomatic observe. Occ op removal

IMPERFORATE ANUS

Quite common cong abnormality. Often ass c̄ Recto–vaginal fistula (in F), Recto–vesical fistula (in M). Occ ass c̄ Perineal fistula; Oesophageal atresia

CLIN: Failure to pass meconium. Later Bile stained vom; Abdo distension

INVESTIGATION: • AXR (c̄ child upside down c̄ lead marker on anal dimple)

RX: Colostomy & pull through or anoplasty

Rectal Prolapse

Cong maldevelopment of perirectal tissues predisposed to by Malnutrition, CF, Constipation, Rectal polyps

CLIN: Projection of rectal mucosa outside anus during defaecation

RX: Correct any constipation. May strap buttocks together between defaecations. Rarely need op

Causes of Constipation (LIST 14 PAED)

A. NEONATES
1. Cong intestinal obst
2. Meconium ileus
3. Hirschprung's disease
4. Spinal anomaly
5. Hypothyroidism
6. HyperCa^{2+}

B. LATER INFANCY & CHILDHOOD
1. Feeding problems:
   a) Poor fluid intake
   b) Low residue diet
2. Bowel lesions:
   a) Hirschprung's disease
   b) Anal fissure
   c) Enterogenous cyst
3. Mismanagement of toilet training
4. Hypothyroidism
5. Pb poisoning
6. Drugs:
   Esp Laxative abuse
7. Excessive vomiting
8. Hypotonia

THE LIVER, BILIARY SYSTEM & PANCREAS

Cystic Fibrosis

Aut. Rec. 1 in 1500 births in UK. Esp Whites

PATHOLOGY: Pancreatic enzyme secretions ↓ → malabsorption, disturbance of bile acid metabolism. Lungs normal at birth, then poor clearing of secretions → resp obst → bronchiectasis, LRTI esp Pseudomonas, Staph & pulm BP ↑ → chr hypoxia. Often fatty liver & occ focal biliary cirrhosis

CLIN: May present neonatally c̄ meconium ileus (bile stained vomit, abdo distension, constipation) or rectal prolapse. Commoner GI symptoms are Diarrhoea; Steatorrhoea; Abdo distension. Appetite often good yet failure to thrive. Variable resp symptoms : Often Cough; Wheeze; LRTI; Clubbing. Often "salty kiss". Occ Nasal obst due to polyps; Haematemesis; Haemoptysis; Pneumothorax; Kyphosis; CCF; Liver ↑; Spleen ↑; Delayed puberty. M are sterile. Rarely Obst J; Liver failure; Diabetes; Cholangitis; Gallstones. In M often inguinal hernia, hydrocoele, undescended testis

INVESTIGATIONS: • Sweat test: Na >70mmol/l
- Duodenal intubation: Enzymes ↓, HCO_3 ↓
- CXR: Many signs eg Ring shadows, patchy consolidation
- AXR: In meconium ileus—multiple fluid levels, mottling

RX: Physio—postural drainage (teach parents) c̄ mucolytic agents, bronchodilators, expectorants.

Antibiotics. ?use prophylactic antibiotics. High protein, high salt, low fat diet inc vits & pancreatic enzymes. For meconium ileus, Gastrografin enema or op

PROG: Improving. Median survival 20yrs

General Investigations for Malabsorption

- Fat balance or Nepholometry
- Sweat test
- XTT
- BG
- Clinitest &/or urine chromatography
- FBC
- Folate
- Fe
- B12
- X-R: Eg Wrists, Ba studies, CXR
- Jejunal biopsy
- Ca, Alk phos
- LFT
- U&E
- Stool C&S: Esp Giardia

Reye's Syndrome

Rare. Esp childhood

CLIN: Flu like illness c̄ apparent improvement followed by persistent vom, encephalopathy, coma. Occ Liver ↑

INVESTIGATIONS:
- AST, ALT ↑
- BG: Occ ↓
- NH_4 ↑
- Liver biopsy: Fatty liver, Mitochondrial dysfunction

RX: Dexamethasone to ↓ cerebral oedema. Supportive therapy

PROG: Poor

Cirrhosis

Rare in childhood. Paediatric causes inc Biliary atresia, α_1-antitrypsin def, Wilson's disease, CAH, CF

Tumours of the Liver

Rare. Commonest are hepatoma & hepatoblastoma

CLIN: Present in infancy or early childhood. Liver ↑↑. Occ J; Ascites. Lung mets

INVESTIGATIONS:
- Ultrasound
- Laparotomy & biopsy
- αFP

RX: X-Rad & Cyt.T

PROG: Poor

DISORDERS OF RESPIRATORY SYSTEM

Cong Malformations

CHOANAL ATRESIA

May be Uni- or bilat

CLIN: Bilat atresia → Mouth breathing, SOB on feeding, Apnoeic attacks, Mucus++ in nasal cavities. Unilat atresia → unilat nasal obst. Chr mouth breathing → deformities of chest, face, nasopharynx

INVESTIGATION:
- Nasopharyngiogram

RX: Relieve obst c̄ op

CONG LARYNGEAL STRIDOR

Common. Usually due to unusually long & curved epiglottis

CLIN: Presents at birth c̄ stridor. Rarely interferes c̄ well being. Recover by 1yr

SUBGLOTTIC STENOSIS

Tracheal narrowing due to fibrous stricture or web

CLIN: Stridor

INVESTIGATIONS:
- Tracheoscopy
- X-R: Soft tissue view of neck

RX: Occ require tracheostomy

Causes of Stridor (LIST 15 PAED)

1. Croup
2. Spasmodic croup
3. Epiglottitis
4. Bacterial tracheitis
5. Foreign body
6. Vascular ring
7. Subglottic stenosis
8. Cong laryngeal stridor
9. Retrosternal goitre
10. Neuroblastoma
11. Diphtheria
12. Infantile tetany
13. Trauma
14. Webs
15. Retropharyngeal abscess
16. Angioneurotic oedema
17. Cysts
18. Papillomata
19. Tracheomalacia
20. Micrognathia
21. Subglottic haemangioma

LUNG AGENESIS

Rare. Ass c̄ Anencephaly. May be unilat

DD: Digphramatic hernia

SEQUESTRATION

An area of pulm tissue c̄ systemic vascular supply. Usually asymptomatic

CYSTICADENOMATOID LUNG

May be ass c̄ polycystic kidney

CLIN: SOB; Cyanosis. Occ LRTI; Pneumothorax

INVESTIGATION: • CXR: Multiple cysts, Honeycomb lung

CONGENITAL LOBAR EMPHYSEMA

Due to defect in bronchial cartilage (Chondromalacia)

CLIN: Present as neonate c̄ resp distress

INVESTIGATION: • CXR: Emphysema

RX: Lobectomy

URTI

Common. Esp winter in UK. Esp lower social classes. Esp 0–3yrs. Mainly viral eg Rhinoviruses → coryza, RSV, Adenovirus (Type 3 → conjunctivitis, Cv LN ↑), Enteroviruses, Parainfluenza & Influenza

GENERAL RX: Push fluids, light diet, tepid sponge if pyrexia

COMPLICATIONS:
1. LRTI
2. Aspiration pneumonia
3. Acute OM
4. Acute sinusitis
5. Retropharyngeal abscess
6. Quinsy
7. Acute-Laryngo–Tracheo Bronchitis (Croup)

HERPANGINA

Usually due to Coxsackie virus. An URTI c̄ ulcers on post pharynx & fauces

CROUP

Inflam of epiglottis & arytenoids → laryngeal obst. Esp due to Parainfluenza virus. Esp 0–4yrs

CLIN: URTI. Then Laryngeal stridor; Fever; Hoarseness; Cough; Resp rate ↑; Resp distress eg intercostal indrawing, use of accessory muscles. Later Cyanosis; PR ↑

RX: Medical emergency. O_2; High humidity; Cool. Be prepared for tracheostomy esp if acute epiglottitis. Occ steroids

SPASMODIC CROUP

Esp 1–3yrs. Occ FH. Usually viral cause. Allergic & psychogenic factors may ppt

CLIN: Usually few signs of infection. Often presents suddenly in evening. PR ↑; Cough; Stridor; Resp distress; SOB ppt by excitement. Occ Cyanosis. Episodes last a few hrs & often recur

RX: Reassure. Steam inhalation often terminates laryngeal spasm. Occ require hospital admission. Rarely tracheostomy

EPIGLOTTITIS

Due to *H.influenzae*. Esp 3–6yrs

CLIN: Fever; Stridor; Painful swallowing; Drooling; Swollen epiglottis (cherry-red epiglottis). Progresses to airway obst in 6–12hrs

INVESTIGATION: • Direct laryngoscopy ± intubation

RX: Medical emergency. Establish airway. Ampicillin or Chloramphenicol. Extubate when swelling subsides

LRTI

ACUTE BRONCHIOLITIS

Disease of infants. Esp winter. Usually due to RSV

CLIN: URTI for 1–2 days. Then progressive SOB; Wheezing or grunting; Severe cough; Resp rate ↑; Mild pyrexia; Rhonchi. Occ difficulty c̄ feeding; Dehydration; Creps; Hyperresonant percussion note (obst emphysema); CCF; Cyanosis

INVESTIGATIONS:
- CXR: Overinflated lung; Patchy consolidation
- Serial astrups: Resp acidosis

RX: O_2 tent; High humidity. Push fluids, occ need IV Rx. Physio. Occ HCO_3 for acidosis; Digoxin for CCF; Antibiotics for 2° infection

PROG: Most recover. Usually no permanent lung damage. ? → ↑ incidence of asthma

Causes of Wheezing (LIST 16 PAED)

1. Acute bronchiolitis
2. Asthma
3. CF
4. TB
5. Foreign body
6. Tracheal web, stenosis, tumour
7. CHD
8. Drugs:
   Eg Cepahlosporins, Erythromycin

ASTHMA IN INFANTS (WHEEZY BRONCHITIS)

Below age of 1yr it is difficult to distinguish asthma from bronchitis due to infection esp viral. Typical asthma symptoms rarely begin before 2yrs old; some therefore prefer term wheezy bronchitis in infants

BACTERIAL PNEUMONIA

STAPHYLOCOCCAL PNEUMONIA: Commonest bacterial pneumonia in infancy. Often complicates CF

Clin: Often preceding URTI. Then Fever; Irritability; Poor feeding; SOB; Exp grunt; Cough. Occ D&V; Signs of consolidation

Investigations:
- CXR
- Sputum C&S
- Blood cultures
- WCC
- Astrup

Rx: Antibiotics eg Flucloxacillin or Fucidin; O_2; Good fluid intake

Complications:
1. Emphysematous bullae & Pneumothorax
2. Lung abscess
3. Septicaemia

PNEUMOCOCCAL PNEUMONIA: Common cause of pneumonia in older children

Clin: Sudden onset of Fever; Malaise; Cough; Resp rate ↑; Exp grunt. Often Dullness; Bronchial breath sounds; Fine creps; Friction rub. Occ Chest pain; Meningism; Febrile convulsion. Rarely cyanosis

Investigations:
- CXR: Often consolidation
- Sputum C&S
- WCC ↑

Rx: Antibiotics eg Benzylpenicillin. Good fluid intake. Occ O_2

LIPOID PNEUMONIA: Can develop if oily substances given nasally or orally. Esp 0–6mths

Clin: Progressive SOB; Cough. Occ 2° infection

Investigation: • CXR: Widespread opacities

Rx: No specific Rx

Atelectasis

Common in young children. 2° to bronchial occlusion eg TB, measles, pertussis, foreign body, asthma. Compensatory emphysema

CLIN: Symptoms depend on 1° cause

INVESTIGATION: • CXR: Lobar collapse/consolidation

DISORDERS OF THE CVS

In developed countries most Ht disease is cong. Elsewhere Rh Ht disease is still common

CHD

Quite common. Cause often unknown. Occ FH. Incidence approx 1 in 200 births

Simple Classification of CHD (LIST 17 PAED)

A. CYANOTIC LESIONS
1. TGV
2. Fallot's Tetralogy
3. TAPVD
4. Single Vent & Tricuspid atresia
5. Ebstein's anomaly
6. Pulm atresia c intact septum
7. Truncus arteriosus
8. Single Vent
9. Double outlet RVent

B. L-R ACYANOTIC SHUNTS
1. VSD
2. PDA
3. ASDs

C. ACYANOTIC CHD WITHOUT SHUNTS
1. PSt
2. AS
3. Coarctation of Aorta
4. Hypoplastic L Ht syndrome
5. Anomalous L coronary artery
6. Vascular rings

GENERAL PATHOGENESIS: Ht develops in 1st trimester. Cardiac malformation usually represents an arrest of development c̄ subsequent attempt by remainder of Ht to compensate. In womb, foetal oxygenated blood from placenta passes from umbilical vein via ductus venosus to R Atrium. R & L Atria communicate via foramen ovale. L Atrial blood supplies body. Ductus arteriosus connects pulm artery to aorta thereby diverting most RVent blood from lung. Blood travels to placenta via umbilical arteries. At birth PVR ↑, Pulm VascR ↓ → Pulm blood flow ↑, Pulm artery O_2 sat ↑, closure of foramen ovale & ductus arteriosus. At 2wks, Pulm VascR = adult level. Pulm VascR will not fall if: Hypoxia eg Chest infection; CNS anomaly → hypoventilation or abnorm circulatory communications eg Large VSD; Aortopulmonary communication

GENERAL CLIN: Four common presentations: Cyanosis, Ht failure c̄ tachypnoea, Disturbances of HtR or rhythm, Murmurs. Ht failure in infancy → feeding problems, resp rate ↑, PR ↑, liver ↑, Wt ↑; ↑ incidence of LRTI

Causes of Cyanosis (LIST 18 PAED)

A. NEONATES
1. CHD:
   a) TGV
   b) Pulm atresia
   c) Tricuspid atresia
   d) Ebstein's anomaly
   e) Obstructed TAPVD
2. Resp centre depression:
   a) Brain defects
   b) Cerebral haem, oedema
   c) Drugs
   d) BG ↓
3. Resp Disease:
   Eg Foreign body, RDS, Choanal atresia, TOF
4. Infections:
   Eg Meningitis

B. 1–12 MONTHS
1. CHD:
   a) Fallot's tetralogy
   b) Double outlet RVent
   c) Single vent c PSt
   d) Non-obst TAPVD
2. Severe chest disease:
   Eg RDS, Atelectasis, Pneumothorax
3. Rarely:
   Eg Methaemoglobinaemia

C. CHILDREN OVER 1 YEAR
1. CHD:
   a) Fallot's
   b) Eisenmenger's
   c) Ebstein's anomaly
2. Resp disease:
   Eg Pulm fibrosis

Cyanotic CHD

TGV

Commonest cause of cyanotic CHD. Aorta arises from morphological RVent & pulm artery from LVent. Survival at birth only possible if patent foramen ovale, PDA, ASD or VSD

CLIN: Presentation depends on type of ass lesion: c̄ norm closure of ductus arteriosus → hypoxia & circulatory fail; c̄ large VSD or PDA, minimal cyanosis; c̄ VSD & PSt mimics Fallot's. At birth, usually Cyanosis; SOB; Loud S2. Occ systolic murmur LSE; Obese

INVESTIGATIONS: • CXR: Egg-shaped Ht,

Pulm plethora, Narrow vascular pedicle
- ECG: ^RVH^
- Echocardiography
- Cardiac catheterisation

RX: Balloon atrial septostomy (Rashkind Op). At 6–9mths Mustard op c̄ baffle to redirect venous return. If TGV & VSD, banding to prevent pulm vascular disease c̄ later Mustard op, removal of band & repair of VSD

PROG: Without Rx 95% die before 1yr. Large VSD ensures longer survival but ↑ pulm vascular disease. Op mort 5–10% c̄ quite good prog for survivors

FALLOT'S TETRALOGY

Common CHD. Classical features are: VSD, RVent outflow tract obst (infundibular PSt), RVH, Overriding of interVent septum by aorta. The severity of the stenosis determines degree of R-L shunt via VSD & hence degree of cyanosis. VSD tends to close & PSt tends to worsen during 1st yr

CLIN: Cyanosis usually by 1yr esp ppt by exercise, emotion. Often squatting following exertion; Systolic murmur; RVent heave; Loud S2; Clubbing. Later Polycythaemia c̄ ↑ risk of cerebral abscess, cerebral thromb, endocarditis. In severe cases hypercyanotic spells c̄ intense cyanosis & LOC

INVESTIGATIONS:
- CXR: "Cor en Sabot", Oligaemic fields, 25% have R sided aortic arch
- ECG: ^RVH^, ^R axis deviation^. Occ L hemiblock
- Echocardiography
- Cardiac catheterisation

RX: Cyanotic episodes: Place child in knee–elbow position, 100% O_2, Morphine, β blocker. Prophylactic Propranolol. 1-stage repair c̄ repair of VSD & relief of outflow obst or 2-stage op ie Aorto–pulmonary communication eg Blalock–Taussig op & definitive repair at 2–5yrs

PROG: Worst if complete pulm atresia. Op mort 10%

TAPVD

Rare. All pulm viens drain directly or indirectly into RAtrium
3 types: Supracardiac, Intracardiac & Infracardiac. Infracardiac type often → obst pulm venous flow

CLIN: Mild cyanosis; SOB; Systolic murmur; RVH; Large Ht. Present early if obst, occ do not present for 2–3yrs

INVESTIGATIONS:
- CXR: Cottage loaf (Snowman) Ht
- Cardiac Catheterisation

RX: Balloon septostomy. Occ able to transplant vein into LAtrium

PROG: Poor

SINGLE VENT & TRICUSPID ATRESIA

1–2% of CHD. Survival depends on ASD & PDA

CLIN: Cyanosis at birth; Variable murmurs

INVESTIGATIONS:
- CXR: Oligaemic fields
- ECG: ^L axis deviation^, ^LVH^
- Echocardiography
- Cardiac catheterisation

RX: Palliative Blalock op c̄ Fontan op (Conduit from RAtrium into RVent outflow tract) at 5yrs

EBSTEIN'S ANOMALY

Rare. Displacement of tricuspid valve leaflets into RVent. Usually ass c̄ ASD or patent foramen ovale

CLIN: Often cyanosed at birth. Later cyanosis may fade as ASD shunt is abolished (↓ pulm VascR). Occ present again in adolescence c̄ Cyanosis; SOB

INVESTIGATIONS:
- CXR: Pear-shaped Ht
- ECG: 80% ^RBBB^, 20% WPW syndrome
- Echocardiography
- Cardiac catheterisation

RX: Repair or replacement of valve

PULMONARY ATRESIA c̄ INTACT VENT SEPTUM

Occ ass c̄ PDA

CLIN: Severe cyanosis; SOB; Continuous murmur

INVESTIGATIONS:
- CXR
- Echocardiography
- Cardiac catheterisation

RX: Palliative op of shunt & valvotomy. Occ radical repair possible

PROG: Poor

TRUNCUS ARTERIOSUS

Rare. A single trunk arises from Ht through a single arterial valve & gives rise to aorta & pulm arteries. Always ass VSD

CLIN: Ht failure; Systolic to & fro murmur at LSE; Ht ↑

INVESTIGATIONS: • CXR: Narrow mediastinum; Pulm plethora; 50% have R sided aortic arch
• Echocardiography
• Cardiac catheterisation

RX: Reconstructive op

PROG: High op mort

SINGLE VENT

May be ass c̄ atresia of AV valve

CLIN: Cyanosis; SOB; Ht ↑; Systolic murmur

INVESTIGATIONS: • CXR: Pulm plethora
• ECG
• Echocardiography
• Cardiac catheterisation

RX: Rashkind's op

PROG: Poor

DOUBLE OUTLET RVENT

Both aorta & pulm artery arise from RVent c̄ VSD allowing LVent blood to reach systemic circulation. Various types. Occ ass c̄ PSt

CLIN: May present like a VSD, Fallot's or an Eisenmenger syndrome

INVESTIGATIONS: • CXR
• ECG
• Angiography

RX: Surgical repair

Acyanotic L-R Shunts

VSD

Commonest form of CHD. Presentation depends on size of defect

PATHOGENESIS: When VSD small, size restricts flow & systemic P is >> pulm P. When VSD large, Vent P equalise & shunt is due to lower pulm VascR. As pulm VascR falls after birth, ↑ blood flow to L Ht often → Ht failure

CLIN: Small VSD often asymptomatic, occ sl RVent impulse & pansystolic murmur. Larger VSDs usually present at 4–6wks. Large VSDs usually → SOB; Ht failure; Failure to thrive; Marked RVent inpulse; Pansystolic murmur; Loud S2; Ht ↑; Liver ↑; Occ Functional murmurs of MSt; PSt; AI (late)

INVESTIGATIONS: • ECG: Occ ˆLVHˆ
• CXR: Pulm plethora
• Echocardiography
• Cardiac catheterisation

RX: Observe small VSD & offer prophylaxis against SABE. Treat Ht failure medically c̄ Dig & diuretics. Surgery if failure of medical Rx, development of pulm BP ↑, pulm vasc obst or infundibular PSt. Emergency surgery is by banding of pulm artery to ↓ pulm blood flow. Elective open Ht surgery to correct VSD is carried out in early childhood

COMPLICATIONS: 1. Eisenmenger's syndrome
2. Recurrent LRTI
3. SABE
4. AI
5. Infundibular PSt

PROG: About 50% close spontaneously. Op mort 5–10%

Cardiac Causes of Heart Failure (LIST 19 PAED)

A. NEONATES
1. Coarctation of aorta
2. Truncus arteriosus
3. Obstructed TAPVD
4. Hypoplastic L Ht
5. Single Vent
6. Severe AS
7. Complete AV canal

B. 1–6MTHS
1. VSD
2. PDA
3. Coarctation of aorta
4. SVT
5. EFE
6. Cardiomyopathies

C. >6MTHS
1. Myocarditis
2. Cardiomyopathies
3. Acquired Ht disease: Eg Rheumatic carditis

PDA

PDA connects L pulm artery c̄ desc aorta. After birth PaO_2 ↑ → PDA closure in 1st wk. Delayed closure may be due to CHD or prematurity

PATHOGENESIS: If duct small, then only sl ↑ in pulm blood flow. Large PDAs → large ↑ in pulm Vasc flow & Ht failure. Very wide PDA may → Eisenmenger syndrome. Spontaneous closure occurs in premature but otherwise is rare

CLIN: Depends on size of PDA. Occ Ht failure; Failure to thrive. Classically, Collapsing pulse; Continuous murmur well heard under L clavicle. Occ only systolic murmur heard. In more severe cases, SOB; Ht ↑; Marked failure to thrive; Loud P2; Rib recession

INVESTIGATIONS:
- ECG: Occ ^LVH^
- CXR: Occ Pulm plethora
- Echocardiography

RX: Close all PDAs electively except some premature cases

COMPLICATIONS: 1. SABE
2. Eisenmenger's syndrome

ASDs

Common CHD. F>M. Ass c̄ Down's syndrome esp cushion defects; Marfan's syndrome; Ellis van Creveld (c̄ single atrium); Holt–Oram syndrome (c̄ Triphalangeal thumb)

PATHOGENESIS: Ostium secundum defects develop in floor of fossa ovalis. Ostium primum defects occur due to incomplete fusion of septum primum c̄ endocardial cushions. In common AV canal there is an AV valve common to both vents due to a combined ostium primum & VSD. Ostium secundum defects are commonest

OSTIUM SECUNDUM DEFECTS: Usually an isolated defect. RVent vol overload in large defect

Clin: Occ asymptomatic. Occ LRTI; SOB; Widely fixed split S2; Mid-systolic murmur & click; Functional mid-diastolic tricuspid murmur. Often ass PSt (systolic thrill & loud pulm systolic murmur). Occ present in adulthood c̄ Ht failure &/or AF

Investigations:
- ECG: ^R axis deviation^, ^rsR^ in ^V1^
- CXR: Occ Ht ↑, Pulm plethora
- Echocardiography

Rx: Surgical repair in childhood

Complications: 1. Lutembacher syndrome: ASD c̄ MSt due to Rh fever
2. SABE

OSTIUM PRIMUM DEFECT: Ass c̄ endocardial cushion defect. L cushion defect are commoner & affect ant leaflet of mitral valve. R cushion defect affect septal cusp of tricuspid valve

Clin: May be asymptomatic but often significant MInc → Ht failure; Failure to thrive; LRTI; Ht ↑

Investigations:
- ECG: ^L axis deviation^
- CXR
- Echocardiography
- Cardiac catheterisation: Goose neck deformity of LVent outflow due to cleft mitral valve

Rx: Surgical repair in childhood

COMMON AV CANAL:

Clin: Present early infancy c̄ Ht failure; LRTI; Ht ↑; Thrills; Systolic murmur

Investigations:
- ECG: Occ ^L axis deviation^, ^LVH^, ^RVH^ or Ht block
- CXR
- Echocardiography
- Cardiac catheterisation: Goose neck deformity

Rx: Surgical repair

Prog: Poor. Op mort 20–25%

EISENMENGER'S SYNDROME

Irreversible pulm Vasc disease due to large defect between systemic & pulm circulation

PATHOGENESIS: Pulm VascR is >systemic VascR → R to L shunt & cyanosis. Age at which shunt reverses varies, underlying ASD often presenting later than a VSD or PDA

CLIN: SOB; Tiredness; Failure to Thrive; Cyanosis (in PDA feet are more blue than hands); Ht ↑; Loud S2. Occ PInc; Angina; Haemoptysis; Syncope; Arrhythmias

INVESTIGATIONS:
- CXR: Prominent central pulm vessels, periph pruning
- ECG: ^RVH^, ^R axis deviation^
- Cardiac catheterisation

RX: No specific Rx except occ Ht & lung transplant

PROG: Poor. Most die before age 35

Acyanotic CHD Without Shunts

PSt

Often isolated. Valvar >Supravalvar, Infundibular. Rubella ass c̄ periph PSt. Infundibular PSt part of Fallot's

CLIN: Often asymptomatic. RVent heave; Ejection systolic murmur in pulm area radiating post; Ejection systolic click; Soft P2. Rarely Cyanosis; R Ht failure

INVESTIGATIONS: • ECG: Occ ^RVH^
- CXR: Post sten dilatation of pulm vessels
- Echocardiography
- Cardiac catheterisation

RX: Surgical correction or balloon valvoplasty

PROG: Low op mort. Good

AS

M>F. May be Valvar, Supravalvar or Subvalvar. Supravalvar ass c̄ idiopathic hyperCa^{2+}. Common bicuspid aortic valve rarely → AS until adulthood

CLIN: Severe AS → SOB; Syncope; Angina; Ht failure. Supravalvar sten ass c̄ abnormal facies; Arterial P L arm >R; Systolic thrill; No click; No early diastolic murmur. Valvar sten ass c̄ norm periph pulses; Systolic thrill; Ejection click; Early diastolic murmur. Subvalvar sten ass c̄ jerky periph pulses; No systolic thrill or click; Early diastolic murmur. Rarely sudden death

INVESTIGATIONS: • CXR: Often norm
- ECG: Severe AS ass c̄ ^LVH^
- Echocardiography
- Cardiac catheterisation

RX: Advise against strenuous exercise. Surgery if severe symptoms

PROG: Good unless severe AS

COARCTATION OF AORTA

Quite common. Ass c̄ Turner's syndrome, Parachute mitral valve, Supravalvar MSt, Subvalvar AS. Two main gps: Pre-ductal & juxtaductal coarctation

PRE-DUCTAL (INFANTILE): Often ass c̄ other CHD

Clin: Neonatal Ht failure. Occ Differential cyanosis; Absent femoral pulses

Investigations: • ECG: ^RVH^
- CXR: Ht ↑, Pulm plethora

JUXTADUCTAL COARCTATION (ADULT): Usually presents in late childhood or adulthood

Clin: Upper limb BP ↑; Decreased or absent femoral pulses. Occ Systolic thrill; LVH; Mid-systolic murmur

Investigations: • ECG: Occ ^LVH^
- CXR: Rib notching

GENERAL RX: Surgical resection of narrowed segment or subclavian flap. Dig & diuretics for Ht failure

COMPLICATIONS: 1. Ht failure
2. Cerebral Haem
3. Endocarditis
4. Aortic rupture

PROG: If surgery delayed after aged 4yrs, BP ↑ may persist

HYPOPLASTIC L HEART SYNDROME

A syndrome ass c̄ hypoplasia of LVent, asc aorta & aortic arch

CLIN: As PDA closes, development of severe Ht failure

INVESTIGATIONS: • CXR
- Echocardiography
- ECG

RX: No effective Rx

PROG: Most die in neonatal period

ANOMALOUS L CORONARY ARTERY

A L coronary artery arising from pulm trunk → perfusion of Ht c̄ venous blood

CLIN: Episodes of pallor, sweating & pain in infancy (?Angina). Ht ↑; No murmurs

INVESTIGATIONS: • ECG: Mimics ant MI
- CXR
- Selective angiocardiography

RX: No specific Rx

PROG: Usually die in infancy

Vascular Rings

Compression of trachea &/or oesophagus by abnormal great vessels eg R aortic arch, Anomalous R subclavian artery

CLIN: May present in infancy c̄ feeding difficulties & stridor or later c̄ dysphagia & repeated LRTI

INVESTIGATIONS: • Ba swallow
- CXR

RX: Where possible divide aberrant vessel

Myocarditis In Childhood

Several causes. May be idiopathic

(Fiedler's myocarditis) or 2° to acute nephritis, Diphtheria

FIEDLER'S MYOCARDITIS

Esp 1–2yrs. Viral cause ?Coxsackie

CLIN: Pallor; Periph cyanosis; Fever; Anorexia; SOB; CCF; Gallop rhythm; Lung creps. Occ Cough; D&V; Oedema; Abdo pain

INVESTIGATIONS:
- CXR: Ht ↑, occ pleural effusions
- ECG
- ESR
- Viral studies

RX: Bed rest; O_2; Dig; Diuretics

PROG: Poor

Vascular Malformations

4 path types of angiomas. Cutaneous angiomata (naevi) are very common cong abnormalities

SOLID HAEMANGIOMATA

Have no blood flow through them. Rx not usually needed

PORT WINE (CAPILLARY NAEVI)

Endothelial channels are present but do not connect c̄ main vascular system. Common. May be unsightly

CLIN: Red or purple. Don't blanch easily on pressure

RX: Occ remove c̄ laser Rx

CAVERNOUS HAEMANGIOMATA (STRAWBERRY NAEVI)

A direct connection between naevus & vascular system

CLIN: Bright red elevated well circumscribed naevi. Often multiple. Occ Regress in early childhood

RX: Occ surgical removal

CIRSOID ANEURYSM

A direct connection between arterial & venous systems. May → local hypertrophy, Ht failure

NEUROLOGICAL DISORDERS

Cong malformations of CNS are common. Many cases of mental handicap, CP & Ep are due to defective CNS development. CNS cong malformations are important causes of SB & neonatal death

Neural Tube Defects

Possibly due to poor maternal vit diet. Ass c̄ low social class, high parity, maternal age ↑

GENERAL RX: For F c̄ h/o NTD birth give good diet inc vit supplements before & during pregnancy. αFP & Acetyl cholinesterase are raised in anencephaly & open defects & potentially allows for therapeutic abortion

ANENCEPHALY

F>M. Incompatible c̄ life. Can be diagnosed prenatally by scan or αFP

SPINA BIFIDA

Failure of closure of lower end of neural tube. Commonest in lumbo–sacral region. Variable severity. Ass c̄ hydrocephalus, talipes, GUS disease

CLIN: Spina bifida occulta is usually asymptomatic, often its site is marked by skin pigmentation or tuft of hair, rarely → lower limb weakness, incontinence

Meningocoele: A portion of dura & arachnoid protrude through defect. Usually asymptomatic

Myelomeningocoele: Involvement of spinal cord &/or cauda equina in defect. Often Hydrocephalus; ↓ power &/or sensation in lower limbs; Incontinence; Orthopaedic anomalies eg Talipes

INVESTIGATIONS:
- Ultrasound of Brain & GUS
- IVU

RX: Cover any defect with skin in 1st 24hrs. If hydrocephalus increasing, insert shunt. Correct any remediable GUS obst. Antibiotics for UTIs. Later physio. Occ require ileal bladder, correction of talipes

PROG: Poor for myelomeningocoele but improving. Many survive into adult life

Microcephaly

Head circumference >2s.d. below mean for age & sex. Occ FH or due to pre-natal X-Rad or infection eg CMV, Toxoplasmosis

CLIN: Small cranium. Occ Ep; IQ ↓

DD: Craniosynostosis

Megalencephaly

Rare. Brain hypertrophy often asymmetric. Often IQ ↓

DD: Hydrocephalus

Porencephaly

An abnormal fluid filled area of brain. May be congenital or 2° to birth injury. Usually → IQ ↓ & CP

Hydranencephaly

Most of the cerebral hemispheres replaced by fluid. Head transilluminates

Craniosynostosis

Premature fusion of one or more cranial sutures. Several types
Sagittal suture fusion → Scaphocephaly ie boat shaped. Coronal suture fusion → Brachycephaly or asymmetric plagiocephaly. Fusion of coronal & one other suture → Acrocephaly which may be ass c̄ syndactyly or Cranio–facial dysostosis (Crouzon's Syndrome ie maxillary hypoplasia, beaked nose, projecting lower jaw)
Severe acrocephaly → exophthalmos; Optic atrophy; Headache; Ep; IQ ↓

RX: Surgical relief to allow brain growth in multiple synostoses

De Lange Syndrome (Amsterdam Dwarfism)

CLIN: LBW; Characteristic facies ie confluent eyebrows, long upper lip, anteverted nostrils, small head; Hirsute; IQ ↓; Dwarfism. Ass c̄ Single palmar crease; Syndactyly; Micromelia

Tuberous Sclerosis

Aut Dom. Ass c̄ mesodermal tumours eg teratoma or hamartoma of kidneys, liver & lung, Rhabdomyoma & Neurofibromatosis

CLIN: IQ ↓; Ep; Butterfly rash of adenoma sebaceum; Phakomata on retina; Shagreen pigmented patches. Occ Areas of depigmentation

INVESTIGATIONS:
- SXR: Multiple Ca^{2+} opacities
- CAT scan

RX: Anticonvulsants

Cerebral Palsy

CPs are disorders of mvt & posture resulting from abnormal structural development or non-progressive lesions of the immature brain. Commonly these motor syndromes are ass c̄ Ep, cognitive &/or sensory defects. Incidence in W.Europe is approx 1/1000 live births & is falling. Incidence higher in lower social classes. CP is commonly divided into types depending on major symptom ie Spastic hemiplegic, quadraplegic or diplegic; Pure or diplegic Ataxic; Choreoathetoid or rigid dyskinetic. Spastic cases are commonest. M>F. Approx 55% pre-natal cause eg CNS malformation; 40% perinatal cause; & 5% post-natal cause eg Encephalitis. Many causes, often multifactorial aetiology, inc Anoxia; Infection eg Rubella; Birth trauma; Familial esp symmetrical spastic & ataxic CP; BG ↓; Cerebral Haem; Prematurity

CLIN: Most present in neonatal period c̄ CNS abnormalities (majority who show CNS abnormalities in neonatal period do not develop CP) esp Ep, Apathy, Poor mobility, Poor feeding. As infants often show poor motor development, stereotype postures, bulbar palsy, brisk

reflexes. As children, most have speech problems, significant minority have Ep, Mental handicap, Hearing or visual loss esp high tone deafness in athetoid cases, Behaviour problems, Constipation
Spastic quadraplegia affects all four limbs (legs >arms), is often symmetrical & is ass c̄ prematurity. Usually Ep, IQ ↓. Rarely spasticity > in arms, termed double hemiplegia. If arms apparently unaffected, termed cerebral diplegia & often → muscle contractures & scissors gait
Spastic hemiplegia is commoner on R side & affects arm >leg. Often sensory loss, Ep
In ataxic CP, signs often suggest a cerebellar cause
Choreoathetosis is often due to birth trauma. Previously kernicterus was an important cause
Rarely, a lead-pipe type rigidity is observed, usually ass c̄ IQ ↓

INVESTIGATIONS: • Abs for Rubella, CMV, Toxoplasma, Herpes
• Aminoacid chromatogram
• Chromosome analysis
• CAT scan
• EEG

PREVENTION: Genetic counselling. Rubella immunisation. NTD screening. Rhesus iso-immunisation prevention. Reduce number of breech deliveries

RX: Ensure good health & social service support. Physio. Anticonvulsant Rx when needed. Try to school normally. Occ serial PoP for equinus deformity of ankle

PROG: 90% live >20yrs. About 75% walk. About 33% have norm or > IQ

Causes of Low IQ (LIST 20 PAED)

A. PRE-NATAL FACTORS
1. Chromosomal abnormalities inc banding:
   Eg Down's syndrome
2. Idiopathic
3. CNS malformations:
   Eg Microcephaly, Craniosynostosis
4. Dysmorphic Sydromes:
   Eg Amsterdam dwarf
5. Foetal infections:
   Eg Rubella, CMV
5. Biochemical disorders:
   Eg PKU, Mucopoly-saccharidoses, Lipidoses
6. Degenerative disorders

B. PERINATAL FACTORS
1. Asphyxia
2. Birth trauma
3. BG ↓
4. Cerebral Haem
5. Prematurity
6. Malnutrition
7. Hyperbilirubinaemia
8. Maternal PKU

C. POST-NATAL FACTORS
1. Meningitis
2. Encephalitis
3. Trauma
4. Asphyxia
5. Metabolic disease
6. Immunisation reaction
7. Infantile spasms
8. Poisons

Prelingual Deafness

Term to describe deafness arising in foetal, perinatal or neonatal period preventing the acquisition of basic speech. Many causes inc Rubella; Cong hypothyroidism; Familial eg Alport's (c̄ nephritis), Pendred's (c̄ goitre), Usher's (c̄ retinitis pigmentosa), Waardenburg's (c̄ hypertelorism); Cong atresia of ear; Perinatal asphyxia; Kernicterus; Aminoglycoside toxicity; Meningitis. Most are causes of nerve deafness

INVESTIGATIONS: • Test infants c̄ Manchester rattle, whispered voice, loud noise, acoustic cradle, Stanford crib-o-gram
• Audiogram in older children

RX: Early diagnosis aids subsequent speech training

Malformations of The Eye

FAILURES OF DEVELOPMENT

Rarely anophthalmia, microphthalmia or absence of part of eye eg lens. A blocked nasolacrymal duct is common → failure of tear drainage

CONGENITAL GLAUCOMA

Usually due to malformation of the angle of ant chamber & canal of Schlemm → blockage to flow of aqueous humour. May → buphthalmia ie enlargement of globe (DD: Intraocular tumour)

MYOPIA

Often FH. Usually presents at puberty. Rarely → juvenile glaucoma

RX: Glasses

CONGENITAL CATARACT

Usually occur in ass c̄ other malformations eg Rubella syndrome, Galactosaemia

Squint

Normally ocular alignment present in full term children by 1mth. Incidence of squint & amblyopia is approx 2–4%. Esp premature; CNS damaged. The majority are esodeviations. Rarely squint 2° to catarct, retinoblastoma, optic nerve anomaly

INVESTIGATION: • Screening tests inc cover test & photoretinoscopy

RX: Initially treat any amblyopia. Occlusion of norm non-amblyopic eye. Correct any refractive error c̄ lens. Then surgery if possible before age 2

Childhood Meningitis

Meningitis commoner in children than adults. Bacterial >Viral. Esp 2–4yrs. *H.influenzae* >Meningococcus >Pneumococcus >TB

CLIN: Usually prodromal illness eg URTI, GE. Then Headache; Drowsiness; Fever; Irritability; Malaise; Bulging fontanelle in younger children; Stiff neck; Ep. Occ Hydrocephalus
Meningococcal meningitis often → petechial rash. May → Septicaemia & acute bilat adrenal haem (Waterhouse-Friderichsen syndrome); DIC; Arthritis; Deafness
H.influenzae often → subdural effusion
Pneumococcus may → Hydrocephalus, Encephalitis

INVESTIGATIONS: • LP: ↑ P, ↑ WCC, ↑ protein, ↓ sugar in bacterial meningitis. Gm -ve rods suggest *H.influenzae*, Gm +ve diplococcus—pneumococcus, Gm -ve diplococcus—meningococcus
• BG
• Serial head circumference
• Occ CAT scan

RX: Prompt Rx. Treat before sensitivities known c̄ Penicillin, Sulphonamide & Chloramphenicol

WATERHOUSE–FRIDERICHSEN SYNDROME

Acute bilat adrenal haem usually 2° to acute meningococcal septicaemia

CLIN: Sudden onset of Malaise; Irritability; D&V. Soon PR ↑; SOB; Semi-coma; Purpuric rash; BP ↓. Often die

RX: IV antibiotics & steroids

Causes of Acute Childhood Encephalopathies (LIST 21 PAED)

1. Infection:
   a) Bacterial eg Meningococcal, H.influenzae, TB meningitis; Cerebral abscess
   b) Viral eg Herpes simplex encephalitis, SSPE
2. Asphyxia
3. Haem
4. Toxic/Metabolic:
   a) Drugs eg TCAD o/d
   b) Toxins eg Pb, Hg, Alcohol excess, HyperNa^{+}
   c) Inherited metabolic disorders eg Galactosaemia
   d) Endocrine eg Diabetes, Thyroid crisis
   e) Metabolic eg Uraemia, Liver failure, HyperCa^{2+}
   f) Reye's syndrome
5. Immunisation encephalopathy (Rare):
   Eg Pertussis
6. Trauma:
   Eg Scalds, NAI

Febrile Convulsions

A seizure occurring c̄ a temperature of >38°C in the absence of detectable CNS infection. In children aged 6mths–5yrs, Ep threshold is lowered by fever. M>F. Certain gps have ↑ risk of subsequent Ep: Convulsion occuring in F <1.5yrs old, M <2yrs old; Fit lasting >30mins; Focal fit; >1 fit in any illness; FH of fits; Underlying neurological abnormality. However most children c̄ febrile fits do not develop Ep

INVESTIGATIONS: • BG
• LP: If <18mths

RX: Admit to hospital. Reduce fever by removal of clothes, tepid sponging, electric fan, Aspirin. IV diazepam, Sodium valproate. Phenobarb & Sodium valproate prophylactically reduce recurrence of febrile fits & should be used in high risk gps. Children <18mths should initially be treated as if they have meningitis

PROG: Excellent in simple febrile convulsions ie fit lasting <15mins c̄ no focal features in a normally developing child

Ataxia–Telangiectasia

Aut Rec. Ass c̄ IgA def

CLIN: Present in early childhood c̄ cerebellar ataxia. Later Telangiectasia esp on ears, cheeks, bulbar conjunctiva; Choreoathetosis. Often Sinusitis; Bronchiectasis. Occ ass c̄ malignancy eg lymphoma

RX: No specific Rx. Treat infections c̄ antibiotics

Retinoblastoma

If bilat usually Aut Dom. Unilat >Bilat. Esp 0–4yrs

CLIN: Tumour presents in one eye (becomes bilat in about 25% of cases) c̄ creamy-yellow nodule on retina. Later "cat's eye" light reflex; 2° glaucoma; Proptosis. Frequently mets via optic nerve & blood. Eventual blindness

INVESTIGATION: • Photoretinoscopy

RX: Early enucleation of eyeball & optic nerve. X-Rad & Cyt.T if metastatic spread. Careful follow up to detect & treat bilat cases

Neuroblastoma

Esp 2–5yrs. A tumour of sympath nervous tissue. Common sites are adrenal medulla, pre-sacral area & post mediastinal dorsal ganglia

CLIN: Malaise; Irritability; Poor feeding; Anaemia. Occ mets to brain → ↑ ICP or proptosis; bone → limb pains; LN; liver → liver ↑. Occ Palpable dumbbell adrenal tumour

INVESTIGATIONS: • CXR
• IVU
• Ultrasound
• Urinary VMA
• CAT scan
• Bone marrow
• Tumour biopsy

RX: Screening of urine for VMA in infancy is carried out in some countries. Surgical removal of tumour c̄ X-Rad ± Cyt.T

PROG: Best if picked up in early stage. Some tumours spontaneously regress. Occ ass c̄ other 1° tumours

GUS DISORDERS

Cong GUS Malformations

BILAT RENAL AGENESIS (POTTERS SYNDROME)

Incompatible c̄ life. Characteristic facies ie low set ears, micrognathia, flat nose, crease on chin. Ass c̄ oligohydramnios. Unilat renal agenesis is usually asymptomatic

RENAL HYPOPLASIA

Bilat hypoplasia → slowly progressive RF; Failure to thrive; Dwarfism & renal osteodystrophy. Unilat hypoplastic kidney often → chr pyelonephritis & kidney often → chr pyelonephritis & BP ↑

FUSION OF KIDNEYS

Variety of forms. Commonest is horseshoe kidney c̄ fusion in midline. May → UTI, Hydronephrosis

DISPLACEMENT OF KIDNEYS

Abnormally placed kidneys may → distortion of ureters & renal vasculature. Occ → UTI, Hydronephrosis

DUPLICATIONS OF RENAL PELVIS & URETER

Common abnormalities. 3 main types: Double pelvis, single ureter; Double pelvis, double ureter (one may end ectopically in urethra or vagina); Double pelvis c̄ one norm ureter, one blind ending ureter. All may be unilat or bilat

CLIN: Occ UTI; Calculus; or Hydronephrosis

INVESTIGATION: • IVU

RX: Implant ectopic ureter into bladder. Unilat hydronephrosis may require nephrectomy

CONGENITAL URETERAL STENOSIS

Rare. → hydronephrosis

URETEROCOELE

A cystic dilatation of terminal intravesical portion of ureter. May be 2° to stricture at ureterovesical junction. May → obst, hydronephrosis, UTI, calculi. Ass c̄ duplex system

INVESTIGATION: • IVU: "Cobra-head" filling defect in bladder

RX: Reconstruction of Uretero–vesical junction

CONGENITAL MEGAURETER

Grossly dilated but not apparently obst ureter. Often → UTI, Calculi. Occ esp in F ass c̄ megacystis

RX: Reconstructive surgery

ABERRENT BLOOD VESSELS

Common. May cause obst at PUJ → hydronephrosis

ECTOPIA VESICAE & EPISPADIAS

A defect in lower abdo wall → bladder open to exterior. In epispadias the urethra lies open on dorsum of penis. Often ass c̄ herniae & other malformations

CLIN: Incontinent. Often UTI. ↑ risk of bladder Ca

RX: Close defect. Often need ileal conduit

PERSISTENT URACHUS

A fistula between bladder & umbilicus. In complete form, urine passed per umbilicus. Incomplete closures may → urachal diverticulum, urachal cyst or blind ending umbilical fistula. Occ ass c̄ Prune belly syndrome (def of abdo musculature, bilat kidney dysplasia, cryptorchidism)

RX: Surgical closure or removal

URETHRAL VALVES

Situated in post urethra. 3 types: Below verumontanum (commonest); Above verumontanum; Partial diaphragm across lumen of urethra

CLIN: Poor stream; Dribbling incontinence; Nocturnal enuresis; Vom; Hesitancy; Palpable bladder. Often UTIs. May → Hydronephrosis, Hydroureter

INVESTIGATIONS: • Micturating cystogram • Urethroscopy

RX: Excise valve

DD: Meatal sten

Cong Causes of Urinary Obst (LIST 22 PAED)

1. Aberrant vessel
2. PUJ stricture
3. Ureteral kink
4. Ureteral stricture
5. Ureteral valve
6. Ureterovesical junction stricture
7. Ureterocoele
8. Vesical diverticulum
9. Contracted bladder neck
10. Urethral valves
11. Urethral diverticulum
12. Urethral stricture
13. Paraphimosis
14. Phimosis
15. Urethral meatal stricture

HYPOSPADIAS

Common. Various types all c̄ abnormal external urethral meatus opening. Glandular >Penile >Perineoscrotal >Bulbous. Ass c̄ cryptorchidism

RX: Surgical repair occ in several stages. Correction of penile curvature (chordee) may be required

DD: Virilisation eg due to Cong adrenal hyperplasia

VAGINAL OCCLUSION

May represent absent vaginal orifice or commonly an imperforate hymen.

Latter may not be recognised until menstruation begins

MALDESCENT OF TESTIS

Most cases where testicle not present in scrotum are due to retractile testes. True undescended testes may lie in line of natural testicular descent or ectopically. Cryptorchidism = testes lying within abdo cavity. Rarely cryptorchidism due to Klinefelter's, Hypopituitarism, Eunuchoidism. Spontaneous descent often occurs in first 3mths esp in preterm. Often ass c̄ Ing H

INVESTIGATIONS: • Testicular venogram
• Chromosomes
• Gonadotrophins

RX: Bring testes down into scrotum by orchidopexy at early age

PROG: Risk of sterility even in unilat cases. ↑ risk of testicular tumour

Childhood UTI

Common. In 0–3mths M>F, 4–12mths M=F, thereafter F>M. In infancy & early childhood often underlying cong malformation. Infantile kidney is very vulnerable to scarring. Esp *E.coli*

PATHOGENESIS: Often urinary tract obst & gross vesico-ureteric reflux → renal scarring esp in 1st yr

CLIN: Fever. Occ Vom; Abdo pain. In infants, diagnosis may be difficult. In older children h/o Dysuria; Frequency; & occ Enuresis, Haematuria

GENERAL INVESTIGATIONS: • Repeated urine C&S (Occ by bladder puncture in infant)
• Occ IVU (If cong morphological abnorm eg Duplex; Incontinence)
• Occ DTPA (Esp if pelviureteric junction abnorm eg loin pain)

INVESTIGATIONS IN INFANTS: • Ultrasound & KUB, DMSA Scan, Micturating Cystogram

INVESTIGATIONS IN OVER ONE YR OLD:
a) **Boys:** Ultrasound & KUB, DMSA. Occ Micturating cystogram
b) **Girls:** (c̄ recurrent UTI): Ultrasound & KUB, DMSA. Occ Micturating cystogram

RX: Prompt Rx c̄ antibiotics of initial infection very important in preventing scarring. Prophylactic antibiotics in infants & those c̄ h/o repeated UTIs. Surgery to relieve any vesicoureteric obst. Regular review

Enuresis

About 20% of 3yr olds are wet at night, falling to about 10% at age 5. If enuresis starts after a period of dryness, a ppt event eg Marital discord, moving house, is likely

INVESTIGATION: • Urine C&S

RX: Usually no Rx indicated until aged >4yrs. Putting the child on potty before going to bed may help. A buzzer alarm triggered by urine is sometimes helpful. Occ Rx of underlying emotional cause is required

Nephroblastoma (Wilms Tumour)

Tumour of early childhood. 2F:1M. Unilat >> Bilat

CLIN: Abdo mass; Failure to thrive. Occ Fever; BP ↑; Haematuria; Hemihypertrophy (Beckwith–Wiedermann syndrome); Aniridia; Microcephaly; Cryptorchidism. Later mets to liver, lungs

INVESTIGATIONS: • IVU
• Ultrasound
• CAT scan
• CXR
• ESR ↑

RX: Nephrectomy & Cyt.T

PROG: 5yr survival 85%

Causes of Hemihypertrophy (LIST 23 PAED)

1. Wilm's tumour
2. Neuroblastoma
3. Silver syndrome
4. Russell syndrome
5. Neurofibromatosis
6. A-V malformation

HAEMATOLOGICAL DISORDERS

At birth, Hb 17±3g/dl, thereafter falling to 11.5 at 3mths. At birth 50–65% of Hb is HbF which is gradually replaced over 1st yr by HbA. WCC at birth is 18,000 ± 7000/mm c̄ 60% polymorphs. By 2wks, polymorphs fall to adult level of 3500–4500/mm but lymphocyte count rises rapidly. Lymphocyte count does not fall to adult level until puberty. In neonatal period macrocytosis is normal

Haemolytic Uraemic Syndrome

Esp in <3yrs old

PATHOGENESIS: Grossly disordered small vessels in kidneys → mechanical fragmentation of RBC (microangiopathic haemolysis). Platelets involved in path but usually little evidence of coagulation

CLIN: Episode of GE or URTI followed by Oliguria or anuria; Anaemia; Purpura. Occ D&V; BP ↑; CRF; Haem; J; Hburia; Cerebral infarcts → Ep, Coma, Blindness

INVESTIGATIONS:
- Platelets ↓
- FBC & film
- Urinalysis
- U&E
- WCC ↑
- Coagulation tests: Occ evidence of DIC

RX: Supportive therapy ie Restore fluid & electrolyte balance; Packed cell transfusions; Low protein, low salt, high cal diet. Peritoneal dialysis or plasma exchange. Streptokinase & Heparin are occ used

PROG: Mort 10–20%

Henoch–Schonlein Purpura

Probably allergic reaction to infection. Esp children

CLIN: Often h/o sore throat or URTI. Malaise; Headache; Anorexia; Fever; Purpura over buttocks, ankles, arms, elbows, forearms, legs & thighs (extensor surfaces >flexor), occ ecchymoses. Occ Painful swollen jts esp large; Flitting arthritis; Abdo colic; D&V; Melaena; Nephritis c̄ proteinuria, haematuria & occ nephrotic syndrome, BP ↑, RF

INVESTIGATIONS:
- FBC
- U&E
- Urinalysis
- Platelets: Norm

RX: Steroids for nephritis

PROG: Most recover in 1–4mths. Some relapse. Worst prog if GN c̄ crescents

DD: Intussusception

Chr Granulomatous Disease

Polymorphs ingest but don't destroy bacteria. Aut Rec but M>F. Norm delayed hypersensitivity & Ab formation

CLIN: LN ↑; Skin sepsis; Osteomyelitis; Pulm infiltrations; Abscess; Liver ↑; Spleen ↑; Discharging sinuses; Effusions. Common infecting organisms are *E.coli*, *Staph pyogenes*, Pseudomonas, Aspergillosis

INVESTIGATIONS:
- Nitroblue tetrazolium test: Polymorphs fail to reduce dye
- WCC ↑
- Hb ↓
- ESR ↑
- Gammaglobulins ↑

RX: Antibiotics

PROG: Fatal by early childhood

Congenital Immunodeficency Syndromes

CONG HYPOGAMMAGLOBULINAEMIA

Usually X-linked rec. Low levels of IgG, IgA & IgM

CLIN: Usually present at 6–12mths (when maternal Abs no longer present). Repeated infections esp bacterial eg OM, Sinusitis, Pneumonia, Pneumocystis, TB. Often Bronchiectasis; Arthritis

INVESTIGATIONS:
- PPE
- CXR
- Ig levels

RX: Antibiotics. Weekly gammaglobulin injections. Avoid immunisations

FAMILIAL (SWISS) AGAMMAGLOBULINAEMIA

Aut Rec. Gross def of IgG, IgA, IgM. Thymic hypoplasia. No plasma cells; Not able to develop delayed type hypersensitivity

CLIN: Recurrent severe infections. Occ malabsorption

INVESTIGATIONS:
- WCC: Severe lymphopenia
- Ig levels

RX: BMT

THYMIC APLASIA (DIGEORGE SYNDROME)

Rare. Complete absence of thymus & parathyroids. Ass c̄ aortic arch anomalies. No delayed type hypersensitivity. Plasma cells present

CLIN: Neonatal tetany; Repeated infections

RX: Implantation of foetal thymic tissue

PROG: Poor. Most die in early childhood

LYMPHOPENIA & THYMIC ALYMPHOPLASIA c̄ NORMAL IMMUNOGLOBULINS

Rare. Aut Rec. Rudimentary thymus. No lymphocytes in tonsil, appendix, Peyer's patches. No delayed hypersensitivity. Norm Igs

CLIN: Repeated infections

RX: Foetal thymus transplant

PROG: Death often in 1st year

Wiskott–Aldrich Syndrome

X linked Rec. Triad of thrombocytopenia, eczema & repeated infections. IgM def. Impaired delayed hypersensitivity. Ass c̄ ↑ RES malignancies

CLIN: Eczema; Asthma; Purpura; Recurrent infections eg OM; Pneumonia; Meningitis

RX: BMT

Reticuloses (Histiocytosis X)

Malignant granulomatous disease of RES. 2M:1F. Esp <4yrs

EOSINOPHILIC GRANULOMA OF BONE

Esp older child, Young adult. Usually solitary lesion

CLIN: Tender swelling esp skull, pelvis or limb. Occ Muscle weakness; Anaemia; Haem; Purpura

INVESTIGATIONS:
- SXR: Occ "Geographical skull"
- FBC
- Platelets ↓
- X-R of swelling
- Biopsy

RX: X-Rad

PROG: Very good if solitary lesion

LETTERER–SIWE DISEASE

Esp infants

CLIN: Fever; Liver ↑; Spleen ↑, LN ↑; Purpura esp thorax; Anaemia. Occ Pulm infiltration; J; Granulomatous ulcers in perineum, ear. Rapidly progressive

INVESTIGATIONS:
- FBC
- Platelets
- WCC ↓
- CXR: Occ honeycomb lung
- Biopsy of marrow or LN

RX: Cyt.T

PROG: Poor

HAND–SCHULLER–CHRISTIAN SYNDROME

Esp young children. Many symptoms due to abnormal cholesterol deposits

CLIN: Classically triad of Exophthalmos, DI & defective membranous skull bones. More commonly Anaemia; Liver ↑; Spleen ↑; Bone pain & swelling; Swollen necrotic gums; Skin rashes esp Xanthoma; Otorrhoea; Infantilism

INVESTIGATIONS:
- FBC
- SXR: "Geographical" skull
- CXR: Honeycomb lung
- Serum cholesterol: Norm

RX: X-Rad & Cyt.T. Pitressin for DI

PROG: Poor

BONES, JOINTS & CONNECTIVE TISSUE DISORDERS

Congenital Abnormalities

ACHONDROPLASIA

Aut Dom

CLIN: Short limbs esp proximally; Depressed nose; Large head; Lordosis; Trunk only sl affected; Waddling gait; Trident hand. Occ Spinal stenosis → incontinence, lower limb weakness

PROG: Many have normal life span

DIASTROPHIC DWARF

Aut Rec

CLIN: Short limbs; Scoliosis; Jt contractures; Dwarfism. Often abnormal facies; Ass cong defects eg cleft palate

CHONDROECTODERMAL DYSPLASIA (ELLIS VAN CREVELD SYNDROME)

Aut Rec

CLIN: Chondrodysplasia; Polydactyly; CHD; Abnormal nails & teeth; Short limbs esp distally

CLEIDOCRANIAL DYSPLASIA

Rare. FH

CLIN: Abnormal or absent clavicles → abnormally mobile shoulders. Often Absent pubic ramus; Characteristic facies; Poor dentition; Hypoplastic maxilla

OSTEOGENESIS IMPERFECTA

Extreme skeletal fragility. Foetal type presenting at birth & Aut Dom type presenting in early childhood

CLIN: Blue sclera; Multiple #; Deformed bones; Otosclerosis in Aut Dom type

INVESTIGATION: • Appropriate X-Rs

RX: Avoid activities likely to cause #s. Occ Surgical insertion of extensible rods

OSTEOPETROSIS (ALBERS-SCHONBERG DISEASE)

Severe Aut Rec form & more benign Aut Dom type. A persistence of 1° calcified cartilagenous matrix c̄ faulty osteoclastic activity. All bones are sclerotic. Aut Rec form presents in infancy whilst Aut Dom form presents later

CLIN: Cong form present c̄ Anaemia; Haem; Failure to thrive; LN ↑; Spleen ↑; Liver ↑; 2° infections; J; Progressive cranial nerve palsies. May → SB; Death in infancy; IQ ↓; Hydrocephalus
In Dom may present c̄ Anaemia; Path #

RX: BMT

ARTHROGRYPHOSIS MULTIPLEX CONGENITA

Rare

CLIN: Extensive fixed joint deformities esp flexion

RX: Occ corrective surgery possible

FAILURES OF LIMB DEVELOPMENT

Not uncommon. May be total absence (Amelia), Partial absence (Ectromelia) or absence of intermediary portion of limb (Phocomelia). Thalidomide in pregnancy was ass c̄ phocomelia

PARTIAL ABSENCE OF VERTEBRAE

Hemivertebrae → Scoliosis; Vertebral body defects or absence → kyphosis (eg seen in mucopolysaccharidoses)

VERTEBRAL FUSION

Common in lumbosacral regions. Klippel–Feil syndrome caused by fusion or absence of Cv vertebrae → short neck, is ass c̄ elevation of scapula (Sprengel's Shoulder)

POLYDACTYLY

Not uncommon. Extra digit often rudimentary. Occ part of dysmorphic syndrome

SYNDACTYLY

Fusion of digits. Not uncommon. Occ inherited. Variable functional def

Childhood Arthritis

Causes of Childhood Arthritis (LIST 24 PAED)

1. Septic Arthritis:
   Eg H.influenzae, Staph aureus
2. Post infective arthritis:
   Eg Meningococcal, Rh fever, Post dysentery
3. Viral arthritis:
   Eg Hep B, Infectious mononucleosis, Mumps, Rubella
4. Juvenile chr arthritis
5. Juvenile spondylitis
6. Juvenile psoriatic arthritis
7. IBD arthritis
8. SLE
9. Henoch–Schonlein pupura
10. Dermatomyositis
11. MCTD
12. Scleroderma
13. Sickle cell anaemia
14. Haemophilia
15. Leukaemia
16. Serum sickness

JUVENILE CHR ARTHRITIS (STILL'S DISEASE)

Aetiology unknown. ↓ incidence of HLA Dw3 & Dw4. Only a minority have a disease mimicking adult Rh Arth. 3 main sub gps: Systemic, Polyarthritic, Pauciarticular (<4jts)

SYSTEMIC TYPE: F=M. Esp 1–5yrs
Clin: Abrupt onset c̄ temperature ↑; Flitting pink maculopapular rash; LN ↑. Occ Liver ↑; Spleen ↑; Pericarditis; Wt ↓; Anaemia. Arthritis usually mild. Later often widespread polyarthritis

POLYARTHRITIC TYPE: F>M
Clin: Acute or insidious onset. Non migratory polyarthritis esp Neck, wrist, elbow, fingers, knee, ankles, toes. Undulant course. Occ Dwarfism

PAUCI–ARTICULAR TYPE: Commonest. Esp 1–5yrs. F=M
Clin: Arthritis esp knee, ankle or elbow. Occ Chr iridocyclitis

GENERAL INVESTIGATIONS:
- FBC: Hb ↓
- ESR ↑
- WCC
- Ig ↑
- ANA +ve esp Pauci–articular
- Rh F: Usually -ve
- X-R jts: Late changes

GENERAL RX: Physio. Occ splints to prevent jt deformities. Bed rest if systemic features. Aspirin or NSAID eg Naproxen. Occ Gold, Penicillamine, Chloroquine or alternate day steroids for systemic illness. Occ orthopaedic surgery eg synovectomy

Special forms of Chr juvenile arthritis:

i) SEROPOSITIVE JUVENILE Rh ARTH: Esp F aged 10–15yrs. Resembles adult Rh Arth c̄ progressive erosive arthritis & nodules. Occ AI; Atlanto–axial subluxation

ii) JUVENILE SPONDYLITIS: Esp M aged 10–15yrs. Usually HLA B27 +ve, FH of Ank Sp
Clin: Asymmetrical large jt lower limb arthritis. Occ iridocyclitis; AI. Later may → Sacroiliitis, Ank Sp

GENERAL COMPLICATIONS:
1. Iridocyclitis can → Cataracts, glaucoma
2. Amyloidosis
3. Permanent jt damage
4. CRF

PROG: Good. Low mort

DD OF SYSTEMIC FORM:
1. Infections
2. Rh fever
3. Post-dysenteric arthritis
4. SLE

DD OF POLYARTHRITIC FORM:
1. Post-dysenteric arthritis
2. Psoriatic arthritis
3. SLE
4. Sarcoid
5. Acro–osteolysis
6. IBD athritis

DD OF PAUCI–ARTICULAR FORM:
1. Infection
2. Post-dysenteric arthritis
3. IBD arthritis
4. Psoriatic arthritis
5. Hypogammaglobulinaemia
6. Synovial disorders

Septic Athritis

Bacterial >Viral. Usually 2° to septicaemia. Esp Staph, Strep, *H.influenzae*, Pneumococcus, Gonococcus. Sickle cell disease ass c̄ septic arthritis due to Salmonella

CLIN: Acute, swollen, hot, painful jt; Fever; Rigors. Occ >1 jt involved. May → jt destruction

INVESTIGATIONS: • WCC: Occ ↑
- FBC
- Blood cultures
- Jt fluid C&S

RX: Antibiotics for 6–12wks. Rest jt in functional position, mobilise as infection clears. Aspirate persistent effusions

DD:
1. Osteochondritis
2. Slipped epiphysis
3. Haemarthrosis
4. Transient hip synovitis

Infantile Cortical Hyperostosis (Caffey's Disease)

Esp infants

CLIN: Fever; Irritability; Tender over affected bones esp long bones, ribs, clavicles, mandibles, scapulae. May have relapsing–remitting course

INVESTIGATIONS: • X-R Bones: Periostitis, New bone, Cortical thickening
- ESR ↑
- Alk phos ↑

PROG: Full recovery in approx 1 year

DD:
1. Multiple osteitis
2. Scurvy

DERMATOLOGY

Ectodermal Dysplasia

X-Linked Rec. Rare

CLIN: Alopecia; Anhidrosis; Depressed nose; Frontal bossing; Abnormal nails & teeth; Chr rhinitis. ↑ Risk of hyperthermia

RX: Care to avoid hyperthermia

Xeroderma Pigmentosum

Aut Rec. Rare. Premalignant → Basal cell Ca, Squamous cell Ca, Malignant melanoma

CLIN: Present in infancy c̄ solar sensitivity → Dry, atrophic, freckled skin. Occ Dementia

Acrodermatitis Enteropathica

Aut Rec. Due to Zinc def. Esp infants

CLIN: Perioral & anogenital dermatitis; Diarrhoea; Alopecia

RX: $ZnSO_4$

Congenital Poikiloderma (Rothmund–Thomson Syndrome)

Aut Rec. Rare

CLIN: Telangiectasia & atrophy of skin; Pigmentation; Reticulate erythema. Occ Dwarfism; Photosensitivity; Hypogonadism

RX: No effective Rx

Focal Dermal Hypoplasia (Goltz Syndrome)

X-linked Dom

CLIN: Areas of thin skin esp scalp, thighs. Occ Hypertrichosis; Malformed nails

Incontinentia Pigmenti (Bloch–Sulzberger Syndrome)

X-linked Dom. F>M. ? → M abortion

CLIN: Present at birth c̄ vesicles on limbs & trunk. Later warts which heal leaving pigmented streaks. Occ CNS, Dental, Skeletal, Ophthalmic lesions

Ehlers–Danlos Syndrome

Aut Dom

CLIN: Elastic, fragile skin; Hyperextensible jts. Minor trauma → Skin tears; Haem; Bruising; Scarring esp Knees

RX: No specific Rx

Tylosis

Aut Dom. Rare. Premalignant →

Oesophageal Ca

CLIN: Diffuse, localised hyperkeratosis of soles & palms

RX: Salicylic acid in paraffin for thickened palms

Keratosis Follicularis (Darier's Disease)

Aut Dom

CLIN: Nails ↑; Hard papules occuring symmetrically esp trunk, neck, face, scalp, axillae

Mongolian Spots

Esp Blacks, Asians

CLIN: Pigmented spot esp lumbo–sacral area. Fade spontaneously

DD: Ecchymosis

Atopy

Hereditary tendency to develop allergic reactions. Common. Liable to develop eczema, asthma, rhinitis, conjunctivitis, urticaria

ATOPIC ECZEMA

Common. Usually FH of atopy. Bottle > Breast fed

CLIN: Onset in early childhood c̄ erythema esp flexures, cheeks, wrists, forehead, ankles. Pruritus → Thickened skin (Lichenification). In wet form: papulo-vesicular rash forms crusts & exudes fluid. In dry form: red, scaly skin. Occ 2° infection esp Staph or Strep. Often h/o asthma or rhinitis. Most remit in childhood, but pregnancy, innoculation, viral infection, emotion may reactivate

INVESTIGATIONS:
- IgE: Usually >180IU/l
- +ve Prick tests to common allergens
- Swab for C&S
- RAST

RX: If possible, remove suspected allergen or irritant eg woollen clothing. Topical steroids; Tar paste; Emollients; Ichthammol & Zn paste (chr eczema). Antihistamines for pruritus. Topical antibiotics for infection. Breast feeding probably of value

COMPLICATIONS:
1. Eczema herpeticum ie Herpes simplex infection c̄ vesicular eruption & fever
2. Vaccinia 2° to innoculation

DD:
1. Seborrhoeic dermatitis
2. Contact dermatitis
3. Pityriasis

Infantile Seborrhoeic Dermatitis

Common. Esp 0–3mnths. Often FH. Ass c̄ greasy skin

CLIN: Red, scaly, non-itchy eruption esp scalp (cradle-cap), retro–auricular areas, groin, axilla, face, trunk. Rarely 2° infection

RX: Zn & Ichthammol ointment. Occ require steroid cream & Clioquinol

PROG: Usually resolve at 3 mths

DD: Atopic eczema

Napkin Dermatitis

CLIN: Red scaly rash in napkin area not involving gluteal folds

RX: Clean napkins c̄ detergent. Change napkin frequently

Pityriasis Rosea

Unknown cause. Esp young adult. Not infectious

CLIN: Sudden onset c̄ solitary macular lesion (Herald patch). 7–10 days later, macular rash c̄ oval well defined scaly lesions esp affecting trunk & proximal limbs. Resolution occurs in 6–10wks. Occ Pruritus

RX: Calamine lotion

PROG: Excellent

Acne Vulgaris

Very common feature of adolescents. May still cause problems in early adulthood. Ass c̄ androgenic syndromes eg Cushing's syndrome

PATHOGENESIS: Increased sebum production probably due to androgens ↑ or abnormal gland response → ↑ bacterial colonisation esp c̄ *Propionibacteria acnes*

CLIN: Onset around puberty. Polymorphic lesions inc non inflam "blackheads" & "whiteheads" & inflam lesions which may become cystic & scar. Often worse if greasy skin. In F often worse premenstrually

RX: Topical preparations eg Benzoyl peroxide, Retinoic acid. If moderate or severe acne also require long term (>6mths) oral antibiotics eg Tetracycline or Erythromycin. Occ hormonal therapy required eg high dose Ethinyloestradiol in F; Cyproterone acetate in M. 13-cis-Retinoic acid is being assessed as a treatment

DD: Acne can occur due to drugs eg Steroids or chemicals eg halogenated hydrocarbons

Scabies

Caused by mite (*Sarcoptes scabiei*)

CLIN: Severe pruritus esp nocte; Burrows; Vesicles; Papules; Excoriations. Esp genitalia, soles, axilla, webs between fingers. Occ 2° infection

RX: Paint all body except head & neck (unless infected) c̄ 25% Benzyl benzoate, twice within 24 hrs. Treat all contacts similarly at same time. Disinfect clothes & bedding

Pediculosis

Due to nits (eggs) in hair. Ass c̄ poor personal hygiene

CLIN: Occ Scalp impetigo; Infected bites → Cv, Occipital LN ↑

RX: Use fine comb to remove nits. Apply pesticide eg 0.5% carbaryl lotion & rinse hair 24 hrs later. Change pesticide every 2–3yrs to prevent development of resistence

INFECTIOUS DISEASES

Mumps

Caused by Paramyxovirus. Esp Winter, spring. Child >Infant, Adult. Spread by droplet spread or oral contact. Moderately infectious. Incub Pd 16–21 days. Prodromal Pd 1–2 days. Infect Pd is from a few days before salivary gland swelling until swelling completely regressed

CLIN: May be asymptomatic. In prodromal Pd Fever; Malaise; Headache; Vom; Sore throat. Then tender swelling of one or both parotid glands; Trismus. Acute illness usually lasts 3 days but swelling may remain for 10 days

INVESTIGATION: • Viral studies on saliva, urine, blood

PREVENTION: A live attenuated vaccine is available but is not part of most countries routine vaccination programme

RX: Good oral hygiene. Antipyretics & tepid sponging to ↓ risk of febrile convulsions

COMPLICATIONS:

1. **Meningitis:** Common c̄ good prog
2. **Orchitis:** Common usually unilat
   Clin: Fever; Malaise; Red painful swollen testis. Occ → testicular atrophy. Rarely bilat → sterility
   Rx: Local support. Steroids reduce pain
3. **Encephalomyelitis:** Rare. May → Cranial nerve palsies; Brain damage; Coma
4. **Others:** a) Oophoritis
   b) Pancreatitis
   c) Nerve deafness
   c) Arthritis esp large jts
   d) Mastitis
   e) Thyroiditis
   f) In pregnancy may → abortion or foetal EFE

Causes of Parotid Swelling (LIST 25 PAED)

1. Mumps
2. Acute suppurative parotitis
3. Salivary duct calculi
4. Sarcoidosis
5. Parotid tumours
6. Sjogren's syndrome
7. Iodine & Phenylbutazone sensitivity reactions

Chickenpox

Caused by Varicella-Zoster virus. Droplet spread. Esp children. Worse in pregnant & immunosuppressed. Incub Pd 15–18 days. Prodromal Pd 0–2 days. Infect Pd 5 days pre-rash until 6 days post-development of vesicles (ie until crusting)

CLIN: Fever; Malaise; Headache; Sore throat; Abdo pain. Then lesions appear in crops, initially as macules, then papules, vesicles & finally pustules which form crusts. All stages are present simultaneously. Rash has centripetal distribution c̄ relative sparing of limbs. Rarely soles of feet affected. Maturation from macules to crusts takes 1–3 days. Supf scar remains

RX: Zoster specific Ig for high risk gps for prevention. Calamine or povidone Iodine paint to sooth; Mouthwash for oral lesions. Promethazine for pruritus. Daily antiseptic baths may help

COMPLICATIONS: These are rare in healthy children but not uncommon in immunosuppressed esp Leukaemics & adults

1. **2° Skin Infection:** Esp Staph or Strep
   Rx: Antibiotics
2. **Varicella Haemorrhagica:**
   Clin: Fever; Haem into vesicles. DIC
3. **Pneumonitis:** May be ass c̄ Varicella haemorrhagica
   Clin: Cough; SOB; Cyanosis; Haemoptysis
   Investigation: • CXR: Large nodular opacities. Some calcify on recovery
   Rx: Acyclovir
4. **Encephalitis:**
   Clin: Usually presents 7–10 days after onset of rash c̄ cerebellar signs
5. **Others:** a) Myocarditis
   b) Thrombocytopenia

DD: Smallpox

Measles

Esp 6mths–5yrs. Due to RNA myxovirus. Spread by direct contact, droplet spread or air. Highly infectious. Incub Pd 7–14 days. Infect Pd from start of prodromal Pd to 4th day of rash. Prodromal Pd 2–4 days

CLIN: In prodromal Pd: Malaise; Fever; URTI. Occ OM; Vom; Conjunctivitis; Tonsillitis. Usually Koplik's spots ie tiny white granules seen on buccal mucosa appear before rash but soon disappear. Dusky red macular rash begins behind ears, spreads to head & trunk, then limbs. Some areas develop confluent larger maculopapules. On recovery brown staining & occ fine desquamation, temperature returns to norm. Rarely Hoarseness; Stridor; Diarrhoea

PREVENTION: Live attenuated vaccine should be given at 15mths. Measles specific Ig should be given c̄ vaccine if h/o Ep

RX: Supportive treatment eg Fluids, bed rest, analgesia

COMPLICATIONS:

1. **Croup**
2. **Viral pneumonitis**
3. **2° Bacterial infection esp pneumonia**
4. **Febrile convulsions**
5. **SSPE**
6. **Post-infectious Encephalitis:**
   Clin: 4–6 days after rash appears. Meningism. Occ Ep; Coma

PROG: In developing countries, measles is ass c̄ high mort esp in malnourished. In UK important preventable cause of childhood death

DD: 1. Rubella
2. Drug rash

Rubella

Caused by Rubella virus. Spread by droplets or direct contact. Esp children & young adults. Incub Pd 14–21 days. Infect Pd from 7 days before until 5 days after rash appears. Prodromal Pd 0–2 days

CLIN: In prodromal pd: Mild pyrexia; Headache; Malaise; Sore throat; Catarrh. Then macular red rash appearing on face & neck & spreading to trunk & limbs; LN ↑ esp sub-occipital; Mild malaise; Conjunctivitis; Pharyngitis. Occ no rash in virologically proven cases

INVESTIGATIONS: • HAI test
• Rubella specific IgM Ab

PREVENTION: Live attenuated vaccine given to girls aged 10–13yrs. Seronegative F in puerperium should be vaccinated & avoid pregnancy for 3mths

RX: Proven rubella in 1st 4mths of pregnancy is an indication for termination

COMPLICATIONS:

1. **Cong Rubella Syndrome:** Severe cong malformations are ass c̄ rubella infections in early pregnancy
2. **Arthralgia, Arthritis:** Esp adults. Esp hands & feet
3. **Encephalitis** (Rare)
4. **Thrombocytopenia** (Rare)

Whooping Cough

Caused by *Bordetella pertusis*. Esp infants & children. Droplet spread. Highly infectious. Epidemics approx every 4yrs. Incub Pd 7–10 days

CLIN: For 7–10 days catarrhal stage c̄ malaise, fever, dry cough, catarrh. Then fever goes & develop paroxysms of cough c̄ frothy sputum & cyanosis during spasms followed by insp whoop. May → exhaustion of child. Paroxysms esp nocte increase for 1–2wks & then usually diminish gradually over 4–6wks. Often no signs between paroxysms

INVESTIGATIONS: • Pernasal swab (Grow on Bordet–Gengou medium): +ve in catarrhal & early spasmodic stages
• WCC: Lymphocytosis

PREVENTION: Isolate infected person from non-immune. Vaccinate children. Vaccine relatively c/i if Birth inj; CNS damage; Personal h/o Ep

RX: Admit child to hospital if severe paroxysms. Hold infant head down during spasms to prevent inhalation. Antibiotics for 2° infection

COMPLICATIONS:

1. **Atelectasis:** Common. May → Bronchopneumonia; Bronchiectasis
   Rx: Physio; Antibiotics
2. **Pressure Effects:** May → Umbilical hernia; Rectal prolapse; Subconjunctival haem; Cerebral haem & brain anoxia (which occ → Ep; CVA; Cranial nerve palsies; Coma); Pneumothorax; Mediastinal emphysema
3. **Encephalopathy:** This rare condition can also occur 2° to vaccination

Scarlet Fever

Caused by GpA Strep. Spread by direct contact or droplet. Incub Pd 1–7 days. Esp 5–10yrs. Esp temperate countries. The incidence & severity of the disease have markedly reduced in the last 100yrs

CLIN: Sudden onset; Follicular tonsillitis; Sore throat; Fever; Malaise; Headache; Vom. Then 1–2 days later punctate scarlet rash which blanches on pressure appears on neck & chest spreading to trunk & limbs; Rash on limbs may be macular; Flushed cheeks. Tonsillar LN ↑. After 4 days desquamation begins. Initially tongue covered by white fur (White strawberry tongue), by 3rd to 4th day peeling → red raw tongue (Red strawberry tongue)

INVESTIGATIONS: • WCC ↑
• Throat swab
• Dick test
• ASOT titre

RX: Penicillin

COMPLICATIONS: 1. OM
2. Peritonsillar abscess
3. Rhinitis
4. GN
5. Rh fever
6. Arthritis
7. Erythema nodosum

Erysipelas

An intradermal Strep infection. Incub Pd 1–7 days

CLIN: Acute onset c̄ Headache, Vom, Fever. Burning pain. Raised erythema c̄ central bulla esp face & lower limb. Often Facial oedema; Conjunctival discharge; Butterfly rash; Supf blisters. Then desquamation, pigmentation. Rarely abscesses

RX: Benzylpenicillin

COMPLICATION: Lymph obst → oedema

Impetigo

Supf skin infection due to Strep or Staph. Highly infectious

CLIN: Rash esp face around nose & mouth. Initially vesicles which then rupture to form golden crusts

RX: Remove crusts & clean skin c̄ antiseptic. In severe case, antibiotics

Roseola Infantum

Uncommon. Esp 0–3yrs. Incub Pd 5–15 days

CLIN: Fever for 4 days; Vom; Irritability. Then temp falls & pink macular rash appears on trunk & spreads to neck, face & proximal limbs. Rash fades after 1–2 days

Infectious Mononucleosis

Common. Esp 15–20yrs. Caused by Ebstein–Barr virus. Subclinical infection common. Low infectivity. Spread by close contact inc kissing. Incub Pd 10–49 days

CLIN: Insidious onset c̄ malaise; Tiredness; Headache; Fever; LN ↑ esp axillary & Cv. Occ Spleen ↑; Palatal petechiae; Pharyngitis; Periorbital oedema; Exudative tonsilitis; J; Skin rash esp c̄ Ampicillin. In Anginose form (esp young M adults): Painful sore throat; Tonsillitis & occ Airways obst; Palatal petechiae. Usually disease continues for 2–3wks but a significant minority suffer from general fatigue & debility for mths

INVESTIGATIONS:
- WCC & Film: Atypical lymphocytes (mononucleosis)
- Paul Bunnell test for heterophil Ab +ve
- LFT

RX: If pharyngeal oedema give steroids. Avoid sports & strenuous exercise until spleen returns to norm

COMPLICATIONS:
1. Depression in convalescent period
2. Haemolytic anaemia
3. Thrombocytopenia
4. Cranial nerve palsies
5. Polyneuritis
6. Meningoencephalitis
7. GN
8. Myocarditis
9. Pericarditis
10. Pneumonitis
11. Rarely: Ruptured spleen; Arthritis; Agranulocytosis

DD:
1. CMV
2. Toxoplasma
3. Rubella
4. Herpes simplex
5. Hepatitis
6. Strep pharyngitis
7. Leukaemia
8. Lymphoma

DUNCAN'S DISEASE

An X-linked immunodef ass c̄ severe infectious mononucleosis. May → malignant lymphoma or agammaglobulinaemia

Diphtheria

Due to *Cornybacterium diphtheriae.* Esp children. Spread by droplet or direct contact. Incub Pd 2–4 days. Infectious until bacilli can no longer be cultured

PATHOGENESIS: Focus of infection usually in throat c̄ liberation of exotoxin

CLIN: Depends on site of infection. Faucial (commonest) → reddening of tonsils, membrane formation, LN ↑. In severe cases swelling of neck, noisy breathing, fever, 2° infection
Laryngeal (usually 2° to faucial diphtheria) → croup
Nasal (esp infants) → chr seropurulent discharge & perinasal exudates
Cutaneous (usually 2° to faucial diphtheria) → ulceration
Occ Neuritis c̄ sequential effects: Palatal paralysis occurs in 3rd wk c̄ nasal voice; In 4th wk eye muscles of accommodation paralysed; In 5th & 6th wks limb weakness & areflexia; In 7th weak pharangeal & or diaphragmatic paralysis

INVESTIGATION:
- Throat & nose swabs c̄ culture

PREVENTION: Immunisation c̄ diphtheria toxoid is given in 1st year (Schick test determines immunity). Booster immunisation should be given to contacts of diphtheria patients

RX: Diphtheria antitoxin in dosages titrated against severity. Erythromycin. Regular assessment of membrane. Throat douching often helps symptomatically. Nurse in isolation until 3 consecutive -ve cultures. Paralysed limbs require physio. Rarely tracheostomy required

COMPLICATION: Myocarditis

PROG: Good

DD:
1. Tonsillitis
2. Infectious mononucleosis
3. Leukaemia

Tinea Pedis (Athlete's Foot)

Common. Usually only affects feet esp between toes. Infection often acquired in swimming baths

CLIN: Itchy excoriated areas between toes liable to bleed. Infection is chronic & reinfection is common

RX: Antifungal ointments. Change socks daily & disinfect c̄ dusting powder. Swimming baths should provide foot baths c̄ disinfectant

DD: Pitted Keratolysis of Feet
Due to Streptomyces
Rx: Topical Fucidin

Tinea Capitis

Scalp ringworm. May be due to Microsporon or Trichophyton species. May cause epidemics in schools

CLIN: Scalp infection → small red papules c̄ loss of hair in affected area. Occ Pustular eruption (kerion)

INVESTIGATIONS:
- Infected hairs may fluoresce c̄ Wood's light
- Skin scrapings

RX: Griseofulvin, Miconazole or Ketoconazole. Rarely require antibiotics & steroids

DD:
1. Seborrhoeic dermatitis
2. Psoriasis
3. DLE

Other Tinea Infections

Due to Microsporon, Trichophyton or Epidermophyton species. Typically cause circular lesions c̄ raised active border & central healing. Can affect body (*Tinea corporis*) or nails (*Tinea unguium*)

RX: Griseofulvin, Miconazole or Ketoconazole

CONG MALFORMATIONS OF LYMPHATIC SYSTEM

Cystic Hygroma

A localised cystic dilatation of lymph vessels

CLIN: Usually presents at birth c̄ a soft fluctuant swelling in neck. Locally invasive

RX: Surgical removal

PROG: Often recur

Milroy's Disease (Cong Elephantiasis)

Familial. Hard oedema of lower limbs c̄ only slight pitting on pressure. Usually no symptoms

PAEDIATRIC ONCOLOGY

Tumours are the commonest form of childhood death. Different spectrum of types & sites in children compared to adults. Commonest causes in UK are leukaemia, brain tumours, neuroblastoma, Wilm's tumour & Rhabdomyosarcoma. Causes of childhood Ca inc Radioisotopes; Radiation; Immunosuppression; Drugs eg maternal diethylstilboestrol → childhood vaginal Ca; Viruses eg Burkitt's lymphoma; Chromosomal abnormalities eg Down's syndrome → ↑ risk of leukaemia; Genetic eg retinoblastoma

Teratoma

Can occur at any site. Tumours contain a variety of differentiated tissue eg enamel, bone. Commonest sites are ovary, testis, sacrum, abdomen, cranium. May be benign or malignant.

Benign may be symptomatic eg local pressure symptoms c̄ mediastinal teratoma

Embryonic Sarcoma

Esp 0–4yrs. Rare. Variable histology. Occur in many sites eg orbits. Variable malignancy; Sarcoma botryoides (embryonic rhabdomyosarcoma) is highly malignant tumour of prostate, vagina or cervix

RX: X-Rad & Cyt.T

Psychiatry

ACUTE ORGANIC PSYCHOSES

Confusional states of sudden onset due to a disturbance of cerebral function. Acute organic psychoses are sometimes termed toxic confusional states or delirium. Delirium is characterised by impairment of consciousness & disorientation in ass c̄ major perceptual abnormalities. Toxic confusional states should imply that a causative toxic agent can be identified

Commonest causes of acute organic psychoses are adverse drug reactions. Esp Elderly, Children

CLIN: May be signs of underlying disease. Usually presents in a few hrs to days esp nocte. Impairment of consciousness is usually mild c̄ short attention span & drowsiness. Initially disorientation in time, later may have disorientation in place & person; Memory ↓ esp short term. Often perceptual abnormalities

Causes of Acute Organic Psychosis (LIST 1 PSY)

A. SYSTEMIC DISEASE
  1. Toxic:
    a) Drugs eg Alcohol, Cannabis
    b) Solvents eg Glue
    c) Heavy metals eg Hg
  2. Metabolic:
    a) Dehydration
    b) Electrolyte or acid/base imbalance
    c) Hypoxia
    d) RF
    e) Liver failure
    f) Vit def eg B1, B3, B12, Folate
    g) Hypoglycaemia
  3. Anoxia:
    Eg Cardio–resp disease, Anaemia, Post-anaesthesia
  4. Infections:
    Eg Septicaemia, Malaria
  5. Endocrine:
    Esp Hypothyroidism, Hyperthyroidism, HypoPT, HPT

B. CNS DISEASE
  1. Head inj
  2. Cerebrovascular disease
  3. Infection:
    Eg Meningitis, Encephalitis, NeuroSy
  4. Epilepsy
  5. SOL:
    Eg Tumour, Abscess

eg hallucinations, illusions which may → person becoming frightened & bewildered. Occ Paranoid ideas; Disturbance of goal directed thought; Mood swings eg between apathy & terror; Violent behaviour

INVESTIGATIONS:
- FBC
- U&E
- BG
- LFTs
- GGT
- WCC
- CXR
- TFTs
- EEG: Usually theta or delta waves c̄ ↓ alpha activity
- CAT scan

RX: Nurse confused patient in a well lit single room c̄ minimum of extraneous noise. Helpful if a small number of people spend a lot of time in contact c̄ patient. Reassurance. Avoid sedation unless behaviour very disturbed. Occ major tranquillisers eg Haloperidol. Treat underlying disorders appropriately

PROG: Usually recover within hours or a few days. Some chr underlying disorders are likely to → recurrences

DD:
1. Chr organic psychosis (dementia)
2. Functional disorders esp affective psychosis in elderly

CHRONIC ORGANIC PSYCHOSIS (DEMENTIA)

A progressive global deterioration of mental function esp intellectual but also involving behaviour & personality. Most cases are due to a diffuse progressive shrinking of the brain of unknown cause. When dementia occurs in people below age of 65yrs it is termed pre-senile dementia. Very common in elderly, approx 10% above 65yrs of age have signs of dementia

Although most cases of dementia are irreversible, it is important to recognise the potentially treatable conditions

Causes of Dementia (LIST 2 PSY)

A. CNS DISEASE
1. Idiopathic atrophic:
   a) Alzheimer's disease
   b) Pick's disease
   c) Huntington's chorea
2. Cerebrovascular disease: Eg Multi-infarcts, Binswanger's disease
3. Head injury:
   a) Late effect of head injury
   b) Subdural haematoma
   c) Punch-drunk syndrome
4. 1° or 2° Tumours
5. Infections: Eg GPI, SSPE, Post-meningoencephalitis, Creutzfeldt–Jakob disease
6. Normal pressure hydrocephalus
7. Obst hydrocephalus

B. SYSTEMIC
1. Metabolic:
   a) Hypothyroidism
   b) HyperCa^{2+}
   c) Hepatic encephalopathy
   d) Dialysis dementia
2. Drugs: Eg Alcohol, Barbiturates, Bromides
3. Vitamin Def: Eg B3, B1, B12, Folate
4. Carcinomatous neuropathy

Causes of Potentially Reversible Dementias (LIST 3 PSY)

1. Subdural haematoma
2. Brain tumour:
   Esp Meningioma
3. GPI
4. Normal pressure hydrocephalus
5. Metabolic disorders:
   Esp Hypothyroidism
6. Vitamin defs
7. Drugs

GENERAL CLIN: Insidious onset. Impairment of memory esp for recent events; Intellectual deterioration inc loss of ability to learn; Change of personality esp apathy; Affective disorders esp depression, anxiety; No clouding of consciousness. Occ Focal CNS signs; Loss of inhibitions; Perseveration; Hallucinations. Early dementia often have some insight & depression. Occ superadded acute confusional episodes. Usually gradual deteriorating course

GENERAL INVESTIGATIONS: • FBC & film
- U&Es
- LFTs
- CXR
- VDRL, TPI, TPHA
- B12
- Serum & RBC folate
- TFTs
- SXR
- ECG
- CAT scan
- Occ LP, Angiography, EEG

GENERAL RX: Identify & treat any reversible cause or acute confusional state. Usually best to nurse in familiar surroundings ie usually at home, c̄ support services eg home helps, health visitors. Obvious dangers within home should be minimised. Try to prevent wandering outside house eg locks on doors, close supervision. Support & explanation to relatives & other carers. May benefit from attendance at day centres. Eventually psychogeriatric placement may be required. Sedatives may be useful

DD:
1. Amnesic Syndromes eg Korsakoff's syndrome
2. Mixed or expressive dysphasia
3. Affective psychosis (*Depressive pseudodementia*): May have intellectual, memory & behavioural problems. Unlike dementia may have periods of functioning at higher levels. Respond to antidepressants

Alzheimer's Disease

Commonest cause of pre-senile & senile dementia. Many believe there are two types, Type 1 usually presenting in 70s & Type 2 at 55–70yrs

PATHOLOGY: Diffuse cerebral atrophy esp frontal, temporal & hippocampal cortex. Histologically senile plaques, neurofibrillary tangles. In Type 2 substantial neuronal cell loss. Deficit in the pre-synaptic component of the cholinergic system

CLIN: General clin of dementia. Often Return of primitive reflexes eg grasp & pout; Apraxia; Agnosia; Dysphasia. Later may develop hypokinesia. Gradual deterioration often → death in 5–10yrs

RX: Cholinergic treatments have not proved useful

Pick's Disease

PATHOLOGY: Asymmetrical atrophy of frontal or temporal lobes c̄ sparing of cortical mantle. Histologically gliosis, neuronal loss & Pick's bodies

CLIN: As for Alzheimer's disease

Creutzfeldt–Jakob Disease

Encephalopathy due to a slow virus

PATHOLOGY: Spongiform degeneration

CLIN: Rapidly progressive dementia. Myoclonus; Focal CNS signs; Extrapyramidal signs

PREVENTION: Disease has been transmitted from affected brain tissue, therefore care in handling brain inc cornea

PROG: Die in a few mths

GPI

Quaternary form of neuroSy

CLIN: Variable presentation. Forms c̄ dementia may have ass mania or euphoria. Argyll–Robertson pupils

RX: Penicillin

PROG: Good

LIAISON PSYCHIATRY

Concerned c̄ the involvement of psychological factors in the diagnosis, management & prevention of illness. The close interaction between mind & body is increasingly recognised

At the 1° care level many people presenting c̄ physical disease also have a psychiatric disorder. Significant minorities of psychiatric inpatients have physical disease & similarly significant minority of medical inpatients have psychiatric disease

Psychological disease esp anxiety, depression & hysteria may present as physical illness. Often people believe that a somatic complaint is a more acceptable basis for a consultation c̄ a doctor. Occ symptoms under voluntary control can be reinforced by psychiatric disorders eg anxiety → PR ↑ → anxiety ↑ → PR ↑↑

Organic disease may present as psychological disorder eg Acute organic psychosis (see LIST 1 PSY); Depression eg Hypothyroidism, Addison's disease; Anxiety eg Hyperthyroidism. Drugs commonly cause psychiatric symptoms

Psychological disorder esp depression may be ppt by organic disease esp amongst those c̄ a previous h/o psychiatric disorder. Depression may be a reaction to physical illness esp chronic. Psychoses eg Schizophrenia may be ppt by physical illness

The presence of psychiatric disorder in medical in-patients is ass c̄ poorer prog esp c̄ Rheumatoid & CVS diseases. This may be due to non-compliance c̄ Rx, anxiety impairing cardio–resp function, or perpetuation of somatic symptoms eg cardiac neurosis

Physical disease may be ppt by psychological factors eg Type A personality → ↑ IHD, recent bereavement → ↑ early mort for surviving spouse

DRUG INDUCED PSYCHIATRIC DISORDERS

Adverse drug reactions are a common cause of psychiatric morbidity. Some drugs cause specific types of psychiatric disorders whilst others produce a spectrum of syndromes in different patients. Esp Very young, Elderly

Causes of Drug Induced Psychiatric Disorders (LIST 4 PSY)

A. ACUTE ORGANIC PSYCHOSIS
1. Tranquillisers & Hypnotics:
   Eg Phenothiazines, Benzodiazepines, Barbiturates
2. Anticholinergics:
   Eg TCAD
3. Antibiotics:
   Eg Sulphonamides, Penicillin
4. Anticonvulsants:
   Eg Phenytoin, Sodium Valproate
5. Dopamine agonists:
   Eg L-Dopa, Bromocriptine
6. Anti-TB drugs:
   Eg Isoniazid, Rifampicin
7. Drug withdrawal:
   Eg Alcohol, Barbiturates, Benzodiazepines, Chlormethiazole
8. Miscellaneous:
   Eg Digoxin, Cimetidine, Aminophylline, β blockers

B. PARANOID OR SCHIZOPHRENIA LIKE PSYCHOSES
1. Hallucinogens:
   Eg LSD, Mescaline, Cannabis
2. CNS Depressants:
   Eg Alcohol, Barbiturates, Anticonvulsants
3. CNS Stimulants:
   Eg Amphetamines, Cocaine, Ephedrine
4. Steroids

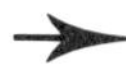

5. Miscellaneous:
   Eg Antimalarials, Bromocriptine, Phenytoin

C. DEPRESSION
1. Anti-hypertensives:
   Eg Methyldopa, Clonidine, Propranolol
2. Major tranquillisers:
   Eg Chlorpromazine, Haloperidol
3. L-Dopa
4. Steroids
5. NSAID & other analgesics:
   Eg Phenylbutazone, Pentazocine, Indomethacin
6. Drug withdrawal:
   Eg Amphetamines

D. MANIA & HYPOMANIA
1. Steroids & ACTH
2. Miscellaneous:
   Eg Salbutamol, L-Dopa

E. HALLUCINATIONS
1. Hallucinogens:
   Eg LSD, Mescaline, Cannabis, "Angel Dust"
2. Psychoptrophic drugs:
   Eg Benzodiazepines, TCAD
3. Anti-parkinsonian drugs:
   Eg L-Dopa, Bromocriptine, Anticholinergics
4. Miscellaneous:
   Eg Indomethacin, Disopyramide, Digoxin

F. DEMENTIA
1. Alcohol
2. Tranquillisers:
   Eg Barbiturates, Bromides, Phenothiazines
3. Anti-parkinsonian drugs
4. Anti-depressants
5. Miscellaneous:
   Eg Insulin → chr BG ↓, Lithium

G. VIVID DREAMS & NIGHTMARES
1. B blockers
2. Fenfluramine
3. Baclofen
4. Anti-hypertensives:
   Eg Methyldopa, Clonidine

H. PERSONALITY CHANGES
1. Barbiturates
2. Benzodiazepines
3. L-Dopa
4. Phenothiazines

GENERAL RX: Discontinue suspected drug wherever possible. Acute organic psychoses & hallucinations generally remit quickly once drug withdrawn. Depression & the paranoid or schizophrenia-like psychoses usually respond to drug removal in <2wks & during this period, drug Rx of the SE may be warranted

DEPRESSIVE DISORDERS

Depression is often an understandable consequence of a provoking life event. Depressive illness represents a state clearly outside the limits of normality. There are two main forms, Neurotic (Reactive) & Endogenous. Depression may also occur as part of an organic illness eg influenza, hepatitis, hypothyroidism

Causes of Organic Depression (LIST 5 PSY)

1. Drugs
2. Infectious diseases:
   Eg Influenza, Infectious hepatitis, Glandular fever
3. Endocrine:
   Eg Hypothyroidism, Addison's disease, Cushing's disease
4. Malignancies:
   Eg Ca pancreas
5. CNS disease:
   Eg Alzheimer's disease, Huntington's chorea, Post head inj, Parkinsonism
6. Vitamin defs:
   Eg PA, Folate def

Neurotic (Reactive) Depression

Often initially presents in young adults

CLIN: Illness ppt by unpleasant life event but symptoms disproportionate to stimulus in intensity &/or duration. Often patient has a predisposing personality c̄ increased sensitivity to minor stress. Miserable; Self pity; Depression; Impaired concentration; Lack of energy. Occ Anxiety; Sleep disturbance esp initial insomnia; Suicidal ideas & attempts; Headache. Less commonly have ↓ appetite & Wt ↓. The symptoms often fluctuate during day usually worsening nocte. The condition often lasts only days or wks but may be chr if the ppt cause persists eg interpersonal conflict

RX: Admit to hospital if: Suicide is likely; Severe depression; Insufficient support can be provided at home. Reassure patients that they will improve. If possible resolve ppt cause eg marital guidance, often c̄ social worker's help. Psychotherapy is often beneficial. Benzodiazepines may be helpful but should not be used long term as danger of dependence

Endogenous Depression & Manic–Depressive Psychosis

Endogenous depression may be part of a manic–depressive illness. F>M. Occ FH. ?Due to a serotonin def upon which is superimposed a catecholamine def coincident c̄ depression & a catecholamine excess coincident c̄ mania. Presenting episode may not occur till middle age

CLIN: Endogenous depression usually has insidious onset. Apathy; Fatigue; Lack of energy; Sad facies; Sleep disturbance esp early wakening; Poor appetite; Wt ↓. Often Feelings of guilt & unworthiness; Suicidal thoughts; ↓ libido; Constipation. Occ Hypochondriacal; Paranoia; Diurnal mood change, usually worse mane; Amenorrhoea. In severe cases (Psychotic depression): Marked loss of interest; Strong suicidal ideas but deed may be prevented by apathy; Delusions of unworthiness; Hypochondriacal delusions eg bowels have rotted. Occ Stupor; Muteness; Unresponsiveness
Occ develop "agitated" depression, when symptoms of anxiety & motor restlessness predominate. In severe cases can → continuous purposeless activity
The duration of an episode varies greatly from hrs to yrs but usually lasts about 6mths
In bipolar form, episodes of depression are interspersed c̄ episodes of mania. Manic phase is characterised by Elevation of mood eg euphoria; Ego inflation; ↑ libido, although performance is usually unaffected; Delusions of grandeur; Distractibilty; Rapid garrulous speech; Flight of ideas; Pressure of thoughts; ↑ energy; ↓ need for sleep; Erratic behaviour. Occ Antisocial behaviour; Incoherent speech; Very good memory. Usually no insight. If symptoms less pronounced termed Hypomania

PROPHYLAXIS: $LiCO_3$ (SE: Tremor, Polydypsia, Polyuria, Wt ↑, RTbA, DI, Thyroid dysfunction) may reduce incidence of attacks esp in bipolar form. Requires monitoring so that therapeutic blood level is maintained. o/d may → confusion & coma

RX: Admit to hospital if: Suicide is likely; Severe depression; Insufficient support can be provided at home. Choice is mainly between antidepressants & ECT. ECT is usually initial Rx in elderly & if prostatic hyperplasia, closed angle glaucoma or CVS disease. Psychotherapy is a useful adjunct to Rx
Many available antidepressants esp TCAD, all have response rate of approx 60% but SE vary. Amitriptyline (SE: Sedation, Anticholinergic effects, Arrhythmias, Confusional states), Viloxazine (SE: N&V). Doxepin (SE: Sedation) & the tetracyclic, Mianserin are less cardiotoxic
The MAOIs (SE: Episodes of BP ↑, headache, meningism & collapse ppt by eg cheese, red wine, yeast, amines; Liver damage; Postural BP ↓) are usually used when TCAD are ineffective. Probably wise to avoid combined use of MAOI & TCAD
ECT is effective in about 80–90% although some have early relapse. It should be carried out following a muscle relaxant anaesthetic, using a pulsed current & a unilat electrode over the non-dominant hemisphere. SE are few in well run units c̄ usually only slight temporary confusion & memory loss following procedure. Usually 6–8 treatments are required
Rarely psychosurgery if prolonged severe depression eg bilat

cingulotractotomy
Manic patients usually require hospital admission occ compulsorily.

Haloperidol or Chlorpromazine for episodes of mania. ECT is often helpful. $LiCO_3$ for prophylaxis

THE DYING PATIENT

Sadness, worry & fear of the future are understandable reactions of the dying & their families. Not uncommonly depression, anxiety or other psychiatric problems result. Often attempts to resolve problems within the patient's life are more beneficial than symptomatic drug Rx

The practice of not informing the patient totally about the illness & its prog is still common. Relatives who keep such a secret may find this burden stressful & require the opportunity to discuss their worries. When secrets are kept, fears may fester in isolation. Usually the patient has already considered the possibility that the illness may be terminal. Often telling the patient about the condition & its prog is helpful to both the patient & the family. Children also are usually aware of the tension surrounding such a secret & often it is better to discuss the situation c̄ them

The frequent necessity to change their normal roles eg going to work, often causes problems & requires counselling

People who are reasonably well but are likely to suffer sudden death esp those c̄ IHD, occ react by becoming disabled by chr anxiety ± depression (eg cardiac neurosis). Psychotherapy may help

People c̄ slow progressive disease often fear that the terminal stages will be very painful & undignified. Such fears can often be reconciled when it is explained that pain can be very well controlled by Rx & if the patient is allowed to discuss his management c̄ the staff. Occ problems in the life of the patient may → a desire to die early. Occ patients near death appear to withdraw from life; this should be explained to the relatives as a norm reaction

Although affective disorders are common in the dying, diagnosis is more difficult because of concurrent symptoms of the underlying disease. Depression can often be reliably detected if excessive guilt or low self-esteem are present; Amitriptyline may benefit. Anxiety is often lessened by reassurance, good symptom control & observing the peaceful death of other patients; Anxiolytics eg Diazepam occ are of value. Paranoid ideas eg that the staff are killing the patient, are not uncommon. Such ideas may be relieved by psychotherapy or require Haloperidol

The drug treatment regime may itself cause psychiatric problems & should be regularly monitored. Appropriate modifications of Rx are often required

The setting of death is important. Many prefer to die at home c̄ care provided by their relatives & appropriate statutory workers inc specialised domiciliary terminal care teams in some areas. The hospice provides an environment tailored to deal c̄ the physical & psychological problems of the terminally ill. Some acute hospitals have specialised teams to advise on the care of the terminally ill

Following death inc SB, it is often helpful for relatives to observe the dead body at peace. This often allows them to accept the reality of death & to start expressing grief. Counselling is often required when the death has been due to suicide or violence. Early in the bereavement period it is useful if the close relatives are relieved of some of their normal duties so that it is easier for them to grieve. Often those who do not appear to grieve, present later c̄ psychiatric illness. It is normal if the bereaved have hallucinations of the deceased, sense the deceased's presence or become preoccupied c̄ the image of the dead person. Recovery from grief may take mths or yrs & may require support & sympathetic counselling

MUTILATING SURGERY

Surgical removal of a body part or function may → serious psychiatric illness eg 25% of mastectomy patients develop anxiety, depression &/or sexual problems within 12–18mths of surgery; Colostomy frequently → sexual problems; Amputation often → anxiety or depression. Predisposing factors are Anxiety &/or depression pre-surgery; Adverse experience of Ca in a close contact; Physical complications post-surgery; Inability to discuss problems Psychiatric problems are often not recognised early because the doctor may not ask specifically about the adaptation to surgery or does not meaningfully discuss expressed worries. Accordingly some non-psychiatrically trained doctors underestimate the prevalence of such problems

CLIN: Depression is of the reactive form often c̄ Depressed mood; Sleep disturbance; Lack of energy or agitation; Guilt; Suicidal ideas. Anxiety is usually ass c̄ ↓ concentration; ↑ tension; Irritability; Panic attacks; Sleep disturbance. Sexual problems inc Impotence; Premature ejaculation; Frigidity; ↓ libido

RX: The use of a specialist nurse or social worker to give information & support both before & after surgery → appropriate use of aids & appliances. Their value in reducing psychiatric morbidity is less certain. Patients find it useful to talk c̄ other people who have undergone & successfully adapted to similar surgery. Follow-up after discharge by a specialist nurse → early pick up of most physical & psychological problems. GPs are also well placed to uncover problems
If possible, surgeons should choose a less mutilating form of op eg lumpectomy rather than mastectomy
Depression usually responds to anti-depressants eg Mianserin. Severe anxiety requires a major tranquilliser eg Thioridazine, whilst more minor states may respond to relaxation techniques. The benzodiazepines should not be used long-term because of the risk of dependence. Sexual problems often respond well to behavioural Rx methods (unless surgery has cut nerves to sex organs). A breast reconstruction may be helpful for F who suffer from body-image problems & accept limitations of plastic surgery

ANXIETY NEUROSIS & PHOBIC STATES

A neurosis is a non-organic distressing mental illness c̄ no severe affective change or thought disorder. Anxiety neuroses are excessive, persistent or inappropriate anxiety responses to personal or social threats. (N.B Anxiety in many situations (even exams!) may improve performance). The anxiety may be learnt from previous experience; particular places or activities may reactivate anxiety eg if present in fire at a cinema may always be anxious about entering cinemas, or if premature ejaculation then anxiety about subsequent performance. Occ FH. Certain personality types eg obsessional, over-dependent, anxiety-prone, are likely to develop neuroses in response to minor stress

CLIN: The acute anxiety state (panic attack) has a sudden onset. Usually obvious ppt factor. Often Palps; Dry mouth; Sweating; Diarrhoea; Freq; Hyperventilation occ → paraesthesiae, tetany; Muscle tension → aches & pains; Terror
In chr anxiety states, often Fearful anticipation; Irritability; Distractability; Feeling of poor memory & concentration (usually no objective evidence); Sleep disturbance; Headaches. Occ Impotence; Frigidity. Overlaid acute episodes. Occ physical symptoms are amplified eg palps. The anxiety may be fixated to one system of the body c̄ symptoms being most

prominent in that system
The phobic neuroses occur in specific situations & patients become anxious when anticipating that they will have to enter that situation. Children often have simple phobias eg path fear of spiders. Often anxiety is provoked by situations where person feels that he is being judged critically (social phobias). Occ agoraphobia where anxiety is caused by crowded places & is often ass c̄ depression &/or obsession
Anxiety neuroses are occ ass c̄ reactive depression. Anxiety may → alcohol abuse in an attempt to relieve symptoms

RX: If stress likely to be short-lived, supportive therapy. Often best to discuss c̄ the patient about worries & try to ensure that the nature of the symptoms are understood. Vigorous attempts to persuade those c̄ phobic symptoms to confront situations which cause anxiety
Drug Rx should be started c̄ caution as dependence on drugs is easily acquired & should be prescribed only for short periods. Benzodiazepines relieve anxiety but if used for mths → withdrawal symptoms of tremor, N, apprehension, insomnia if withdrawn suddenly. TCADs are useful esp when depression & anxiety coexist. Occ β blockers are used to control palps & tremor
Relaxation training which helps ↓ muscular tension is helpful if practiced regularly; thus relaxation gps sometimes of benefit. Success c̄ these techniques may obviate need for drugs. Anxiety management training in which the patient is taught how to induce anxiety & bring it under control, is best undertaken by a clin psychologist. Behaviour therapy is the Rx of choice for chr phobic anxiety states. A planned programme in which the patient is encouraged to frequently return to the ppt situation is preferable to flooding (ie where patient is placed in ppt situation without preparation or desensitisation), where a graduated approach to the reintroduction to the stressful situation is employed. People esp young c̄ personality disorders, may benefit from psychotherapy

DD:
1. Anxiety states due to organic disease eg thyrotoxicosis
2. Reactive depression
3. Obsessional neuroses
4. Alcohol abuse

OBSESSIONAL NEUROSES

An act or a recurring thought which is subjectively thought to be abnormal, is resisted & results in anxiety. Obsessional acts are termed compulsions. Onset esp young adulthood. Occ underlying obsessional (anankastic) personality ie orderly, conscientious, rigidity of views, egotistical, impatient & occ stingy, superior, self-reproachful

CLIN: Obsessional thoughts are of two major types, ruminations & phobias. Obsessional ruminations esp concern recurring doubts eg repeated thought of "have I locked door" after leaving house, or preoccupation c̄ hostile intentions eg mother fearing she will harm child even though she loves it. Obsessional phobias are impulses or ideas which are recognised as absurd but nevertheless generate extreme anxiety
Obsessional acts may be the result of an obsessional thought eg doubting that the door is locked → repeated checking of door. Occ a self-contained ritual is observed eg clothes taken of before bed at set time in specific order. Compulsions often relate to cleanliness eg repeated unnecessary washing of hands
The struggle against obsessional thoughts & acts is never satisfying & → variably severe symptoms of anxiety. Rarely suicide
Obsessional symptoms may occur in organic disorders eg encephalitis lethargica or as part of other psychiatric disorders eg schizophrenia

RX: Psychotherapy is often useful. Short courses of minor anxiolytics may be of benefit. Very rarely, in severe cases, pre-frontal leucotomy is undertaken

PSYCHIATRY OF THE CHANGE OF LIFE

Both sexes may be subject to a "mid-life" crisis. F>M. In F this crisis is often ass c̄ the climacteric (N.B in UK mean age of menopause is 51yrs). Psychological symptoms seem to ↑ in F aged 40–55. Some evidence that incidence increases when periods are becoming irregular & rises again in early menopausal F, thereafter falling in the postmenopausal yrs. However in-patient admissions for middle-aged people are not particularly high

CLIN: Common psychological symptoms in menopausal F are Depression; Headaches; Fatigue; Insomnia; Irritability; Palps; Poor concentration. Distress may be caused by the common physical symptoms of the menopause ie Hot flushes & atrophic vaginitis which may → pruritis, cystitis, dyspareunia Common stresses of middle age eg ill health of parents, adolescence of children, learning to live without children at home, problems at work may ppt psychiatric problems. Often life events at this time may cause the individual to reassess his life & may result in a critical examination of past performance & future hopes. These feelings may be expressed as various forms of crisis behaviour inc Anxiety; Depression; Quests to recapture lost youth; Alcoholism; Hypochondriasis; Change of job, home or sexual partner (1 in 5 UK marriages end in divorce after >20yrs); Religious awakening; Nostalgia ie excessive living in past. Ageing & death are often seen as impending threats

RX: Hormone replacement therapy relieves hot flushes & atophic vaginitis but little evidence that oestrogen relieves depression, insomnia or palps. However hormones do seem to elevate mood. Occ pointing out the advantages of middle-age is helpful eg the end of the inconvenience of menstruation. Psychotherapy can → a better understanding of the mid-life crisis & promote a realistic assessment of life situation. Occ drug therapy eg TCAD or ECT are required

ATTEMPTED SUICIDE

The term attempted suicide may be a misnomer because death is not the intended outcome. Other terms have been used eg parasuicide ie an act deliberately undertaken, which mimics the act of suicide but results in non-fatality. The terms deliberate self-poisoning & deliberate self-injury which describe behaviour without implying intention are probably most suitable. Attempted suicide is very common esp in western world & is a common reason for acute admission to hospital. F>M. Esp 15–24yrs. Esp lower social classes, urban areas, single & divorced, teenage wives, disrupted family relationships. Other risk factors are unemployment & physical health problems eg Ep. The commonest associations amongst the middle-aged & elderly are depressive illness, alcohol abuse, poor physical health & social isolation. In UK about 5–8% have suffered from serious psychiatric illness eg depression, psychopathy, alcohol abuse

CLIN: Most attempted suicides appear to involve little premeditation. Retrospective questioning elicits desire to die, to blot out distressing thoughts, to escape from problems or to inform others of the extent of their distress as the reason for the attempt. Doctors usually explain attempt as a combination of factors often inc cry for help, communication of anger & attempt to influence others perhaps by inducing guilt 90% of cases seen in hospital involve deliberate self-poisoning often ass c̄ high alcohol intake. Substances used reflect availability, thus o/d c̄ Aspirin, Paracetamol & Minor tranquillisers are common

Self-injury is usually by cutting of wrists or forearm. Violent forms of self-injury are rare & suggest true suicidal intention
Approx 20% have 2nd suicide attempt within 1yr & 1–2% have a successful attempt within 1yr

RX: Treat symptoms of acute overdose appropriately. Assess the problems of the patient & assess risk of repetition. Factors which suggest suicidal intent inc admitting suicidal intention, leaving suicide note, premeditation occ inc telling others, preparing for death eg making will, arranging event so that discovery is unlikely. Factors which suggest ↑ risk of further attempts inc alcohol or drug abuse, personality disorder, previous psychiatric Rx, unemployment, low social class, criminal record & living alone
Signs of alcohol or other drug abuse should be actively sought. Interview other relevant sources eg close family members. If underlying psychiatric disorder usually require in-patient psychiatric care & appropriate Rx. Counselling of the patient often c̄ other family members is occ of benefit. Often ↑ home support is arranged eg social worker, CPN

PROG: Special services eg CPN, appear to improve social functioning but may not reduce repetition rate. 50% of all suicides have a h/o deliberate self-injury or self-poisoning

SUICIDE

Suicide is much less common than attempted suicide (approx 15× less in M & 30× less in F), but nonetheless important cause of death. M>F.
Ass c̄ Depression; Alcohol abuse; Personality disorders eg hostile passive dependent people; Poor physical health. Esp Elderly (>45yrs), Divorced, Single, High social class, Unemployed, Urban areas. Commoner in spring. Less common during wartime & if obsessional or hypochondriacal traits. 50% have h/o attempted suicide. Particular risk is during Rx of depression if psychomotor retardation improves before any lifting of mood. 80% of all poisoning deaths occur outside hospital

ACUTE POISONING

Acute poisoning in adults is usually due to drug o/d. Many cases do not reach hospital & about 80% of hospital admissions require only observation in the management of the physical aspects of the o/d. Accidental poisoning in children rarely → morbidity or mort. In adults, drug o/d may involve more than one drug & often involves alcohol; CO poisoning is also an important cause of death. In children, drugs account for the majority of poisonings but household cleaning products are frequently involved

GENERAL RX: Put drugs in child resistent containers & keep household poisons out of reach of children. Avoid prescribing drugs in large quantities esp to at-risk gps. Attempt to prevent further absorption eg Stomach washout; Inducing emesis; Cathartics; Adsorbents eg activated charcoal. Usually these measures are of most value if carried out within 4hrs of o/d. For a few drugs specific antidotes are available. Resuscitation may be required inc ventilation. In severe cases monitor in intensive care. Occ measures to enhance elimination of poison are warranted eg forced alkaline diuresis. The majority of drug o/d merely require regular observation. On recovery, social & psychiatric assessment

Salicylate Poisoning

Usually due to Aspirin overdose. Common

PATHOGENESIS: Salicylates → direct

stimulation of resp centre → resp rate ↑ → resp alkalosis. Also → interference c̄ oxidative phosphorylation → metabolic acidosis. Often HypoK$^+$

CLIN: In mild to moderate intoxication → N&V; Tinnitus; Sweating; PR ↑; Resp rate ↑; Vasodilation. Occ Deafness; Tetany. In severe intoxication (plasma conc >800mg/l), features of moderate intoxication & confusion, BP ↓. Occ Ep, Coma, Pulm oedema; Cerebral oedema; Encephalopathy; BG ↓; Hyperpyrexia; RF; Cardiac arrest. In children, metabolic acidosis, BG ↓ & liver dysfunction are commoner than in adults

INVESTIGATION: • Salicylate level

RX: Gastric lavage or induction of emesis c̄ Ipecacuanha is worthwhile up to 12hrs post ingestion. Activated charcoal may be of value soon after o/d. Correct dehydration, acidosis & electrolyte abnormalities. If [>450mg/l] use forced alkaline diuresis

Paracetamol

Important cause of morbidity & mort esp when combined c̄ dextropropoxyphene (Distalgesic)

PATHOGENESIS: Paracetamol in liver is converted to a toxic metabolite which is usually inactivated by conjugation c̄ glutathione. After large o/d, glutathione is depleted & hepatotoxicity occurs. Large individual variations in resistance to drug toxicity

CLIN: Early N&V. Later may have Upper abdo pain; Liver tenderness. In severe cases liver failure on 3rd–6th day c̄ Encephalopathy; Haem; Resp rate ↑; BG ↓; Cerebral oedema. Rarely ARF

INVESTIGATIONS: • Paracetamol level taken at least 4hrs after ingestion
• LFTs

RX: Treatment depends on plotting level on graph linking Paracetamol concentration c̄ time after overdose. Treat if level above treatment line on graph. N-acetylcysteine & Methionine act by facilitating Glutathione synthesis. They must be given within 8–10hrs of o/d to prevent liver damage, although some protection is afforded until 15–16hrs

NSAID

Not commonly used for self-poisoning

CLIN: Phenylbutazone can → D&V; Ep; Resp rate ↑; Liver failure; Coma; ARF. Mefanamic acid can → Ep; ↓ consciousness. Indomethacin, Fenoprofen & Ibuprofen are relatively safe but may → ARF

RX: Phenylbutazone o/d Rx is difficult as the long T1/2 → prolonged symptoms. Occ Diazepam required for Ep

TCAD

Quite commonly used. The new generation of anti-depressants are generally less toxic in o/d

CLIN: Classical features are Cardiac arrhythmias; Ep; Coma. In mild cases Dry mouth; Dilated pupils; ↓ consciousness. In severe cases may have BP ↓; Temperature ↑ or Hypothermia; Urinary retention; PI; Reflexes ↑; Tone ↑; Resp failure; Skin blisters. Rarely other CNS signs eg extensor plantars, ophthalmoplegia. Most recover consciousness within one day but may become delirious

INVESTIGATIONS: • ECG
• Drug level

RX: Gastric lavage is useful (anticholinergic effect of o/d → ↓ gastric tone). Activated charcoal within 1–2hrs of ingestion. ECG monitoring. Correct acidosis & any electrolyte imbalance. Carefully monitor all comatose eg c̄ Astrup. Adequate O_2. Rarely use anti-arrhythmic drugs

MAOI

Uncommon causes of poisoning

CLIN: Symptoms usually develop about 12hrs after ingestion & inc Muscular rigidity; Sweating; Pyrexia; Resp rate ↑; PR ↑

RX: Supportive Rx. Occ require muscle relaxants or ventilation

Benzodiazepines

Commonly taken in o/d but low toxicity

CLIN: Drowsiness. Occ Dizziness; Cerebellar

syndrome ie ataxia, dysarthria, nystagmus; Hallucinations; Confusion

RX: Supportive treatment

Phenothiazines

Uncommon cause of poisoning

CLIN: ↓ consciousness; Involuntary mvts eg Oculogyric crises; BP ↓; PR ↑. Occ Ep; Arrhythmias

RX: Gastric lavage; Benztropine for dystonic reactions. Supportive Rx

Barbiturates

Before controls on prescriptions, barbiturate o/d was common in UK. Dangerous esp since absorption occurs rapidly

CLIN: May inc Coma; Circulatory failure; Resp failure; Hypothermia; Bullous eruptions

RX: Clear airways; Often require ventilation. Correct any fluid or electrolyte imbalance. Charcoal haemoperfusion may aid elimination

β blockers

CLIN: Small o/d → sinus bradycardia. Larger o/ds may → Confusion; Ep; Coma; PR ↓; BP ↓; Hallucinations; Cardiac arrest

RX: In severe o/d, monitor c̄ ECG in ICU. Gastric lavage if ingestion $<$4hrs previously. Glucagon for severe BP ↓

Digoxin

Uncommon but high mort c̄ large o/d

CLIN: N&V; Drowsiness; Arrhythmias eg SVT, Bradycardia, Ht block

INVESTIGATIONS:
- U&E: Often K^+ ↑
- ECG

RX: Gastric lavage if ingestion $<$4hrs previously. Activated charcoal is useful if $<$1hr since ingestion. Monitor c̄ ECG, treat all arrhythmias except VEs. Occ require pacing. Occ may try haemoperfusion

Bleaches & Disinfectants

Often contain corrosives eg Na^+ hypochlorite, phenol or cresols

CLIN: Oral, pharyngeal & retrosternal burning. Occ Stridor; SOB; BP ↓; Ep; Pulm oedema; Coma

RX: Gastric lavage within 3–4hrs of ingestion unless ingestion of acids or NaOH suspected. Supportive Rx

Paraquat

Uncommon but often fatal o/d

CLIN: Initially N&V; Diarrhoea. Rarely early death from coma, pulm oedema & myocardial toxicity. After 3–4 days often severe ulceration of upper resp & GI tracts → Dysphagia; Dysphonia; Pain on coughing. ARF may occur by 4–5 days. SOB may increase → fatal pulm fibrosis in days or weeks

INVESTIGATIONS:
- Plasma paraquat level
- CXR
- U&E

RX: The outcome of poisoning can be quite well predicted from level of paraquat related to time from ingestion. Empty stomach & give absorbent eg Fuller's earth. Other measures do not seem to influence course

Carbon Monoxide

Incidence has fallen since the replacement of coal gas by methane. CO from car exhausts remains an important cause of death by poisoning

PATHOGENESIS: CO combines c̄ Hb → CarboxyHb → ↓ blood O_2 carrying capacity → tissue anoxia

RX: Remove from poisonous atmosphere. Give 100% O_2

VIOLENT PATIENTS

Violence is not a disease but it may occur in ass c̄ severe life events & psychiatric disorders. Violence to others is often linked c̄ violence to self. Some personality disorders esp psychopathy are prone to violent behaviour. A psychopath is a person c̄ a persistent disorder or disability of mind (whether or not subnormal) which results in abnormally aggressive or seriously irresponsible conduct on the part of the patient & requires or is susceptible to Rx

Common ppt factors are Problems within the home eg marital problems; Sexual jealousy; Institutions where individuals c̄ personality problems congregate eg prisons; Crime

CLIN: Head inj esp frontal may → change in personality & violent tendencies. Schizophrenia occ → violence either due to delusional ideas or disintegration of personality. Paranoid symptoms in affective disorders are unusual causes of violence. Acute confusional states eg post alcohol binge may → violence. Alcohol abuse may also be ass c̄ violence when it → personality change, paranoid psychosis or brain damage

RX: Personality problems require psychotherapy. Discuss problem c̄ family & possibly friends. At scene of violent incident, try to free any victim & prevent further violence. This may be achieved by reassurance & informing the violent person that the reason for his violence is understood. Occ physical restraint inc use of sedatives is required. May require legal compulsory detention. Treat any underlying psychiatric disorder. All murderers require psychiatric assessment (a significant minority subsequently commit suicide). Hospital policies re dealing c̄ violence are useful

SEXUAL DISORDERS

Sexual disorders can be divided into two major gps, problems related to sexual performance & sexual deviations & perversions

Disorders Related to Sexual Performance

The true incidence of sexual difficulties is difficult to determine but they are probably quite common even though few seek professional help

GENERAL CLIN: In M, problems c̄ erection, orgasm or ejaculation are common presenting complaints. In F, lack of sexual enjoyment or loss of libido are commoner presentations. The natural decline in erectile function c̄ age occ → problems

LOSS OF LIBIDO

Loss of libido is usually much more problematic for M, because of social norms. The cause is usually psychological but may occur due to CRF, hyperprolactinaemia or drugs eg antidepressants

IMPOTENCE

Erectile problems can be due to organic or psychogenic causes. Once performance anxiety occurs a vicious circle may be set up compounding problem. Physical causes of loss of erection inc Leriche syndrome; Arterial disease; Diabetes esp in elderly; MS; Spinal inj. Occ surgery eg Abdoperineal resection. Drugs eg TCAD may → impotence. Impotence due to psychological cause is more likely to be intermittent than that due to physical cause

PREMATURE EJACULATION

Due to psychological cause. Often problem compounded by anxiety

INABILITY TO EJACULATE

Ejaculation is under parasympath

control. Inability to ejaculate usually due to psychological factors. Occ due to drugs eg α blockers

IMPAIRMENT OF F GENITAL RESPONSE

Equivalent to M erectile failure. Impairment of vaginal lubrication & vulval tumescence. Often problems of vaginal dryness do not impair sexual relationships. Physical factors inc the Menopause → atrophic vaginitis, vaginal infections → dyspareunia

ORGASMIC DYSFUNCTION: Equivalent to M ejaculatory incompetence. ↑ in F sexual arousal does not reach level to trigger orgasm. Usually psychogenic cause. In surveys many F state that they do not experience orgasm, however many of them do not complain of sexual problem

VAGINISMUS: Spasm of the perivaginal muscles. May cause non-consummation of marriage. Usually psychogenic cause

GENERAL RX OF DISORDERS RELATED TO SEXUAL PERFORMANCE

Counselling inc psychotherapy may be valuable in the Rx of both psychologically & physically caused sexual dysfunction. Usually important to include sexual partner in therapy. Sexual problems often result from: Negative feelings about sex which may have resulted from early socialisation; Ignorance about sex; Poor body image eg post-mastectomy; Resentment & insecurity regarding partner. Most methods involve directed behavioural psychotherapy eg Balint approach, Masters & Johnson method, in which counselling is linked c̄ the couple or patient carrying out specific tasks eg using graded dilators in Rx of vaginismus, or initially concentrating on foreplay without intercourse in Rx of orgasmic dysfunction. Remove any possible ppt drug. Anxiolytics are not usually helpful. Hormonal Rx for menopausal atrophic vaginitis. Occ penile implants for erectile failure

Sexual Deviations & Perversions

Sexual deviation can be defined as a sexual activity or fantasy which is not directed to an orgasm through genital intercourse c̄ a willing member of opposite sex & compatible sexual maturity, persistently & out of the norm of society

HOMOSEXUALITY

M>F. Quite common. Not a disease or perversion. Often difficulties in adjusting to this minority sexual variant are encountered both in the homosexual & his/her family. In some sections of society there are strong norms against homosexuality. Some are exclusively homosexual whilst others are bisexual. It is presumed that early socialisation is important in the development of homosexuality. The admission of homosexuality to others esp family can occur at any age but esp in early adulthood, & often causes psychological stress occ → suicide or other psychiatric disorder

RX: Counselling is aimed at allowing the person ± his/her family (occ inc partner) to understand their sexuality

EXHIBITIONISM (INDECENT EXPOSURE)

A condition in which a man achieves sexual excitement by inappropriately exposing his genitals to others esp women. Exhibitionists usually seek to evoke strong emotional reaction eg shock from others. Often masturbate after the act. Rarely ass c̄ rape

PAEDOPHILIA

Sexual attraction to & interference c̄ children. May be homo- or heterosexual desire. Usually adult M desire for young girls. Interference of adult M c̄ young boys is termed paederasty. Often paedophiles have a poor h/o sexual relationship c̄ adults

FETISHISM

Sexual arousal gained from the use of unusual objects or materials eg rubber. These objects may be only means of achieving sexual excitement. Usually begins in adolescence. May be related to transvestism. Occ clear h/o reason for development of fetish can be deduced

TRANSVESTISM

Sexual gratification derived from dressing up in the clothes of the opposite sex. M>F. Usually begins in adolescence. May occur in hetero- or homosexuals

SADISM

Sexual pleasure derived from inflicting pain esp by beating, whipping or tying partner. M>>F. May occur in hetero- or homosexuals. May → crime

MASOCHISM

Sexual pleasure derived from experiencing suffering. Occurs in M & F. Homo- & Heterosexuals

VOYEURISM (SCOPTOPHILIA)

Sexual gratification derived from watching the sexual practice of others, usually accompanied or followed by masturbation

BESTIALITY

Use of an animal as a means of achieving sexual excitement. Uncommon

GENERAL RX OF SEXUAL DEVIATIONS

If possible interview patient & regular sexual partner. Discuss aim of Rx c̄ the patient eg Is it to develop an ordinary heterosexual relationship?. Try to help patient identify cause of sexual deviancy. Counselling. Occ Oestrogens given to ↓ sexual drive. Important to curb sexual deviancy which harms others

GENERAL PROG

Often poor response to therapy. Much depends on motivation of patient

Trans-sexualism

An inward conviction that the individual has been born into the wrong sex. Rare. No abnormal physical factors. Cause unknown. Often behaviour & dress compatible c̄ the opposite sex. M>F. Usually feeling of having body of wrong sex begins pre-puberty. Occ Depression

RX: Usually do not seek psychological Rx but desire alterations to body image inc "change of sex" op. Electrolysis for undesired hair. Prolonged counselling is required before any drugs eg Oestrogens for breast enlargement or surgery is undertaken

Incest

Sexual intercourse between persons too closely related to contract a legal marriage. Usually refers to the sexual act of an adult family member esp M parent c̄ a child. Difficult to determine prevalence but probably not rare

RX: Although punishable by imprisonment, it is often better for the family if problems can be discussed & advice offered

Rape

Sexual intercourse by a man without the consent of the woman. Often involves violence. Offender often under influence of alcohol. Not uncommon for more than one person to take part in offence. Victim may suffer psychologically eg from feelings of humiliation, disgust of sex interfering c̄ subsequent sexual relationships, anxiety, depression, & physically eg from trauma, STD, pregnancy

RX: Psychological support for victim

PROG: Psychological effects may last years. Rapists often have a h/o crime but few are reconvicted for sexual offences

HYSTERIA

Hysteria is a term used in a number of ways. The WHO define as "Mental disorders in which motives, of which the patient seems unaware, produce either a restriction of the field of consciousness or disturbance of motor or sensory function which may seem to have psychological advantage or symbolic value". F>M. Esp Young adults. Hysterical symptoms are not due to physical abnormality & are produced unconsciously. However follow-up of diagnosed hysterical patients has shown that a significant minority in retrospect had organic disease. Occ hysterical symptoms coexist c̄ physical disease eg hysterical fits occuring in an epileptic

AETIOLOGY: The cause of hysteria is not known but can be explained in terms of role theory. The sick role confers some advantages & therefore is likely to be adopted whenever its adoption outweighs the advantages of health. Hence to many the sick role may be attractive when there is the possibility of financial gain ie "Compensation neurosis", the avoidance of trouble eg fear of prosecution, or the evasion of heavy role responsibilities eg soldiers in war. The traditional dependent role of children & women, theoretically could → manipulative behaviour to compensate for lack of power

Conversion Hysteria

The production of a symptom eg loss of sensation which according to psychoanalytic theory is the conversion of anxiety generated by sexual conflicts into a symbolic form. Others doubt this psychoanalytical theory & use the term more loosely for the unconscious conversion of anxiety into a bodily symptom which usually confers 2° gain eg the "shell shocked" soldier unable to fight due to hysterical paralysis

Dissociation Hysteria

The production of a state, usually amnesia or fugue, which serve to resolve or express some psychological conflict

Hysterical Personality

Hysteria is also used to describe a particular personality

CLIN: May have symptoms of conversion hysteria. Typically dramatic, attention seeking, egocentric, dependent, labile affect, immature, manipulative people N.B The term hysteria is also used by many doctors to describe patients esp F who are considered to be exaggerating symptoms &/or manipulating the doctor/patient relationship. Such patients may also be thought to be hypochondriacs

Mass Hysteria

The effect of suggestion → disturbed behaviour in a large gp of people. Esp Young F; Institutions

CLIN: May → sickness, disturbed behaviour. The particular symptom is determined by the instigators

St Louis Hysteria (Briquet's Syndrome)

Rare familial syndrome occuring in F

CLIN: Usually multiple physical symptoms esp dysmenorrhoea, dyspareunia, for which psychological explanation is strongly resisted. Often results in unnecessary ops

Ganser Syndrome

A syndrome of disturbance of consciousness, hallucinations & a tendency to give approx answers to obvious questions. Often ass c̄ Hysterical conversion symptoms; Impaired memory & attention. Occ malingering is suspected

General Rx

Exclude physical cause. The management strategy depends on underlying theory. If based on role theory then strategy is to demonstrate advantages of relinquishing the sick role. The psychoanalytic Rx would seek to determine unconscious motivation eg by hypnosis & then to remove cause of anxiety. Important not to insinuate that patient's symptoms are not genuine & to allow dignified withdrawal of symptoms

DD

Malingering differs from hysteria in that symptoms are deliberately feigned. Sometimes distinguishing between hysteria & malingering is impossible

HYPOCHONDRIASIS

A neurosis in which the major features are excessive concern c̄ one's general health, in the integrity of functioning of some part of one's body or less frequently one's mind. May coexist c̄ physical disorder when concern is disproportionate. Usually 2° to other psychiatric conditions eg Anxiety, Depression. May be an underlying personality disorder

CLIN: Many possible symptoms, often including Pain; GI symptoms; Palps. Occ Complaints about appearance eg dysmorphophobia

INVESTIGATION: • Exclude genuine physical pathology

RX: For 2° cases treat underlying condition. 1° cases are difficult to treat, behaviour therapy may help

Munchausen Syndrome

Repeated simulation of illness resulting in hospital admission. M>F. May be ass c̄ Psychopathy, Drug or Alcohol abuse, Malingering

CLIN: Variety of described symptoms eg Abdo pain, Chest pain. May use aliases to gain hospital admission

RX: Try to avoid unnecessary ops

AMNESIA

Loss of memory esp inability to remember past experiences

Causes of Amnesia (LIST 6 PSY)

1. Malingering
2. Alcohol
3. Head inj
4. Post-Ep
5. Hysteria
6. BG ↓
7. Severe delirium
8. Transient global amnesia

RX: Treat underlying condition. Narcoanalysis eg c̄ Na^+ thiopentone may be useful

PERSONALITY DISORDERS

Extreme & persistent variation from the normal range of one or more personality traits resulting in suffering for the subject or for others. The term used to describe the personality disorder is the most dominant of these traits. There is no clear cut division between normal & disordered personalities. The personality disorders predispose to psychiatric illness which is often of a corresponding type eg hysterical personality & hysterical neurosis, schizoid personality & schizophrenia. In addition personality disorders are ass c̄ alcoholism, problem drug taking & some forms of sexual deviation

8 types of abnormal personality are described by the WHO:

1. Paranoid: Sensitive; Suspicious; Strong self reference; Prone to develop overvalued ideas; "Idee Fixé". May be Vulnerable or Aggressive
2. Affective: Two forms
   a) Cyclothymic form: Swings of mood from gloomy despondency to elation, confidence &

overactivity. Ass c̄ manic–depressive psychosis
b) Hyperthymic form: Either a persistent gloomy or cheerful mood
3. Schizoid: Shy, reserved, introspective. Often eccentric, sensitive. Ass c̄ Schizophrenia
4. Explosive: Sudden impulsive outbursts of extreme anger. Often irritable, emotionally labile, verbally aggressive
5. Anankastic (*Obsessive–Compulsive*): Conscientious, perfectionist, stubborn, rigid, high ethical standards, insecure, lack of self-confidence, cautious. Ass c̄ Obsessional neurosis
6. Hysterical: Dramatic, attention seeking, egocentric, dependent, labile affect, immature, manipulative, histrionic. Ass c̄ Hysterical neurosis
7. Asthenic: Lacking energy & resilience to cope c̄ life, excessively dependent on others, passive, weak-willed
8. Psychopath (*Antisocial*): Emotionally cold, aggressive, irresponsible, impulsive. Repeated anti-social behaviour not modified by experience

GENERAL RX: Personality disorders are not amenable to radical change. Psychotherapy may allow person to have greater understanding of their undesirable traits & to make some improvements in behaviour

DRUG MISUSE

WHO define drug dependence as "a state, psychic, & sometimes also physical, resulting from the interaction between a living organism & a drug, characterised by behavioural & other responses that always includes a compulsion to take the drug on a continuous or periodic basis in order to experience its psychic effects sometimes to avoid the discomfort of abstinence. Tolerance may or may not be present". The ACMD describe the problem drug taker as "someone who experiences social, psychological, physical or legal problems related to intoxication &/or regular excessive consumption &/or dependence as a consequence of his own use of drugs or other chemical substances"
Drug misuse is increasing in prevalence esp due to ↑ illicit use of drugs esp opiates & cocaine & the ↑ prescription of psychotrophic drugs

AETIOLOGY: Drugs may be taken for a variety of reasons, often multifactorial. Drugs may be taken for direct pharmacological effects eg to obtain +ve effect such as intoxication or hallucinations, or to abolish −ve effects such as pain. Drugs also may be taken as part of a cultural life style, perhaps thereby allowing the misuser to become part of a group. Illicit drug misuse is commoner in young adults & M. Some have linked ↑ prevalence to the worsening social prospects for this sub-gp eg unemployment. However drug misuse is seen in all social strata

GENERAL CLIN: May be a preceding h/o other drug or substance misuse. Occ h/o disturbed family background. The circumstances surrounding drug usage can influence its effect. The route of drug taking can alter effects eg heroin may be injected, inhaled or smoked & be ass c̄ different SE eg IV route ass c̄ abscesses, thromb, HepB. The effect on social functioning is variable, some regular opiate takers have a job & social stability, but many may resort to crime to finance habit &/or descend social scale. Degree of dependence is variable, although long term use is ass c̄ ↑ dependence. Occ drugs, even heroin, can be used irregularly for a long period of time without evidence of loss of control. Often drug misusers may switch from chosen drug, when unavailable, to another even though it may be pharmacologically unrelated. Many of drug misuser's contacts may also be drug misusers
Occ Physical complications eg Hep; o/d; Acute organic psychoses esp paranoid & schizophrenia-like states

RX: Appropriate management of physical complications, acute organic psychoses & o/ds. Usually best to have a problem orientated approach c̄ dependence seen as an interaction between the drug, the individual & his environment rather than a substance-orientated approach. Following assessment, a therapeutic contract should be drawn up between doctor & drug-taker which defines type, purpose & duration of Rx & any relevant stipulations eg regular attendance at OPD, no use of other drugs

Detoxification: Drugs which induce physical dependence, if stopped abruptly, → withdrawal symptoms. These symptoms are controlled by a graduated reduction in dosage of a substitute drug from a similar pharmacological group eg Methadone for opiate dependence, Pentabarbitone for barbiturate dependence. The aim is for the patient to be neither intoxicated or in withdrawal. Usually withdrawal from drugs can be achieved in 2–3wks

Treatment options to be considered by the doctor include:

1. Non-prescribing support: Abrupt cessation of drug taking c̄ supportive measures. Appropriate for withdrawal from stimulant drugs eg Cocaine, Amphetamines
2. Oral drug withdrawal: A graduated reduction of drug dosage → withdrawal. May be inpatient or outpatient procedure. OPD procedure is less easy to monitor eg requires urine testing service & is more subject to non-compliance. If possible avoid tablets as they may be crushed & injected
3. Maintenance prescribing: A temporary measure in response to claims that clinical improvement will result eg due to change in social or legal situation. Should be reviewed regularly by a specialised unit
4. Detoxification c̄ other psychotherapeutic intervention: Drugs are withdrawn in appropriate manner. Psychotherapeutic methods include social skills training, individual & group psychotherapy, marital & family counselling, work rehab. Such Rx should be undertaken by specialised units
5. Therapeutic communities & rehab houses: These facilities are usually run by non-statutory organisations. Their patterns of Rx vary but usually residents are expected to be totally drug free within the community & to develop ways of coping without drugs. Often prolonged programmes for the resident are the norm eg 1–2yrs

If no agreement can be reached c̄ the drug misuser, Rx should be geared to providing the minimum support compatible c̄ safe medical management. Occ underlying psychiatric problems are uncovered, any drug Rx for these conditions should be closely monitored

In the UK, Heroin & Cocaine can only be prescribed to drug addicts by "Home Office" licenced doctors. Any doctor who attends a person & suspects addiction to certain drugs inc Heroin & Cocaine must notify the "Home Office"

GENERAL PROG: The desire to stop illicit drug taking is partly dependent on social factors eg heroin addicts during Vietnam war on returning to USA were usually able to abstain from drug abuse. Some evidence that as people mature they are more able to cease drug misuse. Some drugs esp opiates cause considerable mort & morbidity

Specific Pharmacological Aspects

NARCOTIC ABUSE

Includes Opium, Morphine, Heroin, Methadone. May be administered by various routes

CLIN: Pain relief; Intense pleasure; Relaxation. Between administrations may → Apathy; Clouding of consciousness; Constipation; N; Constricted pupils; ↓ sexual desire. Infections from unsterile injections are common. o/d may → Resp distress; BP ↓; Pulm oedema; Ep; Constricted pupils; Hypothermia; Arrhythmias; RF; Coma. Tolerance & physical dependence often develop. Withdrawal symptoms may be severe c̄ Craving for drug; Drowsiness; Restlessness; Jt pains; Myalgia; Sweating; Abdo pain; Diarrhoea; Rhinorrhoea; Dilated pupils. Withdrawal symptoms are less severe & shorter lasting c̄ Methadone

INVESTIGATION: • Urinary opiate levels

RX: Treat o/d by clearing airway, IV Naloxone. Occ ventilation required. Naloxone is a competitive antagonist & the dose required depends on amount of particular agonist taken. Sudden reversal of o/d can → Tachypnoea; Pupillary dilation; PR ↑; BP ↑; Tremor

COCAINE

Can be inhaled, drunk eg in wine or injected sc

CLIN: Euphoria; ↑ energy; Dilated pupils. Occ "Cocaine Psychosis" ie Tactile hallucinations esp insects crawling over skin (formication) & paranoia; Confusion; Depression. Sniffing of cocaine may → perf of nasal septum. May → psych dependence

INVESTIGATION: • Urinary cocaine levels

AMPHETAMINES

Can be used orally or IV

CLIN: Temporary Euphoria; Insomnia; ↑ energy; Anorexia. Followed by Depression; Irritability; Anxiety. Hence psych dependence occurs quickly. May → "Amphetamine Psychosis" ie paranoia, visual or auditory hallucinations; Stereotype behaviour. Tolerance occurs

INVESTIGATION: • Urinary amphetamine level

RX: Psychosis resolves about 1wk after drug withdrawal. Phenothiazines may be needed to treat psychosis

LSD

Taken orally

CLIN: PR ↑; Dilated pupils. May → Depression ("bad trip") or Ecstasy ("good trip"); Perceptual distortions. Occ "Trips" ("flashbacks") may occur some time after taking drug. Occ ppt psychosis

PHENCYCLIDINE (PCP, ANGEL DUST)

May be inhaled, smoked, eaten or injected

CLIN: Small doses → Intoxication; Analgesia; Restlessness. May → Psychosis; BP ↑; Nystagmus. Larger doses → Ataxia; Muscle rigidity; Ep; Uncommunicativeness. Rarely → Hyperthermia; Ht fail; BP ↑ crisis. Withdrawal symptoms inc Craving for drug; Depression

INVESTIGATION: • Urine levels

RX: Symptomatic Rx eg Haloperidol for psychosis. Desimipramine for withdrawal symptoms

BARBITURATES

May be taken orally or IV. Tolerance develops less rapidly than c̄ opiates

CLIN: May → Ataxia; Nystagmus; Slurred speech; Depression. Injections may → infection eg abscesses, phlebitis, ulcers. Withdrawal symptoms include Insomnia; Anxiety; Tremor; Ep; Delirium; N&V; Hallucinations; Pyrexia. o/d are common & may be fatal esp due to resp depression

CANNABIS (POT, HASH, HASHISH, MARIJUANA, GRASS)

Active component is tetrahydrocannabinol. Usually smoked. Can be taken orally or IV. Very common

CLIN: Acute effects are usually relaxation, ↑ sociability, feeling of well being. Rarely perceptual delusions or hallucinations. Effects of long term use uncertain. Psych dependence common but no tolerance or physical dependence. No strong evidence that cannabis use predisposes to the use of more dangerous ("harder") drugs

SOLVENTS

Commonly abused products are glue, aerosols, petrol, cleaning fluids. Usually solvents are either "huffed" ie applied to a cloth & held to the mouth or "bagged" ie inhaled from plastic bag containing solvent. Esp M teenagers

CLIN: Symptoms vary according to type of solvent
Glues may → acute symptoms of Euphoria; Dizziness; Confusion; Incoordination; N; Coma. Chr effects may occur after <1yr of solvent abuse & inc Lethargy; Anorexia; Moodiness; & rarely neurological symptoms eg periph neuropathy, encephalopathy. A few deaths have occured
Aerosols containing fluorinated hydrocarbons (Freons) may be cardiotoxic & deaths due to arrhythmias may occur

INVESTIGATION: • GLC of blood

RX: Health education. Restrictions of sales of solvents to non-adults. Treat o/d by removing from polluted atmosphere & giving O_2. May need supportive therapy

PROBLEM DRINKING

Alcohol problems are very common esp in the many societies where the "drug" is legal & culturally accepted. Prevalence of drinking is ass c̄ cost of alcohol, cultural norms. Definition of alcoholism can refer to drinking behaviour, behaviour while drinking or consequences of drinking behaviour. The WHO definition is "alcoholics are those excessive drinkers whose dependence on alcohol has attained such a degree that they show a noticeable mental disturbance or an interference c̄ their mental & bodily health, their interpersonal relations & their smooth economic & social functioning, or who show prodromal signs of such developments". M>F. ↓ prevalence c̄ ↑ age in M, but ↑ prevalence c̄ ↑ age in F. Young single people are usually heaviest drinkers. Urban >Rural. Certain high risk occupations eg Brewery workers, Fishermen. Numbers c̄ alcohol problems are difficult to assess, the Lederman formula derives the expected number of heavy drinkers from the mean per capita consumption

AETIOLOGY: Usually multifactorial. Host factors can inc Small genetic effect; Deviant parental lifestyle; Personality disorders eg psychopathy; Pattern of consumption eg more problems if alcohol taken in binges. Environmental factors can inc Cultural norms eg drunkenness is not disapproved of by the Irish; Occupation esp a job milieu that promotes drinking eg journalism, doctors. Agent factors can inc Availability ie price, outlet controls, purchasing controls; Marketing/Promotions

CLIN: There are many alcohol-related problems. Some people pass through a clear sequence of stages ie Pre-alcoholic stage c̄ ↑ in alcohol tolerance; Stage of psychological dependence eg social P to drink or to relieve stress; Stage of physical dependence c̄ loss of control of consumption & withdrawal symptoms if alcohol unavailable. Chr abuse → ↓ alcohol tolerance, ↓ attention to other aspects of lifestyle & often physical, psychiatric & social problems. (Jellinek described 5 sub-gps of drinking problem:

Alpha— Psychological dependence only, symptomatic drinking.

Beta— Drinking appropriate to social upbringing, physical complications without dependence.

Gamma— Physical dependence c̄ loss of control.

Delta— Inability to abstain, physical dependence c̄ loss of control.

Epsilon— Dipsomania, bout drinking)

Most present c̄ symptoms that had not been recognised as related to alcohol eg marital problems, depression, anxiety, lethargy, blackouts, insomnia, gastritis

Physical disease ass c̄ alcohol inc Cirrhosis; Hepatitis; Fatty Liver; Pancreatitis; PU; GI bleed; TB; Mallory–Weiss syndrome; Gastritis; Malabsorption; Diarrhoea; IBS; Pseudo-Cushing's syndrome; BG ↑ or ↓; Obesity; M hypogonadism; Anaemia; Haemochromatosis; Myopathy; Cardiomyopathy; BP ↑; Vitamin defs; Liver Ca; Wernicke's encephalopathy; Amblyopia; Cerebellar degeneration; Periph neuropathy. Large alcohol intake in pregnancy → foetal alcohol syndrome, but smaller intakes probably also → neonatal problems

Ass social problems inc Accidents esp RTA; Crime; Loss of employment; Child abuse inc NAI; Debt. Drinking is generally less socially acceptable in F & attempts to hide evidence of drinking often occur earlier

Intoxication refers to an alcohol induced state of mental & physical inco-ordination. Uncharacteristic disinhibited behaviour ranging from violence to passivity. Occ Lapses of memory; Attempted suicide; Suicide; Fugue states; Ep. Hangovers due to alcohol toxicity & congeners in drinks esp red wines, port, usually → depression, headache, N, dehydration, irritability

Psychiatric problems related to regular excessive consumption inc Marital & family discord; Poor memory; Perseveration; Poor concentration; Wernicke's encephalopathy; Korsakoff psychoses; Dementia; Mood disturbance esp depression; Anxiety. Rarer conditions are Hallucinations;

Cerebellar signs; Morbid jealousy (Othello syndrome ie paranoid delusions & jealousy related to imagined infidelity of spouse)
Withdrawal symptoms occur in cases of physical dependence. Mild symptoms inc Anxiety; Insomnia; Irritability; Anorexia; Sweating; PR ↑. Severe symptoms inc Delirium tremens (ie Disorientation; Confusion; Hallucinations; Terror; Agitation; PR ↑; Tremor; Tachypnoea; BP ↑) occurring about 3 days after stopping drinking; Withdrawal fits usually 1–3 days after last drink; Transient psychotic or affective illness

INVESTIGATIONS:
- FBC
- GGT
- Screening questionnaires eg Michigan alcoholism screening test
- Occ blood alcohol level

PREVENTION: It is difficult to state whether there is a safe level of drinking. Small amounts of alcohol may be cardioprotective. In general, F respond to same dose of alcohol c̄ higher blood levels than M. Health education programmes may benefit but effect of alcohol advertising acts as countervailing force. Licensing controls, increasing cost & control of sales to the young, reduction of sales outlets & possibly curbs on advertising, all ↓ alcohol intake

RX: Discuss lifestyle of problem drinker & determine drinking pattern's relationship to lifestyle. Try to promote trust & agreement that change of alcohol use will be beneficial. Also discuss c̄ partner ± family & friends. Identify problems in maintaining abstinence eg friends usually meet in pub, & agree strategies to handle these problems. Review regularly to assess progress & give encouragement. Self-help gps eg Alcoholics Anonymous may be helpful as they are non-judgemental, offer peer support, offer contact c̄ new social gp c̄ strong identification, & available 24hrs a day. Support from statutory eg social worker, CPN & non-statutory agencies often helpful. Specialised counselling is often helpful for marital problems, sexual problems, depression & phobias
Psychological assessment of drunks is difficult. Close supervision whilst sobering-up is important eg difficult to exclude subdural haematoma
Disulfiram (c/i in advanced liver disease, pregnancy, suicidal depression; SE: Lethargy, Periph neuropathy) acts as a deterrent to alcohol abuse as imbibing alcohol → PR ↑; Tachypnoea; N; Flushing. If possible ensure that administration of drug is supervised. Antidepressants eg Mianserin may aid late depression following abstinence
Withdrawal symptoms require reassurance, regular monitoring, Thiamine. Correction of any metabolic imbalance. Diazepam or Phenytoin for fits. Chlormethiazole for more major withdrawal signs. Hallucinations may require Haloperidol

PROG: Abstinence improves prog of almost all physical problems inc irreversible disease such as cirrhosis. Early detection & advice aids return to problem free drinking. Few c̄ major alcohol problems are eventually able to re-establish problem free drinking. Many problem drinkers do improve, but poor prognostic signs inc poor pre-morbid personality & social isolation

PHENOMENOLOGY

The description of symptoms of psychopathology

Psychopathological Symptoms
(LIST 7 PSY)

A. DISORDERS OF PERCEPTION
1. Sensory distortions:
   a) Changes in intensity eg Hyperaesthesia
   b) Changes in quality
   c) Changes in spatial form eg Macropsia
2. Sensory deceptions:
   a) Illusions ie a perceptual distortion whereby a stimulus is misinterpreted

b) True Hallucinations ie no insight, can't be willed away, in ext space

c) Pseudo Hallucinations ie insight, can't be willed away, in ext space

d) Imagery Hallucinations ie insight, can be willed away, int concept

B. DISORDERS OF THOUGHT

1. Disorders of stream:

a) Tempo eg Flight of Ideas, Retardation, Circumstantiality

b) Continuity eg Perseveration (ie continued repetition of speech or activity), Blocking

2. Disorders of possession of thought:

a) Obsessions

b) Alienation eg Thought insertion, Thought withdrawal

3. Disorders of content: Delusions are incorrigible false beliefs inconsistent c the information available & c the beliefs of the subject's social gp

a) 1° delusion

b) 2° delusion eg based on jealousy, paranoia, love, grandeur, guilt, ill health, nihilism

4. Formal thought disorders eg Schizophrenia:

a) Disorder of heuristic thought ie rational problem solving

b) Disorder of deirestic thought ie inwardly directed fantasy

C. DISORDERS OF MEMORY

1. Amnesia:

a) Psychogenic

b) Organic

2. Distortion:

a) Recall eg Confabulation, Retrospective falsification, Retrospective delusion, "Pathological lying"

b) Recognition eg "Deja-vu", "Dèja vecu", "Jamais-vu", Capgras syndrome

D. DISORDERS OF EMOTION

1. Depression

2. Mania

3. Anxiety

E. DISORDERS OF EXPERIENCE OF SELF

Passivity experiences

F. DISORDERS OF CONSCIOUSNESS

1. Disorientation

2. Delirium

Neurotic disorders are mental disorders without any demonstrable organic basis in which the person may have considerable insight & has unimpaired reality testing in that he usually does not confuse his morbid subjective experiences & fantasies c̄ ext reality. Behaviour may be greatly affected although usually remaining within socially acceptable limits, but personality is not disorganised (WHO) Psychoses are a gp of psychiatric conditions whose symptoms are qualitatively different from normal experience. There is often loss of contact c̄ reality, loss of insight, deterioration of personality. Functional psychoses are of unknown cause, whilst organic psychoses are due to known physical factors affecting brain

DEFENCE MECHANISMS

A set of processes have been formulated to explain certain kinds of experience or behaviour. Originally based on Freudian theory

Denial

Person behaves as though unware of something that he may reasonably be expected to know

Repression

The involuntary removal from consciousness of ideas & urges to action which would cause distress if allowed to enter consciousness. Suppression refers to a conscious action

Projection

Unconscious displacement to another person of thoughts or feelings that are one's own, thereby rendering the original feelings more acceptable

Displacement

Unconscious shifting of emotion from an object or situation to another situation

Regression

Unconscious adoption of behaviour appropriate to earlier stage in individual & social development

Sublimation

The unconscious diversion of undesirable or forbidden impulses into more socially acceptable channels

Rationalisation

Self deception by finding acceptable reasons for conduct which is really prompted by less worthy motives

Reaction Formation

Unconscious adoption of behaviour opposite to that which would reflect true feelings & intentions. Eg prudish attitude to mention of sex may occur in someone c̄ strong but not consciously accepted sexual drives

Identification

Unconscious placing of oneself in the activities or characteristics of another person. May be used to reduce pain of separation or loss

Compensation

Development of personal quality to offset a defect or sense of inferiority

Fixation

Arrest of development of personality at stage short of emotional maturity

SCHIZOPHRENIA

Schizophrenia is not easy to define as there are disputes as to the definition of its boundaries. WHO define as "a gp of psychoses in which there is a fundamental disturbance of personality, a characteristic distortion of thinking, often a sense of being controlled by alien forces, delusions which may be bizarre, disturbed perception, abnormal affect out of keeping c̄ the real situation, & autism. Nevertheless, clear consciousness & intellectual capacity are usually maintained". Common. Peak incidence 25–30yrs. Esp Single; Immigrants. Ass c̄ pre-morbid schizoid personality

AETIOLOGY: Some genetic predisposition shown by twin studies. May be ass c̄ chr Ep. The dopamine hypothesis proposes that schizophrenia is ass c̄ overactivity in certain dopaminergic systems in the brain (?limbic system) & is supported by the inhibition of dopamine transmission by anti-schizophrenic drugs. Psychodynamic theories have postulated that schizophrenia develops as a reaction to or defence against, abnormal communications within the family but little supportive evidence

CLIN: Schizophrenic symptoms tend to change in intensity & nature. Many symptoms can occur & therefore diagnosis based on classical (first rank) symptoms
Generally accepted are Schneider's first rank symptoms: Thought insertion ie experience of thoughts being put into one's mind; Thought withdrawal ie experience of thought being removed from one's mind; Thought broadcasting ie experience of one's thoughts being known to others; Feelings of passivity

ie experience of sensations, emotions or bodily mvts being under ext control; Primary delusion ie delusions arising inexplicably from normal perceptions; Third person auditory hallucinations inc voices discussing or arguing about one, voices commentating on thoughts or behaviour, voices repeating one's thoughts ("Echo de la pensee"), voices anticipating one's thought
Added important diagnostic symptoms inc: Affective change eg blunting of affect, incongruity of affect, mood lability; Formal thought disorder ie lack of causal link between thoughts (asyndetic "Knight's move" thinking), use of imprecise approximations (metonyms), interpenetration of themes, overinclusiveness (ie no boundaries to concept), inability to think abstractly inc "concretism", creation of new words (neologisms)
Rarely Catatonic states ie mutism & immobility c̄ no impairment of consciousness; "Folie a deux" ie transfer of paranoid delusions from psychotic to an associate; Capgras syndrome ie the delusional negation of identity of a familiar person
Often only a few of these principal symptoms may be present. Other less typical symptoms inc: Non-auditory hallucinations; 2° delusions; Time disorientation (in chr schizophrenics)
Clin types ie simple, hebephrenic, paranoid, catatonic, residual, are recognised but overlap between features limits their value
Occ acute episode c̄ clouding of consciousness (oneirophrenia) which may remit spontaneously. Acute episodes may occur in puerperium. Usually chr course, often → decline in social status. Occ Suicide

RX: Assess patient & family. Chlorpromazine & Haloperidol for acute phase. ECT for catatonia & severe depression. Planning & provision of a rehabilitative programme, if possible involving family, friends & workmates (a peaceful supportive atmosphere seems beneficial). Maintenance Rx c̄ depot phenothiazine injections (SE inc: Tardive dyskinesia, Parkinsonism, Atropine like affects, J, Photosensitivity). Specific family education & supervision may be helpful. Change of work to a more sheltered environment may be required, but the multidisciplinary rehabilitation team should try & preserve the drive & initiative of the patient & prevent institutionalisation

PROG: Bad pre-morbid factors are FH of schizophrenia; Schizoid personality; Poor work record; Disturbed family relationships. Poor prog features of illness are Lack of obvious ppt cause; Gradual onset; Flattening of affect; Loss of drive; No affective or catatonic symptoms; Delayed Rx

DD:
1. TLE
2. Drug induced psychosis esp LSD, Amphetamines
3. Dementia
4. GPI
5. Affective psychosis
6. Personality disorders
7. ?Alcohol abuse

Special Forms

SCHIZOAFFECTIVE PSYCHOSIS

The coexistence of schizophrenic symptoms c̄ affective symptoms.
3 forms which are all bipolar ie Anxiety–elation psychosis; Confusion psychosis; Motility psychosis. Typically a relapsing & remitting course is observed (cycloid psychoses)

PARANOIA & PARANOID STATES

Many people c̄ prominent delusions of persecution but without first rank symptoms subsequently develop schizophrenia or an affective psychosis. Prominent paranoid features in schizophrenia are commoner in late onset form esp in F (paranoid schizophrenia)

Causes of Paranoid States (LIST 8 PSYCH)

1. Paranoid personality
2. Acute paranoid reaction
3. Paranoid schizophrenia
4. Affective disorders
5. Organic paranoid states: Eg Delerium, Alcohol abuse, Amphetamines
6. Paraphrenia

GJESSING'S SYNDROME

Very rare. Periodic catatonia ass c̄ changes in nitrogen balance

EROTOMANIA (DE CLERAMBAULT'S SYNDROME)

Delusion of being loved by another person esp stranger of high social status. F>M. May be isolated phenomenon or 2° esp to schizophrenia

RX: Phenothiazines

THE SICK DOCTOR

In general, doctors suffer more mental illness & less physical illness than the general pop. Suicide, cirrhosis, alcoholism, drug dependency & depression are particularly common compared to average. Drug dependency is partly an occupational hazard, drugs being easily available. Suicide rates increase from early middle age esp in the single or divorced & in women. Doctor's wives also have a high incidence of alcohol & drug abuse, & depression

RX: Recognition of or action about the problem may be delayed because of understandable but misplaced support from medical colleagues. Illness may result in reference to the GMC to consider fitness to practice

CULTURE BOUND DISORDERS

Some psychiatric conditions are typically ass c̄ particular cultures eg Amok, Koro

Amok

Esp Malasia, Indonesia

CLIN: Prodromal brooding. Homicidal outbursts for no apparent reason c̄ rapid resolution & apparent amnesia for preceding event. Occ egotistic personality. Often poorly educated

RX: Occ opportunities for intervention & prevention of amok episode

Koro

Esp Chinese in S.E. Asia. May occur in epidemics

CLIN: Panic reaction that penis is disappearing into abdo. Penis may be tied to piece of string

RX: Reassurance & psychotherapy

Chiliastic Syndromes

Demonstrable mental disorder → messianic feelings. Egg in China, the Taiping movement was led by one who claimed to be the younger brother of Jesus; in Melanesia, the Cargo cult Syndrome

Possession Syndrome

Belief that body is possessed or interacting c̄ an alien often ancesteral, spirit. Common traditional belief in some cultures. Syndrome may be present during dreams or ass c̄ religious services

RX: Psychotherapy may benefit

Latah

Esp Malaysian F

CLIN: A state of automatism ppt by stress

Windigo Psychosis

Belief seen amongst some N.Am Indians that patient has become a monster. May cannibalise other tribe members

PSYCHIATRIC DISORDERS AMONGST IMMIGRANTS

Immigration is a stressful life event which may ppt mental illness. The different cultural expression of mental illness may cause diagnostic difficulty eg Asians are likely to present c̄ somatic manifestations of mental illness. Knowledge of the language used to describe illness in varying cultures is important. Misinterpretation of cultural norms can → misdiagnosis eg many rural Indians believe in the "evil eye". The clash of cultures may lead to hostility & resentment which may be diagnosed as mental illness eg as paranoia amongst young Blacks in industrial settings. Psychotic reactions to stress are commoner in non-Western societies & do not necessarily indicate schizophrenic tendencies. Wild excited uncontrolled behaviour is not uncommon in W.Indian immigrants in UK, & is more commonly a reactive excitation rather than mania. Hysterical symptoms are typically culturally specific

Common stressful factors in immigrants are Racial discrimination; Socio-economic deprivation; Loneliness & isolation; Intergenerational conflicts eg differing moral codes, different pattern of family structure; Frustrated ambition

RX: Need to understand cultural setting of symptomatology. If interpreter required, avoid the untrained & the use of children. Rarely repatriation requires consideration

Child & Adolescent Psychiatry

During childhood, psych disorder is commoner in M. Incidence of mental & emotional illnesses rise during adolescence & by late adolescence are commoner in F. In childhood, conduct disorders are common whilst in adolescence depression & attempted suicide are common. Predispositions inc family discord, maternal deprivation, organic brain disorder, non-neurological chr physical illness, illness in close family member, IQ ↓. Higher rates are seen in illegitimate & amongst immigrants

Children often react to psychological disturbance & life stresses c̄ somatic symptoms. Many children attending doctors have psychological problems often in ass c̄ physical disease eg asthma, diabetes

Families who set their children clear consistent rules & enforce them firmly & kindly rarely have problems. Successful Rx of a problem depends on the family's capacity to put advice into practice

The form of presentation is dependent at least as much on the age of the child as on the underlying cause

HYPERKINETIC SYNDROME

Characterised by overactivity, distractability, irritability, restlessness. May be ass c̄ antisocial behaviour, mild CNS signs. May be h/o birth trauma or other early developmental insult. Hyperkinesis may be ass c̄ mental handicap, clumsiness. Not clearly distinguished from persistent overactivity. M>F. Ass c̄ Alcoholism, psychopathy or hysteria in close family members; Maternal depression; Marital dysharmony

CLIN: Overactivity usually decreases c̄ age.

Difficulties at school & c̄ peers are commom. Emotional lability

RX: Distinguish from an active child whose parents perceive as having the syndrome, when re-education of parents is required. Avoid overstimulation, excess fatigue & known ppt factors. Develop regular routine. Ed Psych may help c̄ schooling problems. CNS stimulants eg Dexamphetamine usually benefit but should only be used for short term educational objective. Rx of family members occ indicated

NIGHTMARES

Very common in childhood esp pre-school. May cause anxiety & fear. Commoner in anxious children

RX: Avoid overexcitement during the day. Reassure child before sleep & after the event

NIGHT TERRORS

Uncommon as a persistent symptom. Intense anxiety & screaming at night c̄ amnesia for the episode. Marked autonomic disturbance

RX: Occ require drugs eg Diazepam

ENCOPRESIS

Less common than enuresis. M>F. ?commoner in families preoccupied c̄ toilet training. 1° form represents child who is late in developing faecal continence. 2° form is the regression from previous continence & may represent a severe emotional problem. Constipation c̄ overflow is a third form which may reflect fear of the toilet or conflict between parent & child. Rarely encopresis due to physical cause eg Hirschprung's

RX: 1° & 2° forms usually responds to structured toilet training c̄ positive reward for success. Any ass emotional or social problems require attention. Constipation & overflow require laxatives or suppositories to relieve obst. Then toilet training

TEMPER TANTRUMS

Esp young children. Common cause of parental concern. If persistent may reflect family problems

RX: Reward good behaviour; Give child clear expectations & rules

HABIT DISORDERS

Include Tics, Hair pulling, Breath holding, Stammering, Head banging. Esp 7yrs to puberty

RX: Only require Rx if persistent. Psychiatric & social assessment. Exclude organic factors. Behavioural therapy

GILLES DE LA TOURETTE SYNDROME

Rare. M>F. Onset usually in childhood

CLIN: Tics, initially of face then spreading to body. Then develop involuntary utterances inc barking & obscene words or phrases. Occ Echolalia & Echopraxia ie imitating the speech & action of others

RX: Haloperidol c̄ careful monitoring to ↓ risk of SE; Behaviour therapy

STAMMERING

A disturbance of the rhythm & fluency of speech. M>F. Usually a transient stage in early speech development but occ persist to school age. Cause unknown. Usually not ass c̄ psychiatric disorder but may → anxiety & embarassment

RX: Speech therapy

DYSLEXIA

A centrally determined difficulty in learning to read occuring in the absence of other handicap. Quite common. Esp Low social class. M>F. Urban >Rural. Occ FH; Overt CNS disorder

CLIN: Discrepancy between actual reading performance, & age & intelligence. Variable reading problems eg inability to distinguish letter forms, transposing letters, omissions & additions of words, poor comprehension. Often detected in early school career. Often Poor spelling; Dysgraphia; School failure. Occ → juvenile delinquency

INVESTIGATION: • Psychoeducational tests eg Wechsler intelligence test

RX: Assessment by Ed Psych ± psychiatrist. Speciai tuition. Involve parents in therapy

PROG: Best if Early intervention; Good social background

DD: General reading backwardness eg ass c̄ visual, hearing, motor handicap or mental retardation

Causes of Delayed Speech Development (LIST 9 PSY)

1. Mental Handicap
2. Deafness
3. Emotional deprivation
4. Autism
5. Dyslexia
6. Elective mutism
7. Familial delayed maturation

ELECTIVE MUTISM

A refusal to speak in certain circumstances eg school. Often ass c̄ other – ve behaviour. Cause unknown. Rare

RX: Difficult, but usually spontaneous remission after months or years

SCHOOL PHOBIA

Reluctance to attend school due to fear of separation from mother or less commonly fear of teachers or peers. Esp 11–13yrs

CLIN: May present as obvious separation anxiety or c̄ somatic symptoms eg headache, abdo pain prior to school

RX: Emphasise requirement to return to school immediately. May be useful to involve both parents & the school. Psychotherapy & or behaviour therapy may be of benefit. Underlying family dysfunction may be uncovered & require Rx

DD: Truancy (staying away from school to do something more enjoyable. Ass c̄ poor parental control, poor school performance & delinquency)

PICA

The practice of eating non-nutritious substances eg earth. In infants may represent normal exploratory behaviour. In children occurs esp in mentally handicapped, autistic, emotionally deprived. May → Failure to thrive; Lead poisoning

RX: Keep child away from abnormal items of diet

PROG: Pica usually improves c̄ age

"GROWING PAINS"

Limb pains without identifiable physical cause. Psychological factors are important

PERIODIC SYNDROME

(CHRONIC RECURRENT ABDO PAIN)

Esp 5–14yrs. Parents often poor communicators. Occ life events seem to ppt onset of pain

CLIN: Recurrent episodes of GIT symptoms esp chr recurrent abdo pain & cyclical Vom. No signs between episodes

RX: Exclude organic cause (avoid extensive investigations). Try to reduce ppt stress eg re anxiety over going to school. Occ may try minor tranquillisers

PROG: Tendency to have abdo symptoms as adult. Minor tranquillisers often of no benefit esp in young children

CHILDHOOD NEUROSES

Children usually show diverse combinations of neurotic symptoms rather than classical adult forms. Isolated phobias & rituals are common.

Emotional disorders common between 7yrs & puberty inc phobias, anxiety, unhappiness & poor relations c̄ peers

Childhood Phobia

Common. Esp 4–12yrs

RX: Desensitisation. Occ short term minor tranquillisers may benefit

Anxiety States

CLIN: Overdependent on parents; Timid c̄ other children. Often Disturbed sleep; Nightmares; Headaches; Vom; Abdo pain. May be ppt event eg hospital admission, separation from parents

RX: Discuss worries c̄ child. Parent's management of child may need review. Anxiolytic drugs rarely indicated

Childhood Depression

Usually reactive. May occur 2° to physical illness eg Post Hep

CLIN: Often Abdo pain; Headaches; Anorexia; Difficulty in falling asleep; Weeping. Occ ass c̄ obsession. Suicide is very rare. Bipolar form rarely seen

RX: Psychotherapy; TCAD. Remove ppt factors if possible

CHILDHOOD PSYCHOSES

Rare gp of conditions inc autism, childhood schizophrenia & organic psychoses eg lipidoses

Autism

A syndrome of withdrawal from people & language abnormalities. M>F. Many are mentally handicapped. Partly genetic aetiology. ?due to specific CNS damage

CLIN: Onset before 3yrs. Mutism or abnormal speech eg nominal aphasia, echolalia; Poor understanding of speech; Poor emotional contact c̄ others eg avoidance of eye contact, failure to cuddle; Rituals & routines; Resistance to unfamiliarity. Poor perception of ext stimuli. Occ Lability of mood; Poor pain response; Self-injury; Mobility defect—may be hyperkinetic or ↓ mobility. Often later develop Ep

RX: Special schooling. Try to build on any talents present

PROG: Poor esp if low IQ. Usually improve in later childhood but about 66% remain totally dependent as adults

Childhood Schizophrenia

Rare. Usually presents in adolescence. May be FH. Often pre-morbid schizoid personality

CLIN: Similar to adult. Auditory hallucinations usually less well developed

RX: As for adults

PROG: Probably worse than for adult-onset schizophrenia

CHILDHOOD DEMENTIA

Interference c̄ normal behaviour & personality due to impairment of thought & memory → the loss or slowing down of the acquisition of developmental skills. Rare. Most due to underlying progressive CNS disorder but some treatable causes

Causes of Childhood Dementia (LIST 10 PSY)

A. NON-DEGENERATIVE DISORDERS
   1. Anticonvulsant induced encephalopathy
   2. Leukaemia Rx
   3. Myoclonic Ep
   4. Treatable metabolic disorders: Eg Diet change in PKU children; Some inborn errors in urea cycle
   5. Adverse social condition

B. PROGRESSIVE
   Eg Gangliosidoses, Lipidoses, Ataxia–telangiectasia, Wilson's disease, SSPE, Huntington's chorea, Lesch–Nyhan syndrome

Disintegrative or degenerative psychosis is a term used to describe children who develop dementia after normal development for 2.5yrs. After rapid deterioration lasting 6–9mths, condition stabilises. Motor function usually preserved. No cause usually found

INVESTIGATIONS INC:
- CAT scan
- Psychometric testing
- Lysosomal enzyme assay
- Histochemical analysis of rectal biopsies: +ve in the neuronal ceroid lipofuscinoses
- Brain biopsy: To diagnose Alexander's leucodystrophy, Canavan's disease

RX: Treat any reversible condition. For some conditions genetic counselling is indicated. Special schooling. Usually multidisciplinary support eg from doctor, social worker, Ed Psych is beneficial

ANOREXIA NERVOSA

F>M. Esp adolescents. Parents are usually older than ave. Cause unknown, ?phobic avoidance to food resulting from the sexual & social tensions generated by the physical changes ass c̄ puberty

CLIN: Fear of being overweight & often a distorted body image → activities to reduce wt inc excess dieting, exercise, induction of vomiting following food. As wt falls amenorrhoea & lanugo hair develop. Appetite usually reduces but some have periodic binges followed by induced vomiting (bulimia). Wt may fall to life threatening level

RX: Usually require hospital admission. Insist on eating reasonable meals. Weigh daily & reward wt gain. Individual & family therapy. Chlorpromazine may benefit

PROG: Approx 10% mort

ADOLESCENT TURMOIL

Period of adolescence involves issues such as sexual maturation, gradual increase in independence from parents & forming social relationships which often cause some problem behaviour. Rebellion against parents or other authority, experimentation eg c̄ drugs, anxiety, depression & suicide attempts are all not uncommon. Extreme cases may suffer an identity crisis

Adolescent M esp in towns may develop antisocial behaviour eg truancy, stealing, vandalism

RX: Often a stage of ordinary development which can be dealt c̄ by the family without outside help. Occ Behaviour modification techniques; Discuss possible alterations in parental attitude to child

DEPERSONALISATION

A sensation of dreamlike unreality of the self. Usually occurs as a 1° syndrome in adolescence. 2° causes inc Anxiety states, Fatigue, Acute severe stress, TLE, Schizophrenia, Migraine

JUVENILE DELINQUENCY

M>F. Ass c̄ maternal deprivation, marital disharmony, family discord, criminality in other family members. Less marked ass c̄ low IQ, extraversion, brain damage, XYY chromosome. Commoner in deprived inner cities

CLIN: Some offences usually carried out as part of gang eg gang fights, vandalism, marauding; whilst others which may be performed to prove or comfort individual eg stealing, are carried out alone. Poor, often hostile relations c̄ parents. Often truancy. Many become criminals as adults

RX: Treat whole family. Try to modify lifestyle

PROG: Poor. Family often resistent to help

Psychiatry in the Elderly

The elderly are more likely to suffer from multiple pathology rather than single disease processes. Few illnesses are specific to the elderly age group but many conditions are more prevalent in this age range eg dementia. Psychiatric illness is common in the elderly due to many factors both social eg isolation & biological eg lowered threshold to delirium. Much physical illness in the elderly has psychiatric sequelae

It is difficult to define the normal psychology of aging but deterioration of short term memory, slowness, ↑ cautiousness & rigidity are usually observed

Much psychiatric illness amongst the elderly appears to be unrecognised or regarded as inevitable or unworthy of active Rx. The development of specific psychogeriatric services has helped counterbalance these factors. The aim of the service should be defined in relation to the age distribution of the population, related to the general adult psychiatry service, c̄ close liaison c̄ the geriatric department & social services. A multidisciplinary approach inc psychiatrists, CPNs, social workers, voluntary agencies is advisable

The prevalence of dementia is age-related rising from 5–10% at age 65 to about 20% in those aged >80yrs

Confusion or delirium is common amongst in-patients. It may occur in the demented patient. There are many important causes of confusion in the elderly inc infections, anoxia, metabolic disturbance eg BG ↓, hypothermia, intoxication, MI, tumours, CVA, Ep, subdural haematoma, drug SEs

Depression is common in the elderly & suicide also rises in incidence usually in ass c̄ depressive disease. Although depression amongst in-patients is often unrecognised, symptoms are often marked in the elderly. Delusions & hallucinations are common. Occ a dementia-like picture is seen. Manic–depressive psychosis is observed in the elderly but mania does not increase in incidence c̄ age

Sensory deprivation eg visual or hearing impairment is a common ppt of psychiatric morbidity

Neuroses are common in the elderly but not often a cause of hospital admission. Alcoholism is a common cause of psychiatric & social problems

Schizophrenia rarely presents in old age. Paranoid states are commoner esp in the socially isolated

Legal Aspects

It is in the nature of mental health problems that the views of society & the mentally ill may conflict about the need for & form of Rx. In the UK a series of Acts have laid down guidelines for the principles of consent, compulsory hospitalisation & Rx. In general, informal admission is preferred but the patient's best interests in formal cases should be ensured by a series of legal safeguards

CONSENT TO RX

Consent to medical procedures by a patient must be "informed", a legal concept which has not been well tested in the UK courts. It is generally agreed that the patient must know to what he gives consent ie the general nature & purpose of the Rx, & that the doctor should explain the implications inc the commoner risks. The standard expected is that of a reasonable doctor in the field. However if disclosure of information might cause serious distress or psychological harm this may be grounds for the withholding of information. Obviously in emergencies eg an unconscious patient requiring life saving procedure, treatment may proceed without consent

Detained psychiatric patients are in a unique legal position. It was laid down in the 1983 MHAct, which replaced the 1959 MHAct, that certain treatments required consent even for detained patients. Non-specific Rx eg OT & nursing may be given without formal consent but other treatments (except treaments of special concern) require patient consent or the support of an independent doctor nominated by the MHAct Commission. Sections 57 & 58 cover treatments of special concern requiring informed consent & confirmatory second medical & lay opinions (even amongst non-detained patients). Section 57 provides the most stringent safeguards & concerns Psychosurgery & Rx specified by the Secretary of State eg surgical hormone implants, whilst Section 58 treatments are not considered to present the same degree of hazard & inc ECT & medicines administered during first 3mths of continual detention

COMPULSORY HOSPITALISATION

Compulsory admission &/or detention in hospital is indicated if release from hospital would endanger the patient or other people. The detention order is primarily a medical decision in most countries as detention is usually linked c̄ an appropriate treatment plan

In E&W the 1983 MHAct strengthened the rights of Psychiatric patients.

For detention up to 72hrs, only one doctor's recommendation is required & the form of mental disorder need not be specified but for all longer term orders it must be stated that the patient suffers from one of four categories of mental disorder: Mental illness, Psychopathic disorder, Mental impairment & Severe mental impairment. For longer detentions, an approved psychiatric social worker or a close relative must apply to the hospital administration & two doctors inc at least one psychiatrist must recommend compulsory detention. The social worker must be satisfied that the hospital is the most appropriate way of dealing c̄ the patient's case. If a relative makes an application for detention a social work report by an approved social worker is required

Section 4 allows for emergency admissions for up to 72hrs. As the application can only be granted if the procedures for a Section 2 admission would involve undesirable delay, the patient is protected from the use of this Section except in genuine urgent cases
Under Section 2 (Admission for Assessment) a person may be detained for up to 28 days but an appeal to the MHRT within 14 days can be made by the patient. Discharge can be authorised by the responsible Medical Officer, the hospital manager or the MHRT
Section 3 (Admission for Treatment) allows detention for up to 6mths. Two doctors must state that the patient is suffering from one of the four categories of mental disorder & requires medical Rx to alleviate or prevent deterioration of his condition & that such Rx could not otherwise be provided. The patient may appeal to the MHRT. This Section can be renewed under Section 20(4), where the doctor must state that the patient continues to suffer from mental disorder, that medical Rx in hospitals is necessary, that such Rx is likely to alleviate or prevent deterioration in his condition, that detention is necessary for the health or safety of the patient or for the protection of others & that treatment cannot be provided in any other way. Alternatively for patients suffering from mental illness or severe mental impairment, the doctor must state that if discharged the patient would be unlikely to obtain appropriate care & protect himself against serious exploitation
When a patient is already in hospital & may require psychiatric treatment, the consultant in charge or a nominated deputy may recommend to the hospital administrators that compulsory hospitalisation is necessary for the safety of the patient or others (Section 5(2)). This Section can be used for up to 72hrs. Informal psychiatric patients may be detained for up to 6hrs by an authorised psychiatric nurse whilst a doctor is found to assess under Section 5(2)
Suspected mentally disordered persons found in a public place & considered by a police officer to be in immediate need of care & control may be taken to a place of safety eg police station or hospital (Section 136). The patient can be detained for up to 72hrs during which time there should be an examination by a doctor & any necessary arrangements made
An approved social worker has power under Section 135 to inspect any premises where he has a reasonable cause to believe that a mentally disordered person is not being properly cared for. The social worker can apply to a magistrate for a warrant to remove the person to a place of safety

OFFENDERS c̄ A MENTAL DISORDER

An individual guilty of an imprisonable offence except murder may at the behest of a court be ordered to receive hospital detention & treatment. Under Section 37 a hospital must be willing to receive the case & two doctors of whom at least one is an approved psychiatrist must state that treatment is required in a fashion similar to that required under Section 3. The convict can appeal to a MHRT after 6mths

A court can issue an interim hospital order (Section 38) where a trial of hospital treatment for a period of up to 12wks is ordered & a decision about further placement is then made by the court
Transfers of prisoners to hospital for treatment can be authorised by the Home Secretary on medical advice (Sections 47 & 48)

MENTAL HEALTH REVIEW TRIBUNALS

Provide an appeal procedure for patients subject to long term orders. They hear appeals against compulsory orders & also automatically review all patients who have been detained for 3yrs. They can order immediate or delayed discharge. Patients are entitled to legal representation. The tribunal panel is appointed by the Lord Chancellor & inc a lawyer, doctor & lay member

COURT OF PROTECTION

This court was set up to protect & manage the property of the mentally disordered. A judge can decide, on receiving an application usually from a close relative & two medical recommendations, to appoint a receiver to administer patient's affairs

CHILDREN & THE LAW

In the UK parental consent is usually required for medical care for children aged <16yrs. The rights of children to have a confidential discussion c̄ doctors without parental knowledge have caused legal uncertainties eg when such consultations → the prescribing of contraceptives. When parental consent is refused, it may be necessary to take Care Proceedings

The Child & Young Persons Act 1969 is the most significant legislation affecting the care of children (0–14yrs) & young persons (15–17yrs). Care orders commit those aged up to 17yrs to the care of the L.A Soc Services Dept for a number of different conditions inc exposure to moral danger, poor control by parent, inadequate education, guilt of an offence (not murder), neglect of health by parent, ill-treatment

Under Section 12, the court may impose a supervision order for a period of 1–3yrs. The supervision is carried out by a probation officer or social worker & may inc psychiatric Rx as part of the condition of the order. The offender must consent to any psychiatric Rx

PSYCHIATRY & THE CIVIL LAW

The Civil Law deals c̄ the rights & obligations of individuals to one another. Psychiatrists have special responsibility in the areas of testamentary capacity, fitness to drive, torts & contracts, marriage contracts, receivership & guardianship. The legal concept of abnormal mental state may not match the medical usage of the term

Capacity to Make a Valid Will

A doctor may need to decide whether or not a testator is of sound disposing mind at the time of making the will

Fitness to Drive

Major mental illnesses may →

aggression, disinhibition, suicidal intentions & therefore potentially result in reckless driving

Torts & Contracts

If a tort eg libel, slander, trespass is committed by person of unsound mind any damages awarded against the offender are usually nominal
If a person makes a contract & is of unsound mind at the time, the contract may be non-binding if the contract concerns the "non-necessaries of life". A marriage contract is not valid if at the time of marriage either party was so mentally disordered as not to understand the nature of the contract

Power of Attorney & Receivership

If a patient is unable to manage his possessions by reason of mental disorder, the alternative arrangements of power of attorney & receivership are available
Power of attorney requires the patient to give written authorisation for someone else to act for him during his illness. The patient must comprehend what he is doing
Receivership may be made by an application to the Court of Protection

FITNESS TO PLEAD

English Law requires that a defendant must be in a fit condition to defend himself. A psychiatrist must try to determine if the defendant can understand the nature of the charge, understand the difference between pleading guilty & not guilty, instruct counsel, challenge juries, follow evidence presented in court. If the accused is found unfit to plead, the Home Secretary commits him to a specified hospital

MENTAL STATE AT TIME OF OFFENCE

The mental state of a person at the time of an offence can affect subsequent sentencing &/or be used to absolve the offender of criminal responsibility. Before anyone can be convicted of a crime the prosecution must prove that he carried out an unlawful act (actus reus) & that he had a certain guilty state of mind at the time (mens rea). Children under 10 are deemed incapable of intent. The degree of mens rea required for conviction varies in different types of crime. The defence may argue that a person is not culpable because he did not have a sufficient degree of mens rea & usually suggest that the person was not guilty by reason of insanity or automatism. Diminished responsibilty may be pleaded as defence to the charge of murder & if successful → a conviction of manslaughter

The defence of not guilty by reason of insanity is embodied in the McNaughton Rules. These rules were drawn up by judges & are accepted by the courts as having the same status as statutory law. To establish a defence on the grounds of insanity it must be clearly proved that "at the time of commiting the act, the party accused was labouring under such a defect of reason, from disease of the mind, as not to know the nature & quality of the act he was doing, or, if he did know it, that he did not know what he was doing was wrong"
If a person has no control over an act, he cannot be held responsible for it. When acts of violence have been judged to have been commited as automatisms eg in ass c̄ Ep, concussion, BG ↓, verdicts of not guilty have been returned. This defence is not always

appropriate eg most cases of self-induced intoxication
Diminished responsibilty is based on a much wider definition of mental abnormality than that embodied in the McNaughton Rules. Depression, psychopathy, emotional immaturity & pre-menstrual tension are amongst conditions that have formed the basis of successful pleas. The sentence for a conviction of manslaughter is at the judge's discretion

Neurology

HEADACHE

Tension Headache

Very common. Related to muscular tension

CLIN: Bilat headache like a pressure band. No vom. Pain usually episodic. Occ Continuous

RX: Analgesics. Occ require Diazepam & Amitriptyline

Migraine

F>M. Often FH. Onset usually <40yrs. Definition difficult as attacks vary in intensity, frequency & duration

PRECIPITATING FACTORS: 1. Mild trauma
2. Lack of food
3. Food idiosyncracy eg cheese
4. "Stress"
5. The "Pill"
6. Periods

Prodromal symptoms due to partial ischaemia in intracranial arteries. Headache due to extracerebral vasodilation. 5HT ↑ in prodromal phase & ↓ on headache

CLIN: Prodromal phase precedes headache by 15–30mins, symptoms can include fortification spectra eg Zig-Zag teichopsia, hemianopia, numbness in upper limb, dysphasia, dysarthria, ataxia, vertigo. The headache is ass c̄ pallor, anorexia, N&V, photophobia. Classically unilat, though side can vary in subsequent attacks, but often bilat. Lasts from 2hrs to 5days. Feel "washed out", tired. Occ Post-attack diuresis

INVESTIGATION: • Occ CAT scan esp if late onset, no FH & major neurological signs

RX: Prophylaxis: Avoid trigger foods. Stop pill
Prodromal: Ergotamine
Headaches: Darkened room, analgesics & antiemetics
Specific drugs eg Promethazine, Pizotifen, Clonidine. Rarely Methysergide (SE: Retroperitoneal fibrosis)

Vertebro–Basilar Migraine

Adolescent girls

CLIN: Occipital headache. Prodrome may include vertigo, ataxia, diplopia, bilat paraesthesiae, transient LOC

Hemiplegic Migraine

Rare. Often FH

CLIN: Severe unilat headache 24–48hrs followed by contralat hemiparesis for up to 10 days. May then affect other side. Occ residual neurological defect

Ophthalmoplegic Migraine

Esp children

CLIN: Periorbital headache 2–3 days c̄ IIIn palsy or ophthalmoplegia for up to 10 days

DD: Aneurysm post communicating artery

Amigrainous Migraine

Esp adolescents. Typical prodromata but no headaches. Can simulate stroke. 1–2yrs later classical migraine develops

Symptomatic (Secondary) Migraine

Migraine symptoms caused by a structural lesion. More common in hemiplegic, ophthalmoplegic, strictly unilat & late onset migraine

Migrainous Neuralgia

M>F. Usually no FH. Begins 30–40yrs

CLIN: Clusters of attacks of unilat severe periorbital pain esp early morning lasting 15mins–2hrs. Occ Ipsilat red eye, Lachrymation; Blocked nose; Flushed cheek, Horner's syndrome. Horner's syndrome may persist. Attacks usually daily for 3–6wks

RX: Prophylactic Ergotamine, Methysergide & Propranolol

FACIAL PAIN

Causes of Facial Pain (LIST 1 NEURO)

1. Diseases of teeth, sinuses, ear or throat
   Eg Impacted teeth, Gradenigo's syndrome
2. Atypical facial pain
3. Trigeminal Neuralgia
4. Migrainous Neuralgia
5. Post Herpetic Neuralgia
6. Temperomandibular Arthrosis
7. Temporal arteritis
8. Causes of painful IIIn palsy:
   a) Post communicating artery aneurysm
   b) Diabetes
   c) Ophthalmoplegic migraine
   d) Arteritis
9. Upper Cervical spondylosis
10. Glaucoma
11. Tolosa Hunt Syndrome
12. Ca Nasopharynx
13. Retrobulbar neuritis
14. Glossopharyngeal neuralgia
15. Rarely:
    a) Raeder's paratrigeminal neuralgia
    b) Angina

Atypical Facial Pain

Diagnosis by exclusion. F>M. Esp 20–50yrs

CLIN: Continuous unvarying burning pain in 2nd division Vn area. Depression

RX: Imipramine

Trigeminal Neuralgia

Esp >60yrs. F>M. Usually idiopathic but rarely ass c̄ MS or posterior fossa tumours

CLIN: Electric shock pains in distribution of Vn esp 2nd & 3rd divisions. Numerous triggers eg touching face, washing, cold winds, shaving, chewing. Usually self limiting but may recur

RX: Carbamazepine (SE: Ataxia; Pancytopenia). Occ root section

Post Herpetic Neuralgia

Esp elderly

CLIN: Burning continuous pain esp in 1st division Vn. Corneal scarring

RX: Idoxuridine & topical steroids during acute episode reduce incidence of neuralgia.
N.B Acyclovir does not reduce incidence
Ice packs, vibration, acupuncture, Carbamazepine, nerve blocks have all been tried

Temperomandibular Arthrosis

CLIN: Lower jaw pain occ shooting to ear ppt by chewing, talking

Raeder's Paratrigeminal Neuralgia

Occ due to underlying aneurysm or skull base malignancy

CLIN: Horner's syndrome c̄ no impairment of sweating. Occ Facial pain; Sensory loss. Continuous progression is ass c̄ malignancy

INTRACRANIAL ANEURYSMS

Aneurysms are generally present long before symptoms or signs occur. Aneurysms are frequently seen in circle of Willis at bifurcation pts

GENERAL CLIN OF BLEEDING ANEURYSM: In mild cases—Headache; Photophobia; Neck stiffness; Vom. In severe—Headache & LOC. Later, many possible neurological sequelae eg Hemiplegia, Aphasia

GENERAL INVESTIGATIONS:
- CAT scan
- Angiography
- LP
- SXR

PROG: Approx 50% mort in 1st yr. Approx 50% have a 2nd aneurysmal bleed within 1 year in absence of corrective surgery

Internal Carotid Aneurysm

INFRACLINOID ANEURYSM

Esp elderly. F>M. Aneurysm arises in cavernous sinus

CLIN: Severe retro-orbital pain radiating to nose & forehead. VIn palsy & later IIIn & IVn → unilat ext ophthalmoplegia. Affected pupil is small c̄ no light reflex. Occ Vn 2nd & 3rd division palsy; Corneal reflex ↓. Rarely carotico-cavernous fistula formation

INVESTIGATION: • SXR: Occ Erosion of ant clinoid, Ca^{2+}

RX: Analgesia. Carotid ligation

CAROTICO-CAVERNOUS FISTULA

CLIN: Pulsating proptosis; Tinnitus; Chemosis; Ophthalmoplegia. Vision occ ↓. Retinal haem & microaneurysms

RX: Surgery

SUPRACLINOID ANEURYSM

Arise at origins of post communicating, ant choroidal & rarely ophthalmic arteries

CLIN: Sudden onset of supraorbital pain, IIIn palsy &/or subarachnoid haem

RX: Surgical clipping of aneurysm

Middle Cerebral Artery Aneurysms

CLIN: Subarchnoid haem or rupture into fronto-temporal region ass c̄ hemiparesis

RX: Op if surgically accessible, when stable

Aneurysms in Posterior Fossa

Uncommon

CLIN: Occ Subarchnoid haem; Brain stem signs; Pseudobulbar palsy; Facial hemispasm; Cerebellopontine angle syndrome

Anterior Communicating Artery Aneurysm

CLIN: Subarchnoid haem c̄ no localising signs. Often frontal lobe damage eg personality change. Rarely pressure on optic chiasma

RX: Op if surgically accessible

Mycotic Aneurysms

Local vessel wall dilatations due to infection. Ass c̄ SABE

Microaneurysms

Tiny dilatations at arteriole–capillary junctions. Ass c̄ BP ↑. Intracranial haematomas tend to occur at these sites

Subarachnoid Haemorrhage (SAH)

Usually due to ruptured aneurysm, but occ 2° to bleeding angioma or A-V malformation

CLIN: Severe headache; BP ↑; Vom; Photophobia; Neck rigidity. Later Coma; Bilat plantars ↑. Occ Retinal haem; Papilloedema; Ep. In milder cases Confusion; No LOC; Mild meningism

INVESTIGATIONS:
- CAT
- Occ LP: Bloodstained fluid
- Later angiography

RX: If good recovery; no spasm; single aneurysm then op. Delay surgery if spasm. If multiple aneurysms or no aneurysm detected on investigation, Bed rest 4/52; BP ↓ drugs eg β blocker; Tranexamic acid

ANGIOMAS

Developmental abnormalities of cerebral vasculature. Esp young adults. 3 types: Cavernous, Capillary & Arterial

CLIN: Ep; Headache; Meningism; Other signs of SAH. Occ "Steal" syndromes ie vascular shunts → neurological deficits. Occ cranial bruits. Rarely signs of ↑ ICP

INVESTIGATIONS:
- EEG: Focal abnormality
- SXR
- CAT scan
- Angiography

RX: Surgery if possible. Anti-epileptics. Embolisation of feeding vessels if surgery not possible

PROG: Better than for intracranial aneurysms

Sturge–Weber Syndrome

Capillary malformations affecting only one hemisphere. Skin lesions esp port-wine naevus in Vn area esp 1st division

CLIN: Occ Ep; Mental retardation; Infantile hemiplegia; Hemiatrophy; Hemianopia; Glaucoma. No bruit

INVESTIGATION:
- SXR: Tram line Ca^{2+}

CEREBROVASCULAR DISEASE

Cerebrovascular Accident (CVA)

A stroke is a cerebrovascular disturbance causing focal neurological dysfunction lasting >24hrs
Esp elderly. Incidence increases c̄ age. Infarct commoner than haem

PATH: Cerebral infarction occurs if there is inadequate collateral circulation when a cerebral artery is occluded due to thromb or embolism. Thromb is usually due to atheroma. Embolism can result from atheroma in neck vessels or cardiac lesions eg endocarditis, mural thromb, myxoma
Cerebral Haem is usually due to ruptured intracranial aneurysms, A-V malformation or hypertensive vascular disease. Hypertensive vascular disease is ass c̄ microaneurysms. Small vessel disease of severe BP ↑ may → small

lacunar infarcts & intracerebral haem

PREDISPOSING FACTORS OF CEREBRAL INFARCTION: 1. BP ↑
2. TIA
3. Ht disease including AF
4. Diabetes
5. Hyperlipidaemia
6. Cigs
7. Polycythaemia
8. PVD
9. Trauma
10. Arteritis eg Temporal arteritis
11. Sickle cell disease
12. Leukaemia
13. The "Pill"
14. Hypoglycaemia
15. Cong arterial abnormalities
16. Arterial dissection

CAUSES OF PRIMARY INTRACEREBRAL HAEM: 1. Hypertensive vascular disease
2. Rupture of intracerebral aneurysm
3. A-V malformation
4. Coagulation disorders
5. Thrombocytopenia
6. Drugs: Eg Anticoags; MAOI; Amphetamines
7. Cerebral sarcoid
8. Cerebral amyloid
9. Arteritis
10. SABE c̄ mycotic aneurysm

GENERAL CLIN: Signs depend on the location & extent of the ischaemia, infarct or haem. Each cause a sudden neurological deficit which usually reaches a peak within 6hrs but occ may worsen due to further emboli or haem or extension of thromb. Occ ass c̄ SAH

SPECIFIC CLIN OF CVA:

Internal Carotid Artery Lesion: Spastic hemiplegia; Hemisensory loss; Hemianopia ipsilat to lesion; Dysphasia if dominant hemisphere; Visuospacial disorientation if non-dominant hemisphere; Deviation of head & eyes towards the side of lesion; Amaurosis fugax ("curtain" spreading across visual field—usually unilat). Often bruit

Ant Cerebral Artery Lesion: Eg Lower limb hemiplegia >upper limb; Grasp reflex; Incontinence

Middle Cerebral Artery Lesion: As c̄ int carotid artery but c̄ no involvement of eye ipsilat to the affected artery

Post Cerebral Artery Lesion: Hemianopia ± macular sparing

Vertebrobasilar Artery Lesion: Dysarthria; Dysphagia; Ataxia; Diplopia; Homonymous hemianopia; Nystagmus; Cortical blindness; Intranuclear ophthalmoplegia; Gaze palsy; Cranial nerve lesions; Vertigo; Deafness; Tinnitus; Hemiparesis; Resp failure; N&V; Unilat facial sensory loss c̄ contralat limb motor or sensory loss; Drop attacks; Hiccoughs

Supratentorial Intracerebral Haem: Common sites are basal ganglia & thalamus. Hemiplegia; Dysphasia; Hemianopia; Hemihyperaesthesia; Headache; Vom; Meningism. Initial flaccid paralysis, later spastic

Brainstem Haem: Pons >Medulla. Deep coma; Hyperthermia; Small reactive pupils; No oculocephalic reflex; Quadraparesis

Cerebellar Haem: Occipital headache; LOC; Dizziness; Nystagmus; Ataxia; Brain stem signs esp gaze palsy to side of lesion

INVESTIGATIONS OF CVA: • CAT scan
- Cerebral angiography: If recovered from stroke & fit for vascular surgery
- Arch aortography: Esp if bruit
- FBC, ESR
- BG
- Platelets
- U&E
- ECG
- CXR
- SXR
- Rarely LP

RX OF CVA: In acute episode: Clear airway. Dexamethasone if signs of ↑ ICP. If LRTI—antibiotic/physio. Drain bladder. IV fluids if LOC. Rarely surgery. No anticoags. Careful correction of BP ↑ Steroids if giant cell arteritis
Later: Treat underlying cause eg anticoags for emboli from cardiac lesion where no evidence of cerebral haem. Occ Surgery eg clot evacuation. Supf temporal to middle cerebral artery anastomosis for otherwise inoperable int carotid & middle cerebral artery lesions is being assessed. Physio & rehab. Careful nursing eg to prevent bed sores

COMPLICATIONS OF CVA: 1. DVT
2. PE
3. LRTI
4. UTI
5. Pressure sores
6. Contractures
7. Depression
8. Frozen shoulder

PROG: Worse if LOC. Mort: Haem >Embolus

>Thromb. Overall mort 50% at 6 months. Of survivors 33% fully recover; 33% residual disability; 33% bedridden

DD OF CVA: 1. Tumour
2. MS
3. Hysteria
4. Encephalitis
5. Chr Subdural Haematoma

Multi-infarct Dementia

Rare. A succession of minor vascular events leading to intellectual impairment & eventual dementia. Ass c̄ diminished cerebral blood flow. Stepwise deterioration

RX: Occ vasodilators are helpful

DD: Alzheimer's disease

Transient Ischaemic Attacks (TIA)

A TIA is a cerebrovascular disturbance causing focal neurological dysfunction resolving in <24hrs. 35% TIA are followed by completed stroke

ASS c̄: 1. Anaemia <10g
2. Polycythaemia
3. BP ↓ or BP ↑
4. Cardiac dysrhythmia
6. Carotid stenosis
7. Arterial compression eg Cv spondylosis

CLIN: Abrupt onset. Normally lasts 5–30mins. Signs & symptoms depend on site (see specific clin of carotid & vertebrobasilar CVAs). Occ bruit. Symptoms usually less severe than in CVA

INVESTIGATIONS:
- FBC
- Platelets
- ECG
- CXR
- BG
- ESR
- U&E
- SXR
- Radioisotope &/or Doppler studies
- Carotid Angiography (for signs in carotid territory): In fit esp if bruit
- Angiography if ?subclavian steal syndrome

RX: Treat underlying cause. Stop cigs; Reduce obesity; Control BP. Collar for Cv spondylosis. Dipyridamole & Aspirin or Anticoags >1yr. Carotid endarterectomy for stenosis. Supf temporal to middle cerebral artery anastomosis for otherwise inoperable int carotid & middle cerebral artery lesions is being assessed

PROG: Vertebrobasilar TIA better than int carotid TIA. Slow resolution of TIA & multiple TIA are poor signs

DD: 1. Migraine
2. Focal epilepsy
3. Tumours
4. Aneurysms & Angiomas
5. BP ↓ or BP ↑
6. BG ↓
7. Polycythaemia
8. Hysteria

Subclavian Steal Syndrome

Rare syndrome due to blockage of subclavian artery proximal to vertebral artery origin → cerebral ischaemia on arm exercise

CLIN: Signs of VBI. Bruit; Unequal radial pulses; Unequal BP in arms >15mm Hg

INVESTIGATION:
- Arteriography

RX: Surgery

Lacunar Strokes

Small cystic spaces <15mm in deep brain esp putamen, pons, thalamus. Ass c̄ BP ↑, microaneurysms & atheroma

CLIN: **"Little strokes" eg transient motor weakness, Dysarthria, ataxia. Eventually → pseudobulbar palsy c̄ Dysarthria; Dysphagia; "Marché à petits pas"; Spastic tetraparesis; Emotional lability. Later Incontinence; Dementia**

RX: Control BP

Hypertensive Encephalopathy

CAUSES: 1. Malignant BP ↑
2. Toxaemia
3. Acute GN
4. Phaeochromocytoma
5. MAOI c̄ Tyramine

CLIN: Headache; N&V; Confusion. Occ Nystagmus; Limb weakness; Papilloedema; IIIn palsy; Cortical blindness. Later if untreated, stupor, coma, death

INVESTIGATIONS: • FBC
• U&E
• Urinary VMA
• CAT scan
• LP: Protein ↑; P ↑

RX: Control BP c̄ drugs

DEMYELINATING DISEASES

Multiple Sclerosis

Prevalent in temperate countries. Peak age of onset 30yrs. 3F:2M. Occ familial. ?slow virus c̄ infection before age 15yrs. Ass c̄ HLA-DRw2; High titre measles antibody

PATH: Plaques of demyelination esp of white matter c̄ preserved axons. Oedema reduces axonal conduction

CLIN: Usually onset c̄ symptoms of disease in single site. Commonest presentations are Optic neuritis ie blurred vision, acuity ↓, scotoma; Weakness of one or both legs; Brain stem symptoms eg vertigo, ataxia, diplopia; Sensory loss in lower body esp numbness. Occ Tonic seizures; Dysarthria; Loss of postural sense eg "useless hand"; Lhermitte's sign; Urinary retention; Trigeminal neuralgia; Impotence. Initially in 2/3rds relapsing & remitting course c̄ gradual deterioration eventually (approx 10yrs post onset) becoming progressive. Later Weak spastic legs; Ataxia esp ppt by heat; Impaired postural & vibration sense; Urgency, frequency → incontinence, retention; Impotence; Ataxic nystagmus; Memory loss. Occ Depression; Facial myokymia; 2° infections. Rarely Euphoria; Dementia

INVESTIGATIONS: • LP: Often Cell count ↑, Protein ↑, IgG ↑, Paretic curve
• CAT scan
• Visual evoked potentials
• Magnetic resonance imaging
• To exclude DD eg B12

RX: ACTH—shortens duration of acute relapse. For spasticity give Baclofen. For trigeminal neuralgia give Carbamazepine

PROG: About 15% have a benign course c̄ little progression in 15yrs. Good prog ass c̄ early age of onset, presentation c̄ sensory or motor symptoms, or optic neuritis

DD:
1. SACD
2. Chiari malformation
3. Sarcoid
4. PAN
5. Cv spondylosis
6. Spino–cerebellar degeneration
7. Multiple emboli eg AF
8. Neurosyphilis
9. Behcet's

Devic's Syndrome (Neuromyelitis Optica)

Esp E.Asia, Japan. Can occur as part of MS or acute disseminated encephalomyelitis

CLIN: Bilat optic neuritis followed few mths later by acute transverse myelitis

Schilder's Disease

Rare. Esp childhood. Symmetrical demyelination of cerebral hemisphere white matter

CLIN: Headache; Ep; Hemianopia; Optic neuritis; Cortical blindness; Mental deterioration. Later Dementia; Quadraplegia

PROG: No Rx. Very Poor

SYNCOPE

Transient LOC due to inadequate cerebral blood flow

CAUSES: 1. Vasovagal: Eg Postural hypotension, Heat, Micturition syncope

2. Cardiac: Eg Stokes–Adams, VF, AS, Massive PE
3. Cerebral:
   a) Anoxia
   b) Hypoglycaemia
   c) Hypocapnoea

CLIN: Faint. Pallor; Sweating; Slow pulse

EPILEPSY

An epileptic seizure is an abnormal paroxysmal neuronal discharge & a continuing tendency to seizures = epilepsy. Peak onset 0–15yrs & in >70yrs. May be genetic predisposition

Causes of Epilepsy (LIST 2 NEURO)

1. Idiopathic
2. 1° & 2° Cerebral tumours
3. CVA
4. Trauma:
   Eg RTA, Birth trauma
5. Degenerative disorders:
   a) Pre-senile dementias
   b) Lipidoses
   c) Tuberous sclerosis
   d) Sturge–Weber
6. Infections:
   a) Encephalitis
   b) Meningitis
   c) Brain abscess
   d) GPI or Gumma
7. Metabolic:
   a) Anoxia
   b) Hypoglycaemia
   c) Uraemia
   d) Hepatic coma
   e) Alkalosis
   f) Fever
   g) HypoCa^{2+}
   h) Water intoxication
   i) PKU
   j) Hypomagnesaemia
8. Drugs:
   Eg Lignocaine, Cocaine, Nikethamide, Pb poisoning
9. Cong structural brain abnormality:
   Eg Hippocampal sclerosis
10. Irradiation

Precipitants of Seizures

Seizures may be more common during menstrual period, just before or after waking, c̄ flashing lights, if inadequate anticonvulsant therapy

Types of Seizures

A. GENERALISED SEIZURES

GRAND MAL:

Clin: A generalised seizure. The tonic phase of strong muscular contraction lasts <1min & is ass c̄ LOC, cyanosis, frothing & occ biting of tongue. The clonic phase follows c̄ generalised jerking usually lasting 2–3mins. Then flaccidity, confusion, sleepiness & occ incontinence. Post ictal confusion usually lasts about 1hr. No recall of seizure by patient

PETIT MAL: Esp childhood. Classical form is rare. Pathognomic EEG c̄ synchronous "3 per sec spike & wave" cycle. Atypical forms have irregular "spike & wave" cycles. About 30% later develop grand mal Ep

Clin: Brief "Absence" occ ass c̄ clonic eye mvts. Normal IQ. Atypical forms ass c̄ drop attacks (Akinetic Ep), myoclonic jerks & major seizures

AKINETIC ATTACKS:

Clin: Generalised seizure. LOC, muscle power ↓. Lasts few secs

MYOCLONIC EPILEPSY: Occurs in:

1. SSPE
2. Metabolic disorders eg PKU
3. Batten's disease
4. Tay–Sachs disease
5. Lafora body disease
6. Lennox–Gastaut syndrome
7. Unverricht disease
8. Ramsey–Hunt syndrome
9. Tuberous sclerosis
10. Severe infections
11. Spinocerebellar degenerations
12. Other severe cerebral disorders

General Clin: Sudden uncontrollable jerks

INFANTILE SPASMS: Occur in children between 3–12mths old. A form of myoclonic Ep. Ass c̄ cong & acquired structural CNS disease & metabolic disorders. EEG chaotic

Clin: "Salaam" attacks ie trunk flexed on hip c̄ arms extended & abducted

LENNOX-GASTAUT SYNDROME: Rare. A progressive myoclonic encephalopathy. Onset 3–6yrs of age. EEG irregular "spike wave" cycle

Clin: Myoclonic, Akinetic & Absence attacks

B. PARTIAL SEIZURES

Seizures which start in a small focal area of hemisphere which may or may not become generalised. Partial & generalised seizures often occur in same individual at different times

SIMPLE PARTIAL SEIZURES (Jacksonian): Focus in motor cortex. Upper limb>lower. Ass c̄ structural lesion

Clin: Localised convulsion c̄ progression (march) along body. Upper limb commonest site. May be followed by transient limb weakness (Todd's paralysis). No LOC. Occ Aphasia

SIMPLE PARTIAL SEIZURE (Sensory): Less common than Jacksonian Ep eg Olfactory seizure c̄ focus in ant temporal lobe & sensation of strange smell

PSYCHOMOTOR EPILEPSY: Arise in temporal lobe

Clin: Complex automatic behaviour eg repeated dressing for which there is amnesia after attack

TEMPORAL LOBE EPILEPSY (TLE): Occ due to structural lesion. Ass c̄ simple & complex partial seizures inc psychomotor & sensory forms. However TLE may be also ass c̄ more complex symptoms eg Fugues, Deja vu & jamais vu

AUTONOMIC EPILEPSY: Rare variant

Clin: Epigastric aura c̄ pulse ↑, sweating, vasoconstriction, BP ↓, angor animi (feeling of impending death). Lasts 10–30mins

General Investigations

- EEG
- CAT Scan esp late onset Ep

General Rx

Use single anticonvulsant whenever possible. For grand mal Ep eg Phenytoin; For petit mal Ep, Sodium valproate or Ethosuximide; For myoclonic Ep, Sodium valproate or Clonazepam; For TLE eg Carbamazepine. Monitor serum levels. Often can withdraw drug if attack free for >2yrs

Drug SE & toxic effects include: Phenobarbitone—mood changes, skin rashes, drowsiness; Phenytoin—Hirsutism, gum hyperplasia, osteomalacia, ataxia; Sodium valproate—cong malformations, alopecia. Occ surgery if failure of medical Rx & small circumscribed focus

N.B If h/o Ep can only drive in UK if attack free for >2yrs or if Ep is exclusively sleep associated

Complications

1. Trauma
2. Suffocation
3. Status epilepticus
4. Todd's paralysis
5. Psychiatric & behavioural problems

STATUS EPILEPTICUS

A prolonged seizure. Can occur c̄ any type of seizure. Medical emergency as it may → cardioresp depression, cerebral damage

RX: IV diazepam or thiopentone infusion preferably in ICU

Prognosis

Mean duration of seizures is 10yrs. Worse prog if ass CNS signs, cluster of attacks, more than one seizure type

DD

1. Syncope
2. Cardiac arrhythmias
3. Breath holding attacks in children
4. Cataplexy
5. Night terrors in children
6. Tics
7. Hysteria
8. Transient cerebral ischaemia

MENINGITIS

May be due to bacterial esp Meningococcus, Pneumococcus, *H.influenzae*, TB; Viral esp Echo & Coxsackie or rarely mycoses or amoebic. In new born Gm −ve, Staph & Strep are common. In immunosuppressed, Listeria & Cryptococcus are common. Occ 2° to SABE, OM, Osteomyelitis of skull, Sinusitis. Recurrent attacks commoner c̄ cong defects eg myelomeningocoele, persistence of source of infection eg sinusitis & in immunosuppressed

CLIN: Acute onset. Neck stiffness; Kernig's sign; Photophobia; Vom. Occ Encephalopathy; Cranial n palsy; Infarction; Ep; Papilloedema

INVESTIGATIONS:
- LP: Cells, Protein, Sugar, Culture, Viral studies
- Blood cultures
- BG
- CAT scan

DD OF STERILE MENINGITIS: (WCC ↑ Prot ↑ Sugar ↓ No organism found):
1. Partially treated meningitis
2. TB
3. Fungal meningitis
4. Viral meningitis
5. Cerebral abscess
6. Sarcoidosis
7. Ca
8. Vogt–Koyanagi–Harada Syndrome
9. Behcet's Syndrome
10. SLE
11. Chemical meningitis
12. MS
13. Cholesteatoma

RX: Meningococcus, Pneumococcus: Benzylpenicillin
H.influenzae: Chloramphenicol

COMPLICATIONS:
1. Cerebral abscess
2. Subdural effusion
3. Infarction
4. Arachnoiditis
5. Cranial n palsy
6. Dementia
7. Obst hydrocephalus
8. Intracranial thrombophlebitis
9. Encephalitis
10. Waterhouse–Freidrickson syndrome (c̄ Meningococcus)
11. Deafness

TB Meningitis

Esp India

CLIN: Usually subacute onset eg Malaise, Anorexia for several weeks. Then meningeal symptoms. May be ass c̄ miliary TB. Occ Encephalopathy; CVA; Decerebration; Cranial n palsies; Spinal block; Arachnoiditis; Granuloma; Hydrocephalus

INVESTIGATIONS:
- CSF: Z-N stain. Lymphocytes ↑, Sugar ↓, Protein ↑, Culture
- CXR
- CAT scan

RX: Pyrazinamide, Isoniazid, Rifampicin & Streptomycin in early wks of Rx. Then Pyrazinamide & Isoniazid. Intrathecal drugs unnecessary. Steroids may benefit

Cryptococcal Meningitis

Esp in immunosuppressed

CLIN: Usually subacute onset. Often focal neurological signs. Occ No meningism

INVESTIGATION:
- CSF: Lymphocytes ↑, Protein ↑, Sugar ↓. Indian ink stain

RX: Amphotericin B

Vogt–Koyanagi–Harada Syndrome

CLIN: Uveitis, sterile meningitis, depigmentation, deafness

FOCAL INTRACRANIAL INFECTION

Subdural Empyema

Due to trauma or sepsis 2° to mastoiditis, sinusitis or otitis. Occ complicates a subdural effusion

CLIN: Ac onset. Fever; Headache. Occ ICP ↑. Hemiparesis; Aphasia; Ep

INVESTIGATION: • CAT scan

RX: Surgical drainage. Antibiotics

Intracranial Thrombophlebitis

Rare but potentially fatal condition

CAUSES: 1. Parameningeal infection esp Staph
2. Meningitis
3. Haemodynamic abnormality eg Anaemia; Dehydration; Post partum; Thrombocythaemia

GENERAL CLIN: Fever; ICP ↑; Ep; Consciousness ↓; Focal signs. Occ Meningism

GENERAL INVESTIGATIONS: • CSF: Protein ↑, Sugar norm, RBC ↑, WCC ↑
• Blood culture
• CAT scan
• Angiography

GENERAL RX: Antibiotics

LATERAL SINUS THROMBOPHLEBITIS

Usually 2° to suppurative OM, cholesteatoma & mastoiditis

CLIN: ICP ↑; VIn palsy. Occ IXn, Xn, XIn palsy (Jugular foramen syndrome)

SAGITTAL SINUS THROMBOPHLEBITIS

CLIN: ICP ↑. Paraplegia; Sensory loss in legs; Loss of bladder control; Ep. Occ symptoms of hydrocephalus (although ventricles not enlarged)—if 2° to otitis media or mastoiditis termed otitic hydrocephalus

CAVERNOUS SINUS THROMBOSIS

CLIN: Painful proptosis; Chemosis; Local facial oedema; Retinal haem; Papilloedema; Ophthalmoplegia; Ptosis. Occ Facial pain; Vn 1st div numbness; Meningitis

DD: 1. Orbital cellulitis
2. Orbital, Retro–orbital Ca
3. Malignant exophthalmos
4. Carotico–cavernous fistula
5. Trichinosis

PETROSAL SINUS THROMBOPHLEBITIS

CLIN: Vn & VIn palsies. Occ IXn, Xn, XIn palsies

Cerebral Abscess

CAUSES: 1. Middle ear infection
2. Mastoiditis
3. Frontal Sinusitis
4. Penetrating head injury
5. R to L shunts eg Cyanotic CHD
6. Bronchiectasis

CLIN: Fever & progressive neurological deficit; ICP ↑. Occ Ep; Meningitis

INVESTIGATIONS: • CAT scan
• X-R of sinuses

RX: Antibiotics. Excision drainage

COMPLICATION: Epilepsy

DD: Any SOL

ENCEPHALITIS

Meningitis & encephalitis often occur together. Occ invasion of brain tissue causes more distinctive symptoms. Most cases due to viruses

CAUSES: 1. Herpes simplex
2. Mumps
3. Exanthemata eg Measles, Chicken pox
4. Polio
5. Rabies
6. Arboviruses
7. TB
8. Rarely: Behcet's, Whipple's, Trichinosis, Cysticercosis

GENERAL CLIN: Pyrexia; Consciousness ↓; Ep; Focal CNS sign (May affect brain stem)

Herpes simplex Encephalitis

Commonest cause in temperate climates. Often due to reactivation of latent *Herpes simplex* type 1 virus. The virus reaches the brain via the blood, olfactory mucosa or via Vn. Usually affects temporal lobe

CLIN: Acute onset of "general clin" progressing to coma. Occ Hallucinations; Anosmia; Aphasia

INVESTIGATIONS: • CAT scan
• EEG
• Occ brain biopsy

RX: Acyclovir

PROG: Poor. If survive may be left c̄ severe CNS deficit

Arbovirus Encephalitis

In Americas; Pacific & E.Europe members of Arbovirus gps are important causes of encephalitis

Disseminated Meningoencephalitis

Rare. Occ occurs post infection esp Measles & Vaccinia. Chickenpox usually affects cerebellum. Most recover fully

Subacute Sclerosing Panencephalitis (SSPE)

Rare. Due to measles virus or rarely immunisation. Boys >Girls. Onset in 1st decade

CLIN: Mood changes then IQ ↓. Later Ep & myoclonus. Eventually Dementia; Mutism; Decortication

RX: No useful Rx. Death 2–3yrs post onset

BULBAR PALSY

Bilat LMN lesion of IXn, Xn, XIn, XIIn

Causes of Bulbar Palsy (LIST 3 NEURO)

1. MND
2. Encephalitis
3. Syringomyelia
4. Polio
5. Myasthenia Gravis
6. Medullary tumour
7. Carcinomatous neuromyopathy

CLIN: Dysarthria; Dysphagia; Paralysis of palate; Wasted fibrillating tongue

PSEUDO-BULBAR PALSY

Bilat UMN lesion of IXn, Xn, XIn, XIIn

Causes of Pseudo-Bulbar Palsy (LIST 4 NEURO)

1. MND
2. MS
3. Ischaemia of int capsule
4. Arteriosclerotic parkinsonism
5. Gaucher's disease
6. Brain stem tumours

CLIN: Dysarthria; Dysphagia; Spastic tongue; Emotional lability; Jaw jerk ↑

SARCOIDOSIS

Sarcoidosis may involve any level of the nervous system & muscles & is an uncommon DD of many conditions

NEUROLOGICAL MANIFESTATIONS:

1. Meningoencephalitis
2. Arachnoiditis & Hydrocephalus
3. Cranial nerve palsies esp IIIn, VIn, VIIn
4. Uveitis, Papilloedema, Exophthalmos
5. Progressive multifocal leukoencephalopathy
6. Granuloma
7. Central Alveolar Hypoventilation
8. Polyneuritis, mononeuritis multiplex or mononeuritis
9. Myopathy
10. Myasthenia

CENTRAL ALVEOLAR HYPOVENTILATION

CAUSES: 1. Bulbar polio
2. Brain stem encephalitis
3. Medullary tumour
4. Medullary infarct
5. MND
6. Sarcoid
7. Riley–Day Syndrome
8. Cv cordotomy

CLIN: Resp ↓ esp in sleep. Later Polycythaemia; Pulm BP ↑

INVESTIGATION: • Astrup: $PaCO_2$ ↑, PaO_2 ↓

COMA

Coma may be caused by three mechanisms: Reticular formation damage; Bilat extensive cortical lesions; & Unilat hemisphere lesions c̄ tentorial herniation

Causes of Coma (LIST 5 NEURO)

A. RETICULAR FORMATION DEPRESSION
  1. Drugs:
     Eg Analgesics, Hypnotics, Antidepressents
  2. Cerebellar SOL:
     Eg Tumour, Abscess, Haematoma
  3. Brain stem CVA
  4. Rarely:
     a) MS
     b) Brain stem tumour
     c) Diencephalic lesion

B. LESIONS OF CEREBRAL CORTEX
  1. Cerebral Anoxia:
     Eg Cardiac or respiratory arrest
  2. Metabolic disorders:
     a) Hepatic Failure
     b) Uraemia
     c) Hyperglycaemia
     d) Hypoglycaemia
     e) Hypothyroidism
     f) Addison's disease
     g) Hypopituitarism
     h) Disorders of acid base balance
     i) Hypothermia
  3. Meningoencephalitis

C. UNILATERAL HEMISPHERE LESIONS
  1. Head Injury
  2. Cerebral tumour
  3. CVA:
     Esp Haem
  4. Extradural, Subdural or Sub arachnoid Haemorrhage
  5. Hypertensive encephalopathy
  6. Cerebral abscess

D. OTHERS
  1. Epilepsy
  2. Hydrocephalus
  3. Hypnosis
  4. Cerebral Malaria
  5. Psychogenic

Assessment

1. History: h/o previous illness, drug Rx & circumstances pre-coma
2. Level of consciousness: Response to pain etc (See Head Injury)
3. Brain stem function tests:
   a) Pupillary reaction: Bilat small pupils usually due to pontine lesion or opiate o/d. IIIn palsy suggests med temporal herniation. Preserved pupillary reactions in presence of loss of reflex eye mvts indicates drug coma
   b) Oculo–cephalic response ("Dolls Head" mvt)
   c) Oculo–vestibular (Caloric) responses
   d) Corneal response
   e) Resp pattern: Cheyne–Stokes resp usually due to supratentorial lesion

4. Motor function: Asymmetry suggests focal lesion
5. Tests for meningism
6. Ophthalmoscopy
7. Decortication shown by flexion of arms & extension of legs

Investigations

- BG
- U&E
- Astrup
- Urinalysis
- LFTs
- SXR
- CXR
- CAT scan
- Occ EEG, Tests of endocrine function

Rx

Correct metabolic or endocrine disorders. Dexamethasone for cerebral oedema. Treat underlying cause

HEAD INJURY

Esp <30yrs old. 100,000 cases admitted to hospital/yr in UK. Many head injuries do not require hospital admission

Causes

1. RTA esp front seat. Account for a half of fatal injuries & a fifth of all A&E attendances. Seat belts are protective
2. Accidents at Work
3. Sport esp boxing & horse riding
4. Assaults

Pathology

1° brain damage depends on the direction, rate of application & the severity of the forces, esp acceleration–deceleration, acting on the head. These forces may → local contusion or laceration, neuronal damage, shearing lesions of subcortex & brain stem, contre-coup injuries, haem & cerebral oedema. LOC is ass c̄ structural brain damage

2° brain damage can result from the process of bruising; cerebral haem; hypoxia due to BP ↓, Hb ↓ or resp ↓; ↑ ICP; brain shift; infection

Sharp penetrating injuries may not cause LOC but blunt head injury is usually ass c̄ LOC & post traumatic amnesia (PTA)

Assessment

Severity of head injury determines the management & prognosis. Initial assessment of the conscious state, presence or abscence of a # & focal CNS signs will determine whether the injuries are mild or more severe

Mild Injuries

ASSESSMENT

1. Admit to hospital if a child; # (for 24hrs); Amnesia for >5mins; Focal neurological signs; Severe headache; Disorientation. Take care not to over attribute symptoms to alcohol intoxication. Those not requiring hospital admission should be sent home with a "Head injury card"
2. Scalp lacerations: Can cause large blood loss, may be ass c̄ underlying # or infection. Shave & clean before suturing
3. SXR must be obtained rapidly esp as intracranial infection may occur if # missed. # are ass c̄ intracranial haematomas

   Physical Signs of Cranial Fossa #:

   Ant fossa: Nasal bleeding, orbital haematoma, CSF rhinorrhoea, cranial nerve injuries I-VIn, subconjunctival haem. Immediate & late risk of meningitis

   Middle fossa: Bleeding from ear, orbital haematoma, cranial nerve injuries VIIn-VIIIn & CSF otorrhoea

   Post fossa: Post auricular bruising,

cranial nerve injuries IX-XIn

4. Observations: Pupil size & reactions; Asymmetry in limb responses; Changes in PR, Resp, BP. Assess conscious level
5. Look for ass injuries esp chest, abdo, pelvis, limbs
6. Post traumatic amnesia: The most common evidence of brain damage. The duration of PTA is related to the severity of the brain damage

RX OF MILD INJURIES: Suture scalp lacerations. Give prophylactic antibiotics if orbital haematoma, CSF rhinorrhoea, CSF otorrhoea. Raise depressed #

COMPLICATIONS:

1. **Post-traumatic Syndrome:** Follows mild or moderate injury(ies)
   Clin: Irritable; Poor concentration; Short temper; Loss of confidence; Headache; Vertigo; Hyperacusis. Usually remits in a few wks but occ "accident" neurosis i.e prolongation of syndrome presumed to be due to psychosocial maladjustment occurs
   Rx: Reassure, mild tranquilisers
2. **Chronic Subdural Haematoma:** Usually occurs within 3mths of a mild head injury. Only 50% remember the head injury
   Clin: Headache; Fluctuating consciousness; Mental change eg dementia, confusion. Occ Upward gaze ↓; Mild ptosis; Mild focal signs eg Hemiparesis, Dysphasia, Ep
   Investigations: • CAT scan
   • Isotope brain scan
   Rx: Drain
3. **"Punch Drunk" Syndrome:** A chr encephalopathy due to repeated mild trauma. Esp boxers
   Clin: Personality change; Memory ↓; Dysarthria; Tremor; Ataxia. Occ Parkinsonism

Severe Injuries

Patients with depressed consciousness &/or focal sign

ASSESSMENT

1. Need good history to distinguish primary head injury from those c̄ an underlying cause eg Ep, MI, cerebral infarct, drugs, alcohol
2. Maintain airway: If unconscious, nurse prone c̄ head in dependent position, ET tube & regular suction. Occ require ventilation
3. Fluid & electrolyte balance: May require IV fluids but care not to overhydrate. May need blood transfusion; Ryle's tube aspiration
4. Catheterise if urinary retention
5. Hyperpyrexia is common & may → cerebral oedema
   Rx: Aspirin, ice, fan
6. Observations: These should be performed periodically
   a) Degree of consciousness. 3 parameters used:
   Best motor response: Obey command >Localise pain >Flexion to pain >Extension to pain >No response
   Best verbal response: Normal >Confused >Inappropriate >Groaning >None
   Eye open: Spontaneously >To speech >To pain >None
   b) PR, BP, Resp, Temperature
   c) Pupil reactions
7. Ass injuries
8. Other neuro examination esp for focal signs
9. Avoid drugs eg morphine & other procedures which may mask clin signs

CLIN OF ICP ↑: Headache; Vom; Papilloedema; Occ Cranial n palsies eg VIn

CLIN OF SUPRATENTORIAL COMPRESSION: (Herniation of uncus of temporal lobe through tentorium → midbrain compression) LOC; Pupils ↓ then ↑; IIIn palsy; Hemiparesis; BP ↑, PR ↓; Irreg resp. Often signs of ICP ↑. Rarely Ep

CLIN OF INFRATENTORIAL HAEM: (Compression of cerebellum, pons, medulla, lower Cranial nerves) Irreg resp; BP ↑ PR ↓; Ataxia; Lower cranial n palsies

INVESTIGATIONS: • FBC
• U&E
• Urinalysis
• BG
• Blood & Urine for drug analysis
• SXR
• CAT scan

CAT scans are an essential means of monitoring severe head injury. All such cases should therefore be transferred to a centre c̄ CAT scan & neurosurgical facilities

RX: Maintain airway. Surgery to suture scalp lacerations, elevate depressed #, drain haematomas, repair dural tears

EARLY COMPLICATIONS:

1. **Fall in Conscious Level** May be due to:
   a) Haem—Extradural, Subdural, or intracerebral
   b) Ep
   c) "Distant surgery"
   d) Drugs eg sedatives
   e) Cerebral hypoxia or hypotension
   f) ICP ↑
2. **Infection:** Eg Meningitis, Osteomyelitis
3. **Cerebral Oedema**
4. **Extradural Haem:** Esp middle meningeal artery 2° to # temporal bone. Concussion may be followed by a lucid period of a few hrs before signs. Signs of intracranial compression
   Rx: Urgent drainage
5. **Acute Subdural Haem:** Ass c̄ overwhelming head injury. Patient usually in deep coma
6. **Intracerebral Haem:** Signs of intracranial compression & ICP ↑. Rarely focal signs
7. **SAH**
8. **Early Epilepsy:** Commoner c̄ severe head injury. About 5% of hospital admissions have Ep in 1st wk

LATER COMPLICATIONS:

1. **Physical Sequelae:** Dysphasia; Spasticity. Occ Ataxia. Usually gradually improve
2. **Mental Sequaelae:** Personality change; Depression; Memory defects; IQ usually preserved
3. **Late Epilepsy:** Late Ep occurs in 5% of hospital admissions, about 50% starting in 1st yr. 50% have focal Ep. ↑ chance of development of Ep if: Depressed #; Intracranial haem; PTA >24hrs; Early Ep
   Rx: Anticonvulsants. Occ excise scar

PROG: About 50% of deaths occur before hospital admission. Mortality for coma lasting >6hrs is 50%. About 1/3 of patients who die in hospital have talked

BRAIN DEATH

Present day life-support techniques allow many patients to survive severe brain damage. These techniques are inappropriate if no useful cerebral function can be recovered. Criteria for irreversible brain damage have therefore been drawn up:

1. Deep coma
2. Fixed pupils
3. Absent eye mvts
4. Loss of corneal & gag reflex
5. No spontaneous resp
6. Positive identification of an irremediable structural brain lesion
7. "Flat EEG"
8. Absence of cerebral blood flow
9. Exclude metabolic or pharmacological cause eg Drugs, Hypothermia

Causes of Cerebral Oedema (LIST 6 NEURO)

1. Surgery
2. Trauma
3. Cerebral anoxia
4. CVA
5. Tumours:
   Eg Glioma, Mets
6. Brain abscess
7. SAH
8. Meningitis, Encephalitis
9. Drugs
10. Pb
11. Metabolic:
    Eg Addison's, Hypocalcaemia

HYDROCEPHALUS

The result of excessive CSF P within cerebral ventricles
Ass c̄ spina bifida. In early life ass c̄ malformations, later ass c̄ trauma, SAH & infection

Causes of Hydrocephalus (LIST 7 NEURO)

A. ↑ CSF PRODUCTION
1. Choroid plexus papilloma
2. Bacterial meningitis (?)
3. Vit A ↑ or ↓

B. NON-COMMUNICATING CSF OBSTRUCTION
1. Colloid cyst 3rd ventrical
2. Aqueduct stenosis
3. Tumour
4. Arnold–Chiari deformity
5. Dandy–Walker syndrome

C. COMMUNICATING CSF OBSTRUCTION
1. Meningitis: Eg H.influenzae, TB
2. SAH
3. Trauma
4. Normal pressure hydrocephalus
5. Sarcoid

D. ↓ CSF ABSORPTION
1. CVP ↑
2. Sinus thrombosis
3. Otitic hydrocephalus

GENERAL CLIN IN CHILDREN: Head size ↑; Crackpot skull percussion note; Fontanelle tense; Ep; Optic atrophy; Lid retraction; Cranial n palsy; Spasticity; IQ ↓; ICP ↑

GENERAL CLIN IN ADULTS: Intellectual deterioration; ICP ↑

INVESTIGATIONS:
- SXR
- CAT scan
- Ultrasound scan

RX: Shunt—divert CSF into R Atrium or peritoneal cavity c̄ valve to prevent reflux

Complications of Shunt:
1. Obst of the shunt system
2. Growth of children may → shunt in SVC & thromb
3. Subdural haematoma
4. Infection
5. Epilepsy

PROG: If shunted early & successfully, many children have normal IQ

DD:
1. Subdural Haematoma
2. Hydranencephaly
3. Tumour
4. Macrocephaly

Aqueduct Stenosis

Often cong. Usually presents <20yrs

CLIN: ICP ↑; IQ ↓; Emotional lability; Papilloedema; Cerebellar & pyramidal signs

RX: Shunt

Dandy–Walker Syndrome

Failure of development of 4th ventricle exit foramen → hydrocephalus & cerebellar maldevelopment

Normal Pressure Hydrocephalus

Rare. Communicating hydrocephalus c̄ apparently normal CSF P. Ventricles enlarged. Occ h/o head injury, meningitis or SAH

CLIN: Insidious onset. Memory ↓; IQ ↓; Incontinent; Gait apraxia; Disorientation; Personality change

INVESTIGATION:
- Isotope or CAT encephalography

RX: Shunt

BENIGN INTRACRANIAL HYPERTENSION

Rise of CSF P in absence of SOL c̄ Ventricular size norm or ↓. F>M esp middle aged. Ass c̄ pregnancy, abortion, menopause

CLIN: No focal neuro signs; Headaches; Vom; Papilloedema

RX: Steroids. Self limiting

GENERAL FEATURES OF HEMISPHERIC DISORDERS

Dominant Hemisphere (Usually Left)

1. Dysphasia (A central disorder of speech):
   a) Nominal esp temporal lobe
   b) Expressive—fluent: L post temporal, parietal
   —non-fluent: L frontal
   c) Receptive—Post L hemisphere
2. Dyslexia (A central inability to understand written word): L parieto-occipital ass c̄ R homonymous hemianopia
3. Dysgraphia (Disorder of writing) & Dyscalculia (Central disorder of calculating ability): L parietal lobe
4. Apraxia (Central inability to carry out purposeful mvts): Parietal lobe motor or sensory strips
5. Object & Colour agnosia (Loss of power to recognise the import of sensory stimuli): Dominant Hemisphere
6. Short-term & verbal memory: Dominant Hemisphere

Non-dominant Hemisphere (Usually Right)

1. Visuo-spatial impairment: R Parietal
2. Perception impairment: R parietal
3. Visual memory: Non-dominant hemisphere

INTRACRANIAL TUMOURS

Incidence of 1° tumours 5/100,000/yr in UK. Glioma is commonest adult tumour. Most adult tumours occur above tentorium. The CNS is the 2nd commonest site of childhood tumours; usually occur below the tentorium Aetiology unknown except that immunosuppression → increase in lymphoreticular tumours

PATHOLOGY: a) Gliomas: Are of variable malignancy. In adults esp middle aged M affect cerebral hemispheres. In order of greatest malignancy Glioblastoma >Oligodendroglioma >Astrocytoma. In children the post fossa & 4th ventricle are the common sites. The order of greatest malignancy is Medulloblastoma >Ependymoma >Astrocytoma. The medulloblastoma is the only tumour that commonly metastasises outside the CNS

b) Meningioma: Arise from dural structures. Max incidence 40–50yrs. Usually benign. Occ multiple

c) Pituitary adenomas: Usually benign. Ass c̄ endocrine syndromes

d) Cerebellar Haemangiomata: May be solitary or ass c̄ haemangiomas of retina, kidney or liver. Ass c̄ polycythaemia

e) Craniopharyngioma & Chordoma arise from embryonic remnants

f) Metastases: May occur by extension eg from Ca nasopharynx or via blood. Esp 2° to Ca lung, breast, kidney, thyroid & malignant melanoma

CLIN: 3 major presentations are ICP ↑ ie Headache esp mane, Vom, Drowsiness, Vision ↓; Ep (Often focal); Focal neurological deficit. As disease progresses usually all of the above become manifest & more profound. Chr papilloedema may → optic atrophy

Localising Signs (which are occ present):

a) Unilat hemisphere lesion: Hemiparesis; Homonymous field loss; Dysphasia

b) Frontal lobe: Usually present late. Mood change; Memory ↓ Dementia; Incontinence; Ep; Unilat optic atrophy; Contralat hemiparesis; Presence of primitive reflexes eg Grasp; Anosmia. Foster–Kennedy syndrome of ipsilat optic atrophy & contralat papilloedema is occ seen in frontal or sphenoidal wing meningioma

c) Temporal lobe: TLE; Dysphasia;

Personality change; Contralat upper quadrantic hemianopia

d) Parietal lobe: Focal sensory fits; Aphasia (Global loss of power of expression); Apraxia; Cortical sensation ↓—astereognosis; Body image disturbance; Contralat inf quadrantic hemianopia

e) Occipital lobe: Ep; Contralat hemianopia

f) Central hemisphere: Corpus callosum → dementia, Hemiplegia

g) Sella turcica: Bitemporal hemianopia; Endocrine changes; IIIn–VIn palsies

h) Brain stem: Ataxia; Nystagmus; Dysarthria (Disorder of articulation); Pyramidal tract signs; Lower cranial n palsies; Papilloedema

i) Cerebellopontine angle: Vn, VIIn, VIIIn palsies. Unilat deafness; Vestibular symptoms; Ataxia; Corneal reflexes ↓. Occ hydrocephalus

j) 3rd ventricle & hypothalamus: Hydrocephalus; Hormonal & metabolic changes

k) Cerebellar: Ataxia; Nystagmus; Dysarthria

l) Orbit: Visual loss; Proptosis; Papilloedema; Loss of FEM; IIIn, IVn, VIn palsies

False Localising Signs: 1. VIn palsy
2. In frontal tumours, cerebellar or extrapyramidal signs

INVESTIGATIONS:
- CXR, SXR
- CAT scan
- Angiography
- Surgical biopsy & path staging

N.B SXR may show "copper beaten" skull & erosion of sella when ICP ↑; Displacement of pineal; Ca^{2+}; Hyperostosis & prominent vascular markings if meningioma

RX: Complete surgical removal of meningioma, acoustic neuroma, haemangioblastoma, craniopharyngioma, & cerebellar astrocytoma is usually possible. Partial removal c̄ radiotherapy for medulloblastoma, ependymoma, astrocytoma & pituitary adenoma. Partial removal of glioblastoma & oligodendroglioma. Surgery also used to reduce tumour bulk, slow down progression & control Ep. Dexamethasone to reduce cerebral oedema. Shunt to relieve hydrocephalus

PROG: Glioblastoma very poor prog. Medulloblastoma & ependymoma fair prog. Oligodendroglioma & astrocytoma approx 50% 5yr survival. Meningioma, acoustic neuroma & pituitary tumours have good prog but tend to recur

Neurological Complications of Non-CNS Tumours (LIST 8 NEURO)

A. METASTATIC
1. Intracranial & Spinal mets
2. Meningitis
3. Peripheral neuritis

B. NON-METASTATIC
1. Metabolic:
   a) HypoNa$^+$ eg Bronchial Ca
   b) Hypoglycaemia eg Insulinoma
   c) Muscle weakness eg ACTH producing tumours
   d) HyperCa^{2+} eg Oat cell Ca, Breast Ca, Parathyroid tumours
2. Peripheral neuropathy: Esp Ca lung
3. Encephalomyelitis: Eg oat cell Ca
4. Cerebellar degeneration: Eg Ca lung
5. Myopathy
6. Myasthenic syndrome
7. Dermatomyositis: Eg Ca lung

Neurological Complications of Reticuloses (LIST 9 NEURO)

A. METASTATIC
1. Orbital deposits: Eg Lymphosarcoma
2. Nasopharyngeal deposits: Eg Lymphosarcoma
3. Skull vault & base deposits: Eg Myeloma
4. Intracranial deposits: Eg Leukaemia
5. Spinal deposits: Eg Myeloma
6. Peripheral neuropathy: Esp Lumbar sacral plexus
7. Meningitis

B. NON-METASTATIC
1. Infections: Esp Zoster
2. Intracranial haem, SAH & cerebral infarct: Esp PRV

3. Hypercalcaemia:
   Eg Myeloma
4. Amyloidosis & Carpal tunnel syndrome:
   Eg Myeloma
5. Progressive multifocal leucoencephalopathy
6. Periph neuropathy
7. Dermatomyositis
8. Myasthenic syndrome

Progressive Multifocal Leucoencephalopathy (PML)

Rare disorder. Often terminal. Usually due to reticuloses or leukaemias but occ due to sarcoid or TB. May be due to polyoma virus infection. Diffuse foci of demyelination

CLIN: Rapid downhill course. Hemiplegia; Aphasia; Dysarthria; Ataxia; Visual field defects. Later Coma; Death

INVESTIGATION: • Brain biopsy

RX: Cytosine arabinoside

RESUME OF CRANIAL NERVE SYNDROMES

Cranial Nerve I (Olfactory)

Palsy eg due to meningioma of olfactory groove, head inj → anosmia. Only bilat anosmia usually causes symptoms

Cranial Nerve II (Optic)

Optic nerve disease may → optic atrophy (qv), optic neuritis (qv), visual field defects (qv) & papilloedema (qv)

Cranial Nerve III (Oculomotor)

A complete lesion of the nerve → loss of all eye mvt except abduction, & complete ptosis of upper lid. Pupil is large & unreactive due to paralysis of parasympathetic supply. If lid is elevated may complain of double vision. Partial lesions also occur

Cranial Nerve IV (Trochlear)

Lesions of the nerve may be isolated & → diplopia on looking down. Due to paralysis of superior oblique muscle

Cranial Nerve V (Trigeminal)

The nerve is involved in trigeminal neuralgia (qv). Nerve palsies occ are observed in polio, expanding orbital lesions & brain stem conditions eg syringomyelia, medullary infarct

Cranial Nerve VI (Abducent)

A 6th nerve palsy paralyses the lat rectus muscle & → a convergent squint & diplopia. Nerve palsy may be isolated or occur alongside other palsies as in cavernous sinus thromb. Due to its long course from the pons to the orbit it is often a false localising sign

Supranuclear palsies due to eg midbrain tumours, brainstem encephalitis or cerebrovascular disease cause paralysis of conjugate vision

Cranial Nerve VII (Facial)

Periph lesions can → Facial Palsy (qv). Supranuclear palsies spare the muscles of the upper part of the face. Occ bilat facial palsy occurs eg occ in myasthenia gravis

Cranial Nerve VIII (Acoustic)

Nerve deafness results from lesions of the cochlear division of the nerve or from destruction of the end-organ receptors. Nerve lesions are usually due to tumours eg acoustic neuroma (qv) or trauma. Dysfunction of the vestibular division may → Menière's disease (qv), vestibular neuronitis (qv). Destruction of the vestibular nerve may occur c̄ the aminoglycosides

Cranial Nerve IX (Glossopharyngeal)

Usually involved c̄ other lower cranial nerves in medullary vascular disease or neoplasms in the jugular foramen region. Palsy → loss of gag reflex. Glossopharyngeal neuralgia can simulate trigeminal neuralgia

Cranial Nerve X (Vagus)

The vagal motor nucleus is often involved in medullary tumours, syringobulbia & brainstem infarct. In its periph course the nerve may be damaged at the skull base. The recurrent laryngeal branches may be involved in tumours of the neck or mediastinum. Unilat vagal lesions → unilat palatal paralysis, inability to sustain the sound "EEE" & weakness of voice. Bilat lesions called bulbar palsy (qv). Supranuclear vagal lesions cause pseudobulbar palsy (qv)

Cranial Nerve XI (Accessory)

Nerve palsy → paralysis of trapezius causing drooping of the shoulder. The nerve may be involved in lesions of the medulla or base of skull

Cranial Nerve XII (Hypoglossal)

Commonly involved in MND (qv). Occ involved in tumours or infarcts of the medulla. In unilat lesions the tongue is protruded towards the paralysed side

PARKINSONISM

A syndrome of Tremor, Hypokinesia & Rigidity

Causes of Parkinsonism (LIST 10 NEURO)

1. Idiopathic (Paralysis Agitans)
2. Post Encephalitic
3. Drugs:
   Eg Phenothiazines, Haloperidol, Methyldopa, Reserpine
4. Manganese poisoning
5. Carbon Monoxide poisoning
6. Repeated or severe brain injury:
   Eg Punch-drunk syndrome
7. Rarely:
   a) Neurosyphilis
   b) Cerebral tumour
   c) Behcet's

Idiopathic Parkinsonism (Parkinson's Disease)

M>F. Incidence increases c̄ age. Onset usually in 50's

PATHOGENESIS: Substantia nigra pigmentation ↓. Lewy bodies (intraneuronal inclusions) are found. Cell loss in globus pallidus & putamen. A severe reduction of dopamine in the corpus striatum

CLIN: Usually insidious onset at which time diagnosis may be difficult. Then classical features of coarse "pill rolling" rest tremor of 4–8hz esp of hands relieved by movement; "Cogwheel" rigidity; Hypokinesia c̄ mask like face, slowness, monotonous speech & micrographia. Other signs include Depression; Flexed simian posture; Accelerating gait; Difficulty in initiating or stopping motion; Infrequent blinking. Occ Drooling of saliva; Dysphagia; Heartburn; Constipation; Dysarthria; Blepharospasm. Later Wt ↓; Contractures; Dementia. Rarely oculogyric crises

Other signs include a positive glabellar tap

RX: Rx of choice is a periph Dopa-decarboxylase inhibitor to prevent periph degradation of L-Dopa to dopamine is coupled c̄ L-Dopa (eg as Sinemet) to allow more Dopamine to reach the brain. Alternatives are Amantadine, Anticholinergics,

Bromocryptine. For depression use eg Amitriptyline. Physio & OT
Unfortunately response to L-Dopa usually declines after 1–2yrs & increase in dosage may → Chorea, Dystonia, "On–off" effect, Hallucinations

PROG: Ave survival 10–15yrs if no death due to unrelated cause

DD:
1. Other cause of Parkinsonism (see above) esp drugs
2. Benign essential tremor
3. Arteriosclerotic Parkinson's syndrome
4. Shy–Drager syndrome
5. Steele–Richardson Syndrome
6. Normal pressure Hydrocephalus
7. Wilson's disease
8. Alzheimer's disease
8. Huntington's Chorea
9. Olivopontocerebellar syndrome

Drug Induced Parkinsonism

Certain neuroleptics inhibit dopamine either by blocking receptors or storage mechanisms eg Chlorpromazine, Haloperidol, Metoclopramide, Reserpine & Tetrabenazene.
Parkinsonism indistinguishable from the idiopathic form usually occurs 2–12 wks after the start of Rx
Other involuntary mvts can be induced:

TARDIVE DYSKINESIA: Occurs following long term Rx esp in elderly & may be irreversible. Stereotyped pouting, chewing, grimacing, lip smacking. Occ choreoathetosis

ACUTE DYSKINESIAS: Occur within 4 days of Rx. Dose related. Usually focal eg Trismus, torticollis, blepharospasm, oculogyric crises. Occ generalised eg opisthotonus in children

Rx: Anticholinergics
Akathisia: Uncontrollable motor restlessness

Steele–Richardson Syndrome

Uncommon. Worse prog than Parkinson's disease

CLIN: Supranuclear gaze palsy; Hypokinesia; Rigidity; UMN signs; Retropulsion; Hypertonicity, Dementia

Arteriosclerotic Parkinsonism

Parkinsonian features are sometimes noted in the course of cerebral arteriosclerosis. May be ass c̄ pseudobulbar palsy, corticospinal lesions or dementia

CLIN: Expressionless face; Slowness; Rigidity; Broad based gait; Emotional lability; Hyperreflexia; Bilat extensor plantars. May have stepwise progression due to mild "strokes"

Shy–Drager Syndrome

CLIN: Postural BP ↓; Incontinence; Impotence; No sweating; Cerebellar & UMN signs

INVOLUNTARY MOVEMENTS (DYSKINESIAS)

Tremor

Tremors are involuntary rhythmical oscillations around a fixed point

Causes of Tremor (LIST 11 NEURO)

A. POSTURAL ie on outstretching hands
1. Physiological
2. Exaggerated Physiological tremor:
   a) Anxiety
   b) Thyrotoxicosis
   c) Alcohol
   d) Caffeine
   e) Drugs & metals eg Li, Hg
3. Benign essential tremor
4. Wilson's disease
5. Rarely:
   a) Syphilis
   b) MS
   c) Cerebellar disease
   d) Hereditary peripheral neuropathies

B. REST
1. Parkinsonism
2. Rarely:
a) Cerebral tumour
b) MS
c) Trauma
C. INTENTION
1. Cerebellar disease
2. MS
3. CVA
4. Alcohol
5. Cerebral tumour
6. Drugs:
Eg Phenytoin
7. Spinocerebellar degenerations
8. Brainstem disease
9. Trauma
10. Rarely:
a) Hypothyroidism
b) Non-metastatic effect of Ca
c) Developmental eg Arnold–Chiari

BENIGN ESSENTIAL TREMOR

Common. Aut Dom & sporadic forms. Occurs at any age. Ass c̄ focal dystonias & hereditary periph neuropathies

CLIN: Fine or coarse 6–12hz tremor absent at rest. Usually begins in hand & spreads to involve head, arms & occ legs. Tremor worsened by stress & fatigue, improved by alcohol

RX: Propranolol

Chorea

Chorea is an involuntary irregular forcible strong rapid unpatterned jerk. These fleeting complex mvts are usually exacerbated by voluntary mvts

Causes of Chorea (LIST 12 NEURO)

1. Drugs:
Eg Phenothiazines, L-Dopa, Phenytoin, Amphetamines
2. Sydenham's (Rheumatic) Chorea
3. Huntington's Chorea
4. Senile Chorea
5. Thyrotoxicosis
6. SLE
7. PRV
8. Encephalitis lethargica
9. Hereditary non-progressive Chorea

SYDENHAM'S CHOREA

A focal manifestation of Rh fever. Due to arteritis. F>M. Usual onset 5–15yrs. May recur c̄ "Pill" or pregnancy

RX: Bed rest, Penicillin

PROG: Most recover in 6 mnths

HUNTINGTON'S CHOREA

Uncommon. Aut Dom. Most cases present in middle age

PATHOLOGY: Loss of cortical & striatal neurones

CLIN: Insidious onset eg Personality change, Fidgeting, Depression. Then Chorea; Dementia; Dysphasia; Dyspraxia. In juvenile form Severe rigidity; Ataxia & Ep are common (DD: Parkinsonism). Progressive downhill course

RX: Genetic counselling

Myoclonus

An irreg or rhythmical short lived involuntary muscular jerk originating in the CNS

Causes of Myoclonus (LIST 13 NEURO)

1. Idiopathic Ep
2. Progressive myoclonic Ep:
Eg Lafora body, Lipidoses, Spinocerebellar degenerations, Batten's disease, Unverricht's Disease, SSPE
3. Lennox–Gastaut syndrome
4. Infantile spasms
5. Essential familial myoclonus
6. Metabolic:
a) RF
b) Liver failure
c) Resp failure
d) Alcohol
7. Physiological:
Eg Anxiety or exercise induced

Tics

Abrupt jerky repetitive, stereotyped mvts affecting discrete muscle gps. Can be temporarily suppressed voluntarily. Common in children. In Gilles de la Tourette syndrome, tics ass c̄ swearing & echolalia

Dystonia & Athetosis

Dystonia is a sustained involuntary slow torsion mvt which may be present continually or only during certain actions. If severe may → relatively fixed posture & contractures
Athetosis is closely linked to dystonia. It is a coarse slow irreg writhing involuntary muscular distortion

Causes of Dystonia & Athetosis (LIST 14 NEURO)

1. Idiopathic Torsion Dystonia
2. Drugs & Metals:
   Eg L-Dopa, Neuroleptics, Manganese
3. Hypoxia
4. CVA
5. Encephalitis
6. Wilson's disease
7. Lesch-Nyhan Syndrome
8. Rarely:
   a) Kernicterus
   b) Homocystinuria
   c) Leigh's Disease
   d) Huntington's Disease
   e) Hallervorden–Spatz Disease

IDIOPATHIC TORSION DYSTONIA

Uncommon. Aut Dom, Aut Rec & sporadic forms. Onset usually in childhood

CLIN: Difficulty in running or limp (may be attributed to hysteria) c̄ progression yrs later to deformities of spine & limb. Dystonia may affect resp, speech & swallowing. Later contractures

RX: Benzhexol. Occ stereotactic thalamic surgery

ATHETOID CEREBRAL PALSY

Non-progressive dystonia. May be 2° to kernicterus, birth trauma, birth anoxia

CLIN: Initially hypotonic. Athetosis. Motor development ↓; Speech ↓; IQ ↓. Occ spastic legs

SPASMODIC TORTICOLLIS

A focal dystonia. Head rotated due to clonic or tonic Cv muscle contraction. Esp 30–50yrs. Usually idiopathic but occ due to: Trauma & Infection Cv spine; Neuroleptic drugs; Encephalitis lethargica

CLIN: Local pain; Head rotation; Contraction & hypertrophy of sternomastoid. May → Cv spondylosis

RX: If severe bilat division of upper Cv nerve roots

DD: Hysteria

WRITER'S CRAMP

Difficulty in controlling pen due to spasm of the muscles concerned. Often worsened by stressful ext factors

CLIN: Difficulty in writing. Aching painful hand. Occ tremor. No muscle wasting, sensory loss or reflex changes

RX: Rest. Diazepam

Ballism

Violent involuntary flinging mvts affecting whole limbs. Usually unilat. Often due to subthalamic nucleus lesion

Facial Myokymia

Quivering mvts of the small muscles of the face. Ass c̄ MS & intrinsic brainstem tumours

Palatal Dyskinesia

Due to lesions of red, olive or dentate nucleus

NEUROLOGY OF VISUAL FAILURE

Causes of Loss of Sight
(LIST 15 NEURO)

A. PAINFUL RED EYE
1. Acute Conjunctivitis:
   Eg Staph, Trachoma, Ophthalmia neonatorum, Allergy
2. Acute Iritis:
   Eg Rh Arth, Reiter's Disease, Sarcoid, Behect's
3. Acute Glaucoma
4. Acute Keratitis
5. Episcleritis

B. GRADUAL LOSS OF SIGHT IN NON-INFLAMMED EYE
1. Corneal ulcer
2. Diabetic retinopathy
3. Degenerative disease:
   a) Involutional Macular degeneration eg Tay Sach's disease
   b) Retinitis pigmentosa
   c) Choroido–retinal atrophy
4. Simple glaucoma
5. Cataracts:
   Eg Dystophia myotonica, Wilson's disease, Trauma
6. Lesions affecting optic tracts:
   Eg Meningioma, Pituitary tumours, Aneurysm, ICP ↑, Paget's
7. Hereditary ataxias
8. Toxins:
   Eg Tobacco, Lead, Arsenic, Methanol
9. Syphilis

C. SUDDEN LOSS OF SIGHT IN NON-INFLAMMED EYE
1. Vascular (Ischaemic Optic Neuropathy):
   Eg Central retinal artery occlusion, Temporal arteritis
2. Primary retinal detachment
3. Secondary retinal detachment:
   Eg Retinal & choroidal tumours
4. Retrobulbar neuritis esp MS
5. Methanol
6. Lesions affecting optic pathway:
   Eg Intracranial SOL, Trauma, Aneurysm
7. Hysteria
8. Leber's optic atrophy

Leber's Optic Atrophy

Rare hereditary disease. M>>F. Onset 15–30yrs

CLIN: Sudden onset of acute optic neuritis ie blurred central vision, acuity ↓,eye discomfort, central scotoma. 2nd eye often affected few weeks after 1st. Then optic atrophy. Few recover

Tobacco Amblyopia

M>F. Pipe smokers. Tobacco appears to act through its cyanide content which affects B12

CLIN: Optic atrophy; Acuity ↓; Scotoma

RX: Hydroxycobalamin

PROG: Good

DISORDERS OF SPINAL CORD, SPINAL & PERIPHERAL NERVES

Spinal Compression

Causes of Spinal Compression
(LIST 16 NEURO)

A. VERTEBRAL
1. Cervical spondylosis
2. Spondylolisthesis
3. Disc prolapse
4. 1° or 2° Neoplasm
5. Trauma
6. Vertebral collapse
7. Cong bony anomaly
7. Osteitis:
   Eg TB, Pagets

B. EXTRADURAL
1. Extradural abscess
2. Pachymeningitis:
   Eg Sy, TB
3. Reticulosis, leukaemic or metastatic infiltration

C. INTRADURAL EXTRA-MEDULLARY
1. Neoplasms:
   Eg Meningioma, Neurofibroma, Mets
2. Arachnoiditis
3. Arachnoid cyst

D. INTRAMEDULLARY
1. Neoplasms:
   Eg Glioma
2. Haematomyelia
3. Cyst

E. CRANIOCERVICAL
1. Congenital:
   Eg Chiari Malformation; Basilar impression
2. Atlanto–Axial subluxation:
   Eg Trauma; Rh Arth
3. Arachnoiditis
4. Neoplasms

GENERAL CLIN: Difficulty in walking; Lower limb spasticity; Loss of trunk sensation. Later Loss of bladder control; Retention; Paraplegia

SPECIFIC CLIN FOR CRANIOCERVICAL LESION: Spastic tetraparesis; Syringomyelia; Nystagmus; Ataxia; Occult hydrocephalus; Pain in neck

SPECIFIC CLIN FOR CAUDA EQUINA COMPRESSION: Saddle anaesthaesia; Sphincter disturbance; Flaccid paralysis below knees; Rectal & genital pain

SPECIFIC CLIN FOR HEMISECTION OF CORD (BROWN–SEQUARD SYNDROME): Ipsilat spastic paralysis & loss of position sense; Contralat loss of temperature & pain sense. Ipsilat LMN signs & band of spinothalamic loss

GENERAL INVESTIGATIONS: • X-R spine
• Myelography
• PPE
• Isotope bone scan
• CAT scan

GENERAL RX: Treat early to prevent irreversible cord damage. Operative decompression. Occ radiotherapy

Degenerative Conditions

CERVICAL SPONDYLOSIS

Very common radiological finding of chr Cv spine degeneration esp in elderly

PATH: Disc = Nucleus pulposus & annulus fibrosis. Damage to outer annulus → protrusion of nucleus → nerve root or cord compression. Osteophytes form occ → to compression

PREDISPOSITIONS TO SYMPTOMS:
1. Osteophytes
2. Whiplash inj
3. Cong narrow Cv canal
4. Vascular insufficiency

CLIN: Often asymptomatic. Root symptoms (qv) commonly precede myelopathy. Spastic lower limb(s); Upper limb weakness; Paraesthesiae; Reflexes ↓ at level of lesion; Sphincter disturbance; Sensory level

INVESTIGATIONS: • X-Rs Cv spine
• Myelogram
• CSF: Protein ↑

RX: Rest. Collar. Occ decompressive laminectomy or Cloward's anterior fixation

DORSAL DISC DEGENERATION

Rare. Usually due to straining or lifting

CLIN: Abdo pain & weakness; Back pain. Later paraplegia

RX: Myelogram & mark level of block then dorsal laminectomy

LUMBAR DISC HERNIATION

Common cause of sciatica. Rarely a midline protrusion causes cauda equina compression c̄ neurogenic claudication, incontinence or urinary retention

LUMBAR STENOSIS

Results in intermittent claudication of cauda equina

CAUSES: 1. Congenitally narrow canal eg Achondroplasia
2. Central disc prolapse
3. Spondylosis
4. Spondylolisthesis
4. Multiple disc protrusions
5. Post traumatic arachnoiditis

CLIN: Pain, sensory disturbance & weakness on exercise. Occ Incontinence or Retention

INVESTIGATIONS: • X-R spine
• Epidurography
• CAT scan
• EMG

RX: Surgical decompression

Inflammatory & Infective Disorders

ATLANTO–AXIAL SUBLUXATION

The odontoid peg of the axis is pushed backwards c̄ a risk of cord damage

CAUSES: 1. Rh Arth
2. Developmental abnormality
3. Trauma
4. Ankylosing Spondylitis

CLIN: Usually immediate neuro symptoms of progressive spastic tetraparesis c̄ sensory & sphincter disturbance. Occ VBI. Rarely transient cortical blindness

INVESTIGATION: • X-R Cv spine Flexion/Extension views

RX: Emergency ext fixation then surgical stabilisation of jt

EXTRADURAL ABSCESS

2° to infection, osteomyelitis

CLIN: Back pain & fever c̄ localising signs. Later septic venous thrombosis → paraplegia. Pyramidal signs

RX: Myelography & surgery. Antibiotics

POTT'S DISEASE

TB of a vertebra. Usually ass c̄ paravertebral abscesses

CLIN: Vertebral collapse → cord compression c̄ paraplegia

RX: AntiTB drugs

Causes of Vertebral Collapse (LIST 17 NEURO)

1. Osteoporosis
2. Paget's disease
3. Infections:
   Eg TB; Staph
4. 1° or 2° tumours
5. Myeloma
6. Reticuloses
7. Osteochondritis
8. Histiocytosis

ACUTE TRANSVERSE MYELITIS

Esp young adults. Esp thoracic cord

CAUSES:
1. MS
2. Devic's Syndrome
3. Osteomyelitis
4. Meningitis
5. TB
6. Post vaccination eg Acute disseminated encephalomyelitis
7. Connective tissue diseases
8. Septicaemia
9. Syphilis
10. Radiation Myelopathy

CLIN: Local back pain. Then sensory loss to level of lesion ± hypersensitive band; Flaccid weakness; Urinary retention; Loss of bowel control

INVESTIGATION: • Myelogram to exclude cord compression

RX: If acute disseminated encephalomyelitis or connective tissue disorder use steroids. Treat underlying cause. Occ surgical decompression

ARACHNOIDITIS

CAUSES:
1. Trauma
2. Myelography esp Myodil
3. Previous surgery
4. SAH
5. Infection eg Pyogenic meningitis, TB
6. Idiopathic

CLIN: Often asymptomatic. Occ Painful asc spastic paralysis. Motor & sensory root signs

INVESTIGATION: • Myelogram

RX: Steroids

PROG: Poor if symptoms

SPINAL CYSTS

Include Dermoid, Epidermoid & Arachnoid cysts

CLIN: Occ Backache & root pain

RX: Surgical removal of cyst

SYPHILIS

MENINGOVASCULAR SYPHILIS:

Path: Vascular & perivascular inflam. Endarteritis. Occ Gumma; Spirochaetes

Clin: Varied presentations Eg Meningitis; Cranial nerve palsies; CVA; Transverse myelitis; Optic neuritis; Ep; Meningomyelitis esp dorsal; Amyotrophy; Radiculitis; Spastic paraplegia

Investigation: • LP: CSF Cells ↑, Protein ↑, Glucose norm. FTA, TPHA, VDRL all +ve

Rx: Procaine penicillin for 14 days

TABES DORSALIS: Atrophy dorsal spinal roots & post columns. May coexist c̄ GPI

Clin: 8–20yrs post infection. Sensory symptoms eg Lightning pains usually precede other symptoms by several years. Later symptoms can include Ataxia; Jt position sense ↓; +ve Rombergs; Tabetic crises eg Gastric; Paraesthesiae esp feet; Loss of supf pain sense; Loss or delay of deep pain sense; Charcot's jts; Neuropathic ulcers; Incontinence or retention c̄ overflow; Impotence; Hypotonia; Optic atrophy; Ptosis; Argyll–Robertson pupils; Diplopia; Trigeminal neuralgia

Investigations: • Blood & CSF serology
• CSF: WCC ↑, Protein ↑

Rx: Penicillin. Unlikely that treatment affects course. For lightning pains use Carbamazepine

Developmental Abnormalities

SPINAL DYSRAPHISM

A group of conditions affecting lumbosacral region comprising Spina bifida, Diastomatomyelia, Dermoid cysts, Fatty tumours, Cord tethering & Embryonic tumours. Esp children

CLIN: Weakness & root sensory signs in one or both legs. Then sphincter involvement. Normally presents at puberty

RX: Surgery

SYRINGOMYELIA

Uncommon. A cavitation extending over several segments of the central spinal cord. Majority are ass c̄ cong cervicocranial abnormalities esp Chiari malformations but occ due to Post fossa tumours, Trauma, Arachnoiditis & Spinal cord tumours
Intermittent CSF outflow obst from 4th ventricle → ↑ P in central canal & rupture into cord to form syrinx. As syrinx expands damage to spinothalamic & corticospinal tracts & ant horn cells

CLIN: Insidious onset. Dissociated sensory loss to pain & temperature; Burns; Charcot's jt; Muscle weakness & wasting of hand. Occ Hyperhidrosis; Cyanosis & swelling of fingers; Ulceration. Later Spastic paraparesis
In lesions above C5 (Syringobulbia): Nystagmus; Vertigo; Ataxia; Horner's syndrome; Facial sensory loss; Dysphagia; Dysphonia

INVESTIGATIONS:
- X-R Cv spine
- Myelography: Eg Tonsillar herniation (CSF norm)
- CAT scan

RX: Surgical decompression

BASILAR IMPRESSION

Abnormal skull base due to widened angle between basisphenoid & occipital bone. May occur as an isolated cong defect or ass c̄ Klippel–Fiel syndrome or Osteogenesis imperfecta. The medulla is unusually low & compression of the Cv spinal cord may occur

CLIN: Variable presentations. May → hydrocephalus or syringomyelia. In adults may present c̄ spastic tetraparesis due to high Cv cord compression. Occ → Arnold–Chiari malformation

INVESTIGATIONS:
- SXR: Measure angle
- CAT scan

RX: May require decompressive surgery
N.B Paget's disease → Platybasia c̄ similar widening of angle

Spinocerebellar Degenerations

FAMILIAL SPASTIC PARAPLEGIA

Rare. Esp young adults. M>F. Aut Dom

CLIN: Spastic paraplegia c̄ no sensory or sphincter involvement
Usually pes cavus

FRIEDREICH'S ATAXIA

Onset in teens. Aut Rec. Degeneration of post columns, post root ganglia, spinocerebellar & pyramidal tracts

CLIN: Ataxia; Spastic weakness; Areflexia; Sensation ↓ esp jt position sense; Nystagmus; Pes cavus; Kyphoscoliosis; Heart conduction defects; Dysarthria

PROG: Usually die by early 30s

HEREDITARY SPASTIC ATAXIA (MARIE'S)

CLIN: Ataxia; Optic atrophy; Diplopia; Spasticity

OLIVOPONTOCEREBELLAR DEGENERATION (DEJERINE–THOMAS)

Rare hereditary ataxia. Occ spinal cord dysfunction

Vascular Abnormalities

SPINAL CORD INFARCTION

Occurs following cord compression or occ BP ↓, dissecting aneurysm, vasculitis, syphilis, idiopathic
Usually ant spinal artery occlusion c̄ sparing of post columns (supplied by post spinal arteries)

CLIN: Weakness & numbness of legs; Loss of sphincter control

PROG: Very poor if no improvement within 24hrs

ANGIOMA & A-V MALFORMATIONS OF SPINAL CORD

Esp thoracolumbar cord

CLIN: Backache; Cord compression c̄

myelopathy & progressive paraplegia. Occ SAH

INVESTIGATIONS: • Myelogram: "Bag of Worms"
• Angiography

RX: Surgery &/or Embolisation

Intraspinal Tumours

Types:

A. PRIMARY

1. Extradural:
   a) Neurofibroma
   b) Meningioma
   c) Sarcoma
   d) Neuroblastoma
   e) Chordoma
2. Intradural Extramedullary:
   a) Neurofibroma
   b) Meningioma
   c) Lipoma
3. Intramedullary:
   a) Ependymoma
   b) Other glioma
   c) Dermoids
   d) Teratoma

B. SECONDARY

Esp Breast, Prostate, Lung, Thyroid, Uterus
Commonest tumours in children are Sarcoma, Ependymomas, Dermoids, Neuroblastomas
Commonest tumours in adults are Mets, Meningioma, Neurofibroma, Ependymoma & Sarcoma

INTRAMEDULLARY TUMOURS

Esp cervical cord. M=F

CLIN: Sacral sparing (lat spinothalamic tract spared). Sensory level. Occ Sphincter disturbance. Progressive paraplegia

INVESTIGATIONS: • Myelogram
• CAT scan

RX: Surgical decompression

DD: Syringomyelia

EXTRAMEDULLARY TUMOURS

Neurofibromas occur esp at formen magnum & are occ dumb-bell. Meningiomas esp occur at mid dorsal regions & are most common in females

CLIN: Root pain; Insidious development of spastic paraparesis. Occ Neurofibroma causes cauda equina compression

INVESTIGATION: • Myelogram

RX: Excise neurofibroma or meningioma

CARCINOMATOUS MYELOPATHY

Various types inc spinocerebellar degeneration, subacute necrotic myelopathy & MND-like syndrome

Cervical Disc Lesions

In young usually acute disc prolapse. In old usually chr disc degeneration

CLIN: Local pain; Neck stiffness. May have radiculopathy &/or myelopathy.
Occ Pain in affected root myotome; Paraesthesiae in sensory distribution of affected root; Weakness & wasting.
Reflexes ↓: in C5.6 lesion: Biceps, supinator ↓; C7 lesion: Triceps ↓; C8 lesion: finger jerks ↑

INVESTIGATIONS: • X-R Cv spine
• Myelography

RX: Cervical collar. Analgesia. Heat & intermittent traction. If myelopathy, surgery—either decompressive laminectomy or Cloward op

Brachial Plexus Trauma

Ass c̄ birth trauma, RTA. Symptoms depend on root level. C5.6 (Erb's); C7.8; T1 (Klumpke's) ass c̄ Horner's & wasting of small muscles of hand

RX: Surgical repair (if nerve parted in brachial plexus)

Pancoast's Tumour

Apical tumour of lung ass c̄ upper limb flaccid weakness, pain, muscle wastage & sensory loss. Ass c̄ Horner's syndrome. Occ Lymphoedema

INVESTIGATION: • CXR

Thoracic Inlet Syndrome

Esp middle aged women. Usually due to Cv rib or fibrous band

CLIN: Brachial plexus compression esp T1. Loss of pulse on bracing shoulders; Pain; Raynaud's; Weakness, wasting hand & forearm muscles; Sensory loss

INVESTIGATIONS: • X-R
• EMG

RX: Surgery. Remove rib or band

Neuralgic Amyotrophy

Syndrome usually of unknown cause, occ 2° to immunication

CLIN: Acute onset of pain++ in upper limb then weakness & wasting. No sensory loss. Rarely occurs in lower limb

INVESTIGATIONS: • EMG: Acute denervation

RX: Analgesia; Physio

PROG: Usually complete recovery 6–18mths

Radial Nerve Palsy

Due to nerve compression against humeral shaft

CLIN: Painful weakness of wrist & finger extensors. Sensory loss back of hand between thumb/1st digit. Brachioradialis reflex ↓

RX: Relieve pressure. May need physio. Spontaneous recovery

Ulnar Nerve Lesions

Usually due to damage in condylar groove in elbow due to acute P or OA elbow. Rarely entrapment in wrist or hand due to palmar ganglia or synovioma. Some occupations predispose

CLIN: Weakness & wasting of Flexor carpi ulnaris, flexor digitorum profundus & hand muscles except LOAF. Sensory loss of med $1\frac{1}{2}$ fingers; Claw hand; Radial deviation. If lesion in hand, wasting of hand muscles c̄ no sensory loss

RX: Decompress

Median Nerve Lesion

POST INTEROSSEOUS NERVE LESION

CLIN: Weak finger extension, thumb extension & abduction

ANT INTEROSSEOUS NERVE LESION

CLIN: Weak flexion of terminal phalanges of thumb, 1st, 2nd & 3rd fingers

Carpal Tunnel Syndrome

Causes of Carpal Tunnel Syndrome (LIST 18 NEURO)

1. Idiopathic
2. Pregnancy
3. OA of wrist
4. Trauma'
5. Endocrine:
   a) Myxoedema
   b) Acromegaly
6. "The Pill", Premenstrual
7. Rarely:
   a) Amyloidosis
   b) Mucopolysaccharidoses

CLIN: Hand &/or forearm pain & paraesthesiae esp nocte; Numb swollen hand. Occ LOAF muscles weak. Sensory loss lat $2\frac{1}{2}$ fingers

RX: Diuretics, Steroid injection or decompression

Lumbar Root Syndrome

Usually disc prolapse esp L4,5 S1. Occ malignant infiltration eg Ca cervix

CLIN: Backache often ppt by strenuous activity. Sciatica ppt by cough, straining. SLR ↓. Scoliosis on standing. Reflexes ↓ in L4: Knee jerk ↓, Ant tibial ↓; L5: Dorsiflexed toes; S1: Ankle jerk ↓. Calf weakness (S1). Sensory loss in affected dermatomes

INVESTIGATIONS: • X-R
• Myelogram
• EMG

RX: Board under bed. Bed rest. Lumbosacral corset. Physio. Surgery for failure of medical Rx, cauda equina compression, profound root compression signs

Sciatic Nerve Lesions

CAUSES: 1. Barbiturates
2. Blood dyscrasias, anticoags
3. Trauma eg misplaced im injection

CLIN: Sensory loss over lat knee. Muscle wastage

Femoral Nerve Neuropathy

Esp diabetics

CLIN: Weakness, wastage quadriceps & iliopsoas. Knee jerk ↓. Sensory loss—medial side of leg

Lat Cutaneous Nerve of Thigh (Meralgia Paresthetica)

Esp obese, pregnancy & diabetics. Esp middle aged. F>M. Nerve compressed by inguinal lig

CLIN: Pain, numbness & paraesthesiae on anterolat thigh

RX: Diet. Decompress. Local anaesthetic into inguinal lig

Lat Popliteal Nerve Palsy

Compression round fibula head

CLIN: Paralysis of ant tibial & peroneal muscles. Weak dorsiflexion feet & toes, weak foot eversion. No pain. Paraesthesiae & sensory ↓ over dorsum & outer foot. Ankle jerk normal. Foot drop

RX: Usually spontaneous recovery. Occ decompress

DD: L5 root lesion

Tarsal Tunnel Syndrome

Tibial nerve entrapment by flexor retinaculum

CLIN: Pain, paraesthesiae & later weakness of foot

RX: Decompression

Ekbom's Syndrome

Nocturnal burning & restlessness in feet. No pain

RX: Chlorpromazine

Peripheral Neuropathy

Most are symmetrical but occ asymmetrical eg Mononeuritis multiplex

Causes of Peripheral Neuropathy (LIST 19 NEURO)

1. Metabolic:
   a) Diabetes
   b) Uraemia
   c) Amyloid
   d) Myxoedema
   e) Acromegaly
   f) Porphyria
2. Infections:
   a) Leprosy
   b) Guillain–Barré
   c) Tetanus
   d) Brucellosis
   e) Diphtheria
3. Deficiency states:
   a) Alcoholism
   b) SACD
   c) Pellagra
   d) Beri-Beri
   e) Strachan's Syndrome
4. Idiopathic
5. Malignancy
6. Drugs:
   Eg Vincristine, Isoniazid, Metronidazole, Nitrofurantoin
7. Chemicals:
   Eg Pb, Hg, Thallium, Triorthocresyl phosphate
8. Congenital:
   Eg Charcot–Marie–Tooth, Krabbe's, Refsum's
9. Sarcoidosis
10. Collagen vascular disease
11. Trauma
12. Neuralgic amyotrophy

GENERAL CLIN: Numbness; Paraesthesiae; Burning; Pain or constriction of extremities; Unsteadiness; Weakness; Wasting; Reflexes ↓

CLIN OF AUTONOMIC NEUROPATHY: Anhidrosis; Postural BP ↓; Constipation/diarrhoea; Impotence; Atonic bladder; Syncope

GENERAL INVESTIGATIONS:
- FBC
- ESR
- BG
- GTT
- U&E's
- Urinalysis

- PPE
- CXR
- LFT
- EMG
- Rare eg Urinary porphyrins, Nerve biopsy

DIABETIC NEUROPATHY

Quite common. Types:

1. Symmetrical polyneuropathy: Commonest. Sensory > Motor. Legs >arms. Ankle jerk ↓. Vibration in legs ↓. Occ ulcers, neuropathic jts & sensory ataxia (Pseudotabes)
2. Autonomic Neuropathy
3. Mononeuropathy: Esp IIIn & VIIn; Carpal tunnel syndrome
4. Mononeuritis Multiplex
   DD of Mononeuritis Multiplex:
   1. PAN
   2. Rh Arth
   3. SLE
   4. Leprosy
   5. Sarcoidosis
   6. Carcinoma
   7. Amyloidosis
   8. Vaccinations
5. Diabetic amyotrophy: Asymmetrical painful motor neuropathy esp proximal lower limb muscles

URAEMIA

Can occur in severe CRF or on haemodialysis. Distal symmetric predominantly sensory neuropathy

RX: Dialysis or transplant

AMYLOIDOSIS

Mononeuropathy or slowly progressive distal polyneuropathy

MYXOEDEMA & ACROMEGALY

Carpal tunnel syndrome or rarely sensorimotor polyneuropathy

PORPHYRIA

Predominantly motor polyneuropathy

GUILLAIN–BARRÉ SYNDROME

Usually follows viral infection

CLIN: Usually acute onset of paraesthesiae &/or pain in legs followed by muscle weakness which ascends over 3–4 wks occ → quadraplegia & resp failure. Reflexes ↓. Occ Cranial n palsy eg VIIn. Autonomic neuropathy may occur

INVESTIGATIONS:
- CSF: Protein ↑
- Nerve conduction studies

RX: Occ need tracheostomy. Prompt Rx of any infections. Physio

PROG: 80% fully recover. 5% relapse

DEFICIENCY NEUROPATHIES

Alcohol is a common cause of peripheral neuropathy esp a distal sensorimotor symmetrical form; mediated by vit B def

Beriberi (Thiamine), Pellagra (B6) & SACD (B12) ass c̄ distal predominantly sensory neuropathy

Strachan's syndrome of amblyopia, orogenital dermatitis, sensory neuropathy & deafness may be due to Vit B def

NEOPLASTIC NEUROPATHY

Occurs in Ca & reticuloses. May be direct infiltration or non–metastatic manifestation eg the sensory neuropathy ass c̄ Ca lung which can antedate other signs of Ca

HEREDITARY NEUROPATHIES

PERONEAL MUSCULAR ATROPHY (CHARCOT–MARIE–TOOTH): Aut Dom. Onset usually 10–30yrs

Clin: Pes cavus; Equinovarus; Distal muscle wasting → Bilat foot drop, "Upturned champagne bottle" legs. Later distal arm muscles involved. Occ Tremor; Ht ↑

HYPERTROPHIC NEUROPATHY (DEJERINE–SOTTAS): Aut Rec. Mixed polyneuropathy; Ataxia; Periph nerves thickened

REFSUM'S DISEASE: Aut Rec. Phytanic acid ↑

Clin: Mixed polyneuropathy. Retinitis pigmentosa; Ataxia. Occ Anosmia; Cataracts; Deafness; Ht ↑; Ichthyosis

HEREDITARY SENSORY NEUROPATHY: Rare. Aut Dom & Aut Rec forms

RILEY–DAY SYNDROME: Rare. Aut Rec. Esp Jews. Sensory & autonomic neuropathy

METACHROMATIC LEUKODYSTROPHY: Rare. Aut Rec. Onset in 2nd yr

Clin: Retardation; Ataxia; Areflexia; Tone ↓; Sensory neuropathy

KRABBE'S DISEASE (GLOBOID CELL LEUKODYSTROPHY): Rare. Mental retardation. Sensory neuropathy

TANGIER DISEASE: Rare. Familial. HDL ↑

BASSEN–KORNSWEIG DISEASE: Rare. Aut Rec. Spinocerebellar degeneration. Low density lipoprotein ↓. Retinitis pigmentosa

Collagen Vascular Neuropathy

Rh Arth may be ass c̄ mononeuritis multiplex, distal sensory neuropathy, sensorimotor neuropathy or carpal tunnel syndrome
PAN may be ass c̄ mononeuritis multiplex or occ a symmetrical sensorimotor neuropathy
Less commonly neuropathy due to SLE, Wegener's & Sjogren's

RX: Steroids, Physio

MOTOR NEURONE DISEASE (MND)

M>F. Esp late middle age. Cause unknown

PATH: Progressive degeneration of ant horn cells, corticospinal fibres & medullary motor nuclei

CLIN: 3 major presentations Progressive muscular atrophy—LMN lesion; Amyotrophic lateral sclerois—Corticospinal tract & LMN lesion ie wasting of upper limbs, spasticity in lower limbs; Progressive bulbar palsy—Brain stem innervated muscles affected. Muscle wasting & fasciculation c̄ reflexes ↑ & no sensory deficit. Later Dysphagia; Tongue atrophy

INVESTIGATIONS:
- EMG
- Muscle Biopsy
- Myelogram: To exclude high Cv lesion

RX: Physio. Occ cricomyotomy to aid swallowing

PROG: Average survival 3yrs

MYASTHENIA GRAVIS

In non-thymoma cases (85%) peak onset at 10–30 & 60–70yrs. In cases ass c̄ thymoma peak onset at 40–50yrs. F>M. Ass c̄ other auto-immune disease eg Rh Arth, SLE, PA, Hypothyroidism

PATHOGENESIS: Probable auto-immune cause. Thymus often abnormal due to hyperplasia or thymoma. ↓ number of ACh receptors due to anti-ACh receptor antibody

CLIN: Fatiguability of muscles. May be confined to ocular muscles c̄ ptosis & diplopia or be more generalised c̄ limb, bulbar & resp muscle weakness. In severe cases resp failure

INVESTIGATIONS:
- Tensilon test
- Anti-ACh receptor Ab ↑
- EMG
- CXR
- CAT scan
- Anti-striated muscle Ab: +ve in 90% c̄ thymoma

RX: In ocular & mild generalised cases: anticholinesterases. In young c̄ moderate disease: thymectomy. In elderly c̄ no thymoma: prednisolone &/or azathioprine. If thymoma, thymectomy. Occ plasmapharesis
Myasthenic crisis can be ppt by infection & requires anticholinesterases ± immunosuppressives ± ventilation
Cholinergic crisis requires withdrawal of anticholinesterases ± immunosuppressives ± ventilation

Myasthenic (Eaton Lambert) Syndrome

Usually due to Ca lung. Impaired release of ACh from nerve terminal due to pre-synaptic disorder. Mimics myasthenia gravis

MUSCLE DISORDERS

Duchenne Muscular Dystrophy

X-Linked. Commonest inherited myopathy. ? due to sarcolemmal abnormality

CLIN: Delayed motor development. Often diagnosed at 3–4yrs. Difficulty in walking; Gowers' manoeuvre; Proximal myopathy; Calves ↑. Occ IQ ↓. Later Contractures; Scoliosis; Inability to walk; Ht & resp failure

INVESTIGATIONS:
- CPK ↑
- EMG
- Muscle biopsy
- ECG

RX: Genetic counselling. Physio

PROG: Death usually by age 20

Becker Muscular Dystrophy

Onset 5–25yrs

CLIN: Delayed motor development. Proximal myopathy; Pelvic & shoulder girdle wasting. Rarely Ht involvement

PROG: Death between 30–60yrs

Limb-girdle Muscular Dystrophy

F=M. Aut Rec. Onset in teens

CLIN: Onset in either upper or lower limb. Slowly progressive. Later contractures, scoliosis, cardiac involvement

DD: Spinal muscular atrophy

Facio–Scapulo–Humeral Dystrophy

Aut-Dom. F=M. Onset in adolescence

CLIN: Weakness of face & proximal muscles of limb & trunk. Occ Distal muscle weakness eg foot drop. Often benign course

Ocular Muscular Dystrophy

Very rare

CLIN: Bilat ptosis; No diplopia; Occ Ext ophthalmoplegia. May be ass c̄ limb-girdle weakness

Spinal Muscular Atrophies

WERDNIG–HOFFMAN DISEASE

Onset 0–6mths

CLIN: Hypotonia; Muscle weakness inc resp; Areflexia. Rapid downhill course

KUGELBERG–WELANDER DISEASE

Aut Rec. Onset in childhood

CLIN: Hypotonia & muscle weakness. Later contractures. Variable progression, most die by 30 yrs

Myotonic Disorders

MYOTONIA CONGENITA (THOMPSEN'S DISEASE)

Very rare. Usually Aut Dom. Onset in infancy

CLIN: Myotonia ppt by rest & cold, relieved by exercise. Hypertrophy but no weakness of muscles

RX: Procainamide

DYSTROPHIA MYOTONICA

Aut Dom. Usually onset in adult life

CLIN: Myotonia; Distal muscular atrophy; Ptosis; Cataracts; Atrophy of temporal, masseter & sternomastoid muscles; Facial weakness; Frontal baldness; Gonadal atrophy; Ht conduction defects; Hypoventilation; Bony abnormalities; Mental retardation; Dysphagia; Areflexia

INVESTIGATIONS:
- EMG
- Muscle biopsy
- ECG
- CPK: sl ↑
- SXR: Vault hyperostosis, Small sella

RX: Procainamide or Phenytoin

PROG: Often die early due to cardiac or resp failure

PARAMYOTONICA

Myotonia in cold, generalised muscular weakness

DD: HyperK$^+$ periodic paralysis

Polymyositis/Dermatomyositis

F>M. Usually idiopathic but occ ass c̄ Rh Arth, SLE, Scleroderma or 2° to Ca. May be ppt by sunlight, sulphonamides, viral illness

CLIN: Slowly progressive limb-girdle weakness; Muscle pain & tenderness. May have Dysphagia; Heliotrope rash. Later sc calcinosis; Ht conduction defects; Raynaud's

INVESTIGATIONS:
- CPK ↑ (esp acute phase)
- ESR ↑
- EMG
- Muscle biopsy
- For occult Ca

RX: Steroids ± Azathioprine. Physio

PROG: Usually slow recovery in uncomplicated cases

Polymyalgia Rheumatica

Esp >55yrs. F>M. Closely ass c̄ giant cell arteritis

CLIN: Pain & stiffness shoulder, neck, back. No weakness. Wt ↓; Malaise; Fever. Synovitis in shoulders, hips & knees

INVESTIGATIONS:
- ESR ↑
- FBC
- Biopsy artery if signs of temporal arteritis

RX: Steroids

TEMPORAL ARTERITIS

Esp >55yrs. F>M

CLIN: Severe headache; Tender cranial arteries esp temporal; Pain in face, jaw & mouth; Wt ↓; Malaise; Fever; Depression. Later Visual loss; VBI. Ass c̄ polymyalgia rheumatica. Occ Polyneuritis

INVESTIGATION:
- ESR ↑
- Hb ↓
- Globulin ↑, Albumin ↓
- Temporal artery biopsy

RX: Prompt treatment c̄ steroids. Monitor ESR

Endocrine Myopathies

Occur in hyperthyroidism, hypothyroidism, acromegaly, Cushing's disease, Addison's disease & hypopituitarism

Metabolic Myopathies

McARDLE'S DISEASE

Rare. A glycogen storage disorder

CLIN: Exercise induced muscular pain & stiffness. Myoglobinuria. Occ Contractures

INVESTIGATIONS:
- Muscle biopsy
- CPK ↑

ACID MALTASE DEFICIENCY (POMPE'S DISEASE)

Rare. A glycogen storage disorder c̄ infantile, childhood & adult varieties

CLIN OF ADULT FORM: Limb-girdle weakness; lower limb hypertrophy. Occ Resp involvement

CARNITINE PALMITYL TRANSFERASE DEFICIENCY

Rare. A disorder of muscle lipid metabolism

CLIN: Exercise induced muscle pain, cramp & myoglobinuria

CARNITINE DEFICIENCY

Rare. A disorder of muscle lipid metabolism

CLIN: Limb-girdle weakness. Cardiac failure

PERIODIC PARALYSES

All Aut Dom. Rarely ass c̄ thyrotoxicosis. Attacks of flaccid weakness of voluntary muscle
Due to membrane abnormality. Three types:

A) HYPOKALAEMIC: Onset in teens
Clin: Attacks after prolonged rest, on waking or after heavy meal. Lasts for days. Areflexia & hypoK during episode
Rx: Acetazolamide for prophylaxis. KCl in attack

B) HYPERKALAEMIC: Onset in childhood
Clin: Attacks after exercise. Lasts for hours. Myotonia of eyelids, tongue & small muscles of hand. HyperK$^+$ during attack

Rx: Acetazolamide for prophylaxis. Oral glucose & Insulin during attack

C) SODIUM RESPONSIVE NORMOKALAEMIC:

Clin: Attacks ppt by sleep. Last for days

Rx: Acetazolamide for prophylaxis. NaCl during attack

Paroxysmal Myoglobinuria Syndrome

Rare. Unknown aetiology

CLIN: Severe muscle cramps & tenderness ass c̄ paralysis or weakness & myoglobinuria

Floppy Infant Syndrome

Generalised muscular hypotonia from birth

Causes of Floppy Infant Syndrome (LIST 20 NEURO)

1. Cerebral Palsy
2. Mental retardation
3. Cerebral degenerative disease
4. Werdnig–Hoffman disease
5. Benign congenital hypotonia
6. Nemaline myopathy
7. Central core disease
8. Myotubular myopathy
9. Mitochondrial myopathies
10. Prader–Willi syndrome

Progressive Myositis Ossificans

Familial. Sclerosis then ossification in muscle. Ass c̄ extra toes/digits. Presents early c̄ neck swelling. Then shoulder & pelvic muscles ossify. Occ overlying skin ulcerates. Often terminal aspiration pneumonia

Stiff Man Syndrome

Rare. M>F. Fluctuating stiffness & painful spasms

RX: Diazepam

Malignant Hyperpyrexia

Familial. May occur in isolation or c̄ myotonia congenita, osteogenesis imperfecta & central core disease. Potentially lethal on being anaesthetised

CLIN: In acute episode: BP ↑; Ventricular arrhythmias; Hyperventilation; Cyanosis; Muscle rigidity & fasciculation; High fever. Myopathy

INVESTIGATIONS:
- CPK
- Muscle biopsy

RX: Screen individuals at risk

TOXIC DISORDERS

Lead

Esp from lead paint, pipes, cosmetics, petrol. Ass c̄ Pica

CLIN: Anaemia; Abdo colic; Anorexia; Irritability; Fatigue; Vom; Failure to thrive; Blue lines in gums. Occ Nephritis. Periph motor neuropathy eg Wrist drop. Occ Acute encephalopathy esp children c̄ papilloedema, Ep, coma. Occ Chr encephalopathy c̄ Ep, mental changes, blindness & spasticity

INVESTIGATIONS:
- Blood film: Punctate basophilia
- X-R: Lead lines in bones
- Serum lead
- Serum enzymes eg ALA

RX: EDTA

Glue Sniffing

Esp Teenagers

CLIN: Mild euphoria. Occ Periph neuropathy

Acrylamide

CLIN: Periph neuropathy. Ataxia

Arsenic

CLIN: Periph neuropathy; Desquamation;

Mees lines (nails); GI symptoms

RX: British Anti-Lewisite

Carbon Disulphide

CLIN: Periph neuropathy; TATT; Depression

Chlorinated Naphthalenes

CLIN: Ep; Myoclonus

Manganese

CLIN: Psychoses; Extrapyramidal symptoms—Parkinsonism

Mercury

INORGANIC

CLIN: Stomatitis; Saliva ↑; "Erethism"; Tremor

RX: British Anti-Lewisite, Penicillamine

ORGANIC

CLIN: Pins & needles; Ataxia; Sight ↓

Organophosphates

eg TOCP

CLIN: Anticholinesterase effects eg Headache; Abdo pain; Vom; Sweating; Miosis; Twitching. Periph neuropathy

RX: Atropine

Thallium

CLIN: Colic; Diarrhoea; Painful sensory neuropathy; Weakness; Cranial n palsy. Retrobulbar neuritis; Chorea; Psychosis; Alopecia; Mees lines

RX: Diethyldithiocarbamate

NUTRITIONAL DISORDERS

Beriberi

Vit B1—thiamine def. Two forms:
a) Dry: Periph neuropathy; Muscular weakness; Optic atrophy
b) Wet: CCF ± neuropathy

Wernicke–Korsakoff Syndrome

Thiamine def almost always ass c̄ chr alcoholism

CLIN: Heavy drinking without adequate diet → acute onset of confusion. Occ Tremor; Hallucinations; Ep; Nystagmus; Bilat VIn palsies; Conjugate gaze palsies; Truncal ataxia; Headache; Vom; Polyneuropathy. Then coma

RX: Thiamine. On recovery often suffer from Korsakoff's syndrome—a gross defect of short term memory often c̄ confabulation & retrograde amnesia N.B Cerebellar degeneration & polyneuropathy can occur as isolated conditions ass c̄ chr alcoholism

Pellagra

Vit B2 def—Riboflavin

CLIN: GI disturbances; Dermatitis of hands, feet, face, neck & chest → hyperkeratosis; Insomnia; Depression; Optic atrophy

Vit B6 (Pyridoxine) Def

CLIN: Ep; Periph neuropathy; Sideroblastic anaemia

Subaute Combined Degeneration of Cord (SACD)

Vit B12 def is ass c̄ PA, Gastrectomy, Malabsorption, Vegans

CLIN: +ve Lhermitte's sign; +ve Rhomberg's sign; Spasticity; Loss of vibration & jt position sense; Bilat plantar's ↑; Periph neuropathy; Megaloblastic anaemia; Ataxia; Weakness; Impotence. Later incontinence. Occ Optic atrophy; Nystagmus; Dementia

RX: B12 injections

Protein Def (Kwashiorkor)

Esp Tropics & Subtropics. Esp children

CLIN: Oedema; Pigmentation; Desquamation. Brain development ↓

Ophthalmology

THE INJURED EYE

Effects of Contusion to the Eye

EYELIDS:

Haematoma

SUBCONJUNCTIVAL HAEM

CAUSES: 1. Coughing esp Whooping cough
2. Minor trauma
3. Idiopathic

CLIN: Symptomless. Lasts 2/52. Spontaneous recovery

CORNEAL:

Abrasion

CLIN: Pain; Photophobia; Blurring of vision

INVESTIGATION: • Fluorescein

RX: Pad & bandage

IRIS:

Hyphaema ie blood in ant chamber
Occ → glaucoma

RX: Bed rest

LENS:

Cataract or Dislocation

DD: Marfan's syndrome

VITREOUS HAEM

RETINA:

CLIN: Transient retinal anaesthesia; Oedema (Commotio retinae); Haem. Occ Vision ↓

OPTIC NERVE:

Avulsion or ischaemia → Blindness

Perforating Injuries

EYELIDS

RX: Suture
N.B. Burns → Entropion, Ectropion; Occ 2° infection

CORNEA, SCLERA

INVESTIGATION: • X-R (to exclude foreign body)

LENS

→ Cataract

BLOW-OUT FRACTURES

CLIN: Diplopia; Restriction of eye elevation & depression. Echymoses; Subconjunctival haem

INVESTIGATIONS: • X-R—"Tear-drop opacity", step deformity orbital floor.
• CAT scan

RX: Surgical repair

ERRORS OF REFRACTION

N.B : Concave lenses for myopia (short sight)

Squints

Types of Squint (LIST 1 OPHTH)

1. Concomitant:
   a) Normal in neonates
   b) Congenital
2. Paralytic:
   Ocular nerve palsy i.e IIIn, IVn or VIn lesion
3. Latent:
   Exhibited when tired

CONCOMITANT

Congenital

CLIN: FEM c̄ no diplopia. Supression → Amblyopia

PARALYTIC

Lesion of IIIn, IVn or VIn

CLIN: Loss of FEM. Diplopia—the false image is peripheral & is seen by affected eye

IVn: "Down & out" impossible. Sup Obl muscle palsy

IIIn: Ptosis; Abducted eye—"Down & out"; Dilated pupil

VIn: Convergent squint; Diplopia

LATENT

CLIN: Exhibited when tired

INVESTIGATION: • Cover test

Nystagmus

Causes of Nystagmus (LIST 2 OPHTH)

1. Cerebellar lesions:
   Eg Primary tumours; Mets
2. Lesions of IIIn, IVn,VIn, VIIIn:
   Eg Acoustic neuroma
3. Vestibular lesions:
   Eg Viral labyrinthitis
4. Drugs:
   Eg Sedatives, Alcohol, Phenytoin
5. High cervical cord lesions:
   Eg Post inf cerebellar artery thromb
6. Brain stem lesions

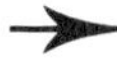

7. Physiological:
   Eg lying or turning over; Optokinetic
8. Lesions within orbit:
   Eg Ocular muscle weakness, Errors of refraction
9. Congenital
10. Wernicke's Encephalopathy

CLIN: In cerebeller lesions slow phase is to side of lesion

Argyll-Robertson Pupil

? Mid-brain lesion

Causes of Argyll-Robertson Pupil (LIST 3 OPHTH)

1. Syphilis
2. Diabetes
3. Alcoholism
4. Mid-brain lesions:
   Eg Multiple sclerosis

CLIN: Loss of light reflex but able to accommodate; Small irregular pupils

Adie's Pupil

Young women

CLIN: Sluggish constriction; Absent reflexes; Large myotonic pupil

Horner's Syndrome

Damage to cervical sympath

Causes of Horner's Syndrome (LIST 4 OPHTH)

1. Cervical adenitis
2. Thyroid operations
3. Aortic aneurysm
4. Syringomyelia
5. D1 lesions:
   Eg Pancoast's Tumour
6. Trauma
7. Cervical cord tumours
8. MS
9. Post inf cerebellar artery thromb

CLIN: Miosis; Partial ptosis; Enophthalmos; Anhydrosis

THE RED EYE

Causes of the Painful Red Eye (LIST 5 OPHTH)

1. Ac Conjunctivitis
2. Ac Iritis
3. Ac Glaucoma
4. Ac Keratitis
5. Episcleritis

Acute Conjunctivitis

Staph >Pneumococcus >*H. influenzae*

CLIN: Red eye "pink"; Discharge; Discomfort; Photophobia. Usually 7/7 course

RX: Irrigate c̄ saline. Hrly bactericidal. Dark glasses

Special more dangerous cases:

a) **OPHTHALMIA NEONATORUM**
Due to Gonococcus
Rx: Penicillin

b) **INCLUSION CONJUNCTIVITIS**
Causes: 1. TRIC agent (Chlamydia)
2. Psittacosis
3. Lymphogranuloma venerium.
4. Adenovirus

Trachoma: Due to TRIC agent.
Commonest cause of blindness from corneal scarring. Esp Middle-East
Clin: Blindness; Ectropion; Entropion
Rx: $CuSO_4$, Sulphonamides

Allergic Conjunctivitis

Due to: Drugs; Cosmetics; Contact lenses; Hay fever; TB

RX: Steroids & Antihistamines

Acute Iritis

DEFINITIONS: Uveal tract = Iris & Ciliary body & Choroid
Iritis : A painful red eye
Choroiditis : Painless eye with impaired vision

Causes of Ac Iritis (LIST 6 OPHTH)

1. Idiopathic—majority
2. Infections:
   a) TB
   b) Gonorrhoea
   c) Toxoplasmosis
   d) Malaria
   e) Toxocara
   f) Syphilis
   g) Weil's disease
   h) Brucellosis
   i) Viral
   j) Exogenous infections
3. Auto-Immune disorders
4. Sarcoidosis
5. Collagen disorders: Eg Rheumatoid arthritis, Still's
6. Sero-negative Arthropathies: Eg Reiter's disease
7. Ulcerative colitis
8. Trauma
9. Behcet's Syndrome
10. Sympathetic Ophthalmites following penetrating wounds may affect other eye

CLIN: Circumcorneal injection c̄ brick red conjunctiva; Tender painful eyeball; Contraction of pupil; Inflam exudation in ant chamber → blurred vision; Hypopyon (fluid level); Keratic ppt; Photophobia; Post synechias (adhesions) of Iris to ant lens can → 2° glaucoma. Relapses are common

RX: Steroids. Atropine (but SE: Glaucoma). Local heat. Pad for photophobia. Treat underlying disorder

COMPLICATIONS: Can → Glaucoma; Cataract

Acute Keratitis

Exogenous form (superficial cornea) eg corneal ulcer >endogenous (deep cornea) eg interstitial keratitis

CORNEAL ULCERS

MARGINAL ULCER
Small; Multiple. Staph infection

CENTRAL ULCER

Causes: 1. Infection 2° to trauma eg Pneumococcus
2. *Herpes simplex* → dendritic ulcer
3. Degenerative conditions eg vit A ↓
4. Overexposure of cornea eg Exophthalmos

GENERAL CLIN: Signs & symptoms of conjunctivitis & mild iritis. Visual loss

GENERAL Rx:

A. Medical: Antibiotics, Atropine, heat pad. No Steroids. Idoxuridine for dendritic ulcer. Paint c̄ Carbolic acid

B. Surgical: Tarsorrhaphy—suturing lids together

COMPLICATION: Very occ → perforation

Interstitial Keratitis

Usually due to congenital syphilis

CLIN: Poor vision; Scarring

RX: Steroids; Atropine; Penicillin. Occ corneal grafts

Episceleritis

Collagen disease

CLIN: Red eye; Dull ache for a few weeks; Often relapses

RX: Steroids, oral Salicylates, heat

Acute Glaucoma

Rise in inter-ocular pressure

PRIMARY ACUTE CLOSED-ANGLE GLAUCOMA

Iris in contact c̄ cornea preventing drainage in Canal of Schlemm. Shallow ant chamber predisposes

CLIN: Severe periorbital pain; Poor vision; Nausea & occ vomiting; "Steamy" cornea due to oedema; Pupil dilated, fixed to light; Ocular tension ↑; Haloes around eyes; Green-grey iris

RX: Pilocarpine—to constrict. β blockers eg Timoptol. Acetazolomide → ↓ aqueous prod. Analgesia, pads, heat. Glycerol in water to dehydrate. If medical Rx fails : Glaucoma Iridectomy

GRADUAL LOSS OF SIGHT IN NON-INFLAMMED EYES

Causes of Gradual Loss of Sight (LIST 7 OPHTH)

1. Corneal ulcers
2. Diabetic retinopathy
3. Degenerative disease:
   a) Involutional Macular Degeneration
   b) Retinitis Pigmentosa
   c) Choroido-Retinal Atrophy
4. Simple glaucoma
5. Cataract (qv LIST 8 OPHTH)

Four commonest (UK) causes of blindness:

Involutional macular degeneration >Glaucoma >Cataract >Diabetes

Simple Glaucoma

PATHOGENESIS: Gradual IOP ↑ overlooked by patient. Later sight ↓. Sclerotic process

CLIN: IOP ↑; Scotoma → blindness; Cupped optic discs. Later optic atrophy

RX: Pilocarpine. Diamox. Neutral adrenaline → ↓aqueous prod. Timoptol. Occ Trabeculectomy or Laser trabeculoplasty

Congenital Glaucoma (Buphthalmos)

"Ox eye". Maldevelopment of drainage angle of ant chamber

RX: Surgery

Cataract

Causes of Cataract (LIST 8 OPHTH)

1. Old age
2. Trauma direct or indirect: Eg Heat, Irradiation
3. Steroids
4. Diabetes
5. HypoPT
6. Cretinism
7. Galactosaemia
8. Homocystinuria
9. Down's Syndrome
10. Dystrophia Myotonica
11. Wilson's disease
12. Glaucoma
13. Rare disorders:
    a) Rubella syndrome
    b) Congenital Hypocalcaemia
    c) Oculocerebrorenal syndrome
    d) Refsum's disease
    e) Laurence-Moon-Biedl syndrome

CLIN: Gradual loss of sight; White opacity in pupil

RX: If irreversible cataract, surgical Rx
a) Intra-capsular extraction (>35yrs)
b) Extracapsular extraction ie needling (<35yrs). Possible as nucleus is relatively soft
If lens removed (Aphakia) require lens implant & use contact lens

Degeneration of Retina & Choroid

INVOLUTIONAL MACULAR DEGENERATION

CAUSES: 1. Old age: Common
2. Tay Sach's disease
3. 2° to Chloroquine
4. Best's disease

CLIN: Bilat central scotoma. Development of subretinal neovascular membrane → macular haem, exudates

Retinitis Pigmentosa

Ass c̄ Laurence-Moon-Biedl; Diabetes; Malabsorption; Cataract; A β lipoprotinaemia; Acanthosis

CLIN: Peripheral vision loss; Night blindness

Choroido-retinal Atrophy

CAUSES: 1. Choroiditis occ 2° to toxoplasmosis
2. High myopia
3. Tabeto-retinal degeneration

CLIN: Vitreous opacities; Vision ↓; Retinal haem

SUDDEN LOSS OF SIGHT IN NON-INFLAMMED EYE

Causes of Sudden Blindness (LIST 9 OPHTH)

A. PAINLESS
1. Vascular causes:
    a) Central retinal artery occlusion
    b) Central retinal vein occlusion
    c) Vitreous Haem
    d) Retinal arteriosclerosis
    e) Temporal arteritis
2. Primary retinal detachment—Trauma
3. Secondary retinal detachment:
    a) Toxaemia
    b) Retinal & Choroidal tumours
4. Methanol
5. Hysteria
6. Retrobulbar neuritis
7. Lesions of optic pathway

B. PAINFUL
1. Migrane
2. Acute Glaucoma
3. Trauma

Retinal Arteriosclerosis

CLIN: "Copper-wire" arteries → "silver-wire". Later retinopathy c̄ haem & hard exudates

If Malignant BP ↑: Papilloedema; Retinal necrosis

If Renal Retinopathy: Oedema; "Fan shaped" exudates; Haem

Diabetic Retinopathy

10-20yrs post onset

CLIN: Micro-aneurysms; "Dot & blot" haem then exudates. Pre-retinal haem; Vitreous haem. Late retinitis proliferans

RX: Photocoagulation. Cataract & vitreous surgery

Central Retinal Artery Occlusion

CAUSES:
1. Spasm
2. Degeneration
3. Embolus
4. Hemiparesis
5. Temporal arteritis

CLIN: Sudden blindness; Narrow arteries → (1-2/7) Cherry red spot → optic atrophy

Central Retinal Vein Occlusion

Often due to venous congestion following arterial P ↑. May be ass c̄ glaucoma

CLIN: Haem; Engorged veins; New anastomotic vessels. Vision ↓↓

Vitreous Haemorrhage

CAUSES:
1. Blood dyscrasia eg anaemia, purpura
2. TB periphlebitis (Eales Disease)—young men
3. SAH ass c̄ sub-hyaloid haem

CLIN: Haem clears slowly. Partial blindness

Causes of Retinal Haemorrhage (LIST 10 OPHTH)

1. Diabetes Mellitus
2. Vascular causes:
   a) Retinal vein thrombosis
   b) Sub-arachnoid haem
   c) Severe anaemia eg PA; Iron deficiency anaemia
   d) Arteritis eg Polyarteritis nodosa
   e) Bleeding diasthesis
3. Raised intracranial pressure
4. Hypertension
5. Trauma

Retinal Detachment

Ass c̄ myopia, trauma

CLIN: Loss of vision in a discrete area preceded by flashes, floating opacities.

Often bilat

RX: Cryotherapy. Scleral plombage

2° Retinal Detachment

CAUSES:
1. Toxaemia
2. Retinal & Choroidal tumours:
   a) Malignant melanoma
   b) Retinoblastoma → glaucoma
   c) Metastases

MELANOMA

Usually uniocular. 2° retinal detachment. Mets to the liver. "A person c̄ a large liver & a glass eye"

RX: Enucleation

RETINOBLASTOMA

Esp infancy. Usually familial; Bilateral

CLIN: White mass. Direct spread to brain

RX: Enucleation

PATTERNS OF VISUAL FIELD LOSS

The Visual Pathway

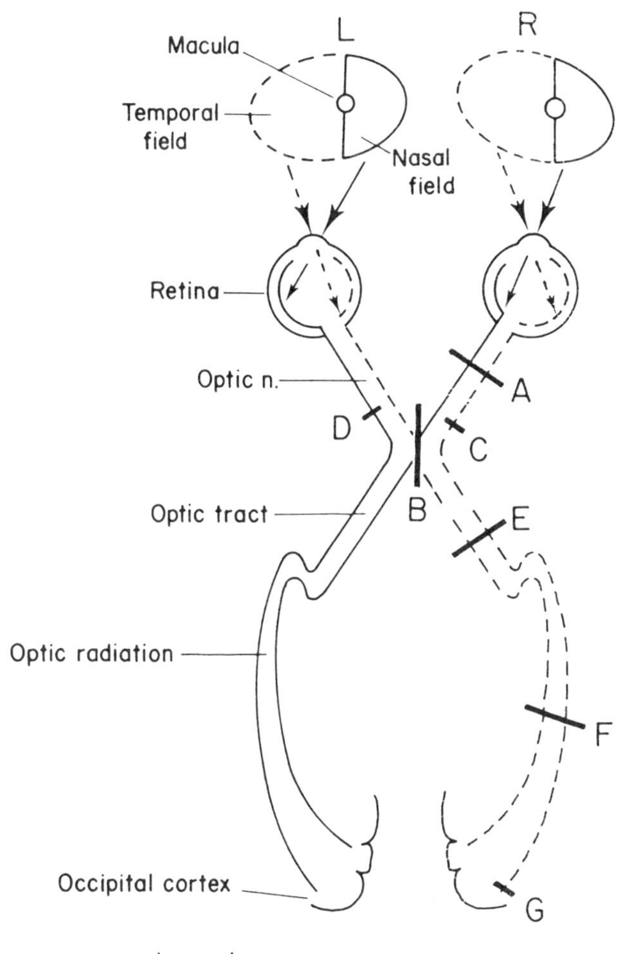

Figure 1 The Visual Pathway

Tunnel Vision

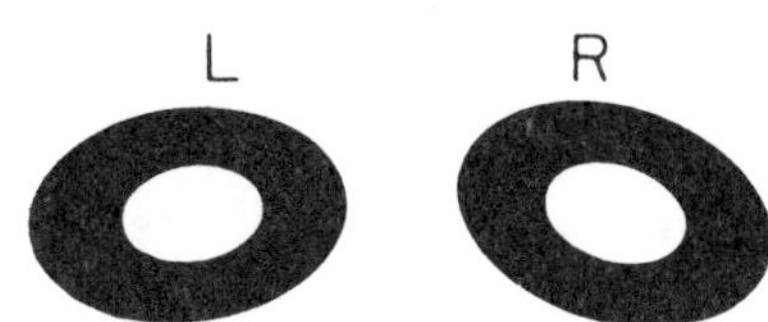

CAUSES: 1. Glaucoma
2. Papilloedema
3. Migraine
4. Retinal disease
5. Tabes
6. Ant calcarine cortex lesion
7. Hysteria

Central Scotoma

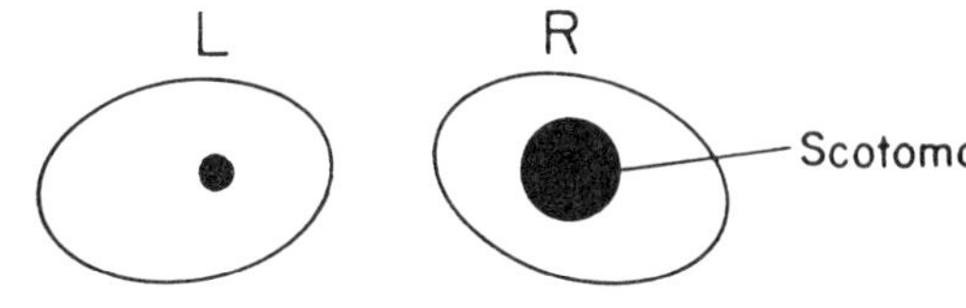

CAUSES: 1. Macular disorders
2. Retrobulbar neuritis esp MS
3. Optic atrophy
4. Occipital pole lesions (Lesion at G Fig 1 above)

Blindness in One Eye

(Lesion at A Fig 1 above)

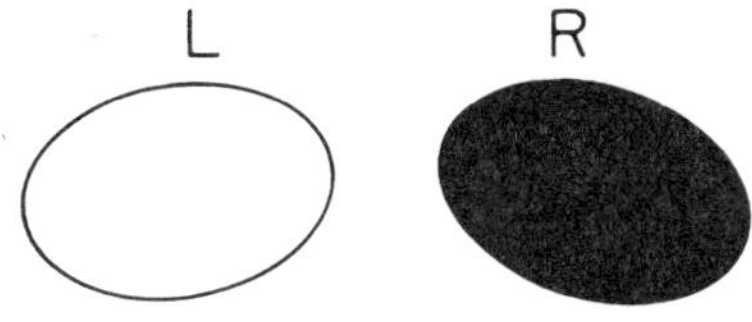

CAUSES:
1. Optic nerve compression eg meningioma
2. Optic nerve glioma
3. Mets
4. Acute retrobulbar neuritis

Bitemporal Hemianopia

(Lesion at B Fig 1 above)

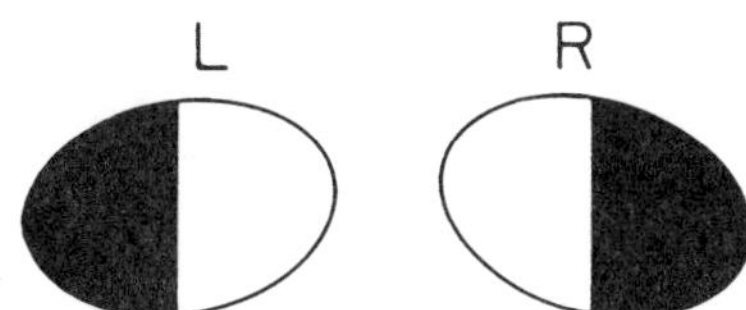

CAUSES: 1. Pituitary tumour
2. Meningioma
3. Carotid aneurysm
4. Trauma

Binasal Hemianopia

(Lesion at C & D Fig 1 above)

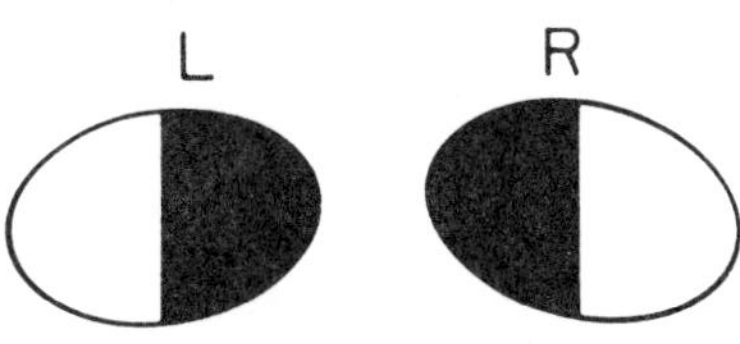

Rare

(Left) Homonymous Hemianopia

(Lesion at E Fig 1 above)

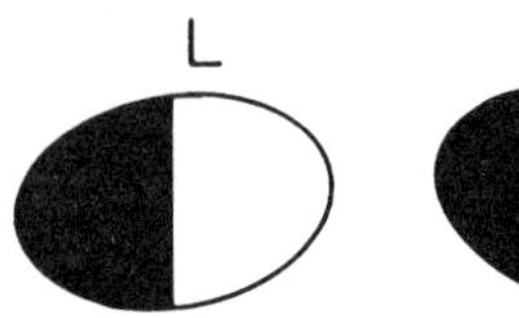

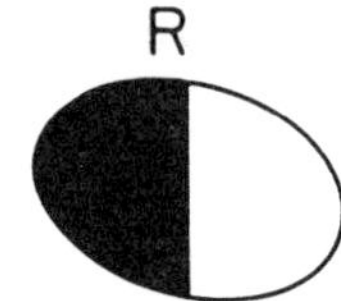

CAUSES: Optic tract lesions usually tumours eg Craniopharyngioma; Meningioma

Special Case:

CAUSES OF HOMONYMOUS HEMIANOPIA c̄ IPSILAT CENTRAL SCOTOMA:

Lesions of lat part of optic chiasma & optic nerve

1. Pituitary tumour
2. Ant communicating artery aneurysm
3. Sphenoidal wing meningioma

(Left) Homonymous Hemianopia

(Lesion at F Fig 1 above)
Special case of homonymous hemianopia c̄ normal pupillary response

Quadrantic Hemianopia

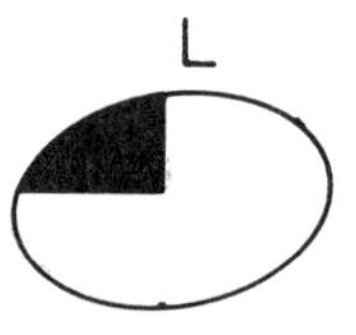

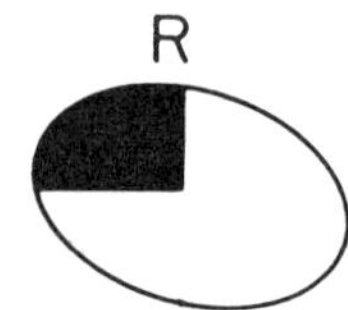

Temporal lobe lesions → upper quadrantinopia
Parietal lobe lesions → lower quadrantanopia

CAUSES: Tumours or abscesses. Rare

LACRIMAL GLAND AND THE EYELID

Causes of Ptosis (LIST 11 OPHTH)

1. IIIn lesion:
   eg Cavernous sinus thrombosis
2. Cervical sympathetic lesion—
   Horner's syndrome
3. Eyelid damage
4. Myasthenia gravis
5. Old age
6. Myopathy
7. Tabes dorsalis
8. Hysteria
9. Congenital

Eyelid Inflammation

EXT STYE (HORDEOLUM)

Pyogenic infection

INT STYE (CHALAZION)

Infection of Meibomian gland → cyst. Feels like hailstones

RX: Incision & Curettage

BLEPHARITIS

Infection of eyelid margin. Occ Staph. Hard to eradicate

RX: Antibiotics ± steroids

Eyelid Displacement

CAUSES:
1. Spasm orbicularis: Infants → eversion; Adults → inversion
2. Atony orbicularis: Infants → inversion; Adults → eversion
3. Scarring eg Trachoma; Burns

SPASTIC ENTROPIUM

CAUSES:
1. Old age
2. VIIn palsy

CLIN: Epiphora (weeping); Infection

RX: Astringents; Surgery ("3 snip" op)

Tumours & Degenerations

XANTHELASMA

CLIN: Creamy deposits sited at med ends of lids

PAPILLOMA

Common. Often viral

DERMOID CYST

CLIN: Cyst at upper inner & outer angles of the orbit

INVESTIGATION: • X-R: Lucent well defined lesion

RODENT ULCER

Basal cell carcinoma. Usually lid margin

CA LACRIMAL GLAND

Rare

RX: Exenteration

PINGUECULAE

Hyaline degeneration of conjunctival collagen

ARCUS SENELIS

Esp old age. White ring just within corneal margin. Vision normal

FAMILIAL DYSTROPHIES

PTERYGIA

Conjunctival flap onto cornea

Lacrimal Gland

SJOGREN'S SYNDROME

F>M. Ass c̄ Collagen diseases eg SLE, Rh Arth

CLIN: Dry mouth & eye. Occ Alopecia

RX: "Artificial tears"

MIKULICZ'S SYNDROME

M>F. Ass c̄ sarcoidosis

CLIN: Swelling of lacrimal & salivary glands; Dry mouth; Ptosis

EPIPHORA

CAUSES: 1. Ectropion
2. Trauma
3. Failure to canalise
4. Infection of lacrimal sac: Ac or Chr dacryocystitis
5. Congenital membranous obstruction

CLIN: Wet eye; Overflow of tears

Exophthalmos

Causes of Exophthalmos (LIST 12 OPHTH)

A. UNILATERAL
1. Dysthyroid disease
2. Intraorbital causes:
   a) Pseudotumour
   b) Granuloma
   c) Tumours eg Meningioma; Neuroblastoma; Retinoblastoma; Melanoma; Lymphoma; Mets
   d) Vascular eg Aneurysm; A-V malformations; Haemangioma; Varices; Caroticocavernous fistula
3. Nasopharangeal & sinus disease:
   a) Mucocoele
   b) Osteoma
   c) Tumours eg Nasopharangeal cancer
4. Intracranial lesions (rare): Eg Meningioma
5. Others:
   a) Neurofibromatosis
   b) Fibrous dysplasia
   c) Congenital glaucoma (Ox eye)
   d) Fungal mass

B. BILATERAL
1. Dysthyroid disease
2. Rarely any of the above can cause bilat exophthalmos esp retinoblastoma

DYSTHYROID DISEASE

MILD FORM: Graves' disease. F>M
Clin: Proptosis; Signs of thyrotoxicosis

SEVERE FORM: M=F. Ave age 50yrs. ? due to EPS
Clin: Proptosis; Signs of thyrotoxicosis. Ophthalmoplegia
Rx: Underlying thyroid condition. Occ Steroids or Tarsorrhaphy

CAROTICOCAVERNOUS FISTULA

CLIN: Pulsating exophthalmos; Conjunctival oedema; Initially painful

ORBITAL CELLULITIS

2° to sinusitis. Occ → Blindness; Meningitis; Cavernous sinus thromb

CLIN: Pain esp if cavernous sinus thromb

RX: Antibiotics

ORBITAL TUMOURS

PRIMARY: Meningioma; Glioma; Pseudotumour

SECONDARY: Ca antrum; Wilm's tumour; Leukaemia; Neuroblastoma

MISCELLANEOUS CONDITIONS

Causes of Papilloedema
(LIST 13 OPHTH)

1. Raised intracranial pressure due to tumours
2. Malignant hypertension
3. Due to obstructed retinal venous drainage:
   a) Tumour
   b) Central retinal vein thrombosis
   c) SVC obstruction
   d) Cavernous, lateral sinus & jugular vein thromb
   e) PRV
   f) Macroglobulinaemia
   g) Hyperlipidaemia
4. Head injury
5. Cerebral anoxia
6. Benign intracranial hypertension
7. Steroid withdrawal
8. Metabolic disorders:
   a) Hypercapnia
   b) Diabetes mellitus
   c) Malignant thyrotoxic exophthalmos
9. Sub-arachnoid haem
10. Meningitis
11. Rare causes:
    a) Lead poisoning
    b) Guillain-Barré syndrome
    c) Vit A poisoning

Causes of Optic Atrophy
(LIST 14 OPHTH)

A. PRIMARY DAMAGE TO NERVE FIBRES
   1. Traumatic:
      a) Trauma
      b) Surgery
   2. Due to pressure:
      a) Paget's disease
      b) Tumours
      c) Aneurysm
      d) Fibrous dysplasia
   3. Lesions of optic tract: Eg CVA
B. POST NEURITIC
   Chronic papilloedema
C. DAMAGE TO RETINA
   1. Choroidoretinitis
   2. Dystrophies
   3. Degenerations
   4. Intra-ocular haem
   5. Central retinal artery occlusion
D. GLAUCOMA
E. RETROBULBAR NEURITIS

Causes of Optic Neuritis
(LIST 15 OPHTH)

1. Multiple sclerosis
2. Freidrich's ataxia
3. Toxins:
   a) Methanol
   b) Tobacco
   c) Lead
   d) Benzene
   e) Clioquinol
4. Giant cell arteritis
5. Diabetes mellitus
6. Infective:
   a) Retinitis
   b) Toxoplasmosis
   c) Syphilis
   d) Typhoid
   e) Mumps
7. Other demyelinating disease—rare:
   a) Schilder's
   b) Devic's
8. Vit B12 deficiency

Hypovitaminosis

VIT A DEF

CLIN: **i) Infants:** Corneal perforation; Blindness; Xerophthalmia
ii) Adults: Night blindness; Skin changes

THIAMINE (Vit B1) DEF:

CLIN: Polyneuritis; Weakness; Reflexes ↓; Palsies; Heart failure

RIBOFLAVIN (VIT B2) DEF:

CLIN: Stomatitis; Vascular keratitis; Retrobulbar neuritis; Scotoma; Optic atrophy

Leprosy

TUBERCULOID FORM:

CLIN: Loss of lashes, eyebrows; Stiff skin; Corneal ulcer

LEPROMATOUS FORM:

CLIN: Ptosis. Patches on lids; Loss of lashes. Episcleral nodules → iritis

Onchocerciasis

Esp Africa & Central Am. Important cause of blindness
Due to Filariasis

CLIN: Corneal infiltrates. Choroido-retinal degeneration → optic atrophy

RX: Diethylcarbamazine

Epidemic Dropsy

Due to Argemone oil poisoning. Esp India. → Glaucoma

Ear, Nose & Throat

The Ear

DEAFNESS

DEFINITIONS:

A. **Conductive Deafness** (CD): Obstruction, defect or lesion of EAM or middle ear which interferes with normal passage of airborne sounds

B. **Perceptive Deafness** (PD): Defect of cochlea or auditory nerve whereby nervous impulses from cochlea to brain are attenuated

Causes of Deafness (LIST 1 ENT)

A. CONDUCTIVE
1. Wax
2. Acute Otitis Media
3. Secretory Otitis Media
4. Chronic Otitis Media
5. Foreign body
6. Otosclerosis
7. Barotrauma
8. Paget's disease
9. Tympanic membrane injuries
10. Meatal infections
11. Rare causes;
    a) Traumatic ossicular dislocation
    b) Cong stenosis
    c) Cancer—Nasopharynx (due to 3), Middle ear, EAM

B. PERCEPTIVE
1. Presbyacusis
2. Infections:
    a) Mumps
    b) Influenza
    c) Rubella syndrome
    d) Herpes
    e) Measles
    f) Infectious meningitis
    g) Cong syphilis
3. Trauma:
    a) Acute & Chronic exposure to loud noise
    b) # of Petrous temporal bone
4. Meniere's disease
5. Drugs:
    a) Aspirin
    b) Quinine
    c) Aminoglycoside antibiotics
6. Acoustic neuroma
7. Otosclerosis—late
8. Rare causes:
    a) Familial eg Alport's syndrome
    b) Multiple sclerosis
    c) Vit B def
    d) Psychogenic
    e) Brain stem lesions
    f) Cong anoxia
    g) Leukaemia
    h) Idiopathic

CLIN:
CD: Bone conduction >Air. Weber's test—sound referred to deaf ear
PD: Air conduction >Bone. Weber's test—sound referred to good ear

INVESTIGATIONS:
- Tuning fork tests
- Audiometry
- X-R IAM

THE AURICLE & EXTERNAL AUDITORY MEATUS

Wax

Secreted by ceruminous glands

CLIN: Occ Deafness; Earache. Rarely Vertigo; Discharge

RX: Soften c̄ eg warm olive oil (for 5 days if very hard). Then syringe

Acute Dermatitis

Usually 2° to Otitis Externa

CLIN: Oedema; Desquamation. Rarely Red auricle

RX: Treat any otitis externa (qv). Topical Betnovate or Zn & 10% Ichthammol

Perichondritis

2° to:
1. Otitis media
2. Haematoma
3. Rarely mastoidectomy

CLIN: Red swollen tender painful pinna

RX: Incision of any abscess. Antibiotics

COMPLICATIONS: 1. Abscess
2. Ear deformity eg "cauliflower ear"

Otitis Externa

Inflam of the skin lining EAM

PATHOGENESIS: Poor aural care eg inadequate drying of ear, scratching, introduction of foreign body, poor syringing → infection. Chemical irritants eg hair dye → local dermatitis

CLIN: Earache worsened by jaw mvt; Deafness; Irritation; Desquamation; Scanty discharge

INVESTIGATION: • Swab

RX: Aural toilet, debridement. If acute: Systemic antibiotics c̄ topical 10% glycerin & ichthammol. If chronic: Daily dressing c̄ topical antibiotic/steroid drops eg Otosporin or Sofradex. Amphotericin B if fungal. Ban scratching & swimming. Prevent water contact c̄ ear for 3/12

PROG: Often recurs if poor aural hygeine

Furuncle

Localised Staph infection of meatal hair follicle. Occ 2° to diabetes

CLIN: Red swollen orifice; Pain; Local tenderness

INVESTIGATIONS:
- Swab.
- Look for diabetes

RX: Analgesia. 10% Ichthammol in glycerine dressing. Local heat. Occ antibiotics

Benign Tumours

EXOSTOSES

Small osteomata of EAM due to prolonged exposure to cold water. Usually bilateral

RX: Occ remove by surgery

PAPILLOMA (SIMPLE WART)

RX: Excision

Malignant Tumours

EPITHELIOMA

Occurs on upper auricle >EAM. Esp elderly

CLIN: Intractable severe pain (late) & bleeding

SPREAD: Direct & via LNs

RX: X-Rad & Surgery

PROG: Poor

RODENT ULCER (BASAL CELL)

Ass c̄ prolonged exposure to sunlight

CLIN: Ulcer c̄ rolled edge & central crusting

SPREAD: Locally invasive

RX: X-Rad or Wide excision

PROG: Good

TYMPANIC MEMBRANE

Tympanic Membrane Injury

CAUSES: 1. Direct trauma
2. Blast, gunfire
3. # temporal bone
4. Otitis Media (OM)

CLIN: Acute transient pain; Deafness; Tinnitus. Rarely Vertigo. Occ Bleeding

RX: Antibiotics

MIDDLE EAR

Otitis Media

ACUTE OTITIS MEDIA

Children >Adult. Winter >Summer

Causes of Otitis Media (LIST 2 ENT)

1. Acute tonsillitis
2. Infections:
   a) Cold
   b) Influenza
   c) Measles
   d) Scarlet fever
   e) Sinusitis
   f) Infantile GE
3. Trauma:
   a) Tonsillectomy
   b) Tympanic membrane trauma
   c) Otitic barotrauma
   d) # temporal bone
4. Post nasal plug

PATHOGENESIS: Infection → inflam, oedema, mucopus → blockage E tube → Tympanic cavity P ↓→ secretion → infection → bulging membrane → rupture → discharge of mucopus

CLIN: Severe throbbing earache; CD; Pyrexia; Profuse purulent discharge. Rarely Tinnitus. Tympanic membrane: Initially lustreless then reddens & bulges, eventually perforates; Cone of light sign lost

INVESTIGATIONS: • Swab
• X-R mastoid (if no resolution)

RX: Early: Analgesia. Penicillin ± broad spectrum antibiotic. If persistence or rapid recurrence perform Myringotomy; Aural toilet. If discharging: Antibiotic, aural toilet

COMPLICATIONS: 1. Acute mastoiditis
2. Labyrinthitis
3. Intracranial abscess
4. Deafness
5. Lat sinus thrombosis
6. VIIn paralysis

SECRETORY OTITIS MEDIA (GLUE EAR)

Common cause of deafness in childhood. Esp 5–7 years

CAUSES: 1. Nasopharyngeal infections & obstructions
2. Otitic barotrauma
3. Acute OM
4. Sinusitis
5. Nasal allergy

PATHOGENESIS: E tube obst →↓ air in middle ear → indrawing of tympanic membrane → middle ear effusion

CLIN: Deafness. Often aural discomfort. Tympanic membrane: Golden in adult; Dull, indrawn c̄ ↑ periph vascularity in children

RX: Treat underlying cause eg antral wash out, adenoidectomy. Myringotomy & insertion of "grommet"

CHRONIC OTITIS MEDIA

2 main types:

A. SIMPLE OR TUBO-TYMPANIC:
Common. Children >Adults

Clin: CD. Often 2° to tonsillitis, adenoids ↑, sinusitis. Mucoid discharge through tear in central part of pars tensa. Relapsing course

Investigations: • Audiogram
• X-R of mastoids

Rx: Ear drops. Aural toilet. Closure of perforation

Complications: 1. Residual deafness
2. Avascular necrosis (requiring reconstruction of ossicular chain)

B. CHRONIC SUPPURATIVE OR ATTICO-ANTRAL:

Definition: A purulent discharge through perf of pars flaccida or post segment of TM. Occ ass c̄ a cholesteatoma in the attic region & a non-pneumatised mastoid process
Children <Adults

Clin: Purulent discharge; Deafness; Earache. Occ Vertigo; Bleeding from granulations

Investigations: • Audiogram
• X-R of mastoids

Rx: **A. Conservative:** Remove cholesteatoma then daily aural toilet
B. Radical: Mastoidectomy to make mastoid antrum, middle ear & EAM into one cavity. Radicalness of operation depends on stage of disease

Complications: 1. Intracranial abscess
2. Deafness
3. Meningitis
4. Labyrinthitis
5. VIIn paralysis
6. Aural polyps
7. Lat sinus thrombosis

Complications of Middle Ear Disease

ACUTE MASTOIDITIS

Suppurative process of mastoid cells ass c̄ bone necrosis. Unusual since advent of antibiotics

CLIN: Persistent, throbbing pain. Mucopurulent discharge. Deafness; Pyrexia; Swelling & tenderness over mastoid process

INVESTIGATIONS: • WCC ↑
• X-R: Loss of cell outline

RX: Antibiotics. If medical Rx fails do cortical or radical mastoidectomy

COMPLICATIONS: 1. Sub-periosteal abscess
2. Neck abscess (Bezold's)
3. Zygomatic mastoiditis

FACIAL NERVE PARALYSIS

Rare. Often transient

RX: Occ mastoidectomy

MENINGITIS

CLIN: Pyrexia; Headache; Neck stiff; +ve Kernig's; Photophobia

INVESTIGATION: • LP

RX: Antibiotics, then mastoidectomy

PETROSITIS (INFECTION OF PETROUS TEMPORAL)

Rare. Involvement of VIn (Gradenigo's Syndrome)

CLIN: Diplopia; Headache; Trigeminal pain; Signs of middle ear infection

RX: Antibiotics, mastoidectomy

EXTRADURAL ABSCESS

CLIN: Ear discharge; Pain; Headache. Occ Temporal swelling. Signs & symptoms of ICP ↑

INVESTIGATIONS: • CAT scan

RX: Antibiotics. Drain abscess. Mastoidectomy

SUBDURAL ABSCESS

CLIN: Signs & symptoms of ICP ↑. Occ Focal epilepsy

INVESTIGATION: • CAT scan

RX: Drainage through burr hole

LABYRINTHITIS

Commonest complication of chronic otitis media. Due to fistula in med wall of middle ear

CLIN: Vertigo; N&V; Nystagmus; Pyrexia. Occ Total hearing loss

RX: Antibiotics, mastoidectomy & remove cholesteatoma

LAT SINUS THROMBOSIS

CLIN: Swinging temp & rigors; Occ

Meningism; Tender ipsilat jugular vein

INVESTIGATIONS: • WCC ↑
• Blood cultures

RX: Antibiotics, mastoidectomy

COMPLICATIONS: 1. Metastatic emboli
2. Cavernous sinus thromb

OTITIC HYDROCEPHALUS

Symptoms of hydrocephalus 2° to sinus thrombophlebitis without enlargement of ventricles

BRAIN ABSCESS

Temporal lobe >Cerebellum by direct spread or via blood

CLIN: Signs & symptoms of ICP ↑. Occ Localising signs eg nominal aphasia

INVESTIGATION: • CAT scan

RX: Antibiotics, drainage through Burr hole, mastoidectomy

Otosclerosis

Sclerotic bone formation fixing stapes footplate & preventing sound waves reaching cochlea
Onset esp 15–30 yrs. Often FH. 2F:1M. Occ pregnancy ppts

CLIN: Bilat (occ unilat) deafness. Tinnitus; Paracusis; Normal tympanic membrane. BC >AC, but BC ↓ late

RX: Stapedectomy & replacement c̄ stapes prosthesis. Hearing aids

INNER EAR

Meniere's Disease

Unknown aetiology. ?due to labyrinthine electrolyte imbalance
Onset 40–60yrs. 50% bilateral eventually

PATHOGENESIS: ↑ Endolymph P → distension of membranous labyrinth & destruction of sensory cells in inner ear

CLIN: Attacks of vertigo, N&V, perceptive deafness & tinnitus lasting 12hrs–4 days. Later PD persists

INVESTIGATIONS: • Audiometry: PD c̄ loudness recruitment
• Caloric tests
• Electronystagmography
• X-R of mastoids

RX: A. Medical: During attack: Bed rest, Stemetil
Between attacks: Serc. Fluids ↓; Salt ↓; Vasodilators

B. Surgical: 1. Insertion of grommet
2. Ultrasonic vestibular apparatus destruction or Decompression of saccus endolymphaticus
3. Labyrinthectomy: In severe unilateral cases
4. Rarely stellate ganglionectomy: To improve blood supply to inner ear

Benign Positional Vertigo

Degeneration of utricular & saccular maculae. Cause unknown. May be 2° to trauma, OA, chr OM

CLIN: Vertigo lasting seconds ppt by putting head in critical positions → nystagmus of brief duration. Fatiguable

Vestibular Neuronitis

? Infection

CLIN: Vertigo. Occ h/o infection. No deafness. Spontaneous recovery

Acoustic Neuroma

Benign tumour arising from sheath of auditory nerve. Ass c̄ neurofibromatosis esp if bilat

CLIN: Slowly progressive deafness usually unilat. Tinnitus. Occ Nystagmus. Later signs & symptoms of Vn, VIIn &/or VIIIn palsies; Ipsilat cerebellar tracts &/or contralat pyramidal tract lesions; ↑ ICP

INVESTIGATIONS: • Audiometry: No loudness recruitment, marked tone decay.
• X-R IAM
• CAT scan ± air meatography

RX: Surgical removal

FACIAL NERVE

Bell's Palsy

CLIN: Unilat facial nerve palsy

RX: ACTH or oral steroids within 24hrs. If no recovery consider Decompression; Dental supports; Tarsorrhaphy; Plastic surgery

PROG: 90% recover but others may have post-gustatory weeping &/or ectropion

Ramsay Hunt Syndrome

Geniculate herpes

CLIN: Vesicles on auricle & ant fauces. Deafness; Dizziness; Facial paresis; Otalgia; Hyperacusis; Ipsilat taste loss

RX: Analgesia

Causes of Facial Nerve Paralysis (LIST 3 ENT)

A. SUPRANUCLEAR & NUCLEAR
  1. CVA
  2. Cerebral tumour
  3. Polio

B. INFRANUCLEAR
  1. Bell's palsy
  2. Trauma:
     a) Surgical procedure
     b) # temporal bone
     c) Birth injury
  3. Acute OM
  4. CSOM
  5. Infection:
     a) Herpes zoster—Ramsay Hunt syndrome
     b) Mononucleosis
  6. Tumours:
     a) Acoustic neuroma
     b) Parotid tumour
     c) Middle ear Ca
  7. Multiple sclerosis
  8. Guillain–Barré Syndrome
  9. Sarcoidosis

EARACHE—OTALGIA

Causes of Earache (LIST 4 ENT)

A. AURAL
  1. Furuncle
  2. Foreign body
  3. Otitis Externa
  4. Acute OM
  5. Chronic OM
  6. Mastoiditis
  7. Acute perichondritis
  8. Neoplasms

B. REFERRED
  1. Dental:
     Eg Impacted lower molars
  2. Post tonsillectomy
  3. Cv spondylosis
  4. Cancers:
     a) Post 1/3 tongue
     b) Fauces
     c) Lat pharynx
     d) Larynx
     e) Hypopharynx
  5. Temporomandibular arthralgia

TINNITUS

Causes of Tinnitus (LIST 5 ENT)

A. LOCAL
1. Presbycusis
2. Otosclerosis
3. Meniere's disease
4. Acute OM
5. Secretory OM
6. Wax in meatus
7. Glomus tumour

B. HEAD & NECK
1. Impacted lower molars
2. High cervical disc lesion
3. A-V aneurysms
4. Temporal lobe lesion
5. Neck wounds
6. Temporomandibular arthralgia

C. GENERAL
1. Fever
2. BP ↑ & atheroma
3. Drugs: Eg Quinine, salicylates, aminoglycosides
5. Alcohol
6. Acoustic trauma

D. IDIOPATHIC

VERTIGO

Causes of Vertigo (LIST 6 ENT)

1. Meniere's disease
2. Vestibular neuronitis
3. Benign postural vertigo
4. Labyrinthitis
5. CSOM
6. Secretory otitis media
7. Drugs: Eg Ethanol, Aminoglycosides, Quinine
8. Vertebro–Basilar insufficiency
9. Tumours: Eg Acoustic neuroma, Labyrinthine neoplasm
10. Geniculate herpes
11. E tube obst
12. Migraine
13. Pontine vascular accident
14. Multiple sclerosis
15. Temporal lobe epilepsy
16. Syringobulbia
17. Cerebellar lesions

The Nose

NASAL INJURIES

Nasal Bones

CLIN: Swelling; Discolouration; Tenderness & deformity. Epistaxis. Occ CSF rhinorrhoea ie # skull

INVESTIGATION: • If CSF rhinorrhoea suspected: Test rhinorrhoea fluid for sugar or occ isotope study

RX: Clean wound. Reduce fracture within 2hrs or at 6–10 days if deformity. PoP splint

Septal Haematoma

Usually 2° to trauma ass c̄ # septum

CLIN: Boggy pink bilat swelling blocking nasal passage

RX: Incise, evacuate, drain & pack. Antibiotics

PROG: Occ cartilage necrosis → deformity

Septal Deviation

CAUSES: 1. Cong ± cleft palate
2. Trauma

CLIN: Nasal obst; Recurrent sinusitis; Headache

RX: A. Medical: Nasal douche
B. Surgical: Septoplasty op of choice. Occ Submucous resection (SMR)

Indications for Surgery:
1. Obst of nasal airway
2. Obst to paranasal sinus drainage
3. To secure haemostasis in epistaxis

Complications: Occ Perf; Epistaxis; Depression nasal bridge

Septal Perforation

CAUSES: 1. Post-op esp SMR
2. Trauma
3. Nose picking
4. Cocaine
5. Tumours eg Rodent ulcer
6. Rare eg Syphilis, Chrome salts
7. Wegener's granuloma

CLIN: May be asymptomatic. Epistaxis; Crusting

RX: Biopsy. Repair

EPISTAXIS

Anatomy: Septum supplied by Ant & Post ethmoidal, Greater palatine, Sphenopalatine & Sup palatine arteries which anastomose in Little's area on the ant septum

Epistaxis is a symptom or a sign not a diagnosis

CLIN: Bleeding. In children usually from Little's area

INVESTIGATION: • Look for underlying cause

RX: Sit upright c̄ head forward. Suck away clots, pack c̄ ribbon gauze soaked in Lignocaine & Adrenaline then apply pressure. Occ post-nasal plugging & antibiotics or surgery is required

Causes of Epistaxis (LIST 7 ENT)

A. LOCAL
1. Spontaneous
2. Trauma:
   a) # Nasal bones
   b) Post-op
   c) Foreign body
   d) Nose picking
3. Acute & chronic Rhinitis
4. Sinusitis
5. Tumours
6. Hereditary telangiectasia

B. GENERAL
1. BP ↑
2. Mitral stenosis
3. Myeloproliferative disease:
   a) Leukaemia
   b) Hodgkins
   c) Lymphosarcoma
4. Anaemia
5. Purpura
6. Haemophilia
7. Infection:
   a) Exanthemata
   b) Influenza
   c) Glandular fever
8. Vit K & C deficiency

RHINITIS

Acute Rhinitis (Common cold)

Viral infection

CLIN: Rhinorrhoea. Fever; Headache; Malaise

RX: Symptomatic

Allergic Rhinitis

Often FH. Ass c̄ nasal polyps
Allergens include pollens (hay fever), house dust mite, cat & dog fur etc

CLIN: Watery rhinorrhoea; Catarrh. Nasal obst; Sneezing fits; Lacrymation; Slight conjunctivitis. Swollen nasal mucosa esp inf turbinates

INVESTIGATIONS: • Skin sensitivity tests
• X-R sinuses

RX: Avoid contact with allergen. Desensitisation. Topical steroid sprays. Anti-histamines. Cautery or diathermy to inf turbinates

Atrophic Rhinitis

Cause unknown. Very rare in UK

CLIN: Dry nose; Crusting c̄ malodour. Occ Headache; Epistaxis; Nasal obst

RX: Syringe daily then use oily spray or Col alk douche. Surgical closure of nares

Vasomotor Rhinitis

CLIN: Watery rhinorrhoea. Catarrh. Nasal obst; Paroxysmal sneezing; Post-nasal drip. Occ Headache

INVESTIGATION: • X-R sinus: Thickening of mucosal lining

RX: Oral ephedrine. Diathermy of turbinates

NASAL POLYPS

Definition: Areas of sinus mucosa distended with fluid protruding into nasal cavity

Ethmoidal

Common. 2° to allergy, chr ethmoiditis or rarely tumour. Ass c̄ cystic fibrosis

CLIN: Nasal obst; Rhinorrhoea; Headache; Sneezing fits; Anosmia

RX: Remove c̄ nasal snare. Ethmoidectomy if recurrence

Antro-choanal

Esp in 15–30 yrs. M>F
Polyp fills antrum & descends into post nasal space

CLIN: Sore throat; Unilat nasal obst & frontal headaches; Facial pain. Rarely Dysphagia; Earache

RX: Remove. Caldwell–Luc op

THE SINUSES

Acute Sinusitis

CAUSES: 1. Bacterial infection 2° to acute rhinitis
2. Trauma
3. Foreign bodies
4. Dental sepsis
5. Deviated septum
6. Nasal polyps
7. Tumours

ACUTE MAXILLARY SINUSITIS

CLIN: Facial pain; Nasal obst & purulent discharge; Fever; Tender over antrum

INVESTIGATIONS: • Nasal swab
• WCC ↑
• Transillumination ↓
• X-R Sinus: fluid level/opacity

RX: Bed rest. Antibiotics eg Erythromycin, Ampicillin. Analgesia. Inhalations. Occ require antral washout

COMPLICATIONS: 1. Spread to other sinuses
2. OM
3. LRTI
4. Chr sinusitis

DD: Ca maxillary antrum (where swelling of cheek occurs, although this sign also occurs in sinusitis ass c̄ dental abscess on tooth root)

ACUTE FRONTAL SINUSITIS

Usually unilat. Often 2° to maxillary sinusitis

CLIN: Supra-orbital morning pain; Local tenderness. Headache

INVESTIGATIONS: • Nasal swab
• WCC ↑
• X-R: Fluid levels

RX: Bed rest. Broad spectrum Penicillin. Analgesia. Frontal sinus trephine & drainage. Treat any ass maxillary sinusitis

COMPLICATIONS:

1. **Orbital Cellulitis or Abscess:**
   Clin: Diplopia; Eyelid oedema; Occ Proptosis
   Rx: Drain, antibiotics
2. **Frontal Bone Osteomyelitis:**
   Clin: Subacute onset. Puffy swelling over frontal bone. Persistent headache
   Rx: Antibiotics. Drain & remove sequestra. Treat early to prevent intracranial sequelae
3. **Cavernous Sinus Thrombosis:**
   Clin: Proptosis; Chemosis; Ophthalmoplegia
4. **Meningitis**
5. **Intracranial abscess**

ACUTE ETHMOIDAL SINUSITIS

Esp infants

CLIN: Pain between & behind eyes; Anosmia; Nasal obst. Occ Purulent epiphora

RX: Antibiotics. Occ drainage

ACUTE SPHENOIDITIS

Uncommon. Difficult to diagnose. Ass c̄ ethmoiditis

CLIN: Central pain occ radiating to temporal region. Occ Purulent post nasal discharge

Chronic Sinusitis

PREDISPOSING FACTORS:
1. Inadequate pneumatisation of sinuses
2. Poor social conditions
3. Atopic reactions
4. Dental sepsis
5. Recurrent infection
6. Poor drainage eg septal deviation
7. Bronchiectasis

CHRONIC MAXILLARY SINUSITIS

CLIN: Nasal obst & purulent discharge; Post nasal drip; Headaches & facial pain. Occ Husky voice

INVESTIGATIONS: • Transillumination ↓
• X-R Sinuses
• Dental inspection
• Nasal swab

RX: Antral puncture & lavage. Occ require Intra-nasal antrostomy or Caldwell-Luc op

CHILDHOOD CHRONIC MAXILLARY SINUSITIS

PREDISPOSITIONS:
1. Adenoids ↑
2. Tonsillitis
3. Repeated viral infections
4. Foreign body
5. Low resistance eg poor diet
6. Bronchiectasis

CLIN: Purulent discharge often bilateral. Nasal obst c̄ mouth breathing. Chr cough esp at night. Tendency to OM & deafness

INVESTIGATIONS: • X-R Sinuses: Occ Fluid level
• CXR
• Swabs
• Transillumination ↓

RX: Trial of Ephedrine drops for 2/52. Antral puncture & wash out (under GA) ± insertion of indwelling catheter. Intranasal antrostomy

CHRONIC FRONTAL SINUSITIS

CLIN: Dull intractable headache

RX: Conservative surgery eg Antrostomy
Radical surgery eg Radical fronto-ethmoidectomy or Obliteration of sinus

CHRONIC ETHMOIDITIS

Usually ass c̄ chr infection in other sinuses

CLIN: Nasal polypi → obst. Nasal discharge; Anosmia; Headache

RX: Occ exenteration of sinus eg intranasal or external ethmoidectomy

Frontal Mucocoele

Esp middle aged

CLIN: Painless swelling above & med to the orbit. Occ Vision ↓; Diplopia

INVESTIGATION: • X-R Sinuses

RX: Intranasal or external excision

Tumours

ANTRAL CARCINOMA

Rarely diagnosed until spread has occured to surrounding structures. Exposure to hardwood dust predisposes to AdenoCa

CLIN: Unilat nasal obst & blood stained discharge. Later Cheek swelling; Epiphora; Proptosis; Diplopia; Facial pain. Swelling or ulceration of hard palate

SPREAD: Direct (early) → cheek, palate, nose, orbit, infra-orbital nerve
LN (Late) → sub-mandibular, deep cervical LN

INVESTIGATIONS: • X-R: Opacity & bony wall destruction
• CAT
• Cytology
• Biopsy

RX: X-Rad, then surgery ± Cyt.T. Review

PROG: 10–15% 5yr survival

ETHMOIDAL CARCINOMA

Usually Squamous cell Ca. Similar clin to antral Ca but invasion of orbit occurs earlier

NASOPHARYNGEAL CARCINOMA

Esp Far East

CLIN: Variety of presentations Neck mass; Unilat deafness; Cv LN ↑; Nasal obst; Epistaxis; Cranial nerve palsies eg diplopia

INVESTIGATIONS: • Biopsy
• X-R Sinuses & Lat soft tissue
• CAT scan

RX: X-Rad. Local implant

PROG: Fair. 25–50% 5yr survival

The Throat

TONSILS & ADENOIDS

The adenoid is lymphoid tissue on post wall of nasopharynx which is maximal in size at about 5yrs

Adenoid Hypertrophy

Esp children 1–5yrs due to repeated URTI

CLIN: Mouth breathing; Snoring; Sleep disturbance. Repeated URTI, LRTI

INVESTIGATION: • X-R: Post nasal space (PNS)

RX: 1–3 yrs Adenoidectomy. If aged >3yrs ?combine c̄ Tonsillectomy

Surgical Complications: 1. Haem
2. Recurrence
3. OM

COMPLICATIONS: 1. Secretory OM
2. Sinusitis

Acute Tonsillitis

Children >>Adults. β haemolytic Strep >Adenovirus, Echo & Flu virus

CLIN: Fever; Sore throat; Dysphagia; Earache; Headache; Malaise; Hyperaemic tonsils; Furred tongue; Cv LN ↑

INVESTIGATIONS: • WCC ↑
• Throat swab

RX: Bed rest, isolate, fluids++, Aspirin, Penicillin

Indications for Tonsillectomy (LIST 8 ENT)

1. Recurrent acute Tonsillitis
2. Quinsy
3. Middle ear infection
4. Cervical LN ↑
5. Dysphagia &/or dyspnoea due to large tonsils
6. Sepsis—carrier or focal
7. Abnormal histology: Eg Cancer
8. Failure to thrive due to recurrent tonsillitis

Contraindications to Tonsillectomy (LIST 9 ENT)

1. Acute URTI
2. Blood dyscrasias
3. Rh fever or nephritis
4. Polio (Very rare)

N.B Cleft palate c/i to adenoidectomy

COMPLICATIONS OF TONSILLECTOMY:

1. Haem—Immediate & delayed
2. Otalgia
3. OM
4. Rarely: Pneumonia, Lung abscess

COMPLICATIONS OF ACUTE TONSILLITIS:

1. Acute OM
2. Quinsy
3. LRTI
4. Acute nephritis
5. Rheumatic fever

DD:
1. Glandular fever
2. Scarlet fever
3. Diptheria
4. Vincent's angina
5. Agranulocytosis

Peritonsillar Abscess (Quinsy)

Pus in peritonsillar capsule 2° to tonsillitis. Esp young adults

CLIN: Starts about a wk after original tonsillitis. Then Fever; Trismus; Dysphagia; Earache

RX: Penicillin. Drainage under LA (Cocaine), then after 6/52 tonsillectomy

DD:
1. Retropharyngeal abscess
2. Parapharyngeal abscess
3. Reticuloses
4. Pharyngeal tumour

Carcinoma of Tonsil

Rare. Squamous Ca >Lymphosarcoma

CLIN: Sore throat; Dysphagia; Otalgia; Tonsil ↑; LN ↑

INVESTIGATIONS:
- FBC
- Biopsy

RX: X-Rad & Surgery

PHARYNX & LARYNX

Acute Pharyngitis

Common. Usually viral eg adenovirus. Ass c̄ nasal infections

CLIN: Dysphagia & malaise; Hyperaemic mucosa

RX: Analgesia

Chronic Pharyngitis

Occ 2° to tooth decay, sinusitis, alcohol, tobacco, nasal polyp, deviated nasal septum

CLIN: Discomfort in throat. No dysphagia

RX: Treat underlying condition. Occ diathermy ± tonsillectomy

DD: Globus hystericus

Retropharyngeal Abscess

Esp infants, young children

CLIN: Fever; Malaise; Dysphagia. Occ Stridor. Bulge to one side of mid-line of post pharyngeal wall

RX: Antibiotics; Incision under GA

Pharyngeal Pouch

Mucosal herniation in Killian's dehiscence. ? 2° to muscular inco-ordination

CLIN: Throat discomfort; Dysphagia; Regurgitation of undigested food; Wt ↓

INVESTIGATIONS:
- Ba swallow
- Oesphagoscopy

RX: Surgery—Excision of pouch or intraluminal cricopharyngeal myotomy

Plummer–Vinson Syndrome (Chronic Hypopharyngitis)

F>M. Esp middle age. Pre-malignant

CLIN: Dysphagia; Wt ↓; Malaise. Angular stomatitis; Glossitis; IDA; Web → post cricoid Ca

INVESTIGATIONS: • FBC
• Oesophagoscopy
• Ba swallow

RX: Iron; Dilatation of web. Observe & long term follow up

Ca Hypopharynx

In M esp pyriform fossa. In F esp post-cricoid area

CLIN: Dysphagia; Wt ↓; Pain in throat; Hoarseness; Earache; Lump in neck. Early spread to Cv LN & neck

INVESTIGATIONS: • Ba swallow
• Oesophagoscopy & biopsy

RX: Laryngopharyngectomy c̄ colonic or gastric interposition. X-Rad for pyriform fossa & post-cricoid tumours

PROG: Poor

Acute Laryngitis

Ass c̄ flu, cold, exanthemata, excessive use of voice, smoking

CLIN: Aphonia (Loss of voice), or dysphonia (A difficulty in speaking); Red tender larynx; Fever; Malaise. Lasts 4–5 days

RX: Rest voice. Treat 1° infection. Stop cigs

Acute Epiglottitis

Usually due to *H. influenzae*. Esp infants

CLIN: Very sore throat; Stridor → resp obst. May kill in hrs

RX: Immediate hospital admission. Antibiotics ± tracheostomy or intubation

Laryngo–Tracheo–Bronchitis

Esp infants

CLIN: Thick tenacious muco-pus → resp distress

RX: Antibiotics; O_2; Humidify. Occ tracheostomy or intubation

Chronic Laryngitis

PREDISPOSING CONDITIONS: 1. Overuse of voice
2. Alcohol, smoking
3. Chr sinusitis
4. Chr bronchitis
5. TB
6. Syphilis

CLIN: Hoarseness but no dysphagia or otalgia. Occ Cough; Nasal obst ± discharge

INVESTIGATIONS: • CXR
• X-R larynx
• WR
• EUA ± Biopsy

RX: Treat underlying cause. Remove any vocal cord polyps or nodules (Singer's nodules)

Leukoplakia (Hyperkeratosis)

Pre-malignant. M>F. Cause unknown. Ass c̄ smoking

CLIN: White patches on larynx

RX: Remove. Observe carefully

Carcinoma of Larynx

Sq cell Ca. 10M:1F

TYPES: Marginal, Supraglottic, Glottic, Subglottic

CLIN: Glottic tumours present earliest. Hoarseness. Later Otalgia; Dry cough; Haemoptysis; Dysphagia; Resp obst

SPREAD: Local & to cervical LN & rarely lung

INVESTIGATIONS: • Biopsy
• Tomography
• CXR

RX: X-Rad (Preserves voice). Occ tracheostomy if airway obst. If recurrence, laryngectomy & block disection of LNs. Speech therapy

Causes of Hoarseness (LIST 10 ENT)

1. Acute laryngitis
2. Chronic laryngitis
3. Tumours of pharynx & larynx
4. Hypothyroidism
5. Hysteria
6. Laryngeal nerve palsy
7. Foreign body
8. Very rarely:
   a) Syphilitic laryngitis
   b) Pharyngeal pouch

Causes of Vocal Cord Paresis (LIST 11 ENT)

1. Carcinoma
   a) Lung
   b) Oesophagus
   c) Mediastinum
   d) Thyroid
   e) Hypopharynx
   f) Nasopharynx
2. Trauma
3. Surgery:
   Eg Post thyroidectomy, Cardiac surgery
4. Pulmonary TB
5. Aortic aneurysm
6. Crico-arytenoid jt ankylosis
7. Medullary infarct
8. Peripheral neuritis
9. Polio
10. Syringomyelia
11. Idiopathic

Tracheostomy

Indications for Tracheostomy (LIST 12 ENT)

1. Resp tract obst:
   Eg Foreign body, Laryngeal Ca, Epiglottitis, Diphtheria
2. Retained secretions:
   Eg 2° to head injury or lung contusion
3. Reduction of dead space:
   Eg Chronic bronchitis & emphysema
4. Respiratory paralysis:
   Eg Myasthenia, Polio, Tetanus, Polyneuritis
5. Radical surgery requirement

TECHNIQUE: GA unless emergency. Hyperextend neck & incise in midline mid-way between cricoid cartilage & suprasternal notch. Insert cuffed tube

POST-OP CARE: Regular suction; Humidify air; Physio; Deflate cuff (5 mins/hr); Antibiotics

COMPLICATIONS: 1. Perichondritis
2. Mediastinal emphysema
3. Obst by crusts
4. Haem
5. Infection
6. Tracheal ulcer & TOF
7. Pneumothorax

SWELLINGS IN THE NECK

Causes of Swellings in the Neck (LIST 13 ENT)

A. MIDLINE SWELLINGS
1. Submental LN ↑:
   Eg Inflam, Mets, Reticulosis
2. Thyroid gland enlargement
3. Thyroglossal cyst
4. Lipoma
5. Sebaceous cyst
6. Sublingual dermoid
7. Subhyoid bursa

B. LATERAL SWELLINGS
1. Salivary gland enlargement:
   Eg Inflam, Sjogren's, Tumour
2. Lipoma
3. Sebaceous cyst
4. LN ↑:
   Eg Inflam, Mets, Reticuloses
5. Branchial cyst
6. Carotid body tumour
7. Sternomastoid "tumour"
8. Neurofibroma
9. Cystic hygroma
10. Subclavian aneurysm
11. Laryngocele
12. Pharyngeal pouch

Thyroglossal Cyst

Embryological remnant that can occur anywhere on thyroglossal tract from foramen caecum to thyroid isthmus. Esp childhood or early adulthood

CLIN: Smooth round tense swelling which moves upwards when tongue is protruded (due to fibrous attachment of thyroglossal tract to hyoid bone). Occ → Infection; Fistulae

RX: Surgical removal

Subhyoid Bursa

Rare. Enlargement of bursa between hyoid & thyrohyoid membrane

CLIN: Soft fluctuant midline swelling below hyoid

Branchial Cyst

Probably an embryological remnant of cervical sinus. Esp young adults

CLIN: Situated deep & ant to sternomastoid. Round tense swelling just below angle of jaw. Occ infection → pain, discomfort. Rarely sinus forms discharging mucus (branchial sinus more often presents at birth opening in ant border of sternomastoid)

INVESTIGATION: • Aspiration of cyst fluid: Cholesterol crystals

RX: Surgical excision

Carotid Body Tumour

Rare tumour. Esp middle aged. May secrete noradrenaline

CLIN: Slow growing painless tumour transmitting carotid pulsation, which arise in the line of carotid sheath at the level of upper border of thyroid cartilage. Palpation may ppt release of sympathomimetics. Rarely → local pressure effects; Mets

RX: Surgical excision

Respiratory System

CHRONIC AIRFLOW LIMITATION

The flow of air in the lung is determined by the lung elastic recoil & airways resistance (AWR). Pathology can be classified according to diseases eg emphysema, chr bronchitis or due to mechanism eg airway narrowing. There is a significant overlap between the various disease processes

Chronic Bronchitis & Emphysema

M>F. Esp UK, Lower social class, Smokers

AETIOLOGY & PATHOGENESIS OF CHR BRONCHITIS & EMPHYSEMA:

1. α_1 anti-trypsin def is an uncommon Aut Rec condition ass c̄ panacinar emphysema which allows ↑ proteolytic activity. Esp affects lower zones presumably due to ↑ blood flow to those areas
2. Smoking → pulmonary alveolar macrophages ↑ → neutrophils ↑ → proteolytic enzymes ↑ → lung destruction. Also cigs inhibit α_1 anti-trypsin
3. Urban dwelling is ass, particularly due to atmospheric pollution
4. Recurrent resp infections esp childhood LRTI may predispose perhaps by affecting lung growth
5. Longitudinal studies have shown that those who start c̄ a low FEV_1, say at age 40, decline faster than others, developing severe airflow limitation by say 55–70yrs
6. Emphysema is ass c̄ loss of elastic recoil & of ↓ diffusing capacity
7. Macleod's syndrome of unilat emphysema is due to childhood bronchiolitis & bronchitis → airway obliteration trapping air distally but no collapse due to collateral ventilation

PATHOLOGY OF EMPHYSEMA:

Emphysema is classified anatomically, it is a permanent abnormal acinar enlargement ass c̄ lung destruction. There are four forms:

A. Proximal acinar: Affects proximal part of acinus. There are 2 types:
   1. Focal emphysema: Ass c̄ coal dust. Gas exchange slightly ↓
   2. Centrilobular emphysema: Ass c̄ cigs, chr bronchitis & inflam of distal airways. Esp upper lobes. Ass c̄ chr airflow obst

B. Panacinar: Affects all the acinus. Esp lower lobes. Esp smokers. Often ass c̄ chr bronchitis

C. Distal acinar: Occurs along septal boundaries, distal acinus, bronchi, vessels & just deep to the pleura. Esp upper lobes. Ass c̄ spontaneous pneumothorax

D. Irregular: Usually localised & 2° to scarring. Ass c̄ TB, Pneumoconiosis,

Eosinophilic granuloma

PATHOLOGY OF SMALL AIRWAY DISEASE: The obst of small airways → mild chr airflow obst. Small airways contribute about 10–20% of total AWR

PATHOLOGY OF LARGE AIRWAYS DISEASE: Chr bronchitis is the major disease of central airways & is defined clinically. Enlarged tracheobronchial glands secrete mucus++. The ratio of gland to wall thickness is increased & correlates c̄ a ↓ FEV. Airway is swollen & thickened. Smooth muscle hyperplasia is seen but is more characteristic of asthma

CLIN: Chr bronchitis & emphysema often occur together. Chr bronchitis is defined as productive cough occurring on most days for 3mths of the year for 2 or more consecutive yrs not due to specific disease such as bronchiectasis
Predominant emphysema is ass c̄ well preserved resp drive & hyperventilation to maintain PaO_2; Marked SOB; Thinness; Overinflated chest; termed "Pink-puffers"
Predominant chr bronchitis has a wide range of symptoms; either the recurrent chest infections or airways obst can predominate. Those c̄ major airways obst are particularly ass c̄ severe resp disability; SOB; Ankle swelling; Productive cough; Cyanosis; Liver ↑; Spleen ↑; Pulmonary BP ↑; Polycythaemia & are termed "Blue Bloaters"

INVESTIGATIONS:
- CXR: In emphysema flattened diaphragms, ↓ vascularity, long thin narrow heart. In chr bronchitis CXR may be norm. Occ signs of pulm BP ↑
- FBC, WCC
- Sputum
- FEV_1, FEV_1/FVC, PEF all ↓
- Astrup: Chr bronchitis PaO_2 ↓, $PaCO_2$ ↑, Resp Acidosis
- Tco ↓
- ECG
- Plethysmograph, He dilution technique: Obst pattern is low FEV_1/FVC, low VC, low PEF, but high RV & TLC. Restrictive pattern is relatively norm FEV_1/FVC & RV/TLC but low PEF & TLC
- V/Q studies: Abnormality in Chr bronchitis >Emphysema

MANAGEMENT: Stop smoking & minimise air pollution. Wt ↓ if obese. Flu vaccine prophylaxis. Prompt antibiotics for exacerbations. Physio. Diuretic for oedema. Bronchodilators esp inhalants eg Salbutamol. O_2 monitored by regular $PaCO_2$ c̄ care not to override hypoxic drive. Encourage exercise between exacerbations. Long term domiciliary O_2 for Cor pulmonale, Polycythaemia & Pulmonary BP ↑. Anticoags for PE & thromb

PROG: Worse if FEV ↓, $PaCO_2$ ↑

Asthma

A disease characterised by recurrent episodes of SOB due to widespread temp narrowing of the lung airways. Common in children esp aged 3–7yrs but few are seriously affected (chr asthma). M>F in childhood. Occ FH. Esp summer when pollen count ↑. Onset usually in childhood but occ in middle aged & elderly (late onset asthma). Atopy predisposes. If allergen eg pollen, house dust mite is known or suspected = extrinsic asthma, if non-allergic = intrinsic asthma. Rarely ass c̄ systemic disease eg PAN, Carcinoid syndrome, Coeliac disease

PATHOGENESIS: Factors causing abnormal narrowing of airways: ↑ smooth muscle tone ie Bronchospsam; ↑ Mucosal thickness 2° to oedema, vascular congestion; ↑ secretions, exudates. In extrinsic form allergen exposure → mast cell sensitisation → mediator release eg histamine, PG & SRS-A → bronchoconstriction
3 main temporal patterns:
1. Irreversible ie little change in the severity of symptoms over time.
2. Brittle ie great variability in the degree of airway obst during the day.
3. Morning dippers ie low PEF on waking

CLIN: Episodes of wheeze, SOB & chest tightness. May be ppt by eg Exercise, Drugs, Fumes, Occupations, Stress, Infection & Foodstuffs. Occ Cough. In children : Occ Pigeon chest, Growth failure. If attack lasts >24hrs (acute severe asthma) → Exhaustion; Cyanosis; Dehydration; PR ↑; & occ death

INVESTIGATIONS:
- PEF
- CXR
- WCC: Occ Eosinophils ↑
- Skin tests

- Bronchial challenge tests
- "Reversibility" c̄ bronchodilator
- In acute severe form: FBC, U&E, Astrup, PEF

RX: Avoid ext allergens. Prophylactic Na^+ cromoglycate ± inhaled steroids eg Beclomethasone. In acute attack: Bronchodilator drugs eg Salbutamol, Ipratropium bromide; Aminophylline; Steroids; O_2. Antibiotics if infection. Route chosen depends on attack severity. Between attacks: May require bronchodilators, steroids. Early morning dippers may be helped by slow release Theophylline. In severe attacks: IV Hydrocortisone & Aminophylline infusions, Nebulised bronchodilators eg Salbutamol, O_2, IV fluids for dehydration, antibiotics if infection. Occ IPPV. Regular monitoring. Later transfer to oral therapy

COMPLICATIONS: Rarely lobar collapse, pneumothorax, steroid SE

PROG: Worse if late onset asthma, chr asthma, atopic. Most childhood asthma does not progress into adulthood

DD: 1. COAD
2. PND

DD IN CHILDHOOD: 1. Bronchiolitis
2. TB
3. Foreign body
4. CF
5. Whooping cough

Occupational Asthma

Asthma induced by agents inhaled at work. Many agents have been described eg Toluene, wood dust. Some are recognised for statutory compensation

CLIN: SOB; Wheeze; Chest tightness; Cough. All ass c̄ work. May occur immediately or 6–8hrs post exposure

INVESTIGATIONS:
- Skin test -ve unless atopic
- Periodic PEF before, during & after work
- Bronchial challenge tests

RX: Avoid cause if possible

PULMONARY EOSINOPHILIA

A group of conditions in which there are CXR pulm infiltrates & a high blood eosinophilia

TYPES: 1. Simple pulmonary eosinophilia (Loffler's syndrome)
2. Prolonged pulmonary eosinophilia
3. Asthmatic pulmonary eosinophilia
4. Tropical pulmonary eosinophilia
5. Hypereosinophilic syndrome
6. PAN

Simple Pulmonary Eosinophilia (Loffler's Syndrome)

Due to transient allergic reaction esp to worms eg Ascaris or drugs eg PAS acid

CLIN: Slight symptoms. Cough ± sputum. Usually no fever. Lasts $<$1mth

INVESTIGATIONS:
- WCC: Sl ↑, Eosinophils sl ↑
- CXR: Transient pulmonary infiltrates
- Stools for ova

RX: Not normally needed, recover spontaneously

Prolonged Pulmonary Eosinophilia

Rare. Allergic reaction lasting $>$1mth

CLIN: Variable severity. Usually cough & fever

INVESTIGATIONS:
- WCC ↑, Eosinophils ↑
- CXR
- Stools for ova

RX: Steroids

Asthmatic Pulmonary Eosinophilia

Commonest type. Esp 30–50yrs. F$>$M. Usually due to aspergillosis occ due to candida & hypersensitivity

Bronchopulmonary Aspergillosis

Allergic response to *Aspergillus fumigatus*. Causes 3 distinct conditions: Aspergilloma; Allergic bronchopulmonary aspergillosis; Septicaemia

ASPERGILLOMA

Colonisation of diseased lung tissue esp TB cavities

CLIN: Occ Haemoptysis; Pneumonia

INVESTIGATIONS:
- CXR & tomography: Cavity c̄ halo. Mass in cavity usually mobile
- Precipitin test +ve

RX: If symptoms resection, selective embolisation or X-Rad

ALLERGIC BRONCHOPULMONARY ASPERGILLOSIS

Colonisation of bronchial tree c̄ allergic response → pulm infiltrate. Often pre-existing lung disease esp asthma. About 2% of atopic asthmatics have type III reaction to aspergillosis

CLIN: Repeated episodes of productive cough occ containing casts or plugs; Fever; Myalgia; Wt ↓; Asthma. Exacerbations esp in winter. Occ plugs in airways → proximal bronchiectasis

INVESTIGATIONS:
- WCC: Eosinophils ↑
- Sputum eosinophilia
- CXR: Transient migratory consolidation, occ local collapse
- Serum IgE ↑
- Bronchography: Proximal bronchi dilated
- Prick test +ve
- Delayed Arthus response
- Precipitin test +ve
- Fungal cultures

RX: Steroids. Occ bronchodilators

SEPTICAEMIC ASPERGILLOSIS

Usually in immunosuppressed patients → mycotic abscesses in lungs, kidneys, brain

RX: Amphotericin

Tropical Pulmonary Eosinophilia

Esp India. Most cases due to filariasis

CLIN: Repeated episodes of Cough; Wheeze; Malaise; Wt ↓. Occ Fever; Chest pain; Haemoptysis; Pneumonia

INVESTIGATIONS:
- CXR: Bilat mottling
- Stool for ova
- WCC: Eosinophils ↑↑
- Filarial CFT +ve
- Sputum eosinophilia

RX: Diethyl carbamazine

Hypereosinophilic Syndrome

Rare. M>F. Infiltration esp of CVS, Lung & CNS

CLIN: Anaemia; Fever; Wt ↓; Malaise; Cough; Pleural effusion; CCF. Occ CNS signs; Liver ↑; Spleen ↑; LN ↑; Pruritis; RF

INVESTIGATIONS:
- FBC
- WCC ↑, Eosinophils ↑↑
- CXR

RX: Cyt.T

PAN

About 1/3 of cases have lung involvement. Variety of symptoms esp cough & wheeze

EXTRINSIC ALLERGIC ALVEOLITIS

An allergic reaction to specific ppt antigens in gas-exchanging areas of lung. Examples are usually occupational or recreational & include Farmer's lung & Bird fancier's lung

CLIN: Symptoms usually time related often 4–8hrs post allergen exposure (Type III reaction). Fever; Malaise; Myalgia; SOB; Dry cough; Tight chest. Occ develop chr symptomatic state c̄ cough, SOB & wt ↓. Occ persistent late insp creps

INVESTIGATIONS:
- CXR: Early nodular shadowing, later upper lobe fibrosis
- Astrup: PaO_2 ↓, $PaCO_2$ norm
- Restrictive V defect

- No eosinophilia
- Ppt Abs: Usually +ve

RX: Removal of antigen. Protect against inhalation eg +ve P helmets. Steroids

DD:
1. Viral or mycoplasmal pneumonia
2. Pulm eosinophilia
3. Sarcoidosis

BRONCHIECTASIS

A permanent bronchial widening & distortion c̄ impaired drainage of secretions usually due to infection
Esp lower lobes although upper lobes when 2° to apical TB. Approx equal nos of uni- & bilat cases. 3 path types: Cylindrical, Saccular & Cystic

Causes of Bronchiectasis (LIST 1 RESP)

1. Infection: Esp children
   Eg Whooping cough, Measles, Bronchiolitis, Aspergillosis
2. Bronchial obst:
   Eg Foreign bodies, Ca, TB, LN ↑
3. Defects in anti-microbial defences:
   Eg CF—Abnormal mucus, Ciliary dyskinesia inc Kartagener's syndrome, IgA def, Hypogamma-globulinaemia
4. Abnormal bronchial wall structures
5. Idiopathic

CLIN: Copious purulent sputum esp in particular postures; Haemoptysis; Recurrent infections; Clubbing; Fever. Occ Chr airways obst; Cor pulmonale; Resp failure; Pleurisy; Growth failure. Ass c̄ sinusitis. Rarely Amyloidosis; Cerebral abscess; Empyema

INVESTIGATIONS:
- CXR
- Sputum cytology
- Bronchography

RX: Physio. Prompt antibiotics for exacerbations & as prophylaxis in severe cases. Occ Surgery if: Recurrent symptoms from localised area; Uncontrolled haem; Aspergilloma

Kartagener's Syndrome

A syndrome of bronchiectasis, sinusitis, situs inversus & OM
Presumably mediated by ciliary motility defect

Causes of Haemoptysis (LIST 2 RESP)

1. Bronchiectasis
2. Lung Ca
3. TB
4. Pulmonary infarct
5. Lung abscess
6. Foreign body
7. Mitral stenosis
8. Chr bronchitis
9. Idiopathic
10. Rarely:
    a) Pneumonia
    b) LVF
    c) Pulm haemosiderosis
    d) PAN
    e) Mycoses eg aspergillosis
    f) Bleeding diatheses

RESPIRATORY FAILURE

There are two types of resp failure:
Type I: PaO_2 <8kPa (60mmHg) c̄ low or norm $PaCO_2$
Type II: PaO_2 <8kPa c̄ $PaCO_2$ >6.5kPa (49mmHg)

PATHOGENESIS: A combination of inadequate ventilation, inefficient gas exchange & poor CO

Causes of Respiratory Failure (LIST 3 RESP)

A. TYPE I
1. Asthma
2. Thromboembolism
3. Pneumonia
4. Lung collapse
5. Acute pulmonary oedema
6. Diffuse alveolitis: Eg Fibrosing alveolitis
7. Large SOL

B. TYPE II
1. Chr bronchitis
2. 1° alveolar hypoventilation
3. CNS respiratory centre depression:
   a) Drugs eg Narcotics, Sedatives
   b) Encephalitis
   c) ICP ↑
   d) Head injury
4. Neuromuscular:
   a) Muscular dystrophy
   b) Polio
   c) Myasthenia gravis
   c) Peripheral neuropathy
5. Kyphoscoliosis Eg Ank Sp
6. Chest injury: Eg Flail chest

CLIN: Cyanosis. SOB if no $PaCO_2$ ↑. If $PaCO_2$ ↑ Headache; Drowsy; Twitching; Warm extremities → Stupor, Coma. Occ Cor pulmonale; 2° polycythaemia; CCF; RF

INVESTIGATIONS:
- Astrup
- CXR
- Sputum
- ECG

RX: Physio, encourage cough. Humidified O_2 (if Type II 20–28%). Occ Antibiotics, Bronchodilators, Diuretic, Mucolytic agent. If somnolence: Nikethamide, Dopram, Intubate & suck, IPPV

CRYPTOGENIC FIBROSING ALVEOLITIS

A syndrome of unknown cause c̄ progressive fibrosis of alveolar walls c̄ a variable excess of interstitial or intra-alveolar cells. Esp late middle aged. M=F. Predisposes to Ca lung.

Ass c̄ eg Rh Arth; Scleroderma; SLE; Polymyositis & Dermatomyositis; CAH; Sjogrens; Raynauds; Ulc colitis; Thyroid disease; RTbA

PATHOLOGY: Desquamative form c̄ mainly inter-alveolar changes & many intra-alveolar macrophages (Type II pneumocytes); Mural form c̄ ↑ wall fibrosis, few macrophages ± necrosis

CLIN: SOB; Clubbing; Late insp creps. Later Cough; Cyanosis; Cor pulmonale. Occ Hepatosplenomegaly; Wt ↓; Haemoptysis. Rarely acute presentation (Hamman–Rich) c̄ pyrexia, cough, SOB, & occ sputum, haemoptysis, chest tightness & cyanosis

INVESTIGATIONS:
- CXR: Honeycomb lung
- Restrictive defect ie FEV_1, FVC, TLC & Tco all ↓
- Astrup: PaO_2 ↓ $PaCO_2$ ↓
- ESR ↑
- ANA, Rh F: Occ +ve
- Lung biopsy
- Broncho–alveolar lavage: ↑ neutrophils

RX: Steroids

PROG: Median survival of chr form 6yrs. Rare Hamman–Rich type usually → death in $<$ 1yr

DD:
1. Sarcoidosis
2. Asbestosis
3. Extrinsic allergic alveolitis

Causes of Diffuse Pulmonary Fibrosis (LIST 4 RESP)

1. Extrinsic allergic alveolitis
2. Pneumoconioses
3. Cryptogenic fibrosing alveolitis
4. Granulomatous disease:
   Eg TB, Sarcoid
5. Collagen diseases:
   Eg Scleroderma, Rh Arth
6. X-Rad
7. Neoplastic infiltration
8. Chr pulm oedema
9. Lipoid pneumonitis
10. Drugs:
    Eg Nitrofurantoin, Busulphan
11. Histiocytosis X
12. Tuberous sclerosis

Causes of Clubbing (LIST 5 RESP)

1. Ca Lung
2. Fibrosing alveolitis
3. Chr suppurative lung disease:
   a) Bronchiectasis
   b) Cystic fibrosis
   c) Lung abscess
   d) Pulm TB
   e) Empyema
4. SABE
5. Cyanotic CHD
6. Mesothelioma
7. PBC
8. Ulc colitis & Crohn's disease
9. Familial
10. Thyrotoxicosis
11. Brachial A-V aneurysm

Drug Induced Respiratory Disease (LIST 6 RESP)

1. Asthma:
   a) Irritant eg Sodium cromoglycate
   b) β blocker eg Propranolol
   c) Aspirin
   d) Allergic/Immunological eg Penicillin
2. Pulmonary Eosinophilia:
   Eg Nitrofurantoin, PAS acid, Sulphonamides, Carbamazepine
3. SLE:
   Eg Hydralazine, Procainamide, Isoniazid, Phenytoin
4. Pulmonary fibrosis:
   Eg Busulphan, Bleomycin, Methotrexate, Cyclophosphamide, Nitrofurantoin
5. Oxygen toxicity
6. Paraquat poisoning
7. Lipoid pneumonia & Oil Embolism
8. Pulmonary Embolism c high oestrogen content pill
9. Pulmonary Oedema:
   Eg Heroin o/d, Methadone o/d, Aspirin o/d
10. Pleural fibrosis:
    Eg Methysergide
11. Mediastinal lymphadenopathy:
    Esp Phenytoin
12. Pulmonary haem:
    Eg Penicillamine, Anti-coagulant o/d
13. Pleurisy c or without effusion:
    Eg Methysergide, Nitro-furantoin, Practolol

N.B Immunosuppressive drugs predispose to opportunistic infections & TB

Oxygen Toxicity

Occurs if continuous inhalation of >40% O_2 is given for >48hrs

PATHOLOGY: High alveolar PaO_2 → necrosis of type I alveolar cells, surfactant inactivation, ↑ in type II cells → fibrosis & scarring

Part of adult resp distress syndrome (ARDS). Vicious circle as high inspired O_2 required to maintain PaO_2 worsens lung damage

ADULT RESPIRATORY DISTRESS SYNDROME

A condition of unknown aetiology c̄ common clin, path & X-R features occuring in seriously ill patients. Predispositions inc Trauma; Gm -ve septicaemia; Shock; Near drowning; Drug o/d; Pancreatitis. Ass c̄ pulm oedema, low PaO_2 & stiff lungs Mechanism: Airway & alveolar collapse/closure → marked $\dot{V}/\dot{Q}$ imbalance c̄ R–L shunt. Stiff lungs, DIC, fat embolism & aspiration pneumonitis may be involved

CLIN: Usually develops 4–24hrs after initial systemic insult. SOB & tachypnoea, cyanosis. Often ass LRTI; Septicaemia; RF; Liver failure; Ileus; Pneumothorax

INVESTIGATIONS: • Astrup: PaO_2 ↓↓
- CXR: Diffuse bilat pulm infiltrates, snowstorm appearance which change only slowly c̄ time

RX: Prevention: Early resus. Treat sepsis. Regular monitoring. IPPV c̄ PEEP. Correct fluid balance. ?Steroids. Antibiotics for proven infection

PROG: Very poor but disease process is reversible

SARCOIDOSIS

A multisystem granulomatous disease of unknown aetiology. Diagnosis is based on histology of non-caseating epithelioid cell granulomas & +ve Kveim test. Esp US blacks. Esp 30–50yrs. F sl>M. Occ FH

CLIN: Commonest presentations are CXR abnormalities (often whilst asymptomatic); Resp symptoms; Erythema nodosum & Ocular sarcoid. The lung & ass LNs are most commonly involved. Occ Cough; SOB; Chest pain; Malaise; Wt ↓. Rarely Pneumothorax, Bronchiectasis; Aspergillosis. Occ Acute uveitis; Parotitis. Rarely Heertfordt's syndrome. Skin sarcoid is quite common—Erythema nodosum >Lupus pernio, sarcoid plaques, nodules. Liver granulomas are common but rarely symptomatic. CNS sarcoid is common late in the disease; many manifestations eg Facial palsy; Periph neuropathy; Meningitis & rarely hypopituitarism, hypothyroidism, DI. Occ supf LN ↑, Spleen ↑, Hypersplenism. Skeletal sarcoid—often febrile arthralgia & bone cysts, rarely chr arthritis. Occ $HyperCa^{2+}$ which may → Nephrocalcinosis, Calculi, RF. Rarely nasal mucosal lesions → dysphagia, SOB; Cardiac involvement eg heart block

INVESTIGATIONS: • Kveim +ve 70%
- CXR: Bilat hilar LN ↑ (Type I), LN ↑ & infiltrates (Type II), Infiltrates ± fibrosis (Type III)
- Serum angiotensin converting enzyme +ve 60%
- Serum Ca^{2+}
- AXR
- Tuberculin test -ve
- LFT
- Lung function tests
- Lung biopsy
- Liver biopsy
- Broncho–alveolar lavage: T lymphocytic alveolitis
- Gallium scanning

RX: Steroids

PROG: 75% who present c̄ acute illness recover spontaneously in <3yrs. Others have progressive organ disfunction (Chr sarcoid) esp pulm fibrosis, chr uveitis, bone cysts & skin lesions (Lupus pernio, sarcoid plaques &/or nodules). Death is often due to resp failure, cor pulmonale, aspergillosis, cardiac & CNS sarcoid

Causes of Bilat Hilar Lymphadenopathy (LIST 7 RESP)

1. Sarcoidosis
2. TB
3. Malignancy:
   a) Hodgkins & Non-Hodgkins Lymphomas
   b) Ca
   c) Leukaemia
   d) Mets
4. Fungal:
   a) Histoplasmosis
   b) Coccidioidomycosis
5. Berylliosis

Causes of Erythema Nodosum (LIST 8 RESP)

1. Sarcoidosis
2. Streptococcal infections
3. Sulphonamides
4. TB
5. Ulc colitis & Crohn's
6. Leprosy
7. Rarely:
   a) Systemic mycoses
   b) LGV
   c) Toxoplasmosis

CHEST INJURIES

Chest trauma is common esp after RTA. Classified into open & closed injuries. Open inj are due to penetrating or perforating inj & are ass c̄ pneumothorax, visceral damage & infection. Closed inj are due to blunt trauma, deceleration & blast inj. Blunt trauma is ass c̄ rib #, flail chest & diaphragmatic rupture. Deceleration inj are ass c̄ visceral ruptures. Blast inj are ass c̄ pulm haematoma, haem & hypoxia

CLIN: Occ Pain; SOB; Haemoptysis; Bruising

INVESTIGATIONS:
- CXR
- ECG
- Astrup
- FBC

GENERAL RX: Clear airway. Adequate analgesia. Physio. Restore blood & fluid balance. Regular monitoring

COMPLICATIONS:

1. **# Ribs:** Common. Esp 7th, 8th & 9th ribs. May be isolated inj
   Clin: Chest pain. Occ infection
   Rx: Analgesia. Physio
2. **Flail Chest:** #s of rib → an isolated segment of ribcage → paradoxical mvt of segment → resp failure, acidosis, CO ↓
   Rx: Analgesia. Support flail, tracheostomy ± PEEP
3. **Pneumothorax:** Ass c̄ # ribs or open chest wound (sucking pneumothorax)
   Rx: Insert intercostal catheter c̄ underwater seal (urgently if a tension pneumothorax)
4. **Surgical & Mediastinal Emphysema:** Ass c̄ ruptured oesophagus, bronchus or trachea; # ribs. Mediastinal emphysema can also occur spontaneously, following valsalva manoeuvre or by tracking from elsewhere. Often ass c̄ pneumothorax, pleural effusion &/or empyema
   Clin: Central chest pain. Occ Hamman's sign; Shock
5. **Haemothorax:**
   Rx: Transfusion, antibiotics & analgesics. Drain. Occ thoracotomy
6. **Lung Contusion:**
   Clin: Occ Haemoptysis
7. **Ruptured Trachea or Main Bronchus:**
   Clin: Acute tension pneumothorax or chr atelectasis & chest infections
   Investigation: • Bronchoscopy
   Rx: Acute: Thoracotomy & repair
   Chronic: Thoractomy & pneumonectomy or bronchial anastomosis
8. **Ruptured Oesophagus:** Rare. → mediastinal emphysema, Acute mediastinitis
   Rx: Thoracotomy & repair. IV relacement therapy
9. **Cardiac Trauma:** esp Tamponade
   Ass c̄ crush, deceleration & blast inj
   Clin: BP ↓; Pulsus paradoxicus
   Investigation: • Echocardiography
   Rx: Thoracotomy or pericardiocentesis
10. **Large Vessel Damage:** Usually fatal
    Rx: Emergency thoracotomy & repair
11. **Ruptured Diaphragm:**
    Clin: Shock; Pain; Haemothorax or Haemoperitoneum
    Rx: Correct shock. Thoracotomy—

reduce abdo contents & repair
12. Damage to Ass Viscera: Eg spleen
13. Traumatic Asphyxia: Severe crush inj → Venous P ↑↑
Clin: Bruising & petechial haem. Occ Sub-Conjunctival Haem

PULMONARY VASCULAR DISEASE

Pulmonary Hypertension

A mean resting Pulmonary artery P of >30/15mmHg

Causes of Pulmonary Hypertension (LIST 9 RESP)

1. ↑ Pulm vascular resistance:
   a) Vasoconstrictive—usually due to Hypoxia,
   eg Chr bronchitis, High altitude, Kyphoscoliosis
   b) Obstructive due to thromboembolism
   c) Obliterative due to arteritis, parasites
   eg PAN, SLE, Scleroderma, Schistosomiasis
   d) Obliterative due to ↓ pulmonary vascular bed
   eg Emphysema
   e) Veno-occlusive disease—1° disease of pulmonary veins
2. Hyperkinetic ie ↑ pulm blood flow:
   Eg L–R shunt due to VSD, PDA
3. Passive ie ↑ L atrial P:
   Eg MSt & LVF
4. 1° Pulmonary BP ↑

GENERAL CLIN: Syncope; Angina; Fatigue; SOB. R Vent heave; Loud P2, S4, early diastolic murmur. Occ CCF; Cyanosis

GENERAL INVESTIGATIONS: • ECG
- CXR: Prominent pulm conus & proximal vasculature c̄ normal or ↓ distal vessels
- Catheterisation

1° PULM HYPERTENSION

Rare. Esp young women. 3 forms: Plexogenic, Thromboembolic & Veno-occlusive

CLIN: Increasing SOB; Angina; Syncope. Occ Haemoptysis. Later CCF; Cyanosis; Giant "a waves"; Functional TI & PInc; R Vent heave; Split S2 c̄ ejection click

INVESTIGATIONS: • CXR
- ECG
- Catheterisation

RX: Anticoagulants

PROG: Poor

Cor Pulmonale

A term denoting R heart disease 2° to chr lung or pulm vessel disease. Often ass c̄ pulm BP ↑

CLIN: SOB; CCF. Occ Angina; Cyanosis; Polycythaemia. RVH; Loud S2; Gallop. Occ TI

INVESTIGATIONS: • FEV_1 ↓
- ECG: ^R Axis deviation^; RVH; ^P^ pulmonale; ^RBBB^
- Pulmonary wedge P

RX: O_2, Rest, Diuretics, Digoxin, Physio

Pulmonary Embolism (PE)

ASS c̄:
1. DVT
2. Age ↑
3. Obesity
4. Immobilisation
5. Pregnancy
6. High oestrogen content pill
7. Post-op
8. Trauma
9. AF
10. MI
11. Cardiac failure
12. Thrombophlebitis migrans eg Ca pancreas
13. Gm -ve sepsis

Termed massive if >50% of major pulm arteries involved

CLIN:
1. Small PE: Asymptomatic or unexplained SOB, pain, fear, PR ↑, fever
2. Medium PE: Pleurisy; Haemoptysis
3. Massive PE: Urge for straining; Pain; CO ↓↓; BP ↓, PR ↑; Collapse; Syncope; SOB; Oliguria; RVF; Pulm BP ↑

4. Chr thromboembolism: Severe pulm BP ↑ (qv). Occ Haemoptysis, Pleurisy

INVESTIGATIONS: • ECG: ^RBBB^, ^T^ inversion. Occ ^S_1, Q_3, $\hat{T}_3$
• CXR: Effusion, Atelectasis, Diaphragm ↑. Oligaemia
• Astrup: PaO_2 ↓ $PaCO_2$ ↑
• Isotope lung scan $\dot{V}/\dot{Q}$ mismatch
• Pulmonary arteriography

RX: A. Prevention: Sub-cutaneous heparin; Leg exercises; Leg cuffs
Early mobilisation post-op
B. Small PE: Anticoags for at least 3mths
C. Medium PE: Opiates. Anticoags
D. Massive PE: Cardiac resus measures. O_2. If resus failing emergency embolectomy. May try thrombolytic agents or heparin
If survive, long-term anticoags
E. Chr thromboembolism: Long term anticoags

PROG: Poor c̄ massive PE. Chr thromboembolism → RVH & occ death

DD: 1. MI
2. Acute bleed
3. Acute Gm -ve shock
4. Pancreatitis
5. Cardiac tamponade
6. Dissecting aortic aneurysm
7. Pneumothorax & lung collapse

Uncommon Pulmonary Vascular Disease

A-V ANEURYSM OR FISTULA

May be ass c̄ telangiectasia elsewhere. Rare

CLIN: Often asymptomatic. Occ Cerebral embolism or Abscess

INVESTIGATION: • Whole lung tomography

RX: Occ surgical repair

GOODPASTURE'S SYNDROME

Lung purpura c̄ glomerulonephritis (GN)

CLIN: Haemoptysis; GN

RX: Plasmapheresis; Steroids

IDIOPATHIC PULMONARY HAEMOSIDEROSIS

Rare. Esp children & young adults. Intrapulm haem of unknown cause. Occ ass c̄ IgA def

CLIN: Anaemia; Haemoptysis; Cough; SOB; Cyanosis; Fever. Occ J; Liver ↑; CCF

INVESTIGATIONS: • CXR
• FBC
• Lung biopsy

RX: Steroids. Fe

PROG: About 50% die in 5yrs

PULMONARY OEDEMA

An increase of extravascular fluid within the lung

Causes of Pulmonary Oedema (LIST 10 RESP)

A. DUE TO ↑ PULM CAPILLARY P
1. LVF
2. MSt
3. Veno–occlusive disease

B. DUE TO ↓ PLASMA COLLOID OSMOTIC P
Hypoalbuminaemia: Eg Cirrhosis

C DUE TO ↑ PULMONARY CAPILLARY PERMEABILITY
1. Pneumonia
2. Toxic fumes
3. Circulating toxins:
Eg Gm -ve Shock, Snake venom
4. DIC
5. Uraemia
6. Radiation
7. Near drowning

D. DUE TO ABNORMAL NEGATIVE P IN PLEURAL SPACE
1. Rx of Pneumothorax
2. Rapid aspiration of pleural effusion

E. DUE TO PULMONARY LYMPHATIC OBST

F. UNKNOWN MECHANISMS
1. High altitude
2. ↑ ICP
3. PE
4. Narcotic overdose
5. Eclampsia

CLIN: SOB; Tachypnoea; Orthopnoea; PND; Cough; Basal creps. Later Cheyne–Stokes resp; Cyanosis; Frothy sputum; Haemoptysis

INVESTIGATION: • CXR: Kerley "B" lines; Bat's Wing appearance

RX: Diuretics. Occ O_2, Digoxin

URTI

Very common. Major cause of absence from work. 6 clinical syndromes: Common cold; Pharyngitis; Pharyngoconjunctival syndrome; Influenza; Herpangina; Croup

Common Cold

Caused by many different viruses

CLIN: Rhinorrhoea & nasal obst; Sneezing; Occ Sore throat; Mild conjunctivitis. Usually recover in <1wk

Influenza

Due to influenza virus A, B, or C. Epidemics esp winter. Rarely pandemics. Highly infectious

CLIN: Sudden onset. Chills; Fever; Headache; Malaise; Muscle aches; Cough; Sore throat. Variable severity. Occ Prostration

RX: Prophylactic "flu" vaccine, however antigenic drift or shift can reduce protection. General supportive measures

COMPLICATIONS: 2° bacterial infections esp Staph & *H.influenza*. Rarely CNS complications eg encephalitis

LRTI

Acute Tracheitis & Bronchitis

Usually 2° to URTI or exacerbation of Chr bronchitis. Esp *H. influenza* & Pneumococcus

CLIN: Variable severity. Irritating dry cough; Airways obst; Mucopurulent sputum; Variable SOB. Occ Fever; Wheeze

RX: Antibiotics; Inhalations. Occ bronchodilators

Pneumonias

Inflam of lung parenchyma due to infection. Usually 1° but occ 2° eg to Ca, Bronchiectasis, Immunosuppression. Esp Elderly. Winter >Summer
Classified according to causal agent or anatomic distribution
Anatomic classification: Lobar pneumonia—infection localised to a lobe; Segmental; Bronchopneumonia—(commonest form) bilat patchy infection

CLIN: Fever; Cough; Mucopurulent sputum; Tachypnoea; Malaise. Signs of consolidation (usually lobar pneumonia)—Chest Mvt ↓; PN dull; Vocal fremitus ↓; Bronchial breathing; Aeogophony; Creps; Whispering pectriloquy. Occ Headache; PR ↓ (commoner if viral cause) or ↑; Pleurisy (commoner if bacterial). Rarely Haemoptysis; Cyanosis. Eventually → Toxaemia; Confusion; BP ↓; Anuria; Oliguria; J

INVESTIGATIONS:
- CXR: Opacification c̄ air bronchogram or bilat patchy shadowing
- Sputum C&S, AFBs
- WCC
- U&E
- Occ Blood gases; Blood cultures; Pleural aspiration; Serology

RX: Bed rest; Correct U&E; O_2; Antibiotics; Analgesics
Choice of antibiotic depends on sputum sensitivity, clin features, h/o pre-existing chest disease & h/o antibiotic allergy.
In most cases where causal agent is

not yet known Ampicillin is Rx of choice. Gentamicin is indicated for severe pneumonia (c̄ Flucloxacillin) & Gm -ve infections. Flucloxacillin is also indicated for penicillin resistant staph. Erythromycin or Tetracycline are indicated for Legionnaire's, Mycoplasma, Psittacosis & Q fever. Failure to respond may indicate inadequate or inappropriate antibiotic, underlying Ca, foreign body, unusual causative organism, host resistance ↓ or complications

Specific types:

PNEUMOCOCCAL PNEUMONIA

Classical type. Common cause of lobar pneumonia. Also cause of bronchopneumonia esp in elderly. Gm +ve

RX: Benzylpenicillin or Ampicillin. Erythromycin if allergy

STAPHYLOCOCCAL PNEUMONIA

Occ 2° to influenza. Can cause multiple lung abscesses

RX: Flucloxacillin & Ampicillin

KLEBSIELLA PNEUMONIA

Unusual. Usually occurs if pre-existing pulm disease. Upper lobe >Lower. Usually bilat. Abscesses are common. Gm -ve

RX: Gentamicin & a Cephalosporin

PROG: 50% mort

LEGIONNAIRE'S DISEASE

Esp elderly, pre-existing lung disease, immunosuppressed. Recently described but now recognised not to be rare. Gm -ve. Incub Pd 2–10days

CLIN: Fever; Profuse sweats; Anorexia; Wt ↓. 2–4 days later Cough; SOB. Later Severe pneumonia; Confusion; Malaise; Myalgia; Abdo pain; Diarrhoea. Occ ARF

INVESTIGATIONS:
- Rise in Ab titre
- ESR ↑↑
- WCC ↑
- U&E: Na^+ ↓
- CXR
- Sputum C&S usually does not isolate
- LFT abnormal
- Serum albumin ↓

RX: Erythromycin

PROG: 10% mort

PSEUDOMONAS PNEUMONIA

Rare except in immunosuppressed, severe pre-existing pulm disease eg CF. Sputum isolation is not proof of pathogenicity. Ass c̄ lower lobe bronchopneumonia

RX: Gentamicin & Carbenicillin parenterally

MYCOPLASMA PNEUMONIA

Esp <35yrs, closed communities. Esp autumn & early winter

CLIN: Usually mild resp symptoms. Fever; Sore throat. Rarely Haemolytic anaemia; Stevens Johnson syndrome; Urticaria; Arthralgia

INVESTIGATIONS:
- Cold agglutinins
- Rising Ab titre

RX: Tetracycline or Erythromycin

Q FEVER

Due to *Coxiella burnetti* ie Rickettsial. Spread by contact c̄ cows & sheep. Incub Pd 2–3wks

CLIN: Fever; Headache; General aches; Cough. Occ becomes chr c̄ likelihood of endocarditis

INVESTIGATION:
- Rising Ab titre

RX: Erythromycin or Tetracycline

PSITTACOSIS/ORNITHOSIS

Due to *Chlamydia psittaci*. Acquired from infected birds either psittacine eg parrots or others eg pigeons. Incub Pd 7–14 days

CLIN: Pneumonia which may be severe c̄ high fever, prostration, headache, photophobia. Usually lasts 1–2wks but occ chr course c̄ Liver ↑, spleen ↑, haemolytic anemia, erythema nodosum

INVESTIGATION:
- CFT. (False +ve WR)

RX: Tetracycline

PNEUMOCYSTIS CARINII

Rare except in immunosuppressed esp in Cyt.T for leukaemia when prophylactic Cotrimoxazole is useful

INVESTIGATIONS:
- Lung biopsy
- Broncho–alveolar lavage

Complications of Pneumonia

1. Empyema
2. Lung abscess
3. Pleural effusion
4. Septicaemia
5. Pulm fibrosis
6. Pulm oedema
7. Resp failure
8. Rarely: Cerebral abscess; Jaundice; DIC; RF; Meningitis; Endocarditis

TUBERCULOSIS

Very important communicable disease due to *Mycobacterium tuberculosis*. Endemic in many countries eg India, Phillipines. Not uncommon in UK. In UK airbourne spread much commoner than bovine. In UK esp elderly, lower social class, immigrants from Indian sub-continent, immunosuppressed, diabetics, alcoholics, post-gastrectomy

PATHOLOGY: Caseating granuloma which heal accompanied by fibrosis ass c̄ calcification

1° Pulmonary TB

The term 1° TB describes the first occasion that the individual is infected. Esp children

Time course of 1° pulm TB:
0/52 infection; 3–4/52 +ve Mantoux; 4–8/52 1° complex (Ghon focus & regional LN ↑); 3–6/12 Pleural effusion; 3–9/12 Bronchial erosion; >12/12 Meningitis/miliary TB; 3yr Bone TB; 5yr Renal TB.

CLIN: Many cases are not clinically apparent & do not progress beyond 1° complex. Occ Anorexia; Wt ↓; Cough. Other complications of 1° TB are local spread in lung; cavitation; segmental collapse; middle lobe syndrome → bronchiectasis in later life

Post 1° TB

Reactivation of 1° TB or reinfection. Wide spectrum of presentations resp features are most common

CLIN OF RESP TB: Cough; Mucoid or purulent sputum; Haemoptysis; SOB; Fever; Malaise; Wt ↓; Chest wall pain. Occ Wheeze; Dyspepsia; Hoarseness; Pleural effusion; Pneumothorax; Cv LN ↑; Lung abscess; Empyema. May spread in lungs &/or to trachea, larynx, mouth, GIT or miliary spread. Later occ Chr pulm fibrosis; Amyloidosis; Resp failure; Aspergilloma

Miliary TB

Widespread dissemination of TB usually c̄ multiple nodules evident in lungs. May occur in 1° or post 1° TB. Measles & whooping cough predispose

CLIN: Fever; Malaise; Wt ↓. Occ Choroidal tubercles; Meningitis; Liver ↑; Spleen ↑. Later Cough; SOB; Cyanosis. Occ occurs in elderly in cryptic form c̄ fewer constitutional symptoms. May → meningitis, pleural effusion, polyserositis, K^+ ↓, blood dyscrasias, DIC

Investigations of Resp TB

1. Tuberculin test—Mantoux test is most sensitive but Heaf test is better suited to surveys. +ve in TB except in miliary TB, TB meningitis, TB in elderly, immunosuppressed, during acute exanthemata & c̄ some chr diseases eg sarcoidosis, Hodgkins. Also +ve if previous BCG
2. CXR: Many possible pictures eg apical opacites, cavitation, fibrosis, calcification, miliary mottling
3. Sputum C&S, AFBs
4. If no sputum: Broncho-alveolar lavage, gastric lavage or laryngeal swabs
5. Occ biopsy eg pleural biopsy

Prevention

BCG VACCINATION

In UK gives about 80% of those immunised protection for up to 15yrs. In high risk countries given at birth. Complications rare

CONTACT TRACING

Gives a significant yield when close contacts of smear +ve patients are identified. All close contacts should be examined but casual contacts only require examination if unusual exposure to a highly infectious disease has occured

CHEMOPROPHYLAXIS

Indicated for infected infants <5yrs old, recent tuberculin converters, long term immunosuppressive Rx, close contacts aged <20yrs. Traditionally use Isoniazid alone

MASS RADIOGRAPHY

Occ indicated to survey closed communities eg common lodging houses or those at special risk eg lab workers

Rx of TB

Combination chemotherapy eg Isoniazid, Ethambutol, Rifampicin, Pyrazinamide for 2mths followed by Rifampicin & Isoniazid for further 4mths. Other drugs include PAS acid & Streptomycin. Careful attention to dose important. Compliance is very important for achieving cure. Steroids are used in severely ill, to reduce inflam rapidly & for hypersensitivity reactions

Rifampicin: Bactericidal. Induces liver enzymes
SE: Orange urine; N&V
Isoniazid: Bactericidal
SE: Periph neuropathy (prevented by Pyridoxine). Occ Fever; Rash
Ethambutol: Bacteriostatic. Not used in very young or elderly
SE: Optic neuritis (Occ irreversible)
Streptomycin: Given IM
SE: Hypersensitivity, Vestibular toxicity. Rarely Deafness; Nephrotoxicity
PAS Acid:
SE: Anorexia; N&V; Hypersensitivity
Pyrazinamide: Bactericidal. Good for TB meningitis
SE: Hepatitis. Rarely Hyperuricaemia; Photosensitivity

DD

1. Pneumonia
2. Lung Ca
3. Lung abscess
4. Pulm infarct
5. Other mycobacterial disease
6. Coccidioidomycosis
7. Histoplasmosis

Other Mycobacterial Disease

Apart from TB & Leprosy there are a number of rare conditions caused by Mycobacteria. They are an unusual DD of TB
M.marinum: Skin granuloma
M.avium: Cv LN ↑
M.kansasii: Cv LN ↑. Lung disease

COCCIDIOIDOMYCOSIS

Due to inhalation of dust borne spores of *C.immitis*. Occurs in 1° & progressive forms. Esp darker skin races

CLIN: Asymptomatic or influenza-like illness. Occ Erythema nodosum or Erythema multiforme. Usually resolves in <2mths but rarely → progressive form c̄ miliary spread or widespread granuloma & abscesses

INVESTIGATIONS:
- CXR: Bilat hilar LN ↑
- Sputum
- Coccidioidin test

RX: In severe 1° or progressive forms—Amphotericin

HISTOPLASMOSIS

Due to inhalation of dust borne spores of *H.capsulatum*. Benign primary, serious acute & chr progressive forms

CLIN: Asymptomatic or influenza like illness. May progress to mimic pulm TB, bronchitis or pneumonia. Granulomas, fibrosis & cavitation are common in chr cases

INVESTIGATIONS: • CXR
• Histoplasmin test
• Sputum C&S

RX: Amphotericin B if symptomatic

PNEUMOCONIOSIS

Pneumoconiosis is pulm disease esp fibrosis due to dust inhalation. Dangerous particles are less than 5μm diameter

Silicosis

Declining incidence in UK. About 150 certifications a year. Esp slate, granite & foundry workers

CLIN: Lung nodules which may progress to PMF. TB may complicate

INVESTIGATION: • CXR: Egg-shell calcification of hilar nodes, nodules predominently upper lobe

RX: Remove from exposure

Coalworkers Pneumoconiosis

Related to degree of exposure to coal dust. Not ass c̄ lung Ca or TB. The commonest pneumoconiosis in W.Europe

PATH: Small nodules are ass c̄ emphysema & simple pneumoconiosis, whilst larger nodules are ass c̄ PMF. PMF is commoner if quartz or silica are plentiful in the coal dust

CLIN: Simple pneumoconiosis is asymptomatic & is a CXR diagnosis.

Occ development of PMF, emphysema which may → cor pulmonale & resp failure. Rarely in Rh F +ve Rh Arth large fibrotic nodules occur which can cavitate (Caplan's syndrome)

INVESTIGATION: • CXR: Nodular opacities, fibrosis esp upper lobes

RX: Prophylactic use of respirators. Regular CXR of workforce. Remove workers from dusty environment on development of simple form

Berylliosis

Acute form causes pulm oedema & miliary mottling on CXR

RX: O_2, Steroids
Chronic form resembles sarcoidosis & may → cor pulmonale

RX: Steroids

Byssinosis

Due to heavy exposure to cotton dust or flax

CLIN: SOB; Cough; Chest tightness on exposure. Likely to develop if pre-existing COAD

RX: Reduce exposure, Bronchodilators

Occupationally Caused Pulmonary Oedema

Pulm oedema & alveolar capillary damage 2° to gases eg Cl^-, SO_4, Ammonia, NO_2 & metal fumes esp cadmium. Cadmium can also cause hepatitis, renal cortical necrosis & emphysema

CLIN: Anxiety; Cough; Frothy phlegm ± blood; SOB; Creps; Respiration ↓. Occ Confusion; Bronchopneumonia; Asphyxia

INVESTIGATION: • CXR: Bats wings shadows

RX: Remove from cause. Observe. Rx for any shock

Non-Fibrotic Pneumoconiosis

Siderosis & Stannosis produce benign nodular CXR changes

Asbestosis

Asbestos includes a group of fibrous silicates c̄ different aerodynamics & hence health risks. Chrysotile is used in the textile industry whilst crocidolite (blue asbestos) was used for marine instalation. Other safer forms are amosite & anthophyllite. Occupational exposure esp in mining, milling, naval & demolition industries. Health effects are dose related.
Asbestosis, a diffuse interstitial pulmonary fibrosis, is the commonest lung effect. Other principal disease problems are pleural disease, mesothelioma & lung Ca

CLIN: Increasing SOB; Cough; Late insp crackles; Clubbing. Occ Cyanosis. Later may develop PMF, Asbestoma, Lung Ca, Pleural effusion or Mesothelioma

INVESTIGATIONS:
- CXR: Basal fibrosis, Shaggy heart border, Calcified plaques esp diaphragms
- Sputum: Asbestos bodies or fibres may be seen
- Lung function tests
- Occ CAT scan, Lung biopsy

RX: Symptomatic Rx. Remove exposure but most cases have been separated from exposure for many yrs. Stop cigs to ↓ risk of lung Ca

Mesothelioma

Large majority of cases ass c̄ asbestos exposure esp crocidolite

CLIN: Chest pain; SOB; Pleural effusions. Occ Ascites

INVESTIGATIONS:
- Biopsy (encourages tumour spread)
- CXR
- CAT scan

PROG: Very poor

LUNG CANCER

Commonest M cause of death from Ca in UK. Very common in UK. Strongly related to cigs hence M>F. Mortality is decreasing in younger M but increasing in F as smoking habits change. Other risk factors are: Air pollution, Urban dwelling, Occupational eg Gas retort workers; Exposure to Radon, coal gas, Nickel, Arsenic, Chromates, Haematite, Asbestos. Passive smoking may be a risk factor

PATHOLOGY: 4 main histological types: Squamous cell (commonest), AdenoCa, Small cell inc Oat-cell, Large cell.
Most lung Ca arises in central airways. Periph tumours are usually adenoCa or large cell Ca. Oat-cell Ca is most rapidly growing & metastasises early. AdenoCa is less ass c̄ smoking & is slow growing. Spread can be direct, via lymph & blood. Common 2° sites are liver, adrenals, bone, brain, kidney, skin

CLIN: Cough; Haemoptysis; Chest pain occ pleuritic; SOB (esp if lymphangitis carcinomatosa); Wt ↓; Anorexia; Malaise; Clubbing. Occ Wheeze; Chest infection; Pleural effusion; Lung abscess; Empyema; Lung collapse. Often symptoms from mets (may be presenting feature) eg SVC obst; Brachial neuritis; Recurrent laryngeal nerve palsy; Horner's syndrome; Bone pain; Liver ↑; Ep
Non-Metastatic Extrapulmonary manifestations include—HPOA; Endocrine syndromes (usually due to Oat-cell Ca) eg inappropriate ADH production, ectopic ACTH production, $HyperCa^{2+}$; Neuropathy; Myopathy; Cerebellar degeneration; Myasthenia; Thrombophlebitis migrans; Pericarditis
High apical tumours (Pancoast's) are ass c̄ brachial neuritis, Horner's syndrome & hoarseness

INVESTIGATIONS:
- CXR ± Tomography: Many appearances eg irregular mass, collapse/consolidation, effusion, abscess, diaphragmatic paralysis, hilar or mediastinal enlargement
- Bronchoscopy ± Biopsy
- Sputum cytology
- FBC: Hb ↓
- U&E
- LFT
- Bone Scan
- Other Biopsies eg pleural, percutaneous
- Mediastinoscopy, CAT scan pre-surgery

RX: Stopping smoking immediately begins to reduce risk of developing lung Ca. Depends on histological type & the stage of disease. Small cell Ca are usually considered unresectable. Other tumours should be considered for surgery if in early stage ie small tumour c̄ no LN or met spread. The value of adjuvent therapy c̄ surgery is unproven. X-Rad is an excellent palliative eg for bony mets, SVC obst, haemoptysis. Combination Cyt.T at present offers little benefit except in small cell Ca where median survival is improved. Palliation c̄ eg Bromptons, Metoclopromide, Chlorpromazine

PROG: Best if Squamous cell, early stage, younger age, no other pulmonary disease or small cell responsive to CyT.T. 3% 5yr survival

Alveolar Cell Ca

Uncommon malignant tumour arising from alveolar or broncho–alveolar epithelium. M=F. Unrelated to smoking. Scar tissue & diffuse lung fibrosis may predispose. Late spread by blood, lymph

CLIN: Variable. Occ Asymptomatic on presentation. Cough; Haemoptysis; SOB; Wt ↓; Malaise. Occ Clubbing; Profuse mucoid sputum

INVESTIGATIONS: • CXR: Irregular nodular shadows >solitary lesion
- Sputum C&S
- Transbronchial biopsy

RX: Resect if solitary lesion. Palliation

Bronchial Adenoma

Uncommon. Pre-malignant tumours. Two major forms: Carcinoid & Cylindromas

CYLINDROMA

Usually occur in large bronchi or trachea. Probably arise from mucous glands. Locally invasive, occ metastasise

CLIN: Haemoptysis; Cough; Infection; Abscess; Obst emphysema. Occ Clubbing

CARCINOID

Usually occur in main bronchi

CLIN: Cough; Small haemoptyses. Occ Chr infection & clubbing; Obst emphysema. May metastasise late. Rarely develop carcinoid syndrome c̄ flushes, facial oedema, BP ↓, PR ↑, fever, abdo pain, diarrhoea, wheezing & dyspnoea

INVESTIGATIONS OF ADENOMA: • CXR
- Bronchoscopy
- Urinary 5HIAA: ↑ in carcinoid syndrome

RX OF ADENOMA: Resect

PROG OF ADENOMA: Good if no mets

Causes of "Coin" Lesion on CXR (LIST 11 RESP)

Coin lesions are vaguely circular opacities c̄ clear surrounding lung

1. Lung Ca
2. Metastasis
3. TB
4. Pulm infarct
5. Rheumatoid Nodule
6. Hydatid cyst
7. Bronchial adenoma
8. Hamartoma
7. Histoplasmoma
8. A-V fistula
9. Wegener's Granuloma
10. Lymphoma
11. Encysted pleural effusion
12. Round atelectasis
13. Coccidiodomycosis
14. Bronchial cyst
15. Sequestered lung segment

Causes of Lobar Collapse (LIST 12 RESP)

1. Complete bronchial obst:
   a) Intraluminal obst eg Foreign body, Mucus plug
   b) Mural eg Lung Ca
   c) Extramural eg LN ↑, Aortic aneurysm
2. Pneumothorax
3. Pleural effusion

LUNG ABSCESS

A localised suppurative lesion of lung parenchyma. Aspiration is the commonest cause

Causes of Lung Abscess (LIST 13 RESP)

1. Aspiration:
   a) Pharyngeal pouch
   b) Oral or pharyngeal sepsis
   c) Oesophageal obst
   d) Near drowning
   e) Bronchiectasis
   f) Impaired consciousness
   g) Alcoholism
   h) Bulbar palsy, Anaesthesia
2. Malignancy
3. Bronchial obst:
   Eg Foreign body, CF, Tumour
4. Infection:
   a) Pneumonia Esp Staph, Klebsiella, Legionella
   b) TB
   c) Amoebiasis
   d) Hydatid disease
   e) Fungi eg Actinomycosis
5. Emboli:
   a) 2° to infected pulm infarct
   b) Septic emboli
6. Infection of cong or acquired cysts

CLIN: Fever; Malaise. Later persistent cough & mucopurulent sputum ± blood. Rarely mets to brain

INVESTIGATIONS:
- CXR
- Sputum
- WCC ↑
- Bronchoscopy

RX: Postural drainage. Antibiotics—use ampicillin & metronidazole if no microorganisms cultured. Surgical excision if failure of medical Rx or complications of bronchopleural fistula or empyema

PLEURAL DISORDERS

Pleural Effusion

Causes of Pleural Effusion (LIST 14 RESP)

A. TRANSUDATES
   1. CCF (R>L)
   2. Nephrotic syndrome
   3. Liver failure
   4. Constrictive pericarditis
   5. Hypothyroidism
   6. Peritoneal dialysis
   7. Meig's syndrome

B. EXUDATES
   1. Infection:
      Eg Pneumonia esp bacterial, TB
   2. Pulm infarct
   3. Trauma
   4. Malignancy:
      Eg Lung, Breast or Stomach Ca mets, Mesothelioma, Lymphoma
   5. Collagen vascular disease:
      Eg Rh Arth, Rh fever, SLE
   6. Sub-phrenic abscess
   7. Pancreatitis
   8. Post MI syndrome
   9. Asbestos exposure
   10. Methysergide
   11. Amoebiasis
   12. Sarcoidosis
   13. Yellow nail syndrome

CLIN: Depends on size of effusion. Occ SOB; Pain on insp; Fever; ↓ Chest mvt; PN dull; Breath Sounds ↓; Vocal fremitus ↓

INVESTIGATIONS: • CXR: Blunting of costophrenic angle if small. Homogeneous shadow c̄ concave upper border. Fluid shifts c̄ gravity unless encysted
- Thoracentesis & Biopsy: Fluid for C&S, Biochem, Cytology. Transudates contain <30g protein/l
- Occ Broncoscopy, Isotope lung scan

COMPLICATIONS OF THORACENTESIS:
1. Pulm oedema
2. Air embolism
3. Haem
4. Pneumothorax

RX: Aspirate large effusions slowly. Treat underlying cause. Malignant effusions, drain & inject Tetracycline, Talc or Bleomycin into pleural space

Empyema

Pus in pleural space. Rare nowadays due to antibiotics

Causes of Empyema (LIST 15 RESP)

1. Severe pneumonia
2. Lung abscess
3. Bronchiectasis
4. Surgery or trauma inc bronchopleural fistula
5. TB
6. Ca
7. Rupture of oesophagus
8. Sub-phrenic abscess
9. Rarely:
   a) Actinomycosis
   b) Amoebiasis

CLIN: High fever; Anorexia; Malaise; Anaemia; Clubbing; Rigors; SOB. May be complicated by: Bronchopleural fistula c̄ cough & blood stained purulent sputum; Discharge through chest wall; Cerebral abscess; Amyloidosis; Lung fibrosis

INVESTIGATIONS: • WCC ↑
- CXR: Pleural effusion may be encysted
- Thoracentesis & biopsy

RX: Antibiotics often inc Metronidazole. Aspirate to dryness c̄ appropriate antibiotic injected into pleural cavity. Chronic empyema may require resection

Pneumothorax

Causes of Pnemothorax (LIST 16 RESP)

1. Primary: Esp young adult males
2. Secondary:
   a) Trauma
   b) Iatrogenic eg Thoracentesis, Surgery, IPPV
   c) Chr bronchitis & emphysema esp rupture of bullae
   d) Asthma
   e) Infections eg Pneumonia, TB, Whooping cough
   f) Congenital cysts & bullae
   g) Bronchial or pleural Ca
   h) Lung abscess
   i) Pulmonary fibrosis or Honeycomb lung eg Histiocytosis X
   j) Occupational lung disease eg Silicosis
   k) Rapid decompression in divers
   l) Pleural endometriosis

CLIN: Sudden chest pain usually on affected side; SOB; Occ Cough; Subcutaneous emphysema. ↓ mvt affected side; ↑↑ PN; Tracheal deviation. Occ Clicking sound related to cardiac cycle (Hamman's sign). If tension pneumothorax: Anxiety; Resp distress; Shock; PR ↑; BP ↓. Mediastinal shift to opposite side. Rarely cyanosis. May become chronic due to formation of bronchopleural fistula

INVESTIGATION: • Insp & Exp CXR

RX: If small—observe. If large—drainage c̄ intercostal catheter attached to underwater seal. Occ require pleurodesis eg c̄ Talc or pleurectomy. N.B Tension pnemothorax requires urgent drainage

Indications for Surgery:
1. Haemopneumothorax
2. Failed medical Rx
3. Recurrent pneumothoraces

COMPLICATIONS:
1. Bronchopleural fistula
2. Empyema
3. Pneumomediastinum
4. Haemopneumothorax

PROG: 20% recur within 1yr

MEDIASTINAL CONDITIONS

Mediastinal Masses

Commonest causes are HH & LN ↑
Most causes are rare

Causes of Mediastinal Masses (LIST 17 RESP)

1. Lymphadenopathy:
   Eg Mets, TB, Sarcoidosis, Reticuloses
2. Cysts:
   a) Bronchogenic
   b) Enterogenous
   c) Pericardial (Springwater)
   d) Hydatid
   e) Meningocoele
3. Tumours:
   a) Thymoma
   b) Dermoid
   c) Teratoma
   d) Neurofibroma
   e) Neurilemmoma
   f) Ganglioneuroma
   g) Neuroblastoma
   h) Mesothelioma
   i) Lipoma
3. Retrosternal goitre
4. Aortic aneurysm
5. Hernia:
   Eg Hiatus hernia, Diagphragmatic hernia
6. Oesophageal lesion:
   Eg Achalasia, Oesophageal pouch, Corkscrew oesophagus, Ca
7. Paravertebral abscess
8. Encysted mediastinal effusion

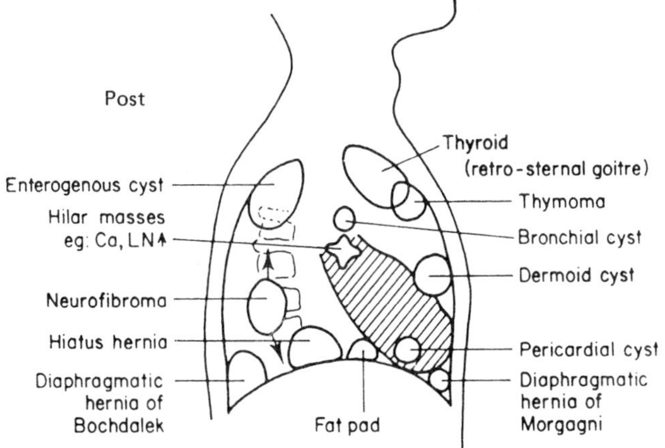

Figure 1 Mediastinal masses - lateral view.

THYMOMA

Uncommon tumour. Ass c̄ Myasthenia gravis, SLE, Thyrotoxicosis, Haemolytic anaemia

CLIN: Occ bronchial or tracheal compression → stridor, wheeze, resp distress

INVESTIGATIONS: • CXR & tomography
• CAT scan

RX: Surgery

Acute Mediastinitis

Usually due to oesophageal rupture

CLIN: Rigors; Fever; Pain; Collapse. Occ Cyanosis, SOB

INVESTIGATIONS: • WCC ↑
• CXR: Mediastinal widening ± Emphysema

RX: Antibiotics & IV feeding &/or surgical repair

Idiopathic Mediastinal Fibrosis

Rare. Esp middle aged

CLIN: Gradual fibrosis → SVC constriction. Swelling of face & neck; Headache; SOB; Giddiness. Occ Epistaxis

INVESTIGATION: • CXR: Mediastinal widening

RX: Surgery to relieve pressure on mediastinum. Occ venous bypass

Causes of Chronic Cough (LIST 18 RESP)

1. Chr bronchitis & emphysema
2. Asthma
3. LVF
4. Ca lung
5. Post nasal drip
6. Chest infection:
   Esp TB, Bronchiectasis, CF, Fungal
7. Sub-phrenic abscess
8. Sarcoidosis
9. Habit cough
10. Smoking

Cardiology

HEART FAILURE

A failure of CO to meet the body's circulatory demand

CAUSES: 1. Loss of myocardium eg MI
2. ↓ Inotropic state eg Cardiomyopathy, drugs & hypertrophy
3. High output states
4. ↑ systolic tension eg BP ↑, dilatation, outflow tract obst
5. Inappropriate PR ↑ or PR ↓

PATHOPHYSIOLOGY: Persistent mechanical overload → hypertrophy & dilatation. Low CO → Renal blood flow ↓, GFR ↓ → Na^+ ↑ → Fluid retention. Impaired contractility & Vent stiffness contribute to Ht failure

Left Ventricular Failure

CLIN: SOB on exertion; Orthopnoea; PND; Frothy sputum & SOB (Pulm oedema); Cough. Occ Haemoptysis; Cyanosis. PR ↑; Ht ↑; Basal creps; Sweating. Occ Pulsus alternans; Triple rhythm; S3; Deviated apex beat; MInc. Often → RVF (CCF)

INVESTIGATIONS:
- ECG: Eg LVH, Ischaemia
- CXR: Ht ↑, Pulm oedema

RX: Diuretics $\pm$ K^+ eg Frusemide. Vasodilators eg Prazosin. Digoxin (↑ inotropic effect). In acute pulm oedema/LVF: Sit patient up; O_2; Diamorphine 10mg IV; Frusemide IV. In cardiogenic shock: Dopamine, ventilate & use balloon pump

Causes of LVF (LIST 1 CARD)

A. PRESSURE OVERLOAD
1. BP ↑
2. AS
3. Coarctation

B. VOLUME OVERLOAD
1. AI
2. MInc
3. PDA
4. VSD

C. MYOCARDIAL DISEASE
1. MI or ischaemia
2. HOCM
3. Myocarditis
4. EMF
5. Idiopathic

D. RESTRICTION OF L VENTRICLE
1. Constrictive pericarditis
2. EMF

Right Ventricular Failure

Causes of RVF (LIST 2 CARD)
1. 2° to LVF
2. MSt
3. Cor pulmonale
4. ASD
5. VSD
6. PSt
7. Pulm BP $\uparrow$
8. TI
9. Amyloidosis
10. Atrial myxoma
11. EMF
12. Constrictive pericarditis

CLIN: Fatigue; Periph oedema; Abdo fullness. Occ Tender liver $\uparrow$; Abdo pain; N; Mild SOB; J; Ascites; Pleural effusion. JVP $\uparrow$; TI; R Vent heave; S3

INVESTIGATIONS: ● ECG: ˆRVHˆ
● CXR: Eg Ht $\uparrow$, Pleural effusion esp R side

RX: Rest, Diuretics $\pm$ K^+. If possible, treat 1° cause. Occ digitalise (not in cor pulmonale)

High Output States

States c̄ a high resting CO

Causes of High Output States (LIST 3 CARD)
A. PHYSIOLOGICAL
1. Anxiety
2. Pregnancy
3. Fever
B. PATHOLOGICAL
1. Anaemia
2. Thyrotoxicosis
3. A-V Fistula
4. Beri-beri
5. Exfoliative dermatitis
6. Carcinoid
7. PRV
8. Cirrhosis

SIGNS: PR $\uparrow$; Bounding pulse; Warm extremities; JVP $\uparrow$; S3; Systolic flow murmurs

TACHYCARDIAS

GENERAL CLIN: Palps. Occ Ht failure; Pain; Lightheadedness

GENERAL RX: Usually treat only if symptomatic

Supraventricular Tachycardias (SVT)

SINUS TACHYCARDIA

Causes of Sinus Tachycardia (LIST 4 CARD)
1. Exercise
2. Anxiety
3. Fever
4. Thyrotoxicosis
5. Acute severe haem
6. CCF
7. Vasodilator drugs: Eg Hydrallazine, Nifedipine
8. Acute MI
9. Severe anaemia
10. Constrictive pericarditis
11. A-V shunts

CLIN: 100–200/min. Gradual slowing on carotid sinus P

RX: Treat underlying condition

ATRIAL ECTOPICS

Usually unimportant. Appear in healthy & c̄ eg Excess caffeine, Cigs, Alcoholism, CCF, PE

ECG: Abnormal ˆPˆ wave. Rarely ˆQRSˆ widened

JUNCTIONAL ARRHYTHMIAS

CAUSES: Can be 2° to Surgery, MI, Dig toxicity, Myocarditis

ECG: Short ˆPRˆ interval or ˆPˆ wave during or after ˆQRSˆ

RX: If bradycardia, occ require pacing. If tachycardia, anti-arrhythmic drug eg Verapamil

PAROXYSMAL ATRIAL TACHYCARDIA

Usually an AV nodal re-entry tachycardia, occ due to a rapid, regularly discharging atrial ectopic focus. Several types eg WPW syndrome

CLIN: 160–260/min. Ppt by activity. Carotid sinus P → stepwise HtR ↓

ECG: a) Rapid rate ˆQRSˆ norm, 1:1 AV response
b) Rapid rate 2:1 AV response. Causes: MI, Digoxin o/d
c) Aberrent vent conduction c̄ 1:1 AV response. DD: VT

RX: Carotid sinus massage. IV Verapamil or Practolol (if previously on Dig or β blockers); If fails, digitalise. If life threatening, electroversion. Maintenance Rx of Digoxin $\pm$ β blocker or Verapamil, Disopyramide, Quinidine or Amiodarone

Special case:

i) WOLFF–PARKINSON–WHITE SYNDROME: A pre-excitation syndrome. Uncommon. Due to accessory AV connection (bundle of Kent) bypassing bundle of His

Clin: Paroxysms of palps. Occ Loud S1; No SVT

ECG: Short ˆPRˆ interval; ˆDeltaˆ wave in wide ˆQRSˆ; Inverted ˆTˆ waves in ˆIII, aVFˆ. Occ AF or Atrial flutter

Rx: Disopyramide or Amiodarone. Don't use Digoxin. Can op to remove or ablate bundle of Kent

ii) LOWN–GANONG–LEVINE SYNDROME: A pre-excitation syndrome. Short ˆPRˆ interval, SVT

ATRIAL FLUTTER

CAUSES: 1. Rh Ht disease
2. IHD
3. CHD esp ASD
4. Thyrotoxicosis
5. Idiopathic
6. Cor pulmonale

Atrial ectopic focus or circular pathway. 260–340/min c̄ often 2:1 conduction slowing on carotid sinus P to eg 4:1

ECG: Saw tooth waves; Varying AV conduction. Occ BBB

RX: Treat underlying cause. Digoxin. Electroversion

ATRIAL FIBRILLATION

Causes of AF (LIST 5 CARD)

1. Rh Ht disease esp MSt
2. Thyrotoxicosis
3. IHD
4. ASD
5. Idiopathic (Lone)
6. Constrictive pericarditis
7. Cardiomyopathy
8. Rarely:
   a) Atrial myxoma
   b) Chest surgery
   c) SABE
   d) Ca lung
   e) Electrocution
   f) Acute viral infection

Multiple atrial ectopic foci. Rate >360/min. May be sustained or paroxysmal

CLIN: Palps. Occ systemic emboli

ECG: Fibrillation waves; ˆQRSˆ norm; Irregular ˆR-Rˆ intervals

RX: Treat underlying cause. Digoxin $\pm$ β blocker or Verapamil. Occ Electroversion. Maintenance Rx Digoxin. Occ Electroversion followed by Quinidine or Disopyramide. Anticoags if AF due to mitral valve disease or thyrotoxicosis

SICK SINUS SYNDROME

A node disorder. Often → Tachycardia–Bradycardia syndrome

CLIN: Palps then syncope or lightheadedness. Marked sensitivity to drugs eg Digoxin & β blockers → marked bradycardia. Risk of arterial embolism

RX: Permanent pacemaker. Antiarrhythmic eg Disopyramide or Amiodarone. Prophylactic anticoags may benefit

Ventricular Tachycardias

VENTRICULAR ECTOPICS

May occur in normal. Frequent or multifocal VEs may be ass c̄ organic Ht disease. Coupled VEs often due to Dig toxicity

ECG: Wide abnormally shaped ˆQRSˆ

RX: Treat if Symptomatic; Multiple; Multifocal; ˆR on Tˆ. Use Quinidine or Lignocaine. If Dig toxicity discontinue drug. Occ maintenance antiarrhythmic Rx eg β blocker

ACCELERATED IDIOVENTRICULAR RHYTHM

Usually 2° to MI. Abnormality in Purkinje fibres

CLIN: Usually well tolerated. Occ Ht failure. Rate 60–120/min

ECG: Paroxysms of broad ˆQRSˆ complexes alternating c̄ norm

RX: Occ Atropine or atrial pacing needed

VENTRICULAR TACHYCARDIA (VT)

Can complicate any form of Ht disease esp IHD. Paroxysmal VT may be due to Dig toxicity, $K^+ \downarrow$, Thyrotoxicosis. May → VF

CLIN: Rate 120–240/min. Rhythm may be regular or sl irregular. Occ LOC; BP ↓; Ht failure

ECG: Fusion & capture beats are pathognomic. Dissociated ˆPˆ waves. ˆQRSˆ widened to >0.14msecs. Rarely ˆRBBBˆ

DIFFERENCES BETWEEN VT & SVT:

1. SVT more regular rhythm, dissociated ˆPˆ waves in VT
2. ˆQRSˆ width > in VT
3. All ˆVˆ leads similar in VT
4. Large ˆR'ˆ in ˆV1ˆ common in SVT
5. No ˆQˆ wave & large ˆSˆ wave in ˆV6ˆ in VT
6. ˆRBBBˆ commoner in SVT
7. Fusion & capture beats only in VT

Rx: If emergency, electroversion. Otherwise Lignocaine IV. If fails, IV Mexiletine or Disopyramide. If stable after 3 days IV therapy start oral Mexiletine or Disopyramide (often not required for VT seen in acute phase of MI). If recurrent episodes use drugs long term eg Mexiletene, Disopyramide, β blocker

Special case:

TORSADE DE POINTES: Usually SE of anti-arrhythmic drugs. Often due to $K^+ \downarrow$, Mg ↓, Bradycardia

ECG:VT c̄ changing polarity. Paroxysms of late premature beats on a long ˆQ-Tˆ interval

VENTRICULAR FIBRILLATION

Irregular depolarisation of ventricles → inco-ordinated contractions. Usually fatal. Usually due to MI but occ seen in AS, complete Ht block, Dig or Quinidine toxicity, hypothermia, or electrocution. Ppt by VT & VEs ˆR on Tˆ beats

RX: Ext cardiac massage, ventilate, defibrillate, IV Lignocaine. Treat acidosis if prolonged resus. Then Mexiletine & Disopyramide

BRADYCARDIA

Bradycardia is a HtR <60/min

Sinus Bradycardia

SA node discharges <60/min. Esp elderly

Sinus Arrest

Failure of SA node to depolarise. Can only be deduced by absent ˆPˆ wave of atrial depolarisation. Period of cardiac standstill ended by an escape beat

Causes of Sinus Bradycardia (LIST 6 CARD)

1. Sleep
2. Athletes
3. Cong
4. Post viral infections
5. Drugs:
   Esp β blockers, Dig
6. Early MI esp inf
7. Hypothyroidism
8. ↑ ICP
9. Rapid rise in BP
10. Obst J
11. Hypopituitarism

Sino–Atrial Block

Disturbance of SA node conduction to atrial muscle. Can be inferred when the block is intermittent & the duration of atrial pause is a multiple of preceding ˆP-Pˆ intervals. Occ abolished by exercise or Atropine. Very difficult to distinguish from sinus arrest

AV Block Above Division of Bundle of His

Often at level of AV node

1st DEGREE BLOCK

ˆPRˆ interval ↑ >0.2secs. An ECG diagnosis. Soft S1

2nd DEGREE BLOCK

Some ˆPˆ waves fail to conduct to ventricles

MOBITZ TYPE I: Wenkebach phenomenon of ˆPRˆ interval gradually ↑ until ˆQRSˆ complex dropped, & cycle starts again c̄ ˆPˆ wave after pause. May be idiopathic or due to ischaemia or Dig toxicity

Rx: IV Atropine occ helps

MOBITZ TYPE II: A fixed ˆPRˆ interval c̄ periodic failure of conduction eg 2:1 or 3:1 block. Often → complete Ht block

Rx: Pacing

3rd DEGREE BLOCK (COMPLETE BLOCK)

No relationship between atrial & vent complexes. Usually Vent rate <50/min. → CO ↓

CLIN: Lassitude; Fatigue; Dizziness esp in exercise; CCF; Awareness of Ht beat if intermittent slow palps; Stokes–Adams attacks (Transient sudden LOC due to ↓ cerebral blood flow) occ → convulsions, incontinence & pallor. Occ cardiac arrest or VF. Slow pulse c̄ ↑ pulse pressure; Cannon waves; Variable intensity of S1. Occ Systolic ejection murmur

ECG: Normal ˆPˆ waves; Variable ˆPRˆ intervals; Slow rate of norm ˆQRSˆ complexes

RX: Atropine for early MI. Usually need pacing. Occ in emergency, IV Isoprenaline

AV Block at Level of Bundle Branches

Damage likelihood RBBB >L AntBBB >L PostBBB. Complete Ht block often follows RBBB c̄ ˆL axis deviationˆ or complete LBBB

LBBB

Ant & Post fascicles. If both blocked = LBBB

Causes of LBBB (LIST 8 CARD)

1. IHD
2. Aortic valve disease
3. LVH:
   Eg Hypertension
4. Cardiomyopathy
5. Myocarditis

ECG: ˆQRSˆ >0.12secs; No ˆRˆ wave in ˆV1ˆ; ˆQˆ waves in ˆV4–6ˆ; ˆTˆ wave usually inverted in ˆV5–6ˆ

L AntBBB (L Ant HEMIBLOCK)

ECG: ˆL axis deviationˆ ie ˆQRSˆ +ve ˆIˆ; –ve ˆIIˆ

DD: Necrosis of inf wall LVent

L PostBBB (L Post HEMIBLOCK)

Causes of Complete Ht Block (LIST 7 CARD)

A. ACUTE
1. Early MI
2. Rh fever
3. Diphtheria
4. Viral & Rickettsial endocarditis
5. Drugs:
   Eg Digoxin, Quinidine, K^+ ↑
6. Cardiac surgery
7. SABE

B. CHRONIC
1. Idiopathic
2. IHD
3. Calcific AS
4. Cong
5. Cardiomyopathy
6. Sarcoid
7. Amyloidosis
8. Sy
9. Collagen vascular disease:
   Eg Ank Sp

ECG: ˆR axis deviationˆ ie ˆQRSˆ –ve ˆIˆ; +ve ˆIIIˆ

DD: 1. RVH
2. Lat wall MI

RBBB

Causes of RBBB (LIST 9 CARD)

1. Benign congenital
2. Pulm BP ↑
3. PE
4. ASD esp ostium secundum
5. IHD
6. Myocarditis
7. Surgery

ECG: ˆQRSˆ >0.12secs; ˆSˆ wave in lead ˆIˆ; ˆRSR'ˆ wave in ˆV1ˆ; ˆTˆ wave inverted in ˆV1ˆ (may occur in norm)

Pacemakers

Various types: Fixed rate; "on demand"; Dual chamber & "synchronous" pacemakers; Programmable

Indications for Pacing (LIST 10 CARD)

A. TEMPORARY
1. Acute MI c complete or bifascicular block
2. Drug eg Dig o/d
3. Tachyarrhythmias resistant to drugs

B. PERMANENT
1. Symptomatic complete Ht block: Eg Stokes–Adams attacks
2. Sick Sinus syndrome: Esp Bradycardia–Tachycardia syndrome
3. Symptomatic 2nd degree AV block
4. Symptomatic bradycardias resistant to drugs

CARDIOACTIVE DRUGS

Digitalis

EFFECTS: 1. Rate & degree of systolic emptying ↑ & venous P ↓
2. Sinus rate ↓
3. AV conduction prolonged, ventricle slowed in AF
4. In large doses, automaticity of subsidiary pacemakers ↑ → dysrhythmias

INDICATIONS FOR USE: AF; Atrial Flutter. Occ Atrial Ectopics; SVT

THERAPEUTIC LEVEL: Approx 0.5–2.5 ng/ml. Digitalising dose of 0.5mg followed at 6hrly intervals c̄ 0.25mg to a total dose of 2–3mg. Maintain on approx 0.25–0.5mg daily. Reduced dose needed in RF, old, children, small. Sensitivity ↑ if: K^+ ↓; Mg^{2+} ↓; Hypothyroid; Hypoxia. Also toxicity in interactions c̄ Verapamil, Quinidine, Amiodarone

CLIN OF TOXICITY: Fatigue; Weakness; N&V. Occ Pulsus bigeminus; Agitation. Rarely Vision ↓

ECG OF TOXICITY: AV or SA node block; Coupled VEs; VT; VF; SVT c̄ 2:1 AV block; Sagging ˆR-Tˆ depression

RX OF TOXICITY: Withdraw drug. Correct any K^+ ↓. If serious arrhythmias, Lignocaine, Phenytoin may benefit. Avoid β blocker as may → Ht failure. Dig Ab may benefit. Occ require pacing

β blockers

ACTION: Sympathetic blockade. β1 blockade → ↓ PR; ↓ CO; ↓ AV node conduction. β2 blockade → ↑ PVR; Bronchoconstriction. β blockade particularly slows HtR during exercise. Some β blockers are relatively cardioselective ie predominantly β1 action

INDICATIONS: 1. BP ↑
2. Angina
3. Following MI
4. Paroxysmal SVT
5. AF (c̄ Dig)
6. Thyrotoxicosis
7. Sinus tachycardia
8. Anxiety

9. HOCM
10. Exercise induced arrhythmias inc VT

TOXICITY: 1. Bradycardia
2. BP ↓
3. Malaise
4. CCF
5. Bronchoconstriction
6. Rarely Rashes; Myalgia; GI upsets

SE: Nightmares; Insomnia; Depression; Raynaud's

Electroversion

INDICATIONS: VT; VF; Atrial flutter; Paroxysmal SVT due to Dig; Life threatening AF; Any symptomatic sustained tachyarrhythmia unresponsive to simple drug Rx
Anticoag cover for mitral valve disease or if h/o emboli

IHD

Most important cause of death in men esp in UK & Scandinavia. M>F esp in middle age. Scotland >England. Rates falling in some countries eg USA

Risk Factors for IHD (LIST 11 CARD)

A. MAJOR
1. M sex
2. Increasing age
3. Cigs
4. BP ↑
5. Familial hyper-cholesterolaemia
6. FH of early IHD

B. MINOR
1. Diet
2. Obesity
3. Diabetes mellitus
4. Physical inactivity
5. Early F menopause
6. Soft water
7. Familial factors
8. Low social class
9. Personality type A
10. Hyperuricaemia
11. Low HDL
12. CS
13. Nephrotic syndrome
14. Hypothyroidism

PATHOGENESIS: Most cases are due to atherosclerosis, a focal deposition of lipids in the arterial intima. Atheroma is due to haemodynamic factors such as BP ↑, turbulence due to Ht mvt & lipometabolic factors. A high saturated fat diet is ass c̄ ↑ IHD. HDL seems to be cardioprotective & is raised by alcohol, exercise & pregnancy. Although there are many risk factors they do not fully account for the occurence of IHD ie many die without known risk factors. The greater the number & severity of risk factors the greater the risk of IHD

1° PREVENTION: Stop smoking. Some evidence that a low fat diet (predominantly unsaturated); Exercise; Mild alcohol intake; Control of BP, are beneficial. Most trials have sought to reduce a range of risk factors simultaneously

Angina

M>F. Incidence increases c̄ age
Ppt by ↑ O_2 demand esp if: HtR ↑; LVent wall tension ↑ (seen if BP ↑ Vent radius ↑). O_2 supply to Ht depends on coronary blood flow & relies on resistance of coronary arterioles, HtR, diameter of coronary vessels, difference between diastolic BP & Vent end diastolic P, O_2 sat, Hb level & 2,3 DPG level in coronary blood. Usually due to atheroma but rarely due to emboli, arteritis, fibromuscular hyperplasia. Angina due to Vent ↑ is seen in AS, HOCM & BP ↑

CLIN: Pain on exertion or due to emotion, relieved by rest. In stable angina the amount of effort to produce pain is reasonably constant, but is ↓ in the cold, c̄ emotional stress & 1–2hrs post prandial. Pain esp retrosternal but may occur in arm, throat, jaw, upper abdo. Occ SOB; Sweating; S3. Pain normally resolves in <10mins at rest, GTN usually provides more rapid relief. Rarely evidence of hyperlipidaemia

INVESTIGATIONS: • ECG ± Exercise ECG:

Norm or occ ^ST^ depression; Flat ^T^ waves

- CXR: Usually norm
- Isotope cardiac imaging
- Coronary angiography

RX: Control BP, stop cigs, diet if obese. GTN inc prophylactic use (SE: Headache, Flushing). Nifedipine ± β blockers. Occ use long acting nitrites. Consider intervention by angioplasty or CABG if intractable pain, young c̄ significant symptoms, L main coronary artery or triple artery disease

PROG: Annual mort approx 4%. ↑ risk of MI & vent arrhythmias

Unstable Angina

A sub gp of angina sufferers c̄ a worse prog. Inc those c̄ angina increasing in frequency or severity, angina at rest >15mins or recurrent angina in early post MI period. Angina decubitus ie pain on lying flat relieved by sitting up, is ass c̄ 3 vessel disease

INVESTIGATION: • ECG: May show ^ST^ elevation at time of pain

RX: Bed rest, β blockers, Nifedipine. Monitor in CCU. Exclude MI. Occ Aspirin. Many respond to medical Rx but some require urgent angiography & CABG. When stabilised proceed to angiography. Occ CABG esp if 3 vessel disease

Myocardial Infarction

Death of Ht muscle due to interruption of blood supply usually due to atherosclerosis. M>F. Esp middle aged & elderly

CLIN: Crushing chest pain usually radiating to L arm ass c̄ sweating, distress, pallor, SOB, anxiety & lasting >20mins. Occ Shock; N&V. May be "silent" esp diabetics, elderly. Occ BP ↑ or ↓; PR ↑ or ↓; S3 or S4; Functional MInc; Pericardial rub &/or pain; Fever after 24hrs; LVF. Many die within 1hr of onset of symptoms

INVESTIGATIONS: • Sequential ECGs: Picture depends on site & time after infarct. ECG initially norm then after few hrs ^ST^ elevation followed by ^Q^ waves & then ^T^ wave inversion c̄ gradual lessening of ^ST^ segment elevation. ^Q^ waves usually persist. In Anteroseptal MI changes in ^I, aVL, V1–3^ c̄ "reciprocal" depressed ^ST^ in ^II, III, aVF^. In Anterolateral MI changes in ^I, aVL, V5–6^ & "reciprocal" changes in ^II, III, aVF^. In Inf MI changes in ^II, III, aVF^ "reciprocal" changes in ^I, aVL, V1–3^. In true post MI large ^R^ in ^V1–2^ c̄ an upright ^T^ in ^V1^

- Sequential cardiac enzymes: CPK-MB max at 24hrs; CPK max at 48hrs; AST max at 48hrs; LDH starts at 48hrs max at 72hrs, elevated up to 9 days
- CXR
- U&E
- Occ Isotope imaging
- Fasting lipid levels

GENERAL RX: Early Rx is beneficial. Admit to CCU if early MI or complications. Bed rest, Diamorphine, O_2. Stop cigs, reduce wt. Occ Anticoags esp transmural MI. Standard Rx for LVF. β blockers within 4hrs of onset appear to reduce size of MI. Leg exercises. Mobilise from 2–3 days in uncomplicated MI

Rehabilitation & 2° prevention: Reassurance. Stop cigs. Regular exercise, ↓ alcohol & ↓ sat fat intake probably beneficial. Control BP. β blockers started 1–6wks post MI → ↓ reinfarction & mort. Long term anticoags may be beneficial. Monitor c̄ post-infarct exercise ECG. Occ CABG esp for 3 vessel disease, L main artery disease, poor angina control

EARLY COMPLICATIONS & THEIR RX

ARRHYTHMIAS:

1. **Sinus Bradycardia:** Common esp early MI & inf or post MI
   Rx: Atropine. Occ Isoprenaline, Pacing
2. **SVT:** Uncommon
   Rx: Carotid sinus massage. Verapamil or β blocker. Occ Digoxin, Electroversion
3. **Paroxysmal SVT & Block:**
   Rx: Stop Dig, Correct K^+, IV Verapamil. Occ β blocker
4. **Atrial Flutter:**
   Rx: β blocker, Digoxin. Occ electroversion
5. **AF:** Quite common esp elderly & those in LVF

Rx: Digoxin $\pm$ β blocker. Occ electroversion

6. **VEs:** Very common. Require Rx if symptomatic
   Rx: IV Lignocaine. If VEs persist continue c̄ Mexiletine. Correct any $K^+ \downarrow$
7. **VT:**
   Rx: Electroversion or Lignocaine. Require long term Rx if recurrent episodes after 1st day
8. **Accelerated Idioventricular Rhythm:** Usually ass c̄ bradycardia
   Rx: Atropine
9. **VF:** Usual cause of sudden death
   Rx: Immediate electroversion then 24–36hrs of Lignocaine
10. **1st Degree AV Block:** Ass c̄ inf MI
11. **2nd, 3rd Degree AV block Ass c̄ Inf MI:**
    Rx: Occ Atropine or pacing
12. **2nd or 3rd Degree AV Block Ass c̄ Ant MI:**
    Rx: Prompt pacing
13. **BBB c̄ Hemiblocks:**
    Rx: Occ pacing
14. **Sinus Arrest:**
    Rx: Usually unsuccessful. Try electroversion &/or intracardiac Adrenaline, Pace

CARDIAC FAILURE: Common
Rx: Diuretics, O_2, Digoxin. Rarely require Dopamine

HYPOTENSION: Common
Rx: Observe. Look for signs of shock. Bed rest

CARDIOGENIC SHOCK: Defined as systolic BP <90mmHg, Oliguria, Metabolic acidosis, & Poor tissue perfusion
Clin: BP →; Oliguria; Cold clammy skin; Confusion; Pallor
Rx: Treat aggressively. Dopamine & vasodilator to reduce afterload & preload, diuretics, O_2. Occ intra-aortic balloon pump, HCO_3

PAPILLARY MUSCLE RUPTURE: Uncommon. Transient acute MInc due to papillary muscle dysfunction is commoner
Clin: Sudden SOB; Acute LVF; BP ↓; Loud apical pansystolic murmur
Rx: Diuretics & afterload reduction. Confirm diagnosis by catheterisation & then surgery
DD: VSD

HYPERTENSION: Usually controlled by adequate analgesia. Occ require β blockers

PERICARDITIS: Quite common
Clin: Chest pain made worse by lying flat & inspiration. Pericardial rub. Usually settles in 1–2 days
Rx: Aspirin. Occ Hydrocortisone

CARDIAC RUPTURE: Uncommon. Rupture of LVent wall → haemopericardium & circulatory arrest. Rupture of septum → VSD c̄ BP ↓, CCF
Rx: Vent wall rupture seldom operable. Repair of VSD is best early
Prog: Poor c̄ LVent wall rupture

RECURRENT CHEST PAINS: Occ due to subendocardial infarct
Rx: β blockers, Nifedipine, Nitrates

LATE COMPLICATIONS & THEIR RX

PULMONARY EMBOLISM:
Clin: Sudden SOB, Ht failure esp R; Syncope; Pleurisy; Haemoptysis
Rx: Anticoags

VENTRICULAR ANEURYSM: May occur c̄ ant or inf MI. Takes months to develop
Clin: May be asymptomatic. Paradoxical mvt of ventricle. Often S3, S4. Ass c̄ CO ↓; Ht failure; Mural thromb c̄ systemic emboli; Recurrent VT
Investigations:
- ECG: Persistent ˆSTˆ elevation esp in ˆVˆ leads
- CXR: Occ Bulging L cardiac border $\pm$ Ca^{2+}, paradoxical mvt
- Echocardiography
- Isotope ventriculography

Rx: Aneurysmectomy $\pm$ CABG

DRESSLER'S SYNDROME: An acute recurrence of pericarditis esp 1–6/52 post MI
Clin: Fever; Pericardial pain; Pleurisy; Pericardial rub
Investigations:
- CXR
- ECG
- ESR ↑
- Echocardiography

Rx: Aspirin, Steroids

PSYCHOLOGICAL SEQUELAE: Neurotic fear of repeat MI can prevent return to appropriate lifestyle. Occ non-organic chest pain symptoms

FROZEN SHOULDER/SHOULDER–HAND SYNDROME:
Rx: Physio

MURAL THROMBI & SYSTEMIC EMBOLI:
Rx: Anticoags

PROGNOSIS

POOR PROGNOSTIC FACTORS:
A. Early: 1. Persistent CCF

2. BP ↓
3. Persistent PR >100
4. Ht ↑
5. Transient AF
6. Late Vent arrhythmias
7. 2nd, 3rd degree block c̄ ant MI
8. New BBB
9. Cardiogenic shock
10. Old age
11. Cardiac rupture
12. Previous MI
13. Ant MI

B. Late:
1. CCF
2. Angina
3. Aneurysm
4. Diabetes Mellitus
5. Ht ↑
6. Thrombi or emboli
7. ST ↓ on exercise ECG

DD of MI & Angina (LIST 12 CARD)

1. Unstable angina
2. Aortic dissection
3. Acute pericarditis
4. Acute oesophagitis
5. Pulmonary embolism
6. Costo–chondritis
7. Cv root lesion
8. Acute cholecystitis
9. Acute pancreatitis
10. PU

Cardiac Arrest

Usually due to asystole or VF

CLIN: LOC; Apnoea; Absent pulses; Pupils dilate after approx 45secs

RX: Ext cardiac massage; Artificial ventilation; Electroversion esp if VF; $NaHCO_3$; Adrenaline & $CaCl_2$ esp if asystole. Monitor c̄ ECG. Later may require anti-arrhythmic drugs

COMPLICATIONS: 1. RF
2. Cerebral damage
3. Resp failure

PROG: Poor esp if asystole or late Rx

MYOCARDITIS

Causes of Acute Myocarditis (LIST 13 CARD)

1. Infections:
   a) Viral eg Coxsackie B, Echo virus, Flu, Chickenpox
   b) Bacterial eg Diphtheria, Clostridium, Staph
   c) Parasitic eg Chagas' disease, Toxoplasmosis
   d) Rickettsial
2. Acute Rh fever
3. Connective tissue disorders
4. Serum sickness
5. Drugs:
   Eg Cyclophosphamide, Daunorubicin
6. Idiopathic (Fiedler's)

Viral Myocarditis

CLIN: Sinus tachycardia disproportionate to systemic illness. Occ Gallop; CCF; Conduction defects; Circulatory collapse; Muscle pain; Pericarditis; Ht ↑

INVESTIGATIONS:
- ECG
- CXR
- Echocardiography
- Viral studies
- Rarely Cardiac biopsy

RX: Bed rest. Standard Rx for Ht failure & any arrhythmias

PROG: Usually good

Diphtheria

CLIN: Sore throat; Bradycardia & CCF. Occ Shock. Early diastolic gallop. Occ late

Stokes–Adams attacks

INVESTIGATION: • ECG: VEs & Ht block common

RX: Antitoxin, antibiotics. Occ pacing

Chagas' Disease

Due to *Trypanosoma cruzi*. Esp Central & S.Am. Many animal reservoirs. Often spread by bite of Triatomid bugs. Occurs in young

CLIN: In acute phase PR ↑; Ht ↑; CCF. Recovery in few mths. Then 10–20yrs later chr, phase c̄ gradual onset of CCF; Ht ↑ & dysrhythmias

INVESTIGATION: • CFT

RX: No effective Rx known

CARDIOMYOPATHIES

Disorder of Ht muscle of unknown cause

3 Types: Congestive (COCM); Hypertrophic (HOCM); Obliterative or Restrictive eg EMF

COCM

Rare. Ass c̄ alcohol & the puerperium. Occ ass c̄ IHD

PATH: Grossly dilated flabby Ht. Some hypertrophy. Poor systolic contractility. High end diastolic P. Low CO, no angina

CLIN: Gradually progressive SOB & Ht failure. Occ Cough; Chest pain. PR ↑; Triple rhythm. Occ MInc; AF

INVESTIGATIONS:
- ECG: Non specific ˆSTˆ changes
- CXR
- Echocardiography
- Angiography

RX: Vasodilators eg Enalapril, Dig & diuretics. Standard Rx for tachyarrhythmias. Anticoags to prevent emboli. Occ surgery for severe MInc. Consider Ht transplant esp in young

HOCM

Marked Vent hypertrophy ± LVent outflow obst. Usually Aut Dom. Can present in young adults

PATH: LVH >RVH esp septum, abnormal muscle architecture. ↑ Vent stiffness → distension ↓. LVent end diastolic P ↑. Often outflow obst & MInc

CLIN: SOB; Syncope; Angina; Palps. Jerky pulse (Pulsus bisferiens). Double apical impulse. Occ S3 or S4, MInc murmur, loud S2. Occ Sudden death

INVESTIGATIONS:
- ECG: LVH, ˆLBBBˆ, ˆQˆ waves, ˆPRˆ interval ↓ (mimics WPW syndrome)
- CXR
- Echocardiography
- "Slit" like cavity on angiocardiography

RX: β blockers or Verapamil. Occ Anticoags; Electroversion; Permanent pacing from RVent. Surgery esp if severe MInc, failure of medical Rx

COMPLICATIONS: 1. AF & systemic emboli 2. VT

Obliterative Cardiomyopathy

EMF

Esp equatorial Africa

PATH: Obliteration of inflow tracts by fibrosis esp Body of L or RVent, post cusp tricuspid & mitral valve

CLIN: RVent involvement → TI, Liver ↑, Ascites. LVent involvement → MInc, emboli. Occ Pericardial effusion; AF

INVESTIGATIONS:
- CXR: Ca^{2+} occ
- ECG
- Cardiac catheterisation: "Dip & Plateau" Vent P pulse

RX: Treat CCF. Surgery

ENDOCARDIAL FIBROELASTOSIS (EFE)

Esp Infants, genetic. May be 2° to coarctation, PDA, aortic atresia

CLIN: Massive Ht ↑. SOB; Resp distress; CCF. Occ Cough; Cyanosis; Gallop rhythm. Usually no murmurs but occ mitral or aortic valve disease. Usually fatal in wks–mths

RX: Rapid digitalisation

EOSINOPHILIC ENDOMYOCARDIAL DISEASE (LOEFFLER'S)

LVent obstructed by eosinophilic mass → LVF & RVF, systemic emboli

RX: Surgery

SPECIFIC CARDIAC MUSCLE DISEASES

Systemic Sclerosis

CLIN: Ht block; Fibrosis → Ht failure

SLE

CLIN: BP ↑; Pericarditis; AI

Amyloidosis

CLIN: Restrictive lesion mimics constrictive pericarditis

Sarcoidosis

CLIN: Ht block. Occ Arrhythmias; Aneurysm

Post Transfusion Haemosiderosis

Complication of multiple transfusion therapy

Haemochromatosis

CLIN: Ht block; CCF, Dysrhythmias

Acromegaly

Cardiomegaly

Friedrich's Ataxia

CLIN: Symmetrical hypertrophy → CCF. Occ Ht block

Duchenne Muscular Dystrophy

CLIN: CCF

ECG: Tall R precordial ˆRˆ waves

Dystrophia Myotonica

CLIN: Ht block, arrhythmias, conduction defects

RX: Pacing

Marfan's Syndrome

CLIN: Occ AI; Aneurysm; Floppy mitral valve; ASD; Conduction defects; Dissecting aneurysm

Pompe's Disease

CLIN: LVH → CCF. Occurs in infants

Hurler's Syndrome

CLIN: Ht ↑; Pericardial effusions; Valvular disease esp MSt; CCF

Morquio–Ullrich Syndrome

CLIN: AI

Beri-beri

CLIN: High CO → CCF, MInc

Carcinoid Syndrome

CLIN: R Ht disease esp TI, TSt, PSt → CCF

Cytotoxic Drugs

Daunorubicin & Doxorubicin can → CCF, dilatation

PERICARDITIS

Causes of Pericarditis (LIST 14 CARD)

1. Acute idiopathic
2. Infections:
   a) Viral
   b) Bacterial eg TB
   c) Fungal
3. MI:
   a) Acute
   b) Dressler's syndrome
4. Malignancy
5. Uraemia
6. Trauma
7. Collagen vascular disease: Eg SLE, Rh Arth
8. Rh fever
9. Post cardiotomy syndrome
10. Hypothyroidism
11. X-Rad
12. Drugs: Eg Hydrallazine, Methysergide, Procainamide
13. Serum sickness
14. Chylopericardium
15. Acute dissection of aorta
16. Hurler's syndrome
17. EMF
18. Reiter's disease

3 path types: Acute fibrinous Pericarditis; Pericarditis c̄ effusion; Constrictive Pericarditis

Acute Fibrinous Pericarditis

CLIN: Sharp chest pain radiating from sternum to L shoulder ppt by coughing, swallowing, inspiration, supine posture. Occ Cough; AF. Friction rub ie a high pitched systolic & early diastolic noise

INVESTIGATIONS:
- ECG: Concave upwards ^ST^ elevation max in ^II^. No reciprocal changes or ^Q^ waves. In subacute phase ^T^ wave inversion
- CXR: Usually norm

DD: Acute MI

Pericarditis c̄ Effusion

Can → cardiac tamponade

CARDIAC TAMPONADE

Impairment of Vent filling due to ↑ intrapericardial P. Can → cardiac arrest

CLIN: Early SOB; Faintness; JVP ↑; N; Pulses paradoxus. Occ Rub; R upper abdo pain or discomfort

INVESTIGATIONS:
- CXR: Globular Ht shadow
- ECG: Low voltage. ^T^ wave changes
- Echocardiography

RX: Pericardial aspiration c̄ ECG monitoring. If recurrence, surgery

Constrictive Pericarditis

A restriction of Vent filling → Venous P ↑ esp on insp, ascites, oedema

SUB-ACUTE FORM

CAUSES: TB; *Coxsackie B*; Staph; Glandular fever; Ca; Traumatic haemopericardium; RF

CLIN: SOB; Pulm oedema; Periph oedema. Ht ↑ then ↓

CHRONIC FORM

Rare. Causes: TB; Viral infections; Ca; Trauma; X-Rad; Rh Arth

CLIN: Sl SOB; Wt ↓; Ascites c̄ little periph oedema; Fatigue; JVP ↑ (Occ ↑ on insp ie Kussmaul's sign); Liver ↑. Occ Mild J; AF; Pulsus paradoxus; Loud early S3; Absent cardiac impulse; Fixed split S2. No Ht murmurs

INVESTIGATIONS:
- CXR: Norm or sl ↑ Ht. Straight L border. Clear lungs. SVC dilated. Occ pericardial Ca^{2+}
- ECG: Low voltage. ^T^ wave inversion. Occ AF
- Echocardiography
- Catheterisation

RX: Pericardiectomy

Specific Causes of Pericarditis

ACUTE IDIOPATHIC PERICARDITIS

Common. Esp young adults. Often h/o URTI

CLIN: Sl fever; Effusion. Occ myocarditis

RX: Aspirin, Prednisolone

POST-CARDIOTOMY SYNDROME

CLIN: 2–4wks after cardiac surgery or trauma develop acute fever c̄ pericarditis & pleurisy. Lasts 1–3/52. May recur

RX: Occ steroids

MALIGNANT PERICARDITIS

Esp Ca lung, Ca breast. Occ Hodgkin's disease

CLIN: Cardiac tamponade

INVESTIGATION: • Bloody aspirate c̄ protein ↑

RX: Triethylene thiophosphoramide injected into pericardium

TB PERICARDITIS

Esp underdeveloped countries

CLIN: Insidious onset, Effusion >dry form. Occ tamponade

INVESTIGATION: • CXR: Occ Ca^{2+} esp in AV fissure & near apex

RX: Anti-TB therapy. Occ pericardiectomy

POLYSEROSITIS

Rare. Affects pleura, peritoneum & synovial jts

CLIN: Constrictive pericarditis. Budd–Chiari syndrome. Occ intestinal obst

HYPERTENSION

WHO definition systolic BP >140mmHg, diastolic >90mmHg

Causes of Hypertension (LIST 15 CARD)

1. Essential primary hypertension
2. Renal: a) Renal artery stenosis
   b) CRF
   c) Acute nephritis
   d) Polycystic disease
   e) Pyelonephritis
   f) Glomerulonephritis
   g) Hydronephrosis
   h) Renin secreting tumours
   i) Diabetes
   j) SLE
   k) X-Rad
   l) Neuroblastoma
3. Endocrine: a) Cushing's syndrome
   b) Conn's syndrome
   c) Acromegaly
   d) Phaeochromocytoma
   e) Adrenal Ca
   f) Hyperparathyroidism
4. Coarctation of Aorta
5. Polycythaemia
6. Hypertensive disease of pregnancy
7. Acute porphyria
8. A-V aneurysm
9. Drugs: Eg Steroids, The "Pill"
10. Neurogenic lesions: Eg Lesions of mid-brain & brain stem
11. ↑ ICP

95% of cases are essential (primary). 1° cases are ass c̄ obesity, excess dietary salt, low K^+ diet, alcohol. Esp Blacks. Familial predisposition. Incidence increases c̄ age. Common & therefore most important risk factor for MI, CVA, Ht failure, RF & PVD. Hypertensives at all ages have a reduced life expectancy. Renal causes account for about 4% of cases

PATH: Imbalance of Renin–Angiotensin system → Aldosterone ↑ & salt & water retention, vasoconstriction → BP ↑

CLIN: Usually no symptoms. BP ↑. Occ S4, LVH, Fundal changes. May → Ht failure; RF; CVA; Eye sight ↓. Malignant accelerated form is particularly likely to → complications inc papilloedema & encephalopathy

INVESTIGATIONS: • Sphygmomanometry: Single estimation quite good predictor. Usually repeat on 3 occasions before deciding on Rx
- CXR: Ht ↑
- Fundoscopy: Haem, exudates, arterial changes. Papilloedema indicates malignant BP ↑
- FBC
- U&E: Urea ↑↑ often indicates Renal artery stenosis
- Creatinine
- ECG: ˆL axis deviationˆ, ˆLVHˆ, ˆSTˆ depression &/or ˆTˆ inversion in ˆV5–6ˆ (strain pattern)
- Urinalysis

- Uric acid: Occ ↑
- Rarely Ultrasound, IVU, Isotope renal arteriogram

RX: Most Rx is instituted to prevent complications. Compliance is related to the simplicity of a regime & lack of SE. Goal is to reduce diastolic BP to <95mmHg. Non drug therapy ie Wt loss if obese, low salt diet, may be indicated in mild BP ↑. Initial Rx is usually c̄ a β blocker &/or a Thiazide (SE: K^+ ↓, Gout). If this is insuf a periph vasodilator eg Nifedipine or Prazosin (SE: Postural BP ↓) can be added. Rarely Frusemide (SE: Hirsutism) is used in place of a Thiazide. In pregnancy, Methyldopa (SE: Impotence, AIHA), Labetalol or Atenolol are usually used. In Ht failure, periph vasodilators are often used β blockers (SE: Periph vascoconstriction) are not recommended in PVD & may mask hypoglycaemic symptoms in diabetics. Enalapril, an angiotensin converting inhibitor, is useful in renal BP ↑ combined c̄ a diuretic
Rx of Hypertensive emergencies eg encephalopathy: Can use Nitroprusside infusion, Labetolol infusion, Diazoxide (SE: Diabetes, rapid BP fall), Hydrallazine or Methyldopa. Too rapid a fall in BP can → MI, CVA or blindness

PROG: Successful Rx of moderate or severe BP ↑ undoubtedly increases life expectancy. Approx risks c̄ BP ↑: CCF ×5; CVA ×100; MI ×2; PVD ×2

PERIPHERAL ARTERIAL DISEASE

Arteriosclerosis

Due to atheroma. Ass c̄ BP ↑; Diabetes; Cigs & Hyperlipidaemias. Common sites are at vessel bifurcations, aorta, medium sized arteries esp supf femoral artery, int carotid artery

CLIN OF LOWER LIMB DISEASE: IC; Absent pulses. Later Rest pain; Ulcers; Gangrene. Femoro–popliteal block → calf IC; Iliac occlusion → thigh IC; Aortic bifurcation occlusion → bilat buttock IC; Block between renal artery & bifurcation → IC & impotence (Leriche syndrome)

INVESTIGATIONS:
- FBC
- BG
- CXR
- ECG
- Angiography if surgery or angioplasty considered

RX: Stop cigs, encourage exercise, diet if obese. Vasodilators unhelpful. Avoid trauma. Chiropody. Surgery or angioplasty indicated if IC is causing significant disability. If rest pain, assess c̄ angiography. Femoro–popliteal obst often requires bypass graft. Aorto–iliac obst often requires graft or endarterectomy (SE: Impotence if pre-sacral nerves cut). Lumbar sypathectomy occ used if moderate IC c̄ cold foot. If gangrene, amputate

Thromboangitis Obliterans (Buerger's Disease)

Rare. Esp young M, heavy smokers

CLIN: Periph ischaemia → rest pain in fingers & toes, foot claudication. Absent periph pulses. Occ previous h/o supf phlebitis

RX: Stop cigs. Sympathectomy. Occ amputation

PROG: Usually improve on stopping smoking

Takayasu's Arteritis (Pulseless Disease)

Rare. Esp young F, Asians. Usually affects aortic arch vessels. Can → ischaemia of arms, CVA. Often absence of periph pulses

INVESTIGATIONS:
- ESR ↑
- Angiography

RX: Steroids, Anti-platelet drugs. Occ surgical bypass

Acute Arterial Ischaemia

Usually due to thromb 2° to atheroma. Occ due to emboli eg in AF, IHD, SABE, Atrial myxoma. If occlusion unrelieved after 6hrs, 2° thromb occurs

CLIN: Sudden onset of pain, pallor & cold.

Loss of pulses. Later Numbness; Paralysis; Muscle swelling; Paraesthesiae. Eventual gangrene

RX: Immediate Heparin infusion. Arterial embolectomy c̄ Fogarty catheter. Occ require angiography. If thromb suspected occ Rx c̄ anticoagulants, analgesia & reflex heating c̄ subsequent elective op. Streptokinase occ used

PROG. Best if early surgery

Indications for Amputation (LIST 16 CARD)

1. Dead limb:
   Eg Trauma, Diabetic gangrene
2. Lethal limb:
   Eg Gas gangrene, Malignant melanoma, Osteogenic sarcoma
3. Useless limb:
   Eg Intractable pain, Flail limb

Special Complications of Amputation (LIST 17 CARD)

1. Haem
2. Sloughing flaps
3. Painful neuroma
4. Phantom limb
5. Osteomyelitis
6. Stump muscle wastage

Digital Ischaemia

RAYNAUD'S PHENOMENON

Due to digital artery constriction. May be 1° or 2°. 1° cases esp seen in young women, occ FH. 2° cases often progress to digital infections & ischaemia

RX: Keep fingers warm. 2° cases may benefit from sympathectomy

Peristent Digital Ischaemia

An ischaemia of digit lasting for days or wks. Esp elderly. May be idiopathic or 2° to PRV, Cv rib

RX: Usually recover spontaneously. Occ require reflex heating. If infection, antibiotics; If gangrene, amputate

FROST-BITE

CLIN: Swelling; Redness; Blistering of digits of hands or feet. Often Infection; Supf gangrene

RX: Reflex heating; Antibiotics; Analgesics; Dextran infusion. Occ surgery for gangrene

ACROCYANOSIS

An arteriolar spasm on exposure to cold → red–blue discolouration. Esp young F

RX: Reassurance. Keep extremities warm. Nifedipine may benefit. Occ sympathectomy

LIVIDO RETICULARIS

A blotchy reticular discolouration of feet & legs. Esp young F. Occ 2° to PAN, PRV

ANEURYSMS

Types: Fusiform; Saccular; False; A-V; Dissecting

AETIOLOGY: Cong eg Berry aneurysm, A-V aneurysm; Trauma; Inflam eg SABE, Sy; Degenerative (commonest) esp atheroma

GENERAL COMPLICATIONS: Rupture; Thromb; Embolism; P on adjacent structures; Infection

Aortic Aneurysm

4 major sites: Asc aorta, Aortic arch, Desc aorta, Abdomen. About 75% occur in abdo. Most aneurysms due to atheroma but aneurysms of asc aorta usually due to Sy, Marfan's or Ank Sp. Ass c̄ BP ↑

CLIN: All may be symptomless
Asc aorta: Occ Chest pain; AI; SVC obst; Obst of R bronchus

Arch: Occ Compress trachea → stridor; Hoarseness; L bronchus obst → wheezing, pneumonia. Erosion of trachea or bronchus can → haemoptysis. Stretching of AV ring → AI
Desc thoracic aorta: Back pain; Vertebral erosion; Oesophageal compression → dysphagia; Oesophageal rupture → haemoptysis
Abdo aorta: Abnormal pulsatile swelling. Occ Abdo pain; Backache; Sciatica. Rupture → Shock, sudden lower abdo & lumbar pain, non-pulsatile tender mass. Occ spontaneous recovery & relapse (leaky aneurysm)

INVESTIGATIONS:
- CXR
- AXR
- Ultrasound abdo & Ht
- CAT scan
- Occ Isotope angiography, Aortography

RX: Risk of abdo rupture is related to the size of aneurysm & therefore op on all aneurysms >6cm diameter. Op mort much higher after rupture. In thoracic aneurysms, risk of rupture is increased if large, enlarging on X-R or symptomatic. Surgery usually requires cardiopulmonary by-pass & prosthetic graft c̄ 10–25% op mort

Dissecting Aneurysm

Result from intimal tear in aortic wall which can rupture externally or into lumen. Haematoma can block orifices of major vessels. Usually 2° to cystic medial necrosis of aortic wall which is ass c̄ Marfan's & Ehlers–Danlos syndromes. Ass c̄ BP ↑

CLIN: Sudden tearing chest pain radiating to arms, neck, abdo. Occ AI; Syncope; Paraplegia; LVF; Anuria; Pericardial rub; Shock; Cardiac tamponade; Loss of periph pulses; L haemothorax; Abdo pain. There is often a h/o a progressive lesion

INVESTIGATIONS:
- CXR: Widened mediastinum
- ECG
- CAT c̄ contrast
- Ultrasound
- Aortography

RX: Control BP c̄ Nitroprusside. Monitor CVP, BP & urine output. If asc aorta involved, immediate op c̄ insertion of graft c̄ cardiopulmonary bypass. If asc aorta not involved, surgery or β blockers

DVT

AETIOLOGY: Alteration in blood coagulation esp post-op due to ↑ fibrinogen, ↑ platelet stickiness, ↓ antithrombin & ↑ blood viscosity due to fluid loss; Vessel wall trauma; Venous stasis esp in Ht failure, prolonged bed rest & pelvic obst

Predisposing Conditions to DVT (LIST 18 CARD)

1. Immobility
2. Obesity
3. Surgery
4. Previous thrombotic disease
5. Pregnancy
6. Malignancy
7. "The Pill"
8. VVs
9. MI
10. CCF
11. Trauma
12. Polycythaemia

PATH: Platelet deposition on endothelium, deposition of fibrin into platelet clumps, trapping of blood cells → occlusion. If tail of clot breaks off → emboli

CLIN: Variable signs, often asymptomatic. Classically Tenderness; ↑ Temperature; Swelling; Redness of affected limb. Rarely cyanosis. May → PE, post thrombotic syndrome (Oedema, VV, Eczema, Ulceration, sc fat necrosis)

INVESTIGATIONS:
- Venography
- Radioisotope scanning
- Doppler ultrasonography
- PT time, APTT: If on anticoags

PREVENTION: Correct avoidable risk factors. Prophylactic sc Heparin or anticoagulation or Dextran infusion for high risk gps. Passive exercises, intermittent calf compression if immobile. Early post-op mobilisation

RX: Anticoagulation for fresh DVTs esp if above knee, unless c/i eg PU, bleeding tendency. Usually continue for 3mths if calf DVT & 6mths if Ilio–femoral DVT. Thrombolytic therapy c̄ Streptokinase or Urokinase is occ used if iliac vein thromb but ↑ SE compared to anticoags esp haem. In pregnancy, Warfarin is c/i & Heparin Rx is used. Thrombectomy if gangrene. Occ vena caval ligation or plication to prevent PE

PROG: ↑ risk of PE if thromb in iliofemoral or pelvic veins

DD:
1. Cellulitis
2. Acute supf thrombophlebitis
3. Rupture popliteal cyst
4. Fracture
5. Osteomyelitis
6. Myositis
7. Bone tumour

VARICOSE VEINS

A vein c̄ incompetent valves eg haemorrhoids, portal BP ↑, varicocoele, legs. Esp occur in supf leg veins

CAUSES: Idiopathic (F>M); 2° to DVT; 2° to Pelvic tumour inc pregnant uterus; Pregnancy

ANATOMY: The low P supf venous system ie the long & short saphenous veins communicate via the medial, central & lat perforator veins c̄ the high P deep venous system. Varicosity at Sapheno–femoral junction is termed "saphena varix"

CLIN: Unsightly swelling. Occ Aching pain; Pigmentation; Eczema; Swelling

INVESTIGATION: • Occ venography

RX: 3 major methods: Supportive bandaging indicated in old, pregnant & unfit. Injection c̄ sclerosant & compression for 6/52 to enable fibrosis to take place. Surgery to remove varicosities & secure incompetent perforators; in Trendelenberg Op, saphenous vein is disconnected from femoral vein & all vein tributaries are ligated & divided. Stripping of veins is achieved by a flexible wire introduced in saphenous vein near med malleolus & passed up to groin. Then vein tied at lower end & stripper at upper end pulled proximally

COMPLICATIONS:
1. Haem
2. Phlebitis
3. Ulcers Esp near malleoli
4. Eczema
5. Rarely malignant change in ulcer (Marjolin's Ulcer)

Superficial Venous Thrombophlebitis

Usually 2° to VVs

CLIN: Tender, red cord-like thickening over vein. Occ pyrexia

RX: Prophylactic Rx of VVs. Support bandage; Elevate leg; NSAID

LEG ULCERATION

Causes of Leg Ulcers (LIST 19 CARD)

1. Venous Ulcer
2. Trauma
3. Ischaemic:
   Eg Atheroma, Buerger's disease
4. Infective:
   Eg Staph, Gumma, "Bairnsdale" (Mycobacteria ulcerans), Osteomyelitis (Marjolin's ulcer)
5. Neuropathic:
   Eg Diabetes, Periph neuropathy, Tabes
6. Neoplastic:
   Eg Sq cell skin Ca, Malignant melanoma
7. Cryopathic:
   Eg Frostbite
8. Self abuse
9. Idiopathic
10. Ass c: Sickle cell disease, Rh Arth. Ulc Colitis (Pyoderma gangrenosum), A-V fistulae

Commonest cause is venous ulceration

CLIN: Ulcer described according to size, shape, floor, edge, base, & exudate. Malignant ulcers usually have heaped up edges

RX OF VENOUS ULCERS: Clean ulcer, elevate leg, dressings, support bandage. Occ Surgery eg Cocketts op (subfascial perforator dissection)

RHEUMATIC FEVER

A systemic illness 2° to a GpA β haemolytic strep nasopharyngeal infection. Esp 5–15yrs. Ass c̄ poverty, overcrowding. Occ FH. Prevalence declining in developed countries, but still common in India & Africa. Risk of Rh fever from strep infection is increased in epidemics

PATH: Aschoff body is pathognomic. Endocarditis, myocarditis, pericarditis, cutaneous nodules

REQUIREMENTS FOR DIAGNOSIS (DUCKETT JONES CRITERIA):
Evidence of previous strep infection plus 2 major criteria or 1 major & 2 minor criteria. Major criteria are: Carditis; Arthritis; Chorea; Nodules; Erythema marginatum. Minor criteria are: Previous Rh fever; Arthralgia; Fever; ^PR ↑^; ESR ↑; WCC ↑. Evidence of previous strep infection are: ASOT ↑; +ve throat culture; Recent scarlet fever

CLIN: Fever 1–4wks post-infection. Occ Carditis c̄ murmurs inc mitral pansystolic, mitral diastolic (Carey Coombs), aortic early diastolic & aortic ejection systolic; Ht ↑; CCF &/or Pericarditis. In carditis, PR ↑ disproportionate to fever, gallop rhythm. Occ Arthritis esp flitting polyarthritis of large jts; Subcutaneous painless non pruritic mobile swellings over extensor surfaces of jts; Arthralgia; Wt ↑; Malaise. Less commonly, Erythema marginatum (Pathognomic). Occ 2–6mths post infection, Chorea. Most cases are active for <3mths. May progress to Rh Ht disease

INVESTIGATIONS:
- WCC
- ESR
- FBC
- C reactive protein
- ASOT
- Throat swab
- CXR
- ECG

RX: Penicillin or Erythromycin for 10 days. Bed rest for 6wks or until carditis or arthritis are non-active. Salicylates relieve pain, fever & arthritis but don't affect course of Rh Ht disease. Dig & diuretics ± steroids for CCF. Haloperidol for chorea. Prevention of recurrences by prophylaxis for at least 5yrs c̄ low dose oral Penicillin. Prompt Rx of Strep pharyngitis c̄ Penicillin prevents Rh fever

COMPLICATIONS: Rh Ht disease occurs in about 1/3 of Rh fever cases. The incidence of affected valves is Mitral >Aortic >>Tricuspid >Pulm mirroring the likelihood of valves being affected during Rh fever episode. MSt is a progressive lesion; MInc if isolated may regress; AI develops in acute attack & persists; AS is a progressive lesion

PROG: Traditionally most morbidity & mort ass c̄ carditis. Worse in underdeveloped countries. Often recurs if no 2° prevention

MITRAL VALVE DISEASE

Mitral Stenosis

Usually present at 20–30yrs. May be isolated or ass c̄ other valve lesions

CAUSES: Rh fever >>Lutembacher's Disease (ASD & MS), Hurler's syndrome, EMF

PATH: Rh endocarditis → chordal fusion, commissural fusion or leaflet thickenening. As valve area reduces, haemodynamics worsen. Haemodynamic changes include: L atrial P ↑; Pulm arterial P ↑; Pulm vascular resistence ↑ c̄ ↓ lower lobe perfusion. In severe cases CO ↓, Pulm oedema

CLIN: Usually present c̄ SOB on exertion. Occ early haemoptysis 2° to bronchial vein rupture. Later Cough; Fatigue; Recurrent bronchitis; PND; Orthopnoea; CCF. Occ Mitral facies; Haemoptysis due to eg pulm infarct, pulm oedema; Thromboembolism; Chest pain; Palps. Rarely Compression of L recurrent laryngeal nerve by large L atrium → hoarseness (Ortner's syndrome); Dysphagia. Symptoms may be ppt by exercise, pregnancy, AF, LRTI. Often AF. Giant "a" waves if pulmonary BP ↑. Tapping cardiac impulse, L parasternal lift (RVH), loud S1, opening snap (soft if calcified valve, closer to S2 if severe), presystolic murmur, apical mid-diastolic murmur (longer if severe). In pulm BP ↑, loud S2. Occ ass c̄ functional valve murmurs eg PI (Graham–Steell murmur), TI. Also signs of any ass valve disease eg aortic valve disease

INVESTIGATIONS:
- ECG: ^P^ mitrale (bifid ^P^ wave) ie L atrium ↑ (unless AF). If pulm BP ↑: ^RVH^, ^R Axis deviation^
- CXR: L atrium ↑, RVH; Kerley's B lines; Upper lobe blood diversion. Rarely pulm haemosiderosis, pulm ossified nodules
- Echocardiography
- Cardiac catheterisation

RX: A. Medical: Diuretics. If AF, Dig & anticoags. If unsuccessful, try cardioversion 6–8wks later esp in young. Long term anticoags

B. Surgery: Indicated may inc: Severe symptoms, Unresponsive AF, Recurrent emboli. If mobile non-calcified valve c̄ no MInc, a closed mitral valvotomy may be indicated. Often require open procedure c̄ valve replacement

COMPLICATIONS:
1. L Atrial thrombus
2. Systemic emboli
3. SABE
4. Pulm infarct, PE
5. Pulm BP ↑
6. Haemoptysis

PROG: Results of surgery good but some restenose esp post valvotomy

DD:
1. L Atrial myxoma
2. L Atrial ball thrombus
3. Cor triatriatum
4. HOCM c̄ obst L vent inflow
5. Functional MSt (Austin Flint murmur) may occur in AI

Mitral Incompetence

May be isolated or ass c̄ other valve lesions. Usually due to Rh Ht disease (usually in ass c̄ MSt) but may occur due to valve prolapse, papillary muscle dysfunction, chordal rupture, annular Ca^{2+} & LVent dilatation

Causes of Mitral Incompetence (LIST 20 CARD)

1. Rh Ht disease
2. Rh fever usually transient
3. Floppy valve syndrome:
   Eg Marfan's, HOCM, IHD
4. Congenital:
   Eg Ostium primum ASD
5. SABE
6. HOCM
7. Rh Arth, SLE
8. Papillary muscle dysfunction or rupture:
   Eg 2° to IHD
9. Functional 2° to LVent dilatation:
   Eg 2° to CCF, BP ↑, COCM
10. EFE
11. Hurler's syndrome

HAEMODYNAMICS: L Atrial P ↑, Pulm capillary P ↑ → Pulm arterial P ↑. Rarely pulm BP ↑

CLIN OF Rh Ht DISEASE: SOB; Fatigue; CCF. Occ PND, Orthopnoea; Haemoptysis; Emboli. Rarely P of large L Atrium → dysphagia or collapsed L lower lobe. Often AF. Apex displaced lat. Soft S1, high pitched blowing pansystolic murmur; S3. Occ Widely split S2; Short mid diastolic murmur; Small vol pulse. Usually signs of other valve lesion esp MSt. Lesion is usually slowly progressive

CLIN OF PAPILLARY MUSCLE DYSFUNCTION: Pansystolic murmur; Pulm oedema, usually severe but may be mild esp 2° to inf MI

CLIN OF MITRAL VALVE PROLAPSE: Usually asymptomatic but may be Fatigue, Palps, Chest pain. Occ Emboli,

SABE. Occ Pansystolic murmur; Mid or late systolic click ± late systolic murmur

CLIN OF CHORDAL RUPTURE: Severe pulm oedema. Systolic murmur heard at LSE (not conducted to carotids) if post leaflet rupture & over spine if ant leaflet rupture

INVESTIGATIONS: • ECG: ˆPˆ mitrale or AF, ˆLVHˆ
• CXR: Occ LVent ↑, L Atrium ↑, Ca^+
• Echocardiography
• Cardiac catheterisation

RX: Prophylaxis against SABE. Mild to moderate symptoms, Dig & diuretics. Anticoags rarely used. If severe symptoms, surgery to prevent irreversible LVent damage. Mitral valve replacement is c̄ mechanical or tissue valves & requires lifelong anticoags or anti-platelet drugs, & regular monitoring

PROG: Early Op mort <5%

TRICUSPID VALVE DISEASE

Tricuspid Stenosis

Rare. Rarely isolated. Usually due to Rh Ht disease. Rarely 2° to carcinoid syndrome

CLIN: JVP ↑; Oedema; SOB; Liver ↑; Hepatic pain on exertion. Giant "a" wave; Shallow "y" descent. Occ AF; Ascites. S1 loud; Occ opening snap accentuated by insp; Diastolic murmur max LSE ppt by insp. Symptoms & signs of other valve disease

INVESTIGATIONS: • ECG: Tall ˆPˆ wave in ˆIIˆ
• CXR: Large R Atrium

RX: If severe symptoms, tricuspid valvotomy

DD: R Atrial myxoma

Tricuspid Incompetence

Causes of Tricuspid Incompetence (LIST 21 CARD)

1. Congenital:
   Esp Ebstein's anomaly
2. Functional due to RVH & Pulm BP ↑:
   Eg MSt, Eisenmenger's syndrome
3. Rheumatic (In ass c mitral valve disease)
4. Traumatic:
   Eg Papillary muscle rupture
5. Carcinoid syndrome
6. EMF
7. SABE:
   Esp drug addicts

CLIN OF EBSTEIN'S ANOMALY (DOWNWARD DISPLACEMENT OF TRICUSPID VALVE INTO RVENT): May be asymptomatic. Often Cyanosis; CCF; Palps. Occ SVT; Gallop rhythm; Opening snap; Systolic & diastolic murmurs at LSE

CLIN OF ACQUIRED TI: Oedema; J; Ascites; Hepatic pain; Pulsatile liver. Large systolic venous waves; Rapid "y" descent; RVent heave; S3; Short mid-diastolic murmur; Pansystolic murmur at LSE ppt by insp

INVESTIGATIONS: • ECG: In Ebstein's anomaly often ˆRBBBˆ & WPW syndrome
• CXR
• Echocardiography
• Cardiac catheterisation

RX: Cong TI use Dig & diuretics. Occ valve replacement. Functional TI due to MSt usually responds to mitral valve Rx eg repair. Acquired TI usually requires annuloplasty or valve replacement

AORTIC VALVE DISEASE

Aortic Stenosis

Causes of Aortic Stenosis (LIST 22 CARD)

1. Congenital esp bicuspid valve
2. Rh Ht disease
3. Degenerative c valvar Ca^{2+}
4. Prosthetic valve malfunction
5. Idiopathic hypercalcaemia (→ supravalvar AS)
6. Idiopathic supravalvar AS
7. HOCM (→ Subvalvar AS)

3 types:
1. Valvar
2. Subvalvar
3. Supravalvar

VALVAR AS

Commonest

HAEMODYNAMICS: Classically anachrotic arterial pulse (but pulse may be norm or ↑ in elderly); LVent P ↑; Vent hypertrophy → diastolic P ↑ → pulm venous P ↑ → LVF. High LVent P can impede coronary blood flow → angina, IHD

CLIN: Symptoms occur late. Occ LVF; Angina; Syncope; Palps; SOB; Sudden death. Anachrotic small vol pulse; Harsh mid systolic ejection murmur ± thrill radiating to carotid arteries. If aortic valve mobile, ejection click & reversed split S2 which are not heard in calcific AS. Often ass c̄ AI

SUBVALVAR AS

Usually due to HOCM

CLIN: No ejection click. Occ Diastolic murmur; Ht ↑; Bisferiens pulse; Double apical impulse; S4

SUPRAVALVAR AS

May be ass c̄ idiopathic hyperCa^{2+}. Often other cong valve defects

CLIN: Characteristic facies ("elfin like"); R arm BP >L arm; Angina; Syncope; IQ ↓. Ejection systolic murmur, no click, no diastolic murmur

GENERAL INVESTIGATIONS:
- ECG: LVH. Occ AF
- CXR: Dilatation of asc aorta. Occ calcified valve esp tight AS
- Echocardiography
- Cardiac catheterisation

GENERAL RX: If symptomatic surgery is normally required. In older or if valve immobile, valve replacement. In young, valvotomy or valve replacement. Prophylactic antibiotics to prevent SABE

PROG: <5% op mort

DD: MInc esp due to post chordal rupture

Aortic Incompetence

Causes of Aortic Incompetence (LIST 23 CARD)

1. Rh Ht disease
2. Arthritides:
   Eg Rh Arth, Ank Sp, Reiter's, SLE
3. Functional AI:
   Eg BP ↑, Atheroma
4. Dissecting Aneurysm:
   Eg BP ↑, Marfan's
5. SABE
6. Trauma
7. Prosthetic valve malfunction
8. Congenital:
   Eg AI c VSD
9. Sy

HAEMODYNAMICS: Wide pulse P; Stroke vol ↑↑; LVent P ↑; Premature mitral valve closure due to high end diastolic LVent P; LVH & dilatation

CLIN: LVF; Palps; Fatigue; Dizziness. Waterhammer pulse; Carotid pulsation (Corrigan's sign); "to & fro" murmur over femoral artery; Capillary pulsation; Apex beat displaced laterally. Occ Syncope; Angina. Diastolic murmur max LSE in exp & leaning forward; Short ejection systolic murmur. Occ Mitral diastolic murmur (Austin Flint). Soft S1; Single S2

INVESTIGATIONS:
- ECG: LVH, ^LBBB^
- CXR: Ht ↑
- Echocardiography
- Cardiac catheterisation
- Coronary angiography
- Sy serology

RX: Antibiotic prophylaxis to prevent SABE. Surgery for acute AI or if LVF. Aortic valve replacement

COMPLICATIONS: 1. SABE
2. Prosthetic valve obst

PROG: Approx 5% op mort. Once symptomatic prompt Rx is needed

DD:
1. Pulm diastolic murmur
2. PDA
3. Ruptured sinus of Valsalva

PULMONARY VALVE DISEASE

Pulmonary Stenosis

Usually congenital but rarely 2° to carcinoid syndrome, Rh Ht disease. Also occurs as part of Fallot's tetralogy

HAEMODYNAMICS: RVent P ↑ → RVH. Post sten dilatation of pulm artery; CO ↓

CLIN: May be asymptomatic. Fatigue; SOB; Angina; Syncope. Periph cyanosis; Giant "a" wave; RVH c̄ thrill. Ejection click; Ejection murmur; P2 soft

INVESTIGATIONS:
- ECG: ˆPˆ pulmonale, RVH
- CXR: Prominent pulm artery, R Atrium ↑
- Echocardiography
- Cardiac catheterisation

RX: Pulm valvotomy

COMPLICATION: SABE

PROG: 2–5% op mort. If op performed before age 20, very good results

Pulmonary Incompetence

Usually 2° to pulm BP ↑ but occ congenital, post valvotomy or 2° to SABE. Functional PI (Graham–Steell murmur) may occur in MSt

HAEMODYNAMICS: ↑ vol load to RVent usually well tolerated

CLIN: Asymptomatic. High pitched blowing early diastolic murmur max in pulm area & LSE

INVESTIGATIONS:
- ECG
- CXR
- Echocardiography

RX: Treat underlying cause

CARDIAC SURGERY

Post-op mort is falling in developed countries. Outcome is influenced by illness severity, extent of procedure, age, state of functioning myocardium, complexity of haemodynamic problem, surgical skill & experience

Types of Replacement Valves

1. Mechanical Valves eg Starr–Edwards, Bjork: Main problem is thromboemboli (incidence reduced by anticoags). Good durability & function
2. Homografts: Uncertain durability but don't require anticoags
3. Heterografts: Usually porcine. Only require anticoags for a few wks. Uncertain durability

INFECTIVE ENDOCARDITIS

AETIOLOGY: In pre-antibiotic era the main cause was *Strep viridans* affecting Rh Ht or cong Ht lesion in young. Nowadays although Strep viridans is still a common cause, many other organisms seen eg other Strep, Staph aureus, Candida & Rickettsial when clin course is usually more acute & older people affected. Also common amongst drug addicts, haemodialysis patients. Occ due to indwelling venous catheters. Paradoxically, trivial lesions of mitral or aortic valves are more commonly affected than those c̄ severe valve disease

PATHOGENESIS: Usually a periph source of infection → transient bacteraemia eg dental extraction, GU procedures, Endoscopy. Usually endocarditis develops on abnormal Ht valve

CLIN: Fever; Rigors; Malaise; Wt ↓; Anaemia; Clubbing. Occ embolic features: Mycotic abscesses; CVA; Sudden blindness; Splenic infarct; MI; Splinter haems. Occ immune complex disease signs: Osler's nodes (Tender subcutaneous nodules); Janeway spots (Red palmar macules); Roth's spots; Conjunctival haem; GN. Occ Cafe-au-lait spots; Spleen ↑; Arthralgia; Psychotic illness. Often murmurs which change during course of illness; CCF. Development of acute AI or MInc are particularly dangerous

INVESTIGATIONS:
- ESR ↑↑
- Blood cultures (usually 6)
- Echocardiography: Can detect vegetations
- WCC
- Urinalysis
- Serum drug levels
- Occ MIC, MBC, Serum cidal levels
- Immunoglobulins

PROPHYLAXIS: 3 principles are identification of at-risk, eradication of sources of bacteraemia in the at-risk & antibiotic cover of at-risk during procedures likely to induce bacteraemia. Usually a dose of antibiotic immediately prior to procedure & one or two after procedure is sufficient

RX: Use bactericidal antibiotics initially IV. Choice according to sensitivity eg *Strep viridans* often use Benzylpenicillin ± Gentamicin. Usually require Rx for at least 1mth. Monitor serum drug levels where appropriate. Cardiac failure Rx is bed rest, Dig & diuretics ± vasodilator. If cardiac failure is intractable or infection persists, cardiac surgery is indicated. Prosthetic endocarditis should be refered to a cardiac centre

PROG: Overall mort approx 30%. Poor prog if elderly, intractable Ht failure, Prosthetic valve, Acute AI, Ht block, periph emboli, failure to identify infective organism, Pseudomonal & fungal endocarditis

Rickettsial Endocarditis

Uncommon cause of SABE

CLIN: Liver ↑; Spleen ↑; Thrombocytopenia; General symptoms & signs of SABE

RX: Long term antibiotics eg Tetracycline & Clindamycin

CARDIAC TUMOURS

Mets much commoner than primary but seldom symptomatic

Atrial Myxoma

Commonest 1° cardiac tumour. L Atrial myxoma commoner than R. Benign but can recur

L ATRIAL MYXOMA

CLIN: Fever; Wt ↓; Occ Arthralgia; Systemic emboli esp large vessels; Syncope. Changing murmurs, often diastolic & systolic murmurs in mitral area. Occ "tumour thud" after S2. May → mitral valve obst c̄ pulm BP ↑

R ATRIAL MYXOMA

CLIN: Mimics tricuspid valve disease. Fatigue; Liver ↑; JVP ↑; Pleural effusions; R Atrium ↑

GENERAL INVESTIGATIONS:

- CXR
- Echocardiography
- ECG
- Cardiac catheterisation

GENERAL RX:

Surgery

Sarcoma

20% of all 1° cardiac tumours

CLIN: "Malignant pericardial disease". Chest pain; Pulsus paradoxus; JVP ↑; Ht ↑. Later Tamponade; Pleural effusions; Cardiac rupture

INVESTIGATIONS:
- CXR
- ECG
- Echocardiography
- Pericardial tap: Blood-stained c̄ malignant cells

RX: Supportive

PROG: Poor

Gastroenterology

ORAL DISEASES

Glossitis

Inflammation of tongue

Causes of Stomatitis (LIST 1 GIT)

1. Infection:
   a) Bacterial eg TB, Sy. Vincents angina
   b) Fungal esp Candida
   c) Viral eg Herpes simplex
   d) Protozoal eg Malaria
2. Drugs eg Methotrexate
3. Deficiencies:
   a) Iron
   b) Folate
   c) Vit B
   d) Vit C
4. Skin diseases:
   a) Pemphigus
   b) Pemphigoid
   c) Stevens-Johnson
   d) Lichen planus
   e) Leukoplakia
5. Idiopathic esp aphthous ulcers
6. Trauma esp Ill fitting dentures
7. Systemic disorders:
   a) Neoplastic eg Ca, Leukaemia
   b) Behcet's disease
   c) Reiter's disease
   d) IBD
8. Other debilitating disorders:
   a) Alcoholism
   b) Malnutrition
   c) Heavy smoking
9. Allergy

Stomatitis

Inflammation of oral mucosa

Cheilitis

Inflammation of lips

CAUSES: 1. PA
2. Chr Alcoholism c̄ poor diet
3. Vit B def

EXFOLIATIVE CHEILITIS

CAUSES: 1. Sun
2. Skin disease esp atopic eczema
3. Lip licking
4. Pipe smoking

ANGULAR CHEILITIS

CAUSES: 1. Old age
2. Poor dentures
3. IDA

Ulcers

1. APHTHOUS

Most unknown cause. Occ B12/folate def; IBD

2. TRAUMATIC

Esp 2° to ragged teeth, ill fitting dentures

3. METHOTREXATE

Ulcers & stomatitis

RX: Reversed by Folinic acid

4. SYPHILIS

Inner, lower lip. Snail track ulcers

5. OTHERS

Bullous disease, Ca, Behcet's, *Herpes Simplex*, TB

Pigmentation

CAUSES:
1. **Melanotic:** a) Racial
   b) Addison's
2. **Peutz-Jegher's Syndrome**
3. **Post-inflammatory**
4. **Drugs:** Eg Quinidine, Pb, Hg, Bi
5. **Acanthosis Nigricans:** Ass c̄ Ca Stomach, Ca oesophagus

Candidiasis

White membranes easily scraped off

CAUSES: 1. 2° to antibiotics
2. Steroids
3. Cyt. T
4. Leukaemia
5. Diabetes

CLIN: Occ → dysphagia. In immunocompromised may → systemic spread

LOCAL RX: Nystatin

Leucoplakia

PREDISPOSITION: 1. Smoking
2. Poor fitting dentures
3. Jagged teeth
4. Chr actinic cheilitis
5. Betel nut chewing
6. Spicy foods
7. Syphilis

CLIN: Persistent white patch on mucous membranes of lips, gums, cheeks, dorsum of tongue. Premalignant → Squamous cell Ca

DD: 1. Candidiasis
2. Lichen Planus
3. White spongue naevus
4. Leucokeratosis

Mucocutaneous Diseases

ERYTHEMA MULTIFORME: eg Stevens-Johnson Syndrome

CLIN: Lip haem, ulceration & crusting. Occ → blisters, erosions & involvement of buccal & gingival mucosa, tongue & palate

LICHEN PLANUS

Lace like bluish white streaks. Violaceous, flat topped polygonal papules

HEREDITARY HAEMORRHAGIC TELANGIECTASIA (OSLER'S DISEASE)

Aut Dom. Multiple telangiectasia esp mucous membranes → epistaxis, IDA. Occ GI bleed

PEMPHIGUS VULGARIS

Epidermal bullae. Erosions, supf ulcers, lip haem c̄ crusts

AMYLOIDOSIS, MYELOMA & WALDENSTROM'S MACROGLOBULINAEMIA

Haem lip papules

MUCOUS MEMBRANE PEMPHIGOID

CLIN: Bullae, ulceration → scarring

SLE

CLIN: In 10–15%, erythema or purpura on palate, buccal mucosa or gums → ulcers

SCLERODERMA

CLIN: Radial furrowing around mouth c̄ limited ability to open

TUBEROUS SCLEROSIS

CLIN: Facial angiofibromas. Ass c̄ Ep, IQ ↓, Adenoma Sebaceum

Other Mouth Lesions

1. Fordyce spots: Ectopic sebaceous glands
2. Geographic tongue: Chr migratory glossitis
3. Scrotal tongue: Congenital
4. Black hairy tongue: Filiform papillae hyperplasia
5. Glossodynia: Unexplained painful tongue

Epulis

Local swelling of gums. 3 types: Periosteal fibrous nodule; Giant cell tumour; Granuloma esp in pregnancy

Carcinoma

MOUTH & PHARYNX

M>F, except post-cricoid Ca F>M, Post tongue F=M

PREDISPOSING FACTORS: 1. Leukoplakia
2. Chr irritation: Smoking; Betel nut chewing; Syphilis; Sepsis; Spices; Sore teeth; Spirits
3. IDA (Plummer-Vinson or Patterson-Brown-Kelly Syndromes) ie Post cricoid Ca c̄ IDA

TYPES: Keratinising squamous cell; Transitional cell; Lymphoepithelioma (not an epithelioma). The latter two esp tongue, tonsil, nasopharynx

SPREAD: 1. Local
2. Lymph
3. Blood (rare, late)

PRESENTATION: Nodule, wart, ulcer, fissure or papilliferous growth

INVESTIGATIONS: • Biopsy
• WR
• CXR
• SXR

RX: X-Rad (c/i Radiation resistent; Recurrence). Surgery. Cyt.T for palliation

COMPLICATIONS: 1. Dysphagia
2. Anorexia
3. Sepsis
4. Bronchopneumonia
5. Haem (jugular vein/carotid artery)

LIPS

9M:1F. Elderly, outdoor types. Lower lip >Upper. Slow growth

SPREAD: Sub-mental, sub-mandibular, int jugular glands

PROG: 80% 5yr survival

DD:
1. Wart
2. Mucous cyst
3. Chr ulcers, fissures
4. Chancre: Upper >>Lower lip
5. Haemangioma, Lymphangioma, Fibroma
6. Herpes simplex
7. Molluscum sebaceum

TONGUE

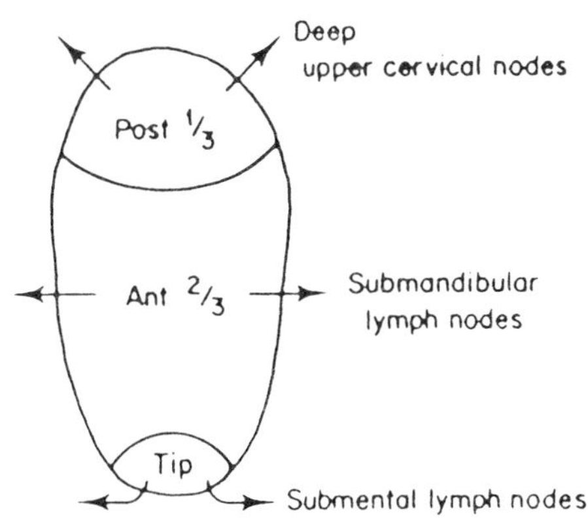

Figure 1 *Lymphatic drainage of tongue*

M>F. Ass c̄ Sy. Post 1/3 Ca usually lymphoepithelioma

CLIN OF ANT 2/3: Initially painless then earache. Bleeding; Ulceration; Ankyloglossia (fixed tongue). Bilat LN spread

CLIN OF POST 1/3: Fast growth. Early LN spread

DD:
1. Benign tumours
2. Ulcers, fissures
3. Circumvallate papilla
4. Lingual thyroid

NASOPHARYNX

Esp Chinese. Squamous cell Ca >Lymphoepithelioma

CLIN: Nasal obstr; Bleeding; Headache; Deafness

SPREAD: To Cv LN

SALIVARY GLAND

Calculi

Common in submandibular gland & duct, rare in parotid. Ass c̄ well kept teeth or the edentulous. Predisposes to Ca

CLIN: Painful swelling ppt by food, Bad taste due to discharge

INVESTIGATION: • X-R: Stone

RX: If in duct remove stone. If in gland, remove gland. Occ post-parotid surgery complication is Frei syndrome ie "post gustatory" sweating, occ requiring tympanic neurectomy

Inflammation

CAUSES:
1. Ass c̄ calculi
2. Post-op
3. Mumps
4. Sjogren's syndrome
5. Sarcoidosis
6. TB
7. Reticuloses
8. Chr recurrent parotitis
9. Dehydration

Post-Operative Parotitis

PREDISPOSITIONS:
1. Dental sepsis
2. NG tube
3. Poor oral hygiene
4. Debilitation
5. Uraemia

CLIN: Hard, enlarged, tender, painful, parotid(s) ± discharge. Occ Suppuration

RX: Sucking sweets. Antibiotics. Occ drainage

Mumps

Incub Pd: 17–21 days. Esp young

CLIN: Usually bilat parotitis. Occ Orchitis; Pancreatitis; Mastitis; Thyroiditis; Oophoritis

Sjogren's syndrome

Esp middle aged F

CLIN: Secretions ↓; Swelling; Dry mouth. Kerato-conjunctivitis sicca. Ass c̄ Rh Arth, Immune liver disease

Sarcoid

Heerfordt's syndrome is parotitis, uveitis & cranial nerve palsy

Mikulicz's Syndrome

Enlargement of all the salivary glands & the lacrimal gland

CAUSES:
1. Sarcoid
2. Reticulosis
3. TB
4. Auto-immune diseases
5. Connective tissue diseases
6. Sjorgren's syndrome

CLIN: Secretory capacity ↓; Swelling on eating

RX: Massage of gland. Exclude any ppt food. Rarely surgery

Chronic Recurrent Parotitis

Esp children

CLIN: Recurrent pain & swelling. Ass c̄ sialectasia, stone or stricture

RX: Remove stones; Sialogogues to encourage drainage; Dilate stricture; Occ surgery

Tumours

MIXED SALIVARY ADENOMA

90% parotid; 90% <50yrs. M=F Mostly benign & slow growing. Usually lower supf pole of parotid. Rarely involves VIIn unless malignant

RX: Wide excision. Preserve VIIn. Post enucleation 25% recur

ADENOLYMPHOMA (WARTHIN'S TUMOUR)

Parotid. Occ bilat. M>F. >50yrs. May be 2° to chr irritation. Derived from lymphoid tissue

RX: Remove

PROG: Excellent

CARCINOMA

M=F. Usually >50yrs

TYPES: Acinic Cell; Mucoepithelioma; AdenoCa; Squamous cell Ca; Anaplastic; Malignant mixed type; Adenocystic (Cylindroma); Mets eg from Nasopharynx

CLIN: VIIn affected; Pain. Present earlier if inside mouth. Local infiltration, rapid growth, spread to LN

RX: Remove gland ± VIIn ± block LN removal ± X-Rad

PROG: Poor but reasonable if survive >3yrs

DD:
1. Sebaceous cyst
2. Lipoma
3. LN ↑
4. Neuroma
5. Adamantinoma of mandible

Adenocystic Ca (Cylindroma)

Commonest tumour of minor glands. Spread along perineural lymphatics. Long survival despite mets

OESOPHAGEAL DISEASE

Causes of Dysphagia (LIST 2 GIT)

A. LUMINAL
1. Foreign body
2. Stomatitis & Glossitis
3. Infections:
   Eg Quinsy; Retropharyngeal abscess; Tonsillitis
4. Plummer-Vinson syndrome

B. CONDITIONS AFFECTING WALL
1. Achalasia
2. Chagas disease
3. Diffuse oesophageal spasm
4. Systemic sclerosis
5. Oesophageal diverticula:
   Eg Pharyngeal pouch
6. Inflammation:
   Eg Oesophagitis due to Candida, Corrosive, PU
7. Stricture:
   Eg Ca, PU
8. Neoplasm

C. EXTRINSIC COMPRESSION
1. Neoplasm:
   Eg Lung; Neck; Mediastinal tumours
2. Enlarged thyroid
3. Aortic aneurysm
4. Enlarged heart:
   Eg Pericardial effusion; Enlarged LAtrium

D. CNS LESIONS (Rare)
1. MND
2. Myasthenia gravis
3. XIn lesions
4. Bilat hemiplegia
5. Polio
6. Dystrophia myotonica
7. MS
8. Polyneuropathy
9. Syringomyelia

E. GLOBUS HYSTERICUS

Sideropenic Dysphagia

Plummer-Vinson or Patterson-Brown-Kelly Syndrome = IDA ± web. Premalignant → post cricoid Ca. F>M

RX: Fe; Dilatation

Achalasia

Unknown aetiology. 3F:2M. Usually 40–60yrs

PATH: Degeneration of ganglion cells of myenteric plexus esp in middle & lower oesophagus → abnormal peristalsis & non-relaxation of sphincter

CLIN: Dysphagia; Retrosternal pain; 2° lung

infection; Wt ↓

INVESTIGATIONS: • X-R: Dilated oesophagus, no gastric air bubble
• Endoscopy & biopsy (not always diagnostic)
• Manometry

RX: Anticholinergic drugs or nitrates. Heller's op ie longitudinal cardiomyotomy

COMPLICATIONS: 1. Pulmonary fibrosis
2. Aspiration
3. Ca
4. Oesophagitis
5. Haematemesis
6. Arthropathy (rare)

DD: 1. Ca Oesophagus
2. Psychogenic dysphagia
3. Ca Stomach
4. Stricture 2° to PU
5. Amyloidosis
6. Chagas' Disease
7. Diffuse oesophageal spasm
8. Systemic Sclerosis

Chagas' Disease

S.Am. Due to *Trypanosoma cruzi*

PATH: Neurotoxins destroy ganglia. Also affects heart → cardiomyopathy & colon → megacolon

CLIN: Fever; LN ↑; Liver ↑; Spleen ↑

RX: Cardiomyotomy

Diffuse Oesophageal Spasm

Spontaneous, localised, non-progressive repetitive contractions of smooth muscle. Ass c̄ hiatus hernia, diverticula & muscle hypertrophy. Sphincter may be involved

CAUSES: 1. G-O relux
2. Ca of Cardia
3. Idiopathic

CLIN: Intermittent substernal pain ass c̄ meals. In 2/3 dysphagia

INVESTIGATIONS: • Endoscopy to exlude Ca
• Manometry
• Ba meal: Beaded or corkscrew oesophagus

RX: Assess dentition. GTN, Long acting nitrates, Ca^{2+} antagonists or Hydrallazine. Occ oesophagomyotomy

Systemic Sclerosis

Failure of peristalsis, gut dilation esp oesophagus

CLIN: G-O reflux → oesophagitis & occ stricture

Swallowed Foreign Bodies

Painful dysphagia. Occ perf c̄ mediastinitis. Rarely perf of aorta

RX: X-R & surgical or endoscopic removal

Perforation of Oesophagus

CAUSES: 1. Foreign body
2. Traumatic
3. Iatrogenic
   a) Endoscopy
   b) Bouginage
4. Spontaneous
5. Mallory-Weiss syndrome (mucosal laceration 2° to vom)

CLIN: Pain in neck, chest & upper abdomen; Dysphagia; Pyrexia. Occ Surgical emphysema

INVESTIGATIONS: • X-R: Free mediastinal gas

RX: Cv perf: Antibiotics, IV drip, drain any abscess
Thoracic perf: Immediate suture

Oesophageal Diverticula

PHARYNGEAL POUCH

Mucosal protrusion in post inf pharyngeal constrictor (Killian's dehiscence) between thyro- & cricopharyngeus. M>F. Esp Old

CLIN: Dysphagia; Regurgitation; Palpable neck swelling

RX: Excision of pouch & myotomy of cricopharyngeus

TRACTION

Fixation to TB glands or pleural adhesions

PULSION

Seen in achalasia

Carcinoma

Common in China, Iran & S.Afr. In UK, causes 2–3% of all deaths from Ca. 3 main sites: post-cricoid, mid-oesophagus (at aortic arch) & supracardial. Squamous cell >>AdenoCa. Esp elderly. M>F. Ass c̄: Carcinogens eg nitrosamines, alcohol, tobacco; Achalasia; Sideropenic dysphagia; Tylosis; Coeliac disease; G-O reflux & chr oesphagitis; Leucoplakia; ? previous gastric surgery; ? Vit A def

CLIN: Dysphagia; Wt ↓; Anaemia. Occ Haematemesis

INVESTIGATIONS: • Ba swallow
• Endoscopy & biopsy

SPREAD: Local to mediastinum; LN to para-oesophageal & tracheo-bronchial LNs; Blood to liver & lungs (late)

RX: X-Rad for high growths ie Squamous cell
Surgery: Resect, insert length of colon. 15% 5 yr survival. Post-op mort high due to wound infection, mediastinitis, empyema, pneumonia
X-Rad & palliative intubation c̄ Mousseau-Barbin or Celestin tube. May → a) Bronchopneumonia b) occlusion by food or growth of Ca c) pressure necrosis of gastric wall

COMPLICATIONS: 1. Obstruction
2. Ulcer
3. Perforation
4. Recurrent laryngeal or phrenic n palsy
5. Empyema or lung abscess
6. Pneumonia
7. Pericarditis
8. SVC obst

DD:
1. Achalasia
2. Peptic stricture
3. Ca stomach
4. Diffuse oesophageal spasm
5. Peptic oesophagitis

Gastro-Oesophageal Reflux

Common in infancy, pregnancy, aged, obese, post gastric surgery. Ass c̄ HH, Scleroderma

CLIN: Regurgitation; Postural pain, Heartburn

INVESTIGATIONS: • Endoscopy & Biopsy
• Isotope scan

RX: A. Medical: Raise head of bed; Wt ↓; No cigs; Avoid ppt factors eg large meals, stooping, Aspirin & NSAID. High dose antacids; Mucaine; Alginates; Metoclopropamide; Cimetidine
B. Surgical: Many types of op eg fundoplication

COMPLICATIONS: 1. Haem
2. Stricture occ Schatzski ring
3. Barrett's Oesophagus: Oesophageal columnar metaplasia, a pre-malignant ulcer

PHYSIOLOGICAL MECHANISMS TO PREVENT G-O REFLUX:
1. Pinchcock action of R crus of diaphragm
2. "Valve-like" effect of angulation at C-O junction
3. Sphincteric action of circular muscle of lower oesophagus
4. "Cork in bottle" action of rugae
5. +ve intra-abdo P

CAUSES OF OESOPHAGITIS 1. G-O reflux
2. Corrosives
3. Irradiation
4. Drugs eg Tetracycline, Emepronium
5. Infection eg candida, herpes

Hiatus Hernia (HH)

PREDISPOSING FACTORS: Obesity; Age; Wasting diseases; Pregnancy; Intra-abdo P ↑ eg cough, constipation, bladder neck obst, corsets; Intra-gastric P ↑ eg DU → pyloric narrowing, pylorospasm in DU or gallstones. Ass c̄ Gallstones, DU

3 TYPES:
1. Sliding (80%):
Clin: Often asymptomatic. Heartburn; Acid reflux; Belching. Occ Ulcers; Fibrosis → Dysphagia; Haematemesis; Anaemia
2. Rolling (10%): Para-oesophageal true hernia
Clin: Flatulent dyspepsia; Distension; SOB; PR ↑. No reflux. Occ Obst; Strangulation; Torsion → pain
3. Combined (10%)

INVESTIGATIONS: • Endoscopy
• Ba meal
• FBC
• Cholecystogram

RX: Nil if asymptomatic
A. Medical: As for reflux oesophagitis. Treat any ass conditions eg constipation
B. Surgical: Indications: Failure of medical

Rx; Large para-oesophageal hernia (liable to bleed or obst); Ulceration; Stricture; Haem

Types of op: Abdo or thoraco-abdo repair ± dilatation, ± V&P

PEPTIC ULCERATION

Epidemiology

In UK, 4DU:1GU

Ass c̄: 1. Smoking, GU>DU
2. Blood gp O (DU)
3. Familial 3x norm in 1st degree relatives
4. Non-secretors (no blood gp substances in mucus)
5. Zollinger-Ellison (ZE) syndrome: → ↑ acid secretion
6. Renal dialysis
7. PRV
8. Ileal resection
9. Hyperparathyroidism (Ca^{2+} → ↑ Gastrin)
10. MEA
11. Aspirin (GU)
12. ? COAD, cirrhosis, CRF
13. ?? steroids, NSAID
14. Stasis post vag (GU)

NB Some immunity in preg, premenopausal & c̄ Oestrogen Rx

Pathogenesis

GU:
1. Biliary reflux
2. ? Gastric stasis
3. ? Mucosal ischaemia
4. Acid secretion norm or ↓

DU: Unknown. In 1/3 acid secretion ↑

General Clin

Pain; Heartburn; Nausea; Vom; Wt loss; Water brash

DU

Usually single. Most in first 2–3 cm of 1st part of duodenum, if not prob ass c̄ disease of pancreas

COMPLICATIONS:
1. Haem
2. Penetration
3. Perf
4. Py.S

GU

Usually single & lesser curvature. Round, punched out c̄ clean base. Often ass c̄ diffuse gastritis

COMPLICATIONS:
1. Haem
2. Penetration
3. Perf
4. Hour glass stomach
5. Malignant 1–5%

Acute PU

CAUSES:
1. Stress eg Burns (Curling's); Post-op; Post-MI; Head injury (Cushing's)
2. Aspirin, NSAID

PATH: Multiple minute mucosal ulceration

COMPLICATIONS:
1. Haem
2. Perf
3. Chr PU

Investigations of Ulcers

- Endoscopy & biopsy
- Ba meal
- FBC
- FOB
- Acid secretion for post-vagotomy & ZE
- Gastrin assay

Rx of Ulcers

MEDICAL RX

Stop cigs → ↑ GU healing. Diet ie small, frequent meals, milk & no fatty foods relieve symptoms. Low dose antacids help symptomatically (Al^{3+} → constipation as $CaxPO_4$ ↓; Mg^{2+} → diarrhoea). Histamine H_1 & H_2 antagonists eg Cimetidine, Ranitidine → PU healing, occ used long term. Occ use other drugs eg Carbenoxolone: GU healing ↑ (SE: Oedema, K^+ ↓, Occ BP ↑); Caved-S: GU healing ↑ (SE less than carbenoxolone); Denol (Bi) → ↑ ulcer healing. High dose antacids → ulcer healing & is Rx of choice for acute PU

ASSESSMENT OF MEDICAL RX: All patients c̄ GU at risk of Ca, therefore endoscope at 8–12 wks to confirm healing

SURGICAL RX

Indications for Surgical Rx (LIST 3 GIT)

A. ABSOLUTE
1. Failure of medical Rx
2. Persistent haem
3. Perf
4. Pyloric stenosis
5. Suspected Ca

B. RELATIVE
1. Combined GU & DU
2. Strong FH

GASTRIC ULCER

1. **Billroth 1:** Commonest op. Partial gastrectomy. Best if ulcer in distal half. 0.5% recurrence rate
   SE: High recurrence of any DU. Higher post-op complications than V&P
2. **V&P:** Theoretically good esp high GU
   SE: Occ GU recurrence
3. **Billroth II:** For high GU

COMBINED GU & DU: 1. Billroth 1 & truncal vagotomy

DUODENAL ULCER:

1. **Billroth II:** Not technically difficult. 75% of stomach removed & gastro-jejunal anastomosis. 3% recurrence rate
   SE: Duodenal stump leakage; Dumping; Bile reflux; Wt ↓; Anaemia; Malabsorption
2. **Tuncal V&P:** Simple op c̄ low mort. Rx of choice in poor risk, emergency, young, & patients c̄ psych history
   SE: High recurrence rate if incomplete Vag. Diarrhoea (2% very bad, occurs in 10%); Dumping; Bile reflux; Malabsorption occurs but less common than c̄ Billroth II
3. **Truncal Vag & Antrectomy:** Low recurrence rate
   SE: Anastamotic leakage; Dumping; Diarrhoea; Bile reflux
4. **Selective Vag & Gastrojejunostomy (GJ):** Used in elderly as technically straightforward. If SE, GJ can be closed. Not suitable for bleeding ulcer. Bypasses duodenum.
   SE: Bile reflux. High recurrence rate
5. **Proximal Gastric Vag (highly selective):** Op of choice c̄ experienced surgeon. Safe as gut not opened & no pyloroplasty needed. Technically difficult. 5–15% recurrence rate
   SE: Uncommon. Rarely diarrhoea; Reflux; Dumping

Complications of Ulcers

BLEEDING

Causes of Haematemesis (LIST 4 GIT)

>80% of episodes due to PU

1. Chronic PU
2. Acute erosions
3. Mallory-Weiss syndrome
4. Varices
5. Tumours esp gastric
6. Drugs esp Aspirin
7. Blood dyscrasias
8. PAN
9. Hereditary telangiectasia (Osler-Weber-Rendu)
10. Uraemia
11. Amyloidosis
12. Idiopathic
13. Polyps
14. Previous upper GIT surgery
15. Recent aortic graft

MANAGEMENT: 1. Bed rest; Lower head of bed; XM; Analgesia; Pass NG tube. Don't feed if bleeding

2. Look for signs of bleeding: PR ↑, BP ↓; Pallor; BP ↓ on transfusion; Blood from NG tube
3. Transfuse if: Acute signs of bleeding; Hb <10gdl; h/o high blood loss; Shock unless due to pancreatitis, perforation
4. Determine cause: Endoscopy, Ba meal. Angiography
5. Surgery if: Repeated haem, Perf or Chr GU & Py.S in >45yrs

Types of op: a) GU: Billroth I or Excision c̄ V&P

b) DU: V&P

c) Acute erosions (avoid op if poss): Partial gastrectomy, Total gastrectomy or Vag & drainage

PERFORATION

Occurs in 10% ulcers esp ant chr DU. 90% M. 5–10% mort

CLIN: Pain ppt by mvt. Occ Vom. Later Shock; Peritonitis & PI

INVESTIGATIONS: • CXR or Erect AXR:

Free gas

RX: A Medical: Analgesia; Drip & suck; Antibiotics

B. Surgical: 1. Op of choice is simple oversewing of ulcer. Many will require subsequent surgery
2. Immediate definitive treatment of ulcer:

Indications: 1. Perf c̄ haem & stenosis
2. ? malignancy
3. If risk of obst
4. Large perf

Types of Op: Vag & drainage or gastrectomy

DD:
1. Perf appendix
2. Ac pancreatitis
3. Ac cholecystitis
4. Perf Ca or diverticula of colon
5. MI
6. Pulmonary disease

PYLORIC STENOSIS (Py.S)

CLIN: Vom++ of bile free undigested stagnant food; Wt ↓; Usually painless. Splash; Visible peristalsis (L to R); Mass

METABOLIC SE: 1. Dehydration
2. Metabolic Alkalosis
3. Scanty urine at first alkaline but then paradoxically acidic
4. Urea ↑
5. HypoCa^{2+} → tetany

INVESTIGATIONS: • U&E
• Ba meal
• Endoscopy

RX: Correct U&E c̄ IV drip; NG tube. Vit C. Then Surgery: Polya or Vag & drainage

DD:
1. Ca stomach
2. Post-op
3. Mucosal diaphragm
4. Adult hypertrophic Py.S
5. Corrosives
6. LN ↑
7. Benign tumours
8. Foreign body
9. Ca pancreas

Complications of Ulcer Surgery

Post-Vag SE (LIST 5 GIT)

1. Diarrhoea
2. Belching
3. Abdominal distension
4. Cardiospasm
5. ? ↑ incidence of gall stones
6. Dysphagia
7. Rarely dumping

Post-Gastrectomy SE (LIST 6 GIT)

1. Dumping syndrome:
   a) Early
   b) Late
2. Stomal ulceration
3. Vomiting
4. Abdo distension
5. Nutritional:
   a) Osteomalacia
   b) Fe, B12, Folate deficiency
   c) Hypoproteinaemia
6. Small stomach syndrome
7. Increased risk of carcinoma in gastric remnant
8. Recrudescence of TB
9. Fistula
10. Osteoporosis
11. Obstruction:
    Eg Stomal oedema, Stomal stenosis, Intusussception

DUMPING SYNDROME

50% immediately post-gastrectomy decreasing to 5% at 5yrs

AETIOLOGY: ? gastric incontinence & gastroduodenal reflux

GENERAL CLIN: Fullness; Nausea; Regurgitation; Dizziness; Flushing; Sweating; Palps & faintness after meals

GENERAL INVESTIGATIONS: • FBC
• BG
• Dumping provocation test meals

EARLY DUMPING: Post-prandial esp ppt by hyperosmolar fluids

Op Cause: Resection> drainage >Highly selective Vag

Rx: Avoid ppt foods. Occ surgery eg convert Polya to Billroth I; Small reversed jejunal loop; Revise pyloroplasty

LATE DUMPING: Occurs 2 hrs post-prandial. Occ due to BG ↓

Rx: Avoid ppt foods

VOMITING OR REGURGITATION

Occurs in 25%. Rarely severe

AETIOLOGY: Common SE of GJ. Gastric outlet obst eg Py.S; Reflux. In Polya, due to afferent loop obst

FOOD VOMITING: Common. If it stops then recurs suspect Ca or stomal ulcer

BILE VOMITING: Occurs in 2%. If severe, Rx: Roux-en-Y & Vag or convert Polya to Billroth I

RECURRENT ULCERATION

AETIOLOGY: 1. Incomplete surgical Rx
2. Inadequate drainage
3. ZE 2% even when complete Vag
N.B Anastomotic (stomal) ulcer commonest after Polya

INVESTIGATIONS: • Fasting Gastrin
• Pentagastrin test
• Insulin

RX: Treat underlying cause eg complete Vag

OBSTRUCTION

AETIOLOGY: 1. Early stomal oedema
2. Stomal stenosis
3. 2° to Polya: Twisting, herniation, or intussusception of loop

RX: Drip & suck ± op

"SMALL STOMACH" SYNDROME

Op Cause: High gastrectomy

CLIN: Post-prandial fullness; Appetite ↓

FISTULA

Duodenal >Gastric >Gastro-jejuno-colic

DUODENAL FISTULA: Mainly leakage after Polya
Rx: If persists >2–3/52, then feeding jejunostomy needed

GASTRIC FISTULA: Anastomotic breakdown after Polya or Billroth I. Dangerous
Rx: Trial of conservative Rx. Close defect at op

GASTRO-JEJUNO-COLIC FISTULA: Usually 2° to Ca or Stomal ulcer. Severe diarrhoea & cachexia
Rx: Excise components of fistula & do high gastrectomy

DIARRHOEA

CONTINUOUS (2%): If Wt ↓ & steatorrhoea suspect nonoperative cause
Rx: Codeine, antispasmodics

EPISODIC:
Op Cause: Truncal Vag >selective Vag
Rx: Anticipatory Codeine or Lomotil. Occ reversed jejunal loop

DYSPHAGIA

AETIOLOGY: Immediate post-Vag oesophagitis

NUTRITIONAL

AETIOLOGY: 1. Poor diet due to small capacity of stomach
2. Rapid throughput of food
3. IF ↓
4. Blind loop syndrome

1. Wt LOSS

2. IDA:
Op Cause: Billroth II >V&P
Rx: Oral Iron

3. VIT B12 & FOLATE DEF:
Rx: B12 injections & folic acid supplements

4. OSTEOMALACIA:
Op Cause: GJ
Rx: Vit D

5. OSTEOPOROSIS:
Op Cause: Resection >Vag

OTHER COMPLICATIONS

1. ↑ chance of malignancy in gastric remnant
2. Recurrence of TB
3. Pancreatitis or pancreatic fistula
4. ? Gallstone formation

TUMOURS OF STOMACH

Benign Tumours

Rare

LEIOMYOMA

Commonest. Present c̄ bleeding. 10% become malignant

HYPERPLASTIC GASTRIC POLYPS

Ass c̄ gastritis. Sl malignant potential

ADENOMATOUS GASTRIC POLYPS

In 50% ass c̄ Ca

RX: Remove

Carcinoma of Stomach

EPIDEMIOLOGY: Commonest in Japan,

USSR, S.Am. Low in USA whites. In UK, 3rd commonest Ca. M>F. Ass c̄ blood gp A & high dietary nitrosamines. Incidence increases c̄ age. Incidence decreasing in the West

PREDISPOSING FACTORS: 1. Achlorhydria, PA 6x
2. Chr gastritis & intestinal metaplasia
3. Benign GU (1%)
4. Partial gastrectomy
5. Gastric polyps (10%)

SITES: Pre-pyloric >lesser curvature >cardia, greater curvature, fundus

TYPES: Almost all AdenoCa. Can be Ulcerative; Polypoid; Diffuse infiltrative (linitis plastica)—"leather bottle stomach"; Mucinous

CLIN: Wt ↓; Epigastric pain; Abdo mass; Anaemia; Anorexia. Occ Py.S. Then Dysphagia; N&V; LN ↑; J; Haem; Ascites; Signs of mets

INVESTIGATIONS:
- Endoscopy & biopsy
- Ba meal
- FOB
- Cytology
- Laparotomy
- Hollander test

SPREAD: 1. Direct: Local spread esp to oesophagus. Transcoelomic spread often to ovaries (Krukenberg)
2. Lymph: Stomach drains to 4 areas & thence to Coeliac nodes. Occ spread to L supraclavicular LN (Troisier's)
3. Blood: Mets to liver via portal venous system

RX: 25% inoperable; 50% palliative or exploratory surgery; 25% "curative" surgery
1. **"Curative Surgery":** Use abdo approach
   a) **Distal Tumours**: Radical sub-total gastrectomy. Remove omentum, LNs & involved organs eg spleen. Then Billroth II
   b) **Proximal Tumours**: Total gastrectomy c̄ removal of omentum, LNs, tail of pancreas & spleen. Then Roux-en-Y
2. **Palliative Surgery:** Poor prog. Bypass op eg Gastrojejunostomy
3. **Inoperable:** Mousseau-Barbin tube; Supportive measures esp analgesia. Occ Cyt.T or X-Rad

COMPLICATIONS: 1. Obst of Pylorus or cardia
2. Haem
3. Perf c̄ peritonitis
4. Fistula esp Gastro-Colic
5. Acanthosis nigricans

PROG: <10% 5yr survival. Worst if linitis plastica type, at cardia, LN involvement or mets

DD:
1. Ca Caecum
2. Uraemia
3. PA
4. GU
5. Benign gastric tumour

GASTRITIS

May be acute or chronic. Chr Gastritis c̄ intestinal metaplasia is pre-malignant

Chronic Superficial Gastritis

Inflam of supf mucosa. Ass c̄ cigs, alcohol, hot food. ? → gastric atrophy

Chronic Atrophic Gastritis

Loss of gastric glands → loss of acid & IF. May → PA & eventually SACD

INVESTIGATIONS:
- Pentagastrin test
- Schilling test
- Intrinsic factor assay

Diffuse Giant Hypertrophic Gastritis (Menetrier's Disease)

M>F. Thick, irreg rugal folds. Ass c̄ hypoproteinaemia & oedema

MALABSORPTION

Causes of Malabsorption (LIST 7 GIT)

A. MUCOSAL LESIONS
  1. Coeliac disease
  2. Tropical sprue
  3. Whipple's disease
  4. Dermatitis Herpetiformis
  5. Intestinal lymphangiectasia

B. INFECTION
  1. Acute GE
  2. Traveller's diarrhoea
  3. Parasites: Eg Tapeworms, Giardia
  4. TB
  5. Blind loop syndrome

C. STRUCTURAL LESIONS
  1. Crohn's disease
  2. Gastric surgery
  3. Intestinal resection: Esp Terminal ileum
  4. Small intestinal diverticula
  5. Fistula
  6. Bowel ischaemia
  7. Systemic sclerosis
  8. Neoplasia: Eg Lymphoma, Leukaemia
  9. Amyloidosis
  10. Intestinal pseudo-obstruction

D. NON-GIT DISEASES
  1. Endocrine:
     a) Addison's disease
     b) Hypothyroidism
     c) Diabetes
     d) Hypoparathyroidism
  2. Malignancy
  3. Extensive eczema or psoriasis
  4. Collagen vascular disease

E. METABOLIC ABNORMALITIES
  1. A-betalipoproteinaemia
  2. Hartnup disease
  3. Hypogammaglobulinaemia

F. DRUGS
  Eg Alcohol, Neomycin, Cholestyramine

G. MALDIGESTION
  1. Pancreatic insufficiency
  2. Alactasia
  3. Zollinger-Ellison syndrome
  4. Cholestasis: Esp Chronic liver disease & biliary tract obstruction

H. RADIATION

Chronic Superficial Gastritis

A gp of disorders characterised by nutritional defs eg Fe, Folate, Vit D, K, & B12 & the following Clin features: Diarrhoea; Wt ↓; Abdo discomfort; Anaemia; SOB; Tiredness; Steatorrhoea

Coeliac Disease (Gluten Sensitive Enteropathy)

AETIOLOGY: ? immunological. Occ familial. Ass c̄ IgA def, HLA-Dw3 & HLA-A8

CLIN: a) Adults
Steatorrhoea; Wt ↓; Abdo pain & swelling; Tiredness; Infertility
b) Child (Usually presents before age of 3)
Failure to thrive; Misery & irritability; Oedema; Glossitis; Alactasia; Bruising & bleeding; Polyneuritis; Bone pain; Tetany. Later Clubbing; SACD; Infantalism; Dwarfism

INVESTIGATIONS:
- Exclude other causes of malabsorption eg CF by sweat test
- Small bowel Ba studies
- Jejunal biopsy, then gluten free diet, then repeat biopsy. Look for subtotal villous atrophy, which responds to the diet

RX: Gluten free diet for life. If severely ill, use steroids

COMPLICATIONS:

1. Malignancy:
a) Lymphoma of Small Intestine Esp Jejunum
Clin: Malaise & malabsorption despite adherence to diet; GI bleeding; Abdo mass; Skin rashes
Rx: Laparotomy ± resection. X-Rad; Cyt.T
Prog: Poor
b) Other Ca in GIT

2. Ulceration: Rare. Occ → stricture
Clin: Malaise; Fever; GI bleed despite adherence to diet
Rx: Steroids, surgical excision
Prog: Poor

3. 2° Pancreatic Insufficiency

Dermatitis Herpetiformis

Skin lesion ass c̄ mild gluten sensitive

enteropathy, HLA-A8. Occ pre-malignant → lymphoma

RX: Gluten free diet. Dapsone

Tropical Sprue

Occurs esp in visitors to tropics. Cause unknown. May remit spontaneously

CLIN: Steatorrhoea; Anaemia; Glossitis & stomatitis; Abdo pain. Occ Oedema; Pigmentation. Variable latent period & course

INVESTIGATION: • Diagnosis by exclusion
- Faeces for parasites
- Jejunal biopsy: Less severe sub-total villous atrophy than Coeliac disease, & eosinophilia
- FBC: Megaloblastic anaemia
- B12 & Folate levels
- Tests for other causes of malabsorption

RX: Tetracycline & Folate for >6/12

Whipple's Disease

Esp middle aged white men. Bacterial causes. Deposits of glycoproteins in macrophages esp of small intestine

CLIN: Wt ↓; Diarrhoea; Migratory polyarthralgia. Often LN ↑; Skin pigmentation; Abdo pain; Anaemia. Occ Fever; Hypoproteinaemia

INVESTIGATIONS: • X-R joints
- Small bowel Ba studies
- GI biopsy: Foamy PAS +ve macrophages

RX: Penicillin & Streptomycin for 2/52 then Tetracycline for 1yr

Intestinal Lymphangiectasia

AETIOLOGY: Adult: 2° to Ca or infection. Child: Hypoplasia of lymph vessels

CLIN: Steatorrhoea; Hypoproteinaemia; Limb oedema

INVESTIGATIONS: • GI biopsy: May show dilated lymph vessels
- Lymphangiogram (technically difficult)

RX: MCT ± laparotomy c̄ resection

Small Bowel Malignancy

CARCINOMA

Very rare. Ass c̄ Coeliac disease, Crohn's disease

LYMPHOMA

A. 1° LYMPHOMA

CLIN: Wt ↓; Fever; Pain; Malabsorption; Clubbing; Abdo mass

INVESTIGATIONS: • Jejunal biopsy
- Sm bowel Ba studies
- Lymphangiography

RX: Surgery. X-Rad. Cyt.T. Steroids

COMPLICATIONS: 1. Perf
2. Ulcer
3. GI bleed

Two special types of 1° Lymphoma:

i) **MEDITERRANEAN:** Occurs esp in Mediterranean, Middle-east & Tropics. Mainly seen in poor young men
Clin: Malabsorption; Abdo pain
Investigations: • Jejunal biopsy
Rx: Steroids & X-Rad or Cyt.T

ii) **ALPHA-CHAIN DISEASE:** M=F. Rare. Pre-malignant. ↑ heavy alpha chains of IgA. Type of Mediterranean lymphoma
Investigations: • Jejunal biopsy: Absent or stumpy swollen villi
- PPE
- Immunology: Detects α chains

Rx: X-Rad & steroids; Cyt.T & steroids or antibiotics

B. 2° LYMPHOMA

Usually 2° to coeliac disease

Intestinal Pseudo-obstruction

Syndrome mimicking mechanical obstruction

Causes of Intestinal Pseudo-obst (LIST 8 GIT)

A. ACUTE
1. Coeliac disease
2. Pneumonia
3. CCF
4. Pancreatitis
5. Idiopathic

B. CHRONIC
1. Systemic sclerosis
2. Amyloidosis
3. Hypothyroidism

INVESTIGATIONS: • X-R: Dilatation, ↓ mobility, ↑ transit time

Systemic Sclerosis

CLIN (GIT): Steatorrhoea; Diarrhoea &/or constipation

INVESTIGATION: • X-R: Dilatation of duodenum, open mouthed diverticula, pseudostrictures

RX: Antibiotics

PROG: Poor

Intestinal Resection

Malabsorption worse if distal resection; long length resected or ileocaecal valve removed

EFFECTS: 1. Loss of bile salts → malabsorption of fats & Vit A, D; Watery diarrhoea & results in formation of oxalate stones. Ass c̄ resection of terminal ileum
2. ↑ Gall stones
3. PU
4. Diarrhoea. Esp ass c̄ loss of ileo-caecal valve
5. Vit B12 def. Ass c̄ resection of terminal ileum
6. Blind loop syndrome. Bacterial overgrowth → malabsorption

RX: Low fat, MCT diet; Vit B12; Cimetidine. Cholestyramine if diarrhoea 2° to bile salt irritation of colon. If large resection may need reversal of a short bowel segment

Giardia lamblia

Ass c̄ agammaglobulinaemia

CLIN: May be asymptomatic. Abdo pain & diarrhoea. Occ → Malabsorption

INVESTIGATIONS: • Duodenal intubation: Trophozoites in upper small bowel
• Stool for cysts

RX: Metronidazole. 2nd line Rx is Mepacrine

Alactasia

CONGENITAL

Rare. Neonates

RX: Lactose free diet

PRIMARY

Many races have adult alactasia

CLIN: Most asymptomatic. Occ Abdo pain & diarrhoea; Rarely steatorrhoea

INVESTIGATIONS: • Jejunal biopsy: No lactase activity
• Lactose tolerance test
• H_2 breath test

RX: Lactose free diet

SECONDARY

Common in children esp c̄ GE

Abetalipoproteinaemia

Rare, inherited. ↓ β-Lipoproteins

CLIN: Steatorrhoea; Retinitis pigmentosa; Acanthocytes; CNS signs eg Ataxia

RX: Vitamin E

Drug Induced Malabsorption

CAUSES: 1. Cholestyramine
2. Neomycin
3. Alcohol
4. PAS acid

CROHN'S DISEASE

F=M. Most common in W.Europe & N.E.USA; Jews. Incidence is increasing. Peak onset 20–60 yrs. Ass c̄ Ank Sp & Ulc colitis amongst family members

AETIOLOGY: Unknown. ? Viral. Ass c̄ low fibre, high sugar diet

PATHOLOGY: Any part of GIT. Terminal ileum >Caecum >Asc colon >Proximal ileum. Transmural disease, usually segmental c̄ skip areas & strictures. Ulcers; Fissures; Mesenteric LN ↑; Granulomas; Fibrosis; Fistulae. Fissures & oedema → cobblestone appearance

CLIN: Commonly Abdo pain; Malaise; Diarrhoea; Wt ↓; Fever; p.r bleed. Occ RIF abdo mass; Clubbing; Urgency & Incontinence. Remitting & relapsing course. Perianal lesions in 75% of cases c̄ colonic involvement eg Skin tags, Anal fissures, Abscesses, Sinuses, Fistulae

INVESTIGATIONS:
- Sigmoidoscopy & Rectal biopsy
- FBC, ESR
- Vit B12
- Double contrast barium studies
- Sinograms
- Exclude TB
- Stool culture
- Yersinia serology
- C-Reactive protein
- Serum immunoglobulins
- Radioisotope scanning c̄ Indium labelled leucocytes

RX: A. Medical:

General: High protein, fibre & calorie diet. B12, Fe, Folate. Occ low fat, lactose-free diet. Occ parenteral feeding
Specific: Steroids &/or Salazopyrine in acute attack. Azathioprine may spare steroids. Metronidazole. Cholestyramine

B. Surgical:

Indications: 1. GIT obst
2. Toxic dilatation
3. Failure of medical Rx
4. Fistula, perianal disease, abscess, perf & large GI bleed
5. Childhood growth retardation
6. To exclude other causes of acute abdo esp appendictis

Ops: Preserve as much bowel as possible. Cover op c̄ steroids
Types: 1. Stricturoplasty
2. Simple resection of diseased segment only
3. Subtotal colectomy & ileorectal anastomosis
4. Panproctocolectomy & Ileostomy

Recurrence of ileal disease is lowest c̄ panproctocolectomy

Intestinal Complications of Crohn's Disease (LIST 9 GIT)

A. COMMON
1. Stricture
2. Fistula
3. Anorectal disorders
4. Abscess
5. Malabsorption
6. Intestinal obst

B. RARE
1. Perf
2. Toxic dilatation
3. Small bowel or colonic Ca
4. Massive haem

C. COMPLICATIONS OF Rx

Systemic Complications (see LIST 11 GIT)

ULCERATIVE COLITIS

F>M. Common in N & S. Europe, US whites, Jews. Ass c̄ Ank Sp. Familial

AETIOLOGY: ? viral, ? auto-immune. ? allergic

PATHOLOGY: Diffuse continuous inflam mucosal disease. Can affect whole colon but in sub gp only rectum (Ulcerative proctitis). Crypt abscesses & pseudopolyps

CLIN: Bloody diarrhoea & mucus p.r. L sided abdo pain & tenesmus. Wt ↓; N&V; Fever; Clubbing
In acute attack: Diarrhoea++; Malaise; Fever; PR ↑; Dehydration
Course: 10% 1 attack only; 10% continuous symptoms; 80% intermittent symptoms. 2 threats to life:
a) Acute severe attack
b) Ca ass c̄ chr active pancolitis for >10yrs

INVESTIGATIONS:
- Sigmoidoscopy & rectal biopsy
- Ba enema
- Colonoscopy
- FBC, ESR, U&E, LFT
- Stool examination
- Radioisotope scanning c̄ Indium labelled leucocytes

RX: A. Medical:

1. Mild attacks ie ass c̄ less than 4 bowel actions per day: High roughage diet; Fe; Oral steroids 4–6/52; Daily steroid enema until sigmoidoscopy norm; Suphasalazine (SE: N&V, headache, rash, fever, haemolytic anaemia. Ass c̄ infertility in M if used >3yrs)

2. Ulcerative proctitis: Sulphasalazine. Steroid enemas. Occ Na^+ cromoglycate
3. Severe attack: Hospital admission essential
   a) Parenteral nutrition: IV fluids, calories, protein
   b) Replacement therapy: Blood, K^+; Fe; Vitamins
   c) Relieve diarrhoea: Codeine, Lomotil
   d) ? antibiotics esp Metronidazole
   e) IV Prednisolone
   f) Steroid enemas
   g) Daily girth measurement to monitor for toxic dilatation

   If improvement, after 5 days of Rx revert to oral steroids; otherwise urgent surgery
4. Maintenance of remission: Sulphasalazine for rest of life

B. Surgical:

Indications: 1. Failure of intensive medical Rx in severe attack: Esp in children; Elderly; & if Extensive colitis
2. Toxic dilatation of colon as ↑ risk of perf
3. Perf
4. Bleeding++: Rare
5. Chr symptoms despite medical Rx
6. Total colitis >10yrs duration as malignancy risk++
7. Suspected Ca
8. Stricture
9. Chr pelvic complications
10. Systemic complications c̄ medical Rx failure
11. Growth retardation in child
12. Multiple GI complications

Types: 1. Panproctocolectomy c̄ permanent ileostomy
SE Ileostomy problems; Impotence; Renal calculi
2. Subtotal colectomy c̄ ileorectal anastomosis
Controversial: Risk of Diarrhoea; Ca; Leak at anastomosis
3. Proctocolectomy c̄ ileoanal anastomosis

Systemic complications (see LIST 11 GIT): Compared to Crohn's disease, Ulc colitis more often affects the liver & biliary tract & is ass c̄ pyoderma gangrenosa

PROG: Following 1st yr survival post-panproctocolectomy, normal life expectancy. Now better survival rates due to improved medical & surgical Rx

DD:
1. Crohn's disease
2. Amoebic colitis
3. Salmonellosis
4. Shigella
5. IBS
6. TB
7. Diverticulosis
8. Campylobacter
9. Cl.difficile
10. Ischaemic bowel disease
11. Lymphomas
12. Acute ileitis c̄ mesenteric adenitis
13. Gonococcal proctitis

Intestinal Complications of Ulc Colitis (LIST 10 GIT)

1. Toxic dilatation
2. Perf
3. Fissure-in-ano
4. Hypokalaemia
5. Infection
6. Large GI bleed
7. Hypoproteinaemia
8. Complications of Rx
9. Colonic Ca: Commoner than in Crohn's
10. Rarely:
    a) Fistula
    b) Strictures Esp 2° to Ca

Extraintestinal Complications of IBD (LIST 11 GIT)

1. Skin lesions:
   a) Erythema nodosum
   b) Erythema multiforme
   c) Pyoderma gangrenosum
2. Ophthalmic:
   a) Uveitis
   b) Conjunctivitis
   c) Episcleritis
3. Hepatic:
   a) Fatty infiltration
   b) Pericholangitis
   c) Cirrhosis
   d) Biliary tract carcinoma
   e) CAH
   f) Gall stones
   g) Sclerosing cholangitis
   h) Amyloidosis
   i) Granulomata

→

4. Skeletal:
   a) Sacroiliitis
   b) Ank spondylitis
   c) Acute arthritis
   d) Osteomalacia
5. Aphthous ulcers
6. Psychiatric
7. Complications of treatment:
   Eg Steroid side effects
8. Clubbing
9. Childhood growth retardation
10. In Crohn's:
    a) Hyperoxaluria & oxalate stones
    b) Ureteric stenosis
    c) Pyelonephritis
    d) Hydronephrosis

MECKEL'S DIVERTICULUM

Remnant of vitello-intestinal duct. 2% pop; 2" long; 2ft from caecum (in ileum)

CLIN: Often asymptomatic. Occ abdo pain. Rarely: Perf & Peritonitis; PU → melaena; Ileo-ileal Intussusception; Umbilical fistula; Raspberry tumour; Vitello-intestinal band → obst, volvulus

APPENDICITIS

Common in western developed countries. In UK, affects 1/6th of pop during lifetime. M=F. Uncommon in infants & aged

AETIOLOGY: 1. Obstruction:
   a) Foreign bodies eg faecolith
   b) Strictures, bands
   c) Inflammation → lymphoid tissue ↑
   d) 2° to Ca caecum or ascending colon

2. Infection eg *E.coli*, *Strep faecalis*. May be 2° to obst

Acute Appendicitis

CLIN: Pain, usually umbilical then RIF, N&V; Constipation >diarrhoea; Anorexia; Fever; Malaise. Occ Frequency & Dysuria

INVESTIGATIONS:
- p.r
- Hb, WCC, U&E
- Urinalysis

RX: Appendicectomy covered c̄ Metronidazole

DD:
1. Mesenteric adenitis
2. Pyelonephritis
3. Ureteric colic
4. Acute cholecystitis
5. Crohn's disease
6. Diverticulitis
7. R. basal pneumonia
8. Diaphragmatic pleurisy
9. GE
10. Herpes
11. TB
12. Gynaecological:
    Eg Acute salpingitis, Torsion, Endometriosis

Acute Appendicitis c̄ Mass

AETIOLOGY: Appendix perf contained by omentum → mass

CLIN: Tender RIF mass; Pain usually for >3/7; Fever; Malaise

RX: Supportive measures eg IV fluids. Surgery: May be emergency or elective. Appendicectomy (if possible) & drainage of any abscess, covered by Metronidazole

DD:
1. Ca caecum
2. Ca colon
3. Crohn's disease
4. Empyema of gall bladder
5. Ovarian cyst
6. TB
7. Psoas abscess
8. Iliac artery aneurysm
9. Renal mass:
   Eg Pelvic kidney, Perinephric abscess or Hydronephrosis
10. Retroperitoneal tumour

Acute Appendicitis c̄ Perforation

CLIN: Malaise; Peritonitis; PR ↑; BP ↓; Abdo

tenderness & rigidity. Late, faecal vomiting

INVESTIGATIONS: • AXR
• Amylase
• Hb, WCC

RX: Drip & suck; Analgesia; Antibiotics. Surgery: Remove appendix; Peritoneal toilet; Catheter

DD:
1. Perf PU
2. Perf diverticula
3. Acute pancreatitis
4. Basal Pneumonia
5. Ruptured ectopic pregnancy
6. Perf gall bladder
7. Sup mesenteric artery occlusion

IRRITABLE BOWEL SYNDROME

Long standing colonic pain & variable bowel habit c̄ no evidence of organic disease. F>M. Esp 20–40 yrs. Ass c̄ abdo pain in childhood, colonic diverticula & migraine

AETIOLOGY:
1. Psychological anxiety
2. ? Low residue diet
3. Abnormal colonic motility
4. ? Food allergy

CLIN: 3 main types:
1. Spastic colon: Pain c̄ intermittent diarrhoea & constipation
2. Bouts of painless, watery diarrhoea (10%)
3. Post prandial upper abdo pain (25%). Mimicks gallbadder disease (hepatic flexure syndrome) or PU (splenic flexure syndrome)

Abdo pain is generally relieved by defaecation

RX: Exclude organic disease. Reassurance. High fibre diet. Antidiarrhoeal agents eg Codeine. For pain use bulk forming agents & antispasmodics eg Isogel, Colofac

DIARRHOEA

Causes of Diarrhoea (LIST 12 GIT)

A. ACUTE
1. Infection:
   a) Food poisoning eg Staph, Salmonella
   b) Viral eg Rotavirus
   c) Bacterial eg E.coli, Campylobacter, Cholera, Cl difficile
   d) Protozoan eg Amoebiasis
   e) Helminthic
2. Drugs:
   a) Pseudomembranous enterocolitis eg Lincomycin
   b) Antibiotics eg Ampicillin
3. Pelvic abscess
4. Ischaemic colitis
5. Allergy
6. Anxiety

B. CHRONIC
1. Post-operative:
   a) Vagotomy
   b) Gastrectomy
   c) Ileal resection
   d) Short circuit operations
   e) Pancreatectomy
2. Bowel diseases:
   a) Inflammatory bowel disease
   b) Tumours: Villous adenoma; Ca colon; Carcinoid tumour; WDHA syndrome; Familial polyposis coli; ZE syndrome
   c) Diverticulitis
   d) IBS
   e) Hirschprung's disease
   f) Intestinal ischaemia
   g) Fistula
3. Other causes of malabsorption leading to steatorrhoea: Eg Coeliac disease, Sprue, Chr pancreatitis
4. Irradiation
5. Metabolic:
   a) Diabetes
   b) Thyrotoxicosis
   c) Alactasia
   d) Pellagra
6. Chronic infections:
   a) TB
   b) Amoebiasis
   c) Actinomycosis
7. Spurious diarrhoea (2° to faecal impaction)
8. Anxiety neurosis
9. Drugs: Eg Purgatives

TWO TYPES:
1. True: a) Steatorrhoea
b) Watery diarrhoea
c) Watery diarrhoea & blood ± Mucus eg Ulc colitis, Ca
d) Mucus eg villous adenoma

c) Blood & mucus eg distal proctitis

2. False: a) Spurious (overflow)
b) Faecal frequency

GENERAL RX: Replace fluids. Correct any electrolyte imbalance. Drugs eg Codeine phosphate

CONSTIPATION

Causes of Constipation (LIST 13 GIT)

1. Low fibre diet
2. Severe dehydration
3. Luminal obstruction:
   a) Ca esp colon
   b) Hirschprung's disease
   c) Adult megacolon
   d) Stricture
   e) Faecal impaction
   f) Late pregnancy
4. Metabolic:
   a) Hypothyroidism
   b) Hypokalaemia
   c) Early pregnancy
   d) Hypercalcaemia
   e) Acute intermittent porphyria
   f) Lead poisoning
5. Drugs:
   Eg Opiates, Anticholinergics, $Al(OH)_3$
6. Painful ano-rectal conditions:
   Eg Fissures
7. Irritable bowel syndrome
8. Depression
9. Spinal cord lesions
10. Prolonged bed rest
11. Chronic purgation

GENERAL RX: p.r exam ± manual removal. High fibre diet. Fluids & exercise. Occ enema

Various Types of Laxatives: a) Surface active agents eg DSS
A stool softener. Used if stools very hard (c̄ stimulant added eg Dorbanex). SE: U&E changes

b) Liquid paraffin
Softens stool. Risk of loss of fat soluble vits, anal soiling & lipoid pneumonia. ? carcinogenic

c) Bulking agents eg Normacol; Isogel
Use c̄ water++. c/i Obstruction; Dysphagia

d) Osmotic agents eg Na^+, K^+, $MgPO_4$ & Lactulose
Nonabsorbed solutes. Useful in acute emergency acting in a few hrs. Lactulose occ used in elderly

e) Stimulant agents eg Castor oil, Anthracene (senna)
Peristalsis ↑. Castor oil acts quicker than Anthracene
Anthracene if overused → dilated colon, pseudostrictures (cathartic colon) & melanosis coli

DIVERTICULAR DISEASE

Common in West. M=F. Common in elderly. 95% of complications occur at sigmoid colon. Early onset R sided diverticulitis common in Japan & Hawaii

AETIOLOGY: Old age often ass c̄ proximal diverticular disease. Low dietary fibre ass c̄ sigmoid diverticular disease

Non-Inflammatory Diverticular Disease

DIVERTICULAR DISEASE OF THE SIGMOID COLON

Due to low fibre diet → hard faeces → intracolonic P ↑ → mucosal herniation at pts of vessel entry

CLIN: Usually asymptomatic. Occ Dyspepsia; Flatulence; Constipation; LIF pain. Occ Blood p.r

DD: 1. Ca
2. IBS
3. Renal colic

DIVERTICULAR DISEASE OF PROXIMAL COLON

Very common in >60yrs. All colon except sigmoid is thin walled c̄ many diverticula

CLIN: Occ asymptomatic. Constipation; Pellet-like faeces

INVESTIGATIONS OF NON-INFLAM DIVERTICULAR DISEASE

- Sigmoidoscopy
- Ba enema
- Colonoscopy
- WCC, ESR (not abnormal)

RX OF NON-INFLAM DIVERTICULAR DISEASE

High fibre diet. Excise if rare giant diverticulum

COMPLICATIONS OF NON-INFLAM DIVERTICULAR DISEASE

1. PERFORATION:
Rx: Drain abdomen c̄ a) Proximal colostomy c̄ exteriorisation of perf or b) partial colectomy

2. BLEEDING:
Clin: Usually sudden & painless
Investigation: • Selective mesenteric angiography
Rx: Bedrest. Occ embolisation. Rarely total colectomy c̄ ileo-rectal anastomosis

Inflammatory Diverticular Disease

ACUTE DIVERTICULITIS

CLIN: Acute onset. Pain over colon esp LIF; Fever; Malaise; Vom; Anorexia. Constipation &/or diarrhoea. Occ Signs of local or general peritonitis

CHRONIC DIVERTICULITIS

CLIN: Alternating constipation & diarrhoea → Obst c̄ Vom, Abdo pain & constipation. Periodic fresh p.r bleeding or melaena. Mimicks & may coexist c̄ Ca colon

INVESTIGATIONS OF DIVERTICULITIS

- Sigmoidoscopy
- Colonoscopy
- Ba enema
- AXR
- ESR, WCC ↑

RX OF DIVERTICULITIS

A. MEDICAL: Bed rest; Drip & suck; Analgesia; Antibiotics. Then Bran

B. SURGICAL:
Indications: a) ? Ca
b) Debilitating symptoms c̄ failure of medical Rx
Resection >Sigmoid myotomy

COMPLICATIONS OF DIVERTICULITIS

1. PERICOLIC ABSCESS:
Rx: Antibiotics. Drain. If faecal fistula forms, colectomy

2. PERITONITIS 2° TO PERF: 30% mort, higher if faecal peritonitis
Rx: Drain. Defunctioning colostomy c̄ exteriorisation, later resection

3. FISTULAE: Eg Vesico-colic fistula → pneumaturia
Rx: Resect involved colonic segment c̄ anastomosis & close bladder defect in one stage op or staged resections
DD: 1. Ca colon
2. Ca bladder
3. Crohn's disease
4. Post X-Rad necrosis
5. Ulcerative colitis

4. OBSTRUCTION: Rare. Seen in chr diverticulitis
Rx: Enema. If medical Rx fails then colostomy & 2–3wks later resect affected segment ± closure of colostomy

5. SUDDEN BLEEDING: Usually self limiting. Rarely Rx hemicolectomy

"Solitary" Diverticula

Asc colon & Caecum >Transverse & sigmoid colon

CLIN: Usually asymptomatic. Occ Abdo pain c̄ mass. Rarely perf

RX: If inflam, hemicolectomy. Excise giant diverticular

DD: 1. Ac Appendicitis
2. Appendix abscess
3. Ca caecum

POLYPS

Types of Polyps (LIST 14 GIT)

1. Hamartomatous:
   a) Juvenile
   b) Peutz-Jegher
2. Benign lymphoid polyposis
3. Metaplastic
4. Pseudopolyposis: 2° to Ulc colitis or Crohn's disease
5. Adenomatous:
   a) Tubular
   b) Villous
   c) Familial polyposis coli
   d) Gardner's syndrome
   e) Turcot's syndrome
6. Canada-Cronkhite syndrome

Hamartomatous Polyps

JUVENILE

Child & young adult. Esp Rectum, distal colon

CLIN: Intussusception & abdo pain; p.r bleed; Rectal prolapse

PEUTZ-JEGHER

Aut dom. Polyps in stomach, duodenum, small intestine >colon, rectum. Ass c̄ mucocutaneous pigmentation. Occ pre-malignant

CLIN: Abdo pain; Anaemia; Intussusception

RX: Ascertain polyp distribution then short segment resection or enterotomy & polypectomy

Benign Lymphoid Polyposis

Inflammatory. Uncommon & asymptomatic

Metaplastic Polyps

Esp rectum. Common. ? viral. Usually asymptomatic

Pseudopolyposis

2° to Ulc colitis & Crohn's

Adenomatous

Vary from small tubular adenomas to large villous papillomas
Pre-malignant esp if: >2cm diameter; Sessile; High degree of dysplasia; Villous; Multiple

CLIN: Usually asymptomatic. Occ p.r bleed. Villous papilloma → mucous diarrhoea c̄ K^+ loss

RX: Excision at colonoscopy. Regular review c̄ Ba enema & endoscopy

Two special conditions:

1. **FAMILIAL POLYPOSIS COLI:** Aut dom. Multiple polyps usually develop when 20–30yrs old. 20% no FH. Highly pre-malignant, Ca taking 10 yrs to develop. Needs screening as usually symptoms occur when Ca already present. Ass c̄ duodenal & gastric polyps
   Rx: Counsel & investigate family. Total colectomy c̄ ileorectal anastomosis. Follow-up c̄ 6 mthly sigmoidoscopies
2. **GARDNER'S SYNDROME:** Rare. Familial polyposis, osteomas, osteosclerosis, bad teeth, sebaceous cysts, lipomas, desmoid tumours esp post-op or in pregnancy. No clear distinction from familial polyposis coli

Canada Chronkhite

Multiple hyperplastic polyps ass c̄ alopecia, nail dystrophy & pigmentation. Very rare. Bad prognosis

Investigations of Polyps

- Sigmoidoscopy
- Colonoscopy
- Double contrast Ba enema
- Biopsy

Ca COLON

Common in USA, S.Am & W Europe. Esp 60–70yrs. F=M. 75% rectum, sigmoid colon. 25% Caecum. Asc colon >transverse, desc >hepatic splenic colon. Often AdenoCa

AETIOLOGY: 1. Low residue diet
2. Neoplastic polyps
3. Ulc colitis
4. Familial polyposis coli
5. Colonic urinary diversion
6. ? High fat diet → high bile acids
7. ? Low cruciferous vegetable diet
8. Abnormal gut bacterial flora
9. Post-cholecystectomy (small risk)

CLIN: A. Ca R colon: May present c̄ IDA only. Colicky abdo pain & vague dyspepsia related to food; Malaise, weakness, anaemia & Wt ↓; Occ mass in RIF c̄ tenderness due to Ca, abscess, or 2° to obst. Rarely perf → peritonitis, fistula. Late Bowel obstruction (but this may be early if Ca near the ileocaecal valve); Ascites; Signs & symptoms of mets esp J

B. Ca L colon: Alteration in bowel habit eg alternating diarrhoea & constipation; Large bowel obstruction; Abdo pain & distension. Occ Perf → peritonitis; Mass in LIF due to pericolic abscess; Vesico-colic fistula; Blood & mucus p.r. Late, Gastrocolic fistula; Signs & symptoms of mets

INVESTIGATIONS: • p.r
• Sigmoidoscopy
• Ba enema
• Colonoscopy & biopsy
• LFT
• Liver scan
• CEA
• Laparotomy

SPREAD: Local & Lymph >Blood >Transcoelomic. Liver mets common

RX: If Op not indicated: Supportive treatment eg Analgesia
Surgical: Bowel prep inc pre-op antibiotics. Correct anaemia; Catheterise; Drip
1. Palliative surgery eg limited resection or bypass op ± Cyt.T
2. Curative surgery:
   a) No obst: Wide excision c̄ end to end anastomosis & remove LNs
   b) c̄ obst: Either emergency resection or defunctioning colostomy. Occ double-barrelled (Paul-Mikulicz) colostomy
   c) c̄ peritonitis: Colostomy & drainage. Occ resection attempted

COMPLICATIONS: 1. Obstruction L>R
2. Perf
3. Fistula
4. Haem, L>R. Uncommon

PROG: Overall, 50% 5yr survival. Related to grade & stage

DD: A. R colon: 1. Mass in RIF (LIST 15 GIT)
2. Gall stones
3. Piles
4. Polyps
5. IBD
6. Appendicitis
7. IBS

B. L colon: 1.Ulc colitis
2. Crohn's
3. Polyps
4. Diverticulitis
5. Piles
6. Ischaemic colitis
7. Sigmoid volvulus
8. Endometriosis
9. IBS
10. Impacted faeces

Causes of Mass in Right Iliac Fossa (LIST 15 GIT)

1. Appendix abscess
2. Neoplastic:
   a) Ca Caecum
   b) Ca Colon
   c) Ovarian tumour
   d) Renal tumour
   e) Carcinoid tumour
3. Crohn's disease
4. Infection:
   a) TB
   b) Amoebiasis
   c) Schistosomiasis
   d) Actinomycosis
5. Empyema of gall bladder
6. Ectopic pregnancy
7. Intussusception
8. Fibroid
9. Psoas abscess

ISCHAEMIA OF GUT

Four special features of gut predisposing to ischaemia: High GI venous P; Avalvular portal system; Sensitivity to arterioles to catecholamines; Ends of capillaries vulnerable to low flow

SYSTEMIC EFFECTS. 1. Exudate of protein → hypovolaemia, BP ↓, haemoconcentration
2. Platelet stickiness ↑ → emboli
3. Mucosal cell barrier breakdown → bacteraemia, septicaemia, endotoxin shock

Acute Small Bowel Ischaemia

AETIOLOGY: a) Arterial embolism 2° to Rh Ht disease or mural thromb post MI or AF.
b) Arterial thromb 2° to atheroma; polycythemia.
c) Prolonged low flow 2° to CO ↓; Digoxin; Haemoconcentration & ass c̄ DIC.
d) Venous thromb

ACUTE MESENTERIC OCCLUSION

Sup mesenteric >inf mesenteric or coeliac artery

CLIN: Sudden, severe abdo pain colicky then continuous. Shock. Then ileus

RX: A. Medical: Correct fluid deficit, use CVP; Gentamicin & Metronidazole; Heparin
B. Surgical: Urgent laparotomy; Embolectomy or aortomesenteric graft. 24hrs later re-op & resect non-viable small bowel loops. Delay in Rx → mesenteric infarction

MESENTERIC INFARCTION

Very dangerous esp if CCF & in old. Better prog if due to non-occlusive ischaemia

CLIN: Severe, diffuse abdo pain; Ileus; Vom & diarrhoea; Hypovolaemic shock. Then peritonitis & occ melaena

RX: A. Medical: Rx as above
B. Surgical: Massive bowel resection

Investigation of Small Bowel Ischaemia

- PCV
- U&E
- WCC
- LDH
- Amylase
- AXR: "Thumbprinting"
- Angiography
- Peritoneal tap: Blood

Prog of Small Bowel Ischaemia

Very poor. Worst in aged, occlusive disease & c̄ infarct

Chr Intestinal Ischaemia

Occlusion/sten of >2 visceral trunks esp middle aged c̄ atheroma

CLIN: Epigastric post prandial pain "mesenteric angina"; Wt ↓ due to fear of eating; Constipation, later malabsorption → diarrhoea. Occ central abdo bruit

INVESTIGATIONS:
- Endoscopy
- Cholangiography
- Ba studies
- Pancreatic function tests
- If above −ve, then angiography c̄ lat views

RX: Side to side aortomesenteric anastomosis

COMPLICATION: Mesenteric infarction

Coeliac Axis Compression Syndrome

May not be a clin entity. F>M. Postulated intermittent compression by diaphragm causing upper abdo ache ppt by food & relieved by lying down. Ass c̄ epigastric bruit

RX: ?? Angiography & decompression op

Colonic Ischaemia

Esp elderly. Less common than small bowel ischaemia. Ass c̄ Atheroma; "Pill"; Diabetes; Previous colonic surgery & rarely PAN; Trauma inc arteriography; Hernia; or Volvulus

ISCHAEMIC COLITIS

10× commoner than gangrenous ischaemic colitis

CLIN: Mild fever; Abdo pain & bloody diarrhoea. N&V; L abdo tenderness

INVESTIGATIONS: • WCC
• Sigmoidoscopy
• AXR
• Ba enema: "Thumbprinting"

RX: IV drip, analgesia, antibiotics. If stricture may need colonic resection

COMPLICATIONS: 1. Stricture (in 50%): may resolve spontaneously
2. Gangrene

GANGRENOUS ISCHAEMIC COLITIS

CLIN: Severe sudden abdo pain; Peritonitis; Shock

RX: Correct hypovolaemia; Antibiotics. Resect necrotic bowel, double barrelled colostomy & later anastomosis

Focal Intestinal Ischaemia

Ass c̄ PAN; Rh Arth; SLE; Dermatomyositis; Wegener's; Crohn's

CLIN: Variable. Stricture; Perf; Haem; Ulcer

BOWEL OBSTRUCTION

Causes of Mechanical Bowel Obst (LIST 16 GIT)

Commonest are: Hernia, Ca Colon & Adhesions

A. LUMINAL
1. Faecal impaction
2. Foreign body
3. Meconium ileus
4. Gall stones
5. Food residue
6. Parasites: Eg Ascaris
7. Pedunculated tumour

B. BOWEL WALL
1. Cong atresia
2. Crohn's disease
3. Ulcerative collitis
4. Diverticulitis
5. Benign & Malignant tumours
6. TB
7. Hirschprung's disease
8. Strictures: Eg Inflammatory, Neoplastic, Traumatic, Post radiation

C. OUTSIDE BOWEL WALL
1. Internal or external herniae: Esp strangulated
2. Adhesions
3. Volvulus
4. Bands: Eg Meckel's diverticulum, Ladd's bands
5. Intussusception
6. Tumours: Eg Ovarian

Common causes at different age gps:
Neonatal: Cong atresia, volvulus, Hirschprung's, meconium ileus
Infants: Intusussception, Hirschprung's, strangulated hernia
Young & middle aged: Strangulated hernia, adhesions, Crohn's
Elderly: Strangulated hernia, Ca, diverticulitis, impacted faeces

MECHANISMS:

A. Simple obst: Proximal bowel dilates c̄ fluid loss (worse for higher lesions). Initially ↑ peristalsis. Ischaemia → ulceration then perf. Bacterial toxins formed which on relief of obst → septicaemia & shock. Distal bowel is collapsed & empty

B. Closed loop obstruction: Accelerated version of simple obst. Ass c̄ sigmoid volvulus, obst hernia & torsion of small bowel
Clin: Gangrene; Perf; Infection (commoner than c̄ simple obst)

C. Strangulation: Transudate of bacterial toxins c̄ 2° peritonitis. Later gangrene & perf
Clin: Pain; Constipation (absolute); Vom; Distension. Usually dehydration & fever. Strangulation is difficult to distinguish from simple obst, often more toxic & occ signs of peritonitis

GENERAL INVESTIGATIONS: • Erect & supine AXR
• WCC
• Check hernial orifices
• Sigmoidoscopy
• Hb, U&E, XM

RX: Usually op except if: PI; Impacted faeces; Sigmoid volvulus (try sigmoidoscopy ± flatus tube decompression); Occ if many previous ops
Pre-op: Drip & suck; Correct U&E; Occ antibiotics
Surgery: Relieve obst eg divide adhesions. Assess bowel viability by observing peristalsis, colour, pulsation. Cover in hot warm pack & reassess. Decompress bowel. If resection needed for small bowel obst, resect & anastomose at op; For large bowel obst resect; colostomy & later anastomosis
Post-op care: Drip & suck; Analgesia; U&E regularly to monitor. Gradually introduce fluids

Volvulus

Twisting of bowel round mesenteric axis. Sigmoid colon, caecum, small bowel >Gall bladder, stomach

AETIOLOGY:
1. Abnormally mobile &/or loaded loop of bowel
2. Fixed apex of loop eg due to adhesions
3. Loop c̄ narrow base

SIGMOID VOLVULUS

4M:1F. Esp elderly. USSR, Scandinavian, African blacks >>UK. Ass c̄ constipation

CLIN: Sudden colicky pain c̄ gross distension of sigmoid colon. Can → gangrene, perf & peritonitis. Occ Recurrent mild attacks

INVESTIGATIONS:
- AXR: Dilated++ air filled bowel loop
- Sigmoidoscopy

RX: Rectal tube via sigmoidoscope to untwist & deflate. If fails, laparotomy c̄ decompression. Then elective resection of redundant sigmoid loop. If gangrene excise necrotic bowel c̄ double barrelled colostomy (Paul-Mikulicz procedure). Later colostomy closure

CAECAL VOLVULUS

Usually ass c̄ caecum having a long mesentery

CLIN: Acute pain c̄ distension R side

INVESTIGATIONS:
- AXR: Absent caecal gas on R. Distended bowel retains haustral pattern

RX: Untwisting c̄ decompression by caecostomy. Post-op adhesions may be beneficial

SMALL INTESTINAL VOLVULUS

Common in Africa. Usually small bowel loop fixed at apex by adhesions or by Meckel's remnant

CLIN: Acute intestinal obstruction. Occ → gangrene

RX: Untwist at op. Treat underlying cause

STOMACH VOLVULUS

Rare. Occ ass c̄ PU, Ca stomach, Diaphragmatic defect

CLIN: In acute form, severe abdo pain & distention. Vom

RX: Decompress & reduce volvulus at op

Paralytic Ileus (PI)

Causes of PI (LIST 17 GIT)

Commonest post-op

1. Post abdominal operation
2. Hypokalaemia
3. Peritonitis
4. Retroperitoneal haem
5. Ureteric colic
6. Diabetic coma
7. Fractures of spine or pelvis
8. Uraemia
9. Drugs:
   Eg Anticholinergics
10. Mesenteric ischaemia

AETIOLOGY:
1. ? Intrinsic nerve paralysis eg peritonitis
2. Autonomic nerve disfunction eg # pelvis, renal colic
3. Metabolic eg K^+ ↓, Urea ↑, diabetic coma
4. ↑ sympath activity eg post-op
5. ? Bowel distension

CLIN: Abdo distension; Constipation; Vom. PI normal for 1–2/7 post-op. Often have concurrent or 2° mechanical ileus

DD FROM MECHANICAL ILEUS:
1. PI rarely lasts >3/7
2. PI no BS; Mechl noisy BS
3. PI no pain; Mechl colic
4. AXR: PI diffuse distension c̄ fluid levels; Mechl localised

PROPHYLAXIS: NG tube; Correct U&E;

Gentle bowel handling at op

RX: Drip & suck until flatus passed & BS returns. Correct U&E. Occ Analgesia; Chlorpromazine

Endometriosis of Bowel

Found in 1/3 of pelvic ops for endometriosis, although often mild. Esp in appendix, caecum, sigmoid, rectosigmoid area, rectovaginal septa. Rarely ileum

CLIN: Lower abdo colicky pain c̄ bowel habit alteration ppt by periods. Occ fibrosis → stricture & obst

RX: Bilat oophorectomy. In young hormone Rx. Rarely resection of stricture needed

MEGACOLON

Chr colon dilatation ass c̄ severe constipation

TYPES: A. Congential:
1. Hirschprung's
2. Anal canal sten

B. Acquired: 1. Idiopathic
2. Laxatives
3. Chagas disease
4. Scleroderma

Hirschprung's Disease

8M:1F. Loss of colonic autonomic ganglia. Esp neonates, children. Most serious in neonates

CLIN: Abdo distension; Constipation; Vom. Failure to thrive. No overflow incontinence

INVESTIGATIONS:
- AXR
- Ba enema: Narrowed distal colon
- Anorectal P studies
- Rectal biopsy: Histochemistry ıse
- Balloon distension test

RX: Resect aganglionic segment., Abdomino-perineal pull-through anastomosis, preserving sphincter

Idiopathic Megacolon

Esp older children, adults. Ass c̄ mental handicap, poor development of bowel habit & personality disorders

CLIN: Abdo distension++; Impacted faeces; Constipation; Lax sphincter → faecal soiling

RX: Empty rectum by enemas, suppositories or stimulant cathartics. Occ anal dilatation. Teach good bowel habit. In adults, occ require colectomy & ileorectal anastomosis

FAMILIAL MEDITERRANEAN FEVER

Aut Rec. Esp Jews, Arabs, Armenians, siblings. Onset childhood to middle age

CLIN: Episodic pyrexia c̄ abdo pain ± rigors usually lasting 1–3/7. Occ Monoarthritis; Pleuritic pain; Skin rashes

INVESTIGATIONS:
- ESR
- WCC
- PPE

RX: Colchicine

COMPLICATIONS: Amyloidosis → spleen ↑; Proteinuria, ARF

CARCINOID TUMOURS & SYNDROME

Carcinoid Tumours

Derived from argentaffin cells. Appendix (25%) >Ileum >Rectum >Other sites eg Lung. Slight malignant potential

CLIN: Usually asymptomatic. Occ present as acute appendicitis; Bowel obst or Intussusception. If liver mets may → carcinoid syndrome

RX: Resect tumour

Carcinoid Syndrome

Occurs in 5% of tumours esp mid gut c̄ large liver mets

AETIOLOGY: Due to release of:

1. 5HT → ↑ gut motility; Diarrhoea; Cardia complications
2. Kallikrein → Vasodilation; Flushing; Asthma; Diarrhoea
3. Prostaglandins → Diarrhoea; ? facial flushing

CLIN: Liver ↑ ± abdo mass. Often initially watery diarrhoea & abdo pain. Then (occ yrs later) flushing of face neck ppt by alcohol, foods, emotion, histamine. Occ Telangiectasia; Pigmentation; Sclerodermatous & Pellagroid eruptions. In 50% PSt or TI → Ht failure. Occ Asthma

INVESTIGATIONS: • Urinary 5HIAA
• Plasma 5-HT

RX: A. Medical: 5-HT antagonists eg Methysergide for diarrhoea. H_1 & H_2 blockade for flushing
B. Surgical: (Often better than medical Rx). Resect or enucleate liver mets or infuse Cyt.T into hepatic artery & ligation/embolisation of hepatic artery

PROG: Median survival 6yrs. Better if appendix primary site

EOSINOPHILIC GUT INFILTRATION

Often cause unknown, in some due to allergy eg to Herring parasite; Collagen diseases. Rare. Lesions anywhere in GIT. All ages.
Type 1 c̄ blood eosinophilia: Infiltration & ulcers esp sm bowel
Type 2 without eosinophilia: polyps esp stomach

CLIN: Abdo pain; D&V. Occ Asthma; Malabsorption & Protein losing enteropathy. Polyps may → obst & intussusception

RX: Steroids. If obst, surgery

PNEUMATOSIS CYSTOIDES INTESTINALIS

Air containing cysts in submucosa, subserosa of Jejunum, Ileum >Colon. Rare. In infants ass c̄ Py.S, GI obst & colitis. In adults ass c̄ colitis, small bowel ischaemia, COAD & asthma

CLIN: Often symptomless or mild diarrhoea c̄ episodic colic. Occ Blood & mucus p.r; Steatorrhoea; Pneumoperitoneum (usually c̄ no peritonitis)

INVESTIGATIONS: • AXR
• Ba studies: Filling defects
• Sigmoidoscopy

RX: 70% O_2 therapy for few days. Occ resect bowel

PSEUDOMEMBRANEOUS ENTEROCOLITIS

Old, neonates >young, fit

AETIOLOGY: *Cl.difficile* 2° to antibiotics esp Lincomycin, Clindamycin or cross infection. Occurs 2/7 to 4/52 after starting Rx

CLIN: Rapid onset of diarrhoea ± blood; Colicky abdo pain; Dehydration & shock. Occ Perf of colon; Toxic megacolon

INVESTIGATIONS:
- Sigmoidoscopy: Shows white or yellow plaques. (N.B. rectum may be spared)
- Biopsy
- AXR
- *Cl.difficile* toxin in faeces
- Faecal culture for *Cl.difficile*
- Ba enema (in fit): Distinctive plaques

RX: Urgent. Isolate patient. Stop causative antibiotics, start oral Vancomycin or Metronidazole. Rehydrate; Plasma expanders eg Dextran. Monitor c̄ CVP

PROG: Has improved c̄ specific antibiotic Rx

SOLITARY ULCER OF RECTUM

May be single or multiple ulcers ↑ Usually <40yrs

AETIOLOGY: ? hamartoma. ? iatrogenic. ? anorectal motor dysfunction

CLIN: Constipation; Blood & mucus p.r; Tenesmus; Lower abdo pain. Occ Difficulty in defaecation → straining++

INVESTIGATIONS: Sigmoidoscopy & biopsy shows proctitis & ulceration. Specific histology

RX: Treat constipation

CARCINOMA OF RECTUM

M>F. Increased incidence c̄ age. 3× risk in first degree relatives. Accounts for approx 50% of all large bowel Ca

AETIOLOGY: 1. Ulc colitis
2. Polyps
3. Familial polyposis
4. Low residue diet
5. Alcohol esp brewery workers

TYPES: Ulcerative; Stenosing; Polypoidal. 99% AdenoCa of which 10% are colloidal. 1% anaplastic

CLIN: Commonly bleeding p.r c̄ mucous; Alteration in bowel habit; Tenesmus & lower abdo colic (esp lower 1/3 Ca); Obst (esp annular tumours); LN ↑. Rarely Wt ↓; Malaise; Abdo mass; Perf. Later Fistulae → vaginal discharge, pneumaturia; J; Bone pain

INVESTIGATIONS:
- p.r
- Sigmoidoscopy & biopsy
- Ba enema
- Liver scan

SPREAD: Direct into lumen & adjacent organs. Via Lymphatics. Blood esp to liver. Transcoelomic (if within peritoneum)
Duke's classification: Stages A–D:
A: Confined to rectal wall
B: Penetrating wall
C1: LN near pedicle not involved
C2: LN near pedicle involved
D: Mets

RX: A. Medical: If inoperable or post-op recurrence: Analgesia, supportive measures. Occ Cyt.T eg 5-FU, CCNU; X-Rad

B. Surgical:
Pre-op: Empty & sterilise bowel. Catheterise
1. Palliative Ops (All ± Cyt.T & X-Rad):
Colostomy for obst. Diathermy of Ca. Excision of rectum eg ant resection
2. Potentially curable Ops (All ± Pre- or post-op X.Rad):
a) Lower 1/3 rectum (within 7cm of

anal verge) & large tumours of middle 1/3: Abdoperineal resection c̄ colostomy. Occ a local excision & anastomosis through the anal canal is possible

b) Middle 1/3. Choice of ops: Abdoperineal or ant resection

c) Upper 1/3 rectum (>12 cm from verge): Ant resection c̄ rectocolic anastomosis. Rectal stump washout c̄ Hg perchloride (to ↓ suture line recurrence). Use stapling gun

Post-op: Drip & suck; Analgesia; Catheter; Perineal drainage tube; Colostomy care. Regular follow up

Post-op Complications: 1. Urinary retention

2. PI
3. Wound complications:
   a) Infection
   b) Sinus
   c) Hernia
   d) Abscess
   e) Faecal fistula esp 2° to anastomotic breakdown Rx: proximal colostomy
4. Faecal/flatus incontinence
5. Small bowel hernia → obst
6. Ca recurrence esp at suture line
7. Impotence
8. Ureteric injury occ → fistula
9. Complications of colostomy:
   a) Herniation
   b) Retraction
   c) Stenosis
   d) Prolapse
   e) Perf (from enema tube)
   f) Sloughing
   g) Lat space obst

PROG: 50% 1yr survival; 30% 5yr survival

DD:
1. Tumours:
   a) Benign eg Lipoma
   b) Malignant eg Sigmoid colon, Ovary, Uterus, Cervix, Prostate, Pelvic mets
2. Inflammation:
   a) Diverticulitis
   b) Endometriosis
   c) Crohn's
3. Infection:
   a) Amoebic dysentry
   b) Lymphogranuloma inguinale
4. Faeces

HAEMORRHOIDS

Causes of Lower GI Bleeding (LIST 18 GIT)

1. Haemorrhoids: Commonest
2. Anal fissure
3. Ruptured perianal haematoma
4. Polyps
5. Carcinoma: Eg Colonic, Rectal, Anal
6. Ulcerative colitis
7. Crohn's disease
8. Diverticular disease
9. Ischaemic colitis
10. Solitary ulcer of rectum
11. Infective colitis
12. Endometriosis
13. Radiation colitis
14. Vascular abnormalities: Eg Angiodysplasia
15. Meckle's diverticulum
16. Conditions causing upper GI bleeding: Eg PU, Varices, Tumours

DD of Multiple Perianal Fistulae (LIST 19 GIT)

1. Crohn's disease
2. Lymphogranuloma venereum
3. TB
4. Hydradinitis suppurativa
5. Actinomycosis
6. Infected perianal dermoid

Haemorrhoids are varicosities of sup haemorrhoidal veins. Ext haemorrhoids is an obsolete term

Internal Haemorrhoids

Ass c̄ Pregnancy; Straining; Low residue diet; Pelvic tumours; CCF; Portal BP ↑
Piles occur at positions 3,7 & 11 o'clock (in lithotomy position). Three degrees:
1st degree: Confined to anal canal. Don't prolapse
2nd degree: Prolapse on defaecation, reduce spontaneously
3rd degree: Persistent prolapse

CLIN: Fresh p.r bleeding ± mucus ± pruritis ani

INVESTIGATIONS: • p.r
• Sigmoidoscopy
• Proctoscopy
• Occ Ba enema

RX: Exclude underlying causes eg Ca

A. Regulate bowel habit: High fibre diet. Occ glycerol supps

B. Injection "submucosal sclerotherapy": For 1st degree & small 2nd degree piles. May require further injection after 2/52

Complications: 1. Pain
2. Ulcer
3. Haem
4. Prostatic abscess
5. Haematuria

C. Elastic band ligation: For large 2nd degree piles

D. Cryosurgery

E. Infra-red coagulation

F. Surgery:

Indications: 1. 3rd degree
2. 2nd degree c̄ severe prolapse
3. Failure of conservative Rx

Methods: a) Excision & low ligation: 3–6wks to heal
b) Anal stretch (Lords procedure)
c) Submucous excision

Post-op: Analgesia, Bath after b.o & redress wound, stool softeners

Complications of Haemorrhoidectomy:
1. Haemorrhage:
a) 1°: Few hrs later eg due to slipped ligature
b) 2°: 7–10 days later from pedicle. May be internal bleed
Rx: 1. Transfuse. Secure bleeding pt or pack round a rectal tube
2. Acute retention
3. Infection
4. Recurrence
5. Stricture:
Rx: May need dilation

COMPLICATIONS OF INT HAEMORRHOIDS: 1. Anaemia
2. Thrombosed prolapsed pile
3. Perianal haematoma
4. Skin tag (sentinel pile)

Thrombosed Strangulated Pile

Ext haemorrhoidal vein thromb. Prolapsed pile gripped by sphincter

CLIN: Pain. Occ → Gangrene & Ulceration

RX: Bed rest; Elevated bed; Ice compress; Laxative; Analgesia. Usually resolves in 2–3 wks. Occ Resect or Anal stretch

Peri-anal Haematoma

Inf haemorrhoidal vein rupture. Covered by skin

CLIN: Acute onset; Blue lump at anal verge; Pain. May resolve → skin tag or rupture → blood loss, ulcer. Resolve at 4–6 wks

RX: Evacuate haematoma

ANAL & PERIANAL DISORDERS

Anal Fissure

Causes of Anal Pain (LIST 20 GIT)

1. Strangulated int haemorrhoids
2. Perianal haematoma
3. Anal fissure
4. Ano-rectal abscess
5. Anal carcinoma
6. Pruritis ani
7. Proctalgia fugax
8. Pilonidal sinus
9. Other ano-rectal infections:
   a) Fungal eg Candida
   b) Bacterial eg Erythrasma
   c) Viral eg Herpes
10. Lichen planus
11. Psoriasis

Tear or ulcer at anal verge following constipated stool passage Ass c̄ pelvic floor weakening at childbirth & Crohn's disease

SITES: Post mid line >Ant mid line >Multiple

TYPES: 1. Acute, supf
2. Chr, deep: Ass c̄ sentinel pile or anal

polyp or hypertrophied anal papilla

CLIN: Acute, severe pain esp on p.r; Slight bleeding; Constipation

RX: Acute supf: Regulate bowel, dilate UA, LA ointment
Chr deep: Lat or Post sphincterotomy & removal of any polyp or sentinel pile ± skin graft. Occ anal stretch performed

Ano Rectal Abscess

PREDISPOSING CAUSES: 1. Anal fissure
2. Perianal haematoma
3. Anal gland infection
4. Injection Rx
5. Crohn's disease
6. Ca
7. Ulc colitis
8. Actinomycosis

CLASSIFIED BY SITE:

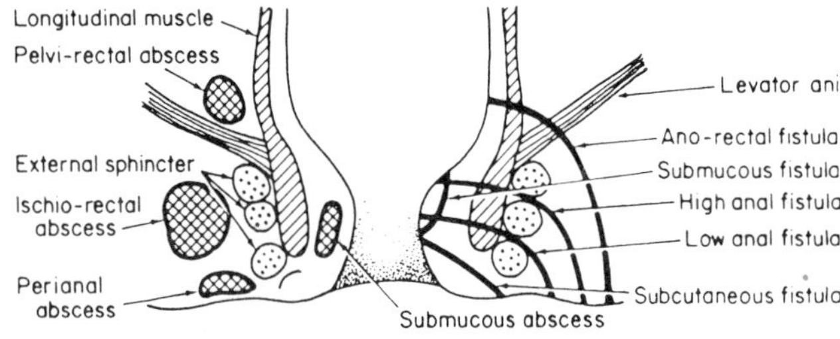

Figure 2 Sites of ano-rectal abscesses

PERIANAL ABSCESSES

Commonest. Usually infection of hair follicle; sebaceous, sweat or anal gland; or perianal haematoma

CLIN: Throbbing deep buttock pain. Red, hot, tender, supf perianal lump c̄ cellulitis

ISCHIORECTAL ABSCESS

Between anal canal & sphincters medially & obturator muscle laterally. May involve other ischiorectal fossa by tracking behind rectum forming a horse-shoe. Usually infection from anal glands, fissure, foreign body or perianal abscess

CLIN: Deep buttock pain ppt by sitting & defaecation. Occ Fever

SUBMUCOUS ABSCESS

Infection of submucosa of anal canal from fissure, anal glands or after injection Rx of piles

CLIN: Mild buttock pain ppt by defaecation. Occ Fever; Toxaemia

PELVI-RECTAL ABSCESS

Rare. Between levator ani & pelvic peritoneum. Ass c̄ Ca rectum; Ulc colitis; Crohn's; Appendicitis. Often follows pelvic cellulitis

COMPLICATION OF ANO-RECTAL ABSCESS

1. Fistula-in-ano
2. Chr abscess formation eg Hidradenitis suppurativa: Multiple abscesses arising from sweat glands

RX OF ANORECTAL ABSCESS

Early op for drainage. Look for & Rx fistulae

Fistula-in-Ano

CAUSES: Anal gland infection >Crohn's >Ulc colitis, Ca, TB

CLASSIFICATION: Subcutaneous, submucous, low anal, high anal, ano-rectal

CLIN: Recurrent discharging abscesses. Malaise

RX: Define course of fistula
a) Subcutaneous, submucous, low anal: Lay open & allow to granulate
b) High-level: Do not divide anorectal ring as → faecal incontinence. Lay open lower part & tie upper part of tract. At 2nd op, when sphincter fixed by scarring, remove upper part

Pilonidal Sinus

Sc track containing hair. M>F esp dark haired young adults. Sacrococcyx >>Axilla, Umbilicus, Fingers (esp in barbers).
? developmental but probably 2° to foreign body

CLIN: Usually asymptomatic. Infection → pain & abscesses c̄ discharge

RX: a) Pilonidal sinus: Antibiotics, shaving & toilet; or lay open track allow to granulate then depilatory cream; or phenol injection; or excise & primary suture
b) Pilonidal abscess: Drain & lay open

Other Anorectal Infections

SYPHILIS

Primary chancre & 6–8wks later perianal condylomata lata

ERYTHRASMA

Due to Corynebacterium. Pruritis ani++

RX: Erythromycin

THREADWORMS

Pruritis ani esp nocte

RX: Piperazine to all close contacts

VIRAL WARTS (CONDYLOMATA ACUMINATA)

RX: Podophyllin

FUNGAL

Esp in diabetics & immunosuppressed

RX: Nystatin or Amphotericin B

Pruritis Ani

CAUSES: 1. Infections:
- a) Scabies
- b) Monilia
- c) Threadworm
- d) Fungi
- e) Lice
- f) Fistula
- g) Erythrasma

2. Anorectal disorders:
- a) 3rd degree pile
- b) Fissure
- c) IBD
- d) Ca

3. Excess sweating
4. Poor cleanliness
5. Idiopathic
6. General:
- a) Diabetes
- b) J
- c) Drugs
- d) Anxiety
- e) Hodgkins

RX: Correct general or local cause. Local Hydrocortisone, Zn oxide, Calamine or Antihistamines

Proctalgia Fugax

Recurring paroxysm of intense rectal pain esp nocte. ? Psychogenic

Anal Stricture

CAUSES: 1. Cong
2. Traumatic esp post haemorrhoidectomy
3. Post X-Rad
4. Ca
5. Crohn's; Ulc colitis
6. Lymphogranuloma inguinale (F>M)

RX: Treat underlying cause. Often repeat dilatations

Anorectal Prolapse

RECTAL MUCOSA PROLAPSE

May occur in child. Ass c̄ prolapsed pile or incompetent sphincter

RX: Ligature & excision of prolapse. In child self-limiting

COMPLETE RECTAL PROLAPSE

Esp elderly F. Ass c̄ lack of rectal fixation, sphincter dysfunction & proctitis

CLIN: Anal discomfort & incontinence

RX: a) Thiersch wire op in frail
b) Abdo op to fix rectum in pelvis eg Polyvinal sponge to induce fibrosis

DESCENDING PERINEUM SYNDROME

Marked descent of perineum on straining ass c̄ incontinence

RX: Avoid excessive straining eg Glycerol supps

Anal Canal Carcinoma

Rare. F>M. Squamous cell Ca

CLIN: Bleeding; Ulceration; Pain

SPREAD: Direct & by lymph to rectum, vagina & LN

RX: Abdoperineal resection ± block dissection of LNs

Anal Margin Carcinoma

Very rare. M>F. Squamous cell Ca

CLIN: Bleeding; Ulceration

SPREAD: To anal canal & perineum

RX: Local excision or abdoperineal resection. Occ X-Rad

Adenocarcinoma Anus

Rare. Highly malignant

CLIN: Woody hard plaque. Bleeding

SPREAD: To groin & rapidly metastasises

RX: Abdoperineal resection

PROG: Poor

HERNIA

A protrusion of part or all of a viscus through its covering into an abnormal situation
Inguinal >Femoral >Umbilical >Incisional >Ventral >Epigastric >Obturator; Spigelian; Lumbar; Gluteal; Sciatic; Perineal

PREDISPOSING FACTORS: 1. Cong defects
2. Surgical incisions
3. Muscle weakness:
Eg 2° to obesity, pregnancy, polio, wasting disease
4. ↑ abdo P:
Eg Chr cough; Constipation; Pregnancy; Urinary tract obst; Vom; Abdo Ca c̄ ascites

VARIETIES: 1. Reducible
2. Irreducible
3. Obstructed: Bowel obst but no effect on arterial supply
4. Strangulated: Bowel c̄ its arterial supply obst. Femoral >Ind Ing >Umbilical >Others

Clin of Strangulation: Sudden severe pain. Vom; Distension; Constipation; No cough impulse

Inguinal Hernia

2 TYPES

a) Indirect (Ind Ing): Through int inguinal ring across inguinal canal
b) Direct (Dir Ing): Through post wall of inguinal canal
60% of inguinal herniae on R side; 20% on L; 20% bilat

ANATOMY

Ext ring: "V" shaped split in ext oblique muscle above & lat to pubic tubercle
Int ring: "U" shaped split in transversalis fascia about 1cm above mid-pt inguinal lig
Inguinal Canal
4cm long. Goes downwards & medially from int to ext ring. Carries spermatic cord in M & round ligament in F
Relations of Inguinal canal:
Ant: Skin, supf fascia, Ext oblique, Int oblique (lat 1/3 only)
Floor: Inguinal & lacunar ligaments
Roof: Int oblique & Transversus Abdominus
Post: Medially conjoint tendon (Int oblique & Transversus abdominus). Laterally transversalis fascia; Lat umbilical lig & inf epigastric artery
Contents of canal:
Spermatic cord (Vas deferens, testicular artery, pampiniform plexus, artery of vas), cremasteric br of inf epigastric artery, ilio-inguinal nerve, genital br of genito-femoral nerve & occ processus vaginalis. Also lymph vessels & autonomic nerves

INDIRECT INGUINAL HERNIA

Usually cong eg persistent processus vaginalis; Patent canal of Nuck in F. May extend through ext ring occ reaching scrotum

COVERINGS: Peritoneum; Fat; Int spermatic fascia; Cremasteric fascia & muscle; Ext spermatic fascia; Supf fascia; Skin

DIRECT INGUINAL HERNIA

Acquired except very rare congenital Oglivie hernia

COVERINGS: Peritoneum; Transversalis fascia; Conjoint tendon; Ext oblique aponeurosis; Supf fascia; Skin

INDIRECT & DIRECT INGUINAL HERNIA

"Pantaloon" or "saddle bag" hernia. Dual sacs around inf epigastric artery

DIFFERENTIATION BETWEEN DIRECT & INDIRECT INGUINAL HERNIAE

Ind Ing: Lat to inf epigastric artery; Controlled by digital P over int ring; Protrudes towards scrotum; Usually cong; Common in young
Dir Ing: Med to inf epigastric artery; Not controlled by digital P; Usually acquired; Rare in young; Rarely strangulates; Appears immediately on standing & disappears on lying

CLIN OF INGUINAL HERNIA

Lump in groin; Groin discomfort; Occ pain. If irreducible may be impossible to know if direct or indirect

DD OF INGUINAL HERNIA

1. Femoral hernia
2. Saphena varix
3. Encysted hydrocele of cord
4. Femoral aneurysm
5. Incomplete testicular descent
6. Inguinal LN
7. Ectopic testis
8. Psoas abscess
9. Skin lipoma
10. Lipoma of cord

RX

UNCOMPLICATED:

A. Medical: Truss indicated if unfit or unwilling for op c̄ easily reducible hernia

B. Surgical: Preferred Rx

a) Ind Ing in young: Herniotomy if post wall of canal normal
b) Ind Ing in healthy adult: Normal post wall, but int ring wide. Herniotomy & herniorrhaphy ie sew conjoint tendon to inguinal lig
c) Large Ind Ing, Dir Ing & recurrent Herniae: Weak post wall. Herniotomy (not if Dir Ing) & hernioplasty
d) Large scrotal Herniae in elderly: Remove cord & testis, obliterate canal

OBSTRUCTION OR STRANGULATION:

Require op
Reduce hernia by opening ext oblique & dividing ext ring ± adhesions. Resect nonviable bowel. Repair hernia. If signs of peritonitis do laparotomy

Femoral Hernia

Hernia through the femoral canal except in rare cases eg Narath's hernia. F>M. Always acquired. Esp middle-aged & elderly

ANATOMY

Boundaries of canal:
Ant: Inguinal ligament
Lat: Femoral vein
Post: Pectineal ligament (Astley Cooper)
Med: Lacunar lig & pectineal part of Inguinal lig & in 10% aberrant obturator artery
Contents of canal:
1. Fat
2. Lymph channels
3. Lymph gland of Cloquet
Coverings: Peritoneum; Fat; Transversalis fascia & fascia lata; Cribriform fascia; Fat; Skin

CLIN: Lump below & lat to pubic tubercle. Obst & strangulation common → tense tender irreducible lump c̄ oedema, abdo pain & vom
If Richter's hernia, no symptoms of obst as only part of bowel lumen is strangulated. Necrosis may occur

RX: Always op. Different types of op eg supra- & sub- inguinal Herniorraphy. Resect any nonviable bowel

Umbilical Hernia

EXOMPHALOS

Embryonic anomaly c̄ failure of mid-gut to return to abdo cavity. Bowel is in translucent sac protruding through ant abdo wall

COVERINGS: Amnion, Wharton's jelly, extra-coelomic peritoneum. Risk of peritonitis

RX: Protect sac c̄ dressings then surgery

CONGENITAL UMBILICAL HERNIA

Obliterated incomplete umbilicus. Esp Blacks. Almost always close spontaneously in <2yrs, otherwise op at 3yrs old

PARA-UMBILICAL HERNIA

Esp obese, multiparous, middle aged F.

Occ irreducible or strangulate. Often contains omentum & occ transverse colon & small bowel

RX: Mayo's Op: Excise umbilicus & sac. Overlap flaps of rectus sheath & suture

Epigastric Hernia

M>F. Small mid-line irreducible hernia in linea alba. Contains extraperitoneal fat

CLIN: Often asymptomatic. Occ Abdo pain mimicking PU or cholecystitis

RX: Mayo's op

Obturator Hernia

F>M. Esp >50yrs. Hernia through obturator canal between pubic ramus & obturator membrane

CLIN: Often intestinal obst. Occ Lump upper, medial thigh. Pain in inner knee from P on geniculate br obturator nerve

RX: Reduce sac c̄ its contents & excise. (Herniorrhaphy impossible)

Spigelian Hernia

Rare. Hernia through arcuate line into post rectus sheath

CLIN: Tender mass. Occ Strangulates

RX: Op

DD: Dir Ing

Gluteal Hernia

Rare. Through greater sciatic notch. Occ → obstruction

RX: Op

Sciatic Hernia

Rare. Through lesser sciatic notch. Occ → obst &/or sciatic nerve pain

RX: Op

Incisional Hernia

Occur through op scar. Strangulation is rare. Examples are lumbar hernia post nephrectomy & perineal hernia post abdoperineal resection

RX: Repair hernia or if unfit truss

Lumbar Hernia

Rare. Usually incisional but occ through inf lumbar triangle or sup lumbar space

GALL BLADDER & BILIARY TRACT DISEASE

Gallstones

70–80% asymptomatic. F>M. Esp elderly. 15% of UK adults have gall stones. USA, W.Europe >Africa

ASS FACTORS:
1. Obesity
2. Diabetes
3. ↑ Triglycerides
4. Haemolytic anaemia
5. Resection of terminal ileum
6. Crohn's disease
7. Low fibre diet
8. Drugs:
   a) Clofibrate
   b) Oestrogens inc "Pill"
9. ? HH & diverticular disease (Saint's triad)

TYPES:
1. Cholesterol: Contain >95% cholesterol
2. Pigment: Mainly contain $CaCO_3$, Ca^{2+} Phosphate, or Ca^{2+} Palmitate
3. Mixed: Contain >70% cholesterol

AETIOLOGY: 1. Cholesterol stones: Ass c̄ ↑ bile salt & ↑ hepatic cholesterol synthesis indicated by ↑ 7 α-OHlase & ↑ 3-OH-3-methyl-glutaryl-CoA levels. When bile is saturated c̄ cholesterol & in contact c̄ seeding agent eg biliary mucus or Ca^{2+} bilirubinate, microcrystals form & if gall bladder emptying is poor, stone develops

2. Pigment stones: Form c̄ excess blood breakdown products but most patients do not have overt haemolysis. In UK ass c̄ chr haemolytic anaemia eg sickle cell. In China pigment stones are found in bile duct

CLIN PRESENTATIONS: Cholecystitis; Biliary colic; Cholangitis; Pancreatitis. Can be silent

RX: Elective cholecystectomy (if silent)

Cholecystitis

ACUTE CHOLECYSTITIS

Acute inflam of gall bladder almost always ass c̄ gallstones

AETIOLOGY: Obst of gall bladder neck or occ cystic duct by stone causing bile to concentrate, inflamming gall bladder. Occ obst of blood supply → gangrene. Rarely 2° to Infection eg Typhoid or Polyarteritis

SEQUELAE:
1. Resolution
2. Contracted gall bladder (Chr cholecystitis)
3. Mucocoele: Obst c̄ expansion of gall bladder c̄ no infection
4. Empyema: Obst c̄ expansion of gall bladder c̄ 2° infection
5. Perforation → Abscess & Cholecysto-duodenal fistula or rarely Peritonitis
6. Gangrene
7. Gall stone ileus
8. Stone in CBD: Occ c̄ J
9. Pancreatitis

CLIN: Abdo pain & tenderness; Fever; Nausea; Dyspepsia. Occ referred pain to back & R shoulder. Rarely J (CBD stone); Palpable mass if mucocoele or empyema. +ve Murphy's sign. Occ Signs of peritonitis

INVESTIGATIONS:
- AXR
- WCC
- Amylase
- Ultrasound of gall bladder
- Oral cholecystogram (Not in acute phase or if J)

RX: A. Medical:
1. Conservative: Bed rest; Analgesia; Antibiotics eg ampicillin 90% settle but if stones left 50% chance that op will be necessary within 20yrs. Therefore later surgery unless poor op risk
2. Dissolution therapy: CDCA or UDCA dissolve cholesterol stones. Indicated in relatively well c̄ lucent stones & functioning gall bladder. Takes >6mths. Often recur when drugs stopped

B. Surgical:
1. Early elective cholecystectomy c̄ op cholangiogram: if gallstones have been confirmed, following pre-op preparation & patient is good risk
2. Elective cholecystectomy c̄ op cholangiogram at 6–8/52: Following conservative Rx if gallstones not confirmed in acute episode
3. Urgent op: If failure of medical Rx
   a) Cholecystotomy c̄ ext drainage: If perf; Empyema
   b) CBD opened & T-tube drainage: If J; Rigors; Pancreatitis

DD:
1. PU
2. Ac pancreatitis
3. MI
4. Ac diverticulitis
5. R lung disease
6. Ac appendicitis
7. Pyelonephritis
8. IBS

Courvoisier's Law

When J, if gall bladder palpable, J is unlikely to be due to stone

Chronic Cholecystitis

Chr fibrosis of wall of gall bladder due to repeated inflam. Ass c̄ stones

CLIN: Dyspepsia; Flatulence; Recurrent abdo pains; Belching; Nausea; +ve Murphy's. Occ Fever; J

RX: Cholecystectomy. If op cholangiogram shows stones then explore CBD, T-tube drainage for 10/7 & remove if T-tube cholangiogram normal

Biliary Colic

Impaction of stone in gall bladder outlet or duct system for short period relieved by passage of stone along duct or back into gall bladder. Not a true colic

CLIN: Constant severe pain for several hrs esp post prandial, usually in R hypochondrium radiating to R scapula. Vom; Sweating. Rarely diarrhoea. If obst unresolved → acute cholecystitis or mucocoele

RX: Bed rest; Analgesia; Treat sequelae. Often need op

Mucocoele

Due to distension of gall bladder c̄ mucus following obst without infection. Ca^{2+} may be secreted in lumen causing "limey bile"; or in wall causing pre-malignant "porcelain gall bladder"

Fistula Formation

Due to formation of tracts at sites of adhesion between gall bladder & duodenum, colon or stomach. Usually stone passed p.r but occ → obst (gall stone ileus)

Stones in Common Bile Duct (Choledocholithiasis)

Found in 15% of patients c̄ stones in Gall Bladder. Occ 2° to abnormal cystic duct junction. Stones may be free in CBD or impact, disimpact, reimpact or pass

ANATOMY: CBD 8cm long. Union of cystic & hepatic ducts. 3 parts:
1st part: In free edge of lesser omentum in front of portal vein & to R of hepatic artery
2nd part: Behind 1st part duodenum
3rd part: In groove on post pancreas in front of IVC
CBD opens into 2nd part of duodenum c̄ pancreatic duct, surrounded by sphincter of Oddi

CLIN: May be asymptomatic but usually symptoms. Impaction → obst & biliary colic. If obst unrelieved, then Obst J in <2/7. If infection, cholangitis develops c̄ fluctuating fever (Charcot's), pain, rigors, J & malaise ± shock, toxaemia, liver abscesses, ARF. If partial or intermittent obst, duct dilates & cholestatic syndrome develops c̄ pruritus ± J. If impaction at ampulla → pancreatitis & cholestasis. If prolonged obst, 2° biliary cirrhosis develops
Post cholangitis → BP ↓, lethargy

INVESTIGATIONS:
- Urobilinogen: ↑ in Obst J
- Stercobilinogen: ↑ in Obst J
- Bilirubin
- Alk phos: ↑ in cholestasis
- WCC
- FBC
- Blood cultures
- AXR
- Ultrasound
- ERCP
- HIDA Scan
- Percutaneous transhepatic cholangiography
- Oral cholecystography or IV cholangiogram (if ERCP fails)

RX: A. Medical: Bed rest; Analgesia; Antibiotics; ± IV drip. Then ERCP (>90% success rate), esp if J or prev cholecystectomy, to remove stones eg by sphincterotomy & Dormier basket. If stones can't be removed, irrigate through nasobiliary tube for 3/7 c̄ dextrose or Mono-octanoin (to dissolve stone), then nasobiliary cholangiogram to see if CBD is clear. If not clear, surgery

B. Surgery: Pre-op: VitK 2–3/7 to ↓ bleeding tendency
At op: Cholangiography; Explore duct system; Remove stones eg c̄ Dormier basket. If ampulla stenosis do sphincterotomy. If CBD patent, Gall bladder may be removed. Put T-tube into CBD. Put a drain into gall bladder region. Occ bypass op needed
Post-op: Restrict fluids till b.o. T-tube Cholangiogram at 10/7: If CBD patent then remove T-tube. If not patent retain large T-tube to allow fistula to form to allow percutaneous removal of stone at 2/12 or if cholesterol stones, irrigate c̄ mono-octanoin within 8 days of op to dissolve stone

COMPLICATIONS:
1. Biliary cirrhosis
2. Liver failure
3. Portal BP ↑
4. Pancreatitis
5. Liver abscess
6. Septicaemia
7. ARF

Sclerosing Cholangitis

Rare. Chr extrahepatic periductal fibrosis c̄ inflammation

ASS c:
1. Biliary surgery
2. Gall stones

3. Ulc colitis
4. Crohn's
5. Retroperitoneal fibrosis
6. Reidel's thyroiditis
7. Pseudotumour orbit
8. Schistosomiasis

CLIN: Mild intermittent J & pruritus

INVESTIGATION: • ERCP shows intrahepatic bleeding of ducts

RX: Rifampicin for infection.
? Azathioprine

COMPLICATIONS: 1. 2° biliary cirrhosis
2. Liver failure
3. Peri-cholangitis ie Chr intrahepatic periductal fibrosis

PROG: Poor

Complications of Biliary Surgery

DUCT SYSTEM

a) Bile leakage: Common in small amounts
b) Ext biliary fistula: Profuse loss of bile. If no obst, usually resolves

Rx: Correct U&E; Protect skin. If no closure by 4/52 then op

c) Biliary peritonitis: Resus then reop. Poor prog
d) Benign stricture: J; Pain; Fever. Occ → biliary cirrhosis, hypersplenism, portal BP ↑

Rx: Excise stricture & anastomose or Choledocho-jejunostomy

VASCULAR

a) Mistaken ligation R hepatic artery → liver necrosis
b) Portal vein trauma. Rarely → portal vein thromb

T-TUBE PROBLEMS

a) Blockage
b) Kink
c) Too long occ → obst; pancreatitis
d) May fall out of CBD
e) Pulled out too early → bile leakage

Post Cholecystectomy Syndrome

Persistent or recurrence of "biliary" symptoms

CAUSES: 1. Residual or reformed stones: Commonest cause
2. Wrong diagnosis eg PU
3. Benign ductal stricture
4. Pancreatitis
5. Ventral hernia
6. Adhesions
7. Cystic duct stump syndrome: If duct remnant >1cm, ↑ risk of cholangitis or stone formation
8. Biliary dyskinesia: Abnormal bile duct P causing biliary colic c̄ no J or fever
9. Painful neuroma
10. Benign papillary stenosis

Biliary Tract Neoplasms

BENIGN

a) Papilloma: Mucus secretion occ → partial obst
b) Adenoma: May be pre-malignant
c) Fibroma; Neuroma: Very rare. Occ → obst

RX: Excise tumour. Anastomose duct

MALIGNANT

a) EXTRA HEPATIC BILE DUCT Ca:
Elderly. May be ass c̄ sclerosing cholangitis & chr ulc colitis. AdenoCa >>Sarcoma >Rhabdomyosarcoma (Children)

Clin: Pruritus; Cholestatic J (may fluctuate); Abdo pain; Wt ↓; Liver ↑; Diarrhoea; Anorexia; Steatorrhoea. Bleeding → anaemia. Necrosis → temp relief of J

Rx: Palliative
a) Bypass tumour by CBD into jejunum
b) Excise tumour (often impossible)
c) ERCP or Percutaneous insertion of drainage tube

b) GALL BLADDER Ca: 4F:1M. Occurs in <0.5% of cholelithiasis cases overall, but commoner if chr cholecystitis or porcelain gall bladder. AdenoCa 90%; Squamous 9%; Rarely carcinoid

Clin: Mass in R upper abdo; Obst J; Wt ↓. Usually preceded by symptoms of cholecystitis
Spreads to liver (early), bile ducts & duodenum

Rx: Usually inoperable. Cholecystectomy

c) AMPULLARY Ca: Usually arise from distal 1/3 CBD or ampulla. AdenoCa

Clin: Cholestatic J (may fluctuate); Slight wt ↓; Occ Abdo pain; LN spread (80%).
Late: Pancreatic insuff eg steatorrhoea & diabetes. Small bowel obst; Haem; Ascites; Splenoportal thromb c̄ spleen ↑

Rx: Whipple op ie removal of duodenum,

proximal 2/3 of pancreas & distal stomach

Prog: Poor

INVESTIGATIONS OF BILIARY TRACT NEOPLASMS: • FBC, ESR
• WCC
• Bilirubin
• Alk phos isoenzymes
• PT time
• LPX: ↑ in 65% c̄ biliary obst
• Ultrasound
• PTC: Often diagnostic
• ERCP

THE PANCREAS

Acute Pancreatitis

F>M. Esp >40yrs. Functional recovery after attack

Causes of Acute Pancreatitis (LIST 21 GIT)

1. Biliary tract disease:
   a) Stones
   b) Stenosis
   c) Tumour
   d) Spasm
2. Alcohol
3. Abdo trauma
4. Penetrating PU
5. Metabolic:
   a) HPT
   b) HyperCa^{2+}
   c) Severe hypertriglyceridaemia
6. Infections:
   a) Mumps
   b) Typhoid
   c) Coxsackie
7. Vascular:
   a) Malignant BP ↑
   b) PAN
8. Chronic Renal Failure
9. Hypothermia
10. Acute Liver Failure
11. Idiopathic (25% of cases)

PATHOLOGY: Oedema alone in mild cases. Often fat necrosis; vascular damage. In severe cases haem & necrosis occ → gangrene & abscess. Rarely pseudocyst formation

CLIN: Variable symptoms. Usually sudden severe persistent pain radiating to back ass c̄ vom & fever. Occ Abdo mass; J; Tetany; Glycosuria
In severe cases Malaise++; Shock; BP ↓. Occ Cyanosis; Bruising of loins (Grey Turner's sign) or periumbilical area (Cullen's sign); ARF; DIC; Effusions; Diabetic coma; Peritonitis; Ileus

INVESTIGATIONS: • Amylase: >1875 IU/l is diagnostic. Peaks at 48hrs
• WCC ↑
• ESR
• Bilirubin slight ↑
• Glucose ↑
• Lipids ↑
• Serum Ca^{2+} ↓
• Methaemalbuminaemia: ↑ in haem pancreatitis
• Serum Mg
• Fibrinogen, FDPs
• CXR; AXR: Occ Pleural effusions; Stones. Rarely sentinel loop
• Ultrasound
• CAT scan
• ? ERCP
• Peritoneal lavage; Laparotomy: If diagnosis uncertain

RX: A. Mild attacks: Rest; Analgesia; Bland diet; No alcohol; Anticholinergics; Antacids. Observe for complications

B. Severe attacks: Bed rest; Analgesia (not morphine); Avoid food; Replacement therapy eg Drip & suck under CVP control, blood; O_2. Observe closely. ? Antibiotics; ? Aprotonin (Trasylol); ? Glucagon; ? Anticholinergics. If HypoCa^{2+}, give 10% Ca^{2+} gluconate; If HypoMg, give $MgSO_4$; If shock, steroids. In severely ill, peritoneal lavage. If attack lasts >1wk, parenteral nutrition, plasma

C. Uncertain diagnosis: Pre-op resus. Laparotomy: Drain abscess, & remove stones as necessary. If J, explore CBD & perform ext biliary drainage

D. Complications: Op to remove necrotic material; drain abscess, pseudocyst. If small bowel obst may need gastroenterostomy

E. After recovery: Investigate & where

possible treat aetiology eg gallstones

COMPLICATIONS: 1. Recurrent attacks ie Acute Relapsing Pancreatitis
2. Pancreatic abscesses
3. Peritonitis
4. ARF
5. DIC
6. Pseudocyst: Unusual
7. Ascites
8. Pleural effusions

PROG: Usually recovery in <14 days. If haem pancreatitis 50% mort

DD:
1. Acute cholecystitis
2. Perf DU
3. MI
4. Acute intestinal obst
5. Ruptured aortic aneurysm
6. Diabetic pre-coma
7. Ruptured ectopic pregnancy
8. Porphyria
9. Other causes of peritonitis

DD of Hyperamylaseaemia: 1. Cholecystitis
2. Perf PU
3. ARF
4. MI
5. Parotitis
6. Hepatitis
7. Intestinal obst
8. Morphia Rx
9. Ruptured aortic aneurysm
10. Idiopathic S-type hyperamylaseaemia

Chronic Pancreatitis

Permanent pathological changes & impaired function post attack. Esp USA, France & Tropics. M>F

Causes of Chronic Pancreatitis (LIST 22 GIT)

1. Alcohol: Common
2. Idiopathic
3. Gallstones: Rare
4. CBD stricture
5. ? Chr protein malnutrition (in E.Africa)
6. Cystic fibrosis
7. Hereditary pancreatitis
8. HPT

PATHOLOGY: Protein ppt in ducts → duct obst. Then atrophy, fibrosis c̄ eventual calcification & calculi. Occ pseudocysts, abscesses. Progressive fibrosis may → obst CBD, duodenum & portal vein.

Calcific pancreatitis strongly ass c̄ alcohol

CLIN: Recurrent episodic epigastric pain radiating to back ppt by alcohol or fatty foods not relieved by vom or alkali. Pain is of variable severity & frequency. Mild fever. Occ Nausea; J; Wt ↓; Diarrhoea; Malabsorption; Anaemia; Diabetes. Occ Asymptomatic. If due to alcohol usually h/o >5yrs heavy drinking c̄ heavy binge 18–48hrs pre-attack. Occ seen in moderate drinkers

INVESTIGATIONS:
- FBC
- ESR
- WCC
- Amylase: may be normal
- Pancreatic function tests:
  a) Secretin-CCK-PZ test: ↓ HCO_3 output, ↑ lactoferrin
  b) Lundh test (test meal): Trypsin ↓
  c) Faecal fats
  d) PABA/C-14 excretion index
  e) Pancreolauryl test
- X-R:
  a) AXR: Occ calcification, ileus
  b) Ultrasound esp for pseudocyst & cyst
  c) ERCP: "chain of lakes" duct appearance
  d) CAT scan esp ? Ca
  e) Biliary tract radiography
  f) Ba studies
  g) Rarely: Selenomethionine scan; Angiography

RX: A. General: Correct predisposing factors eg no alcohol; remove stones; sphincterotomy; low fat diet

B. In mild attacks: Analgesia; Anticholinergics

C. In severe attacks: Bed rest; Analgesia; Drip & suck; Antibiotics

D. If pancreatic insufficiency: Insulin; Low fat, high protein diet; Pancreatic replacement therapy; Occ Cimetidine

E. Surgical Rx:

Indications: 1. If Med Rx fails due to severe, chr pain
2. Uncontrolled bleed
3. Complications: Cyst, Abscess, J

Types of Op: a) Sphincterotomy for reflux
b) Relief of local duct obst at head of pancreas: Sphincteroplasty & dilatation
c) If multiple strictures may do pancreatico-gastrostomy
d) Sub-total Pancreatectomy for pain: High mortality

e) Coeliac ganglion block for pain

COMPLICATIONS:

1. **Pancreatic Cyst:**
   Clin: Persistent pain & occ small bowel obst; Obst J (2° to CBD obst); Haematemesis (2° to portal or splenic vein obst → oesophageal varices)
2. **Pancreatic Ascites:** Rare. Due to ruptured cyst
3. **Pancreatic insufficiency:** Eg Diabetes, Steatorrhoea
4. **Metastatic fat necrosis:** Rare eg tender ankle nodules
5. **Pancreatic Abscess**

PROG: Quite good, if no alcohol & compliance c̄ Medical Rx

DD:
1. Ca head of pancreas
2. Pancreatic cyst
3. CBD stones
4. Ca ampulla of Vater

Pancreatic Cysts

20% of pancreatic cysts are true cysts, 80% are pseudocysts due to fluid collection in lesser sac

AETIOLOGY: True:
1. Congenital
2. Hydatid
3. Ca
4. Retention of secretions usually due to calculi

False (Pseudocysts):
1. Trauma
2. Ac pancreatitis
3. Perf post GU

CLIN: Abdo mass; Often pain. Occ Obst J; Haem

INVESTIGATIONS:
- Ultrasound
- CAT scan
- Rarely: Angiography, Ba meal

RX: Excise true cysts. Drain false cysts into stomach

Pancreatic Tumours

BENIGN

1. **CYSTADENOMA:** Commonest benign tumour. F>M. Occ calcify
   Clin: Occ Diabetes. Rarely pre-malignant
2. **ZOLLINGER–ELLISON TUMOUR:** Alpha cell tumour (Gastrinoma). 60% malignant. May be ass c̄ a parathyroid adenoma &/or MEA
   Clin: Recurrent, multiple PU, diarrhoea
   Investigations:
   - Pentagastrin test
   - Fasting serum Gastrin

Causes of Hypergastrinaemia (LIST 23 GIT)

1. ZE syndrome
2. Antral G-cell hyperlasia
3. Retained & isolated antrum
4. DM
5. Post vagotomy
6. CRF
7. Short bowel syndrome
8. Rh Arth
9. Cimetidine

Rx: H_1 & H_2 block eg Cimetidene. Occ remove tumour c̄ either gastrectomy or truncal vag & long-term Cimetidine. Occ direct embolisation

3. **INSULINOMA:** 90% benign. Secrete insulin. Beta cell tumour
   Clin: Spontaneous hypoglycaemia relieved by sugar. Sweating; Abdo pain; Confusion. Occ Ep; Tremor; Diarrhoea; Hunger & Wt ↓; Coma
   Investigations:
   - Prolonged fast c̄ serial BG & Insulin levels
   - Angiography

Causes of Hypoglycaemia (LIST 24 GIT)

1. Reactive (Post-glucose ingestion):
   a) Post gastrectomy; "Dumping" syndrome
   b) Idiopathic
   c) Early diabetes
2. Starvation
3. Endocrine:
   a) Hypothyroidism
   b) Hypopituitarism
   c) Insulinoma
   d) Addison's disease
   e) B-cell hyperplasia
4. Drugs: Eg Insulin; Oral hypoglycaemics; Salicylates
5. Sensitivity to:
   a) Alcohol
   b) Leucine
   c) Galactose
   d) Fructose
6. Tumours:
   a) Hepatoma
   b) Fibrosarcoma
   c) Ca lung esp Oat-cell
7. Liver disease:
   a) Glycogen storage disease
   b) ALF

Rx: Excision. Direct embolisation at angiography

4. WDHA SYNDROME: Usually due to islet cell tumour producing VIP. Rare. 50% malignant

Clin: Watery diarrhoea (WD), Hypokalaemia (H), Achlorhydria (A). Occ Flushing; HyperCa^{2+}; Tetany

Investigation: • Fasting VIP level ↑

Rx: Excise tumour. If mets, Cyt.T eg Streptozotocin

5. GLUCAGONOMA: Islet cell tumour. Rare

Clin: Necrolytic migratory erythema; Diabetes; Diarrhoea; Anaemia; Stomatitis; Vulvitis

Investigation: • Glucagon level ↑

Rx: Excise tumour

6. SOMATOSTATINOMA: Very rare tumour producing somatostatin

Clin: Diabetes; Steatorrhoea

MALIGNANT

CARCINOMA OF THE PANCREAS

M>F. Esp Polynesians, Jews, US Blacks. Esp in >50yrs

AETIOLOGY: 1. Smoking
2. Diabetes

PATHOLOGY: Head >Body >Tail. 20% periampullary. Usually AdenoCa

CLIN: Often difficult to diagnose, variable presentation. Abdo pain occ radiating to back; Malaise; Wt ↓; Diarrhoea; Depression, Anxiety; Thrombophlebitis migrans (25%). Occ Haem. Later, Ca Head → Painless progressive obst J (which occ remits due to necrosis); Palpable gall bladder &/or liver (due to mets or Biliary cirrhosis). Ca Body → Glycosuria; unstable Diabetes

SPREAD: a) Direct: CBD (obst J); Duodenum (Haem); Portal vein (Portal BP ↑, Ascites); IVC (bilat leg oedema)
b) Lymph
c) Blood: to liver & lungs
d) Transcoelomic

INVESTIGATIONS:
- FBC, ESR
- FOB
- Amylase: Occ ↑
- Secretin-PZ-CCK test
- ERCP
- Ultrasound ± percutaneous pancreatic cytology
- CAT scan
- Ba meal
- Laparotomy

RX: If J give Vit K pre-op
A. Potentially Curative Op: Pancreatico-duodenectomy (Whipple's op) remove distal stomach, duodenum, proximal 2/3rds of pancreas
B. Palliative:
a) Total pancreatectomy & replacement therapy
b) Biliary bypass op eg Cholecysto-jejunostomy
c) X-Rad

PROG: 10% Op mortality. 5% 5yr survival. Periampullary Ca best prog

THE LIVER

Jaundice

DEFINITION: >17μmol/l (>0.9mg/100ml) bilirubin in blood

Causes of Jaundice (LIST 25 GIT)

A. UNCONJUGATED HYPER-BILIRUBINAEMIA
1. Haemolytic Jaundice: Eg Thalassaemia; Sickle cell disease; Septicaemia; Drugs; Hereditary spherocytosis; Cardiac failure
2. Familial non-haemolytic (LIST 26 GIT): Eg Gilbert's disease

B. PARENCHYMAL LIVER DISEASE: Conjugated hyperbilirubinaemia
1. Cirrhosis
2. Viral Hepatitis
3. Alcohol
4. PBC
5. Familial conjugated (LIST 26 GIT)
6. Ca
7. CAH
8. Drugs: Eg Paracetamol
9. Metabolic: Eg Wilsons disease, Haemochromatosis

C. EXTRAHEPATIC BILIARY OBST: Obst J
1. Gall stones
2. Ca esp Pancreas or mets
3. Chr pancreatitis
4. CBD stricture
5. Cong
6. Sclerosing cholangitis
7. Drugs
8. Infection: Eg Hydatid cyst

B & C are both due to interference c excretion of Bilirubin glucuronide

B generally causes hepatocellular J while C generally causes cholestatic J

Causes of Familial Non-Haemolytic Jaundice (LIST 26 GIT)

A. UNCONJUGATED
1. Gilbert's syndrome
2. Crigler-Najjar syndrome
3. Primary "shunt" hyper-bilirubinaemia
4. Familial neonatal hyper-bilirubinaemia

B. CONJUGATED
1. Dubin-Johnson syndrome
2. Rotor syndrome

CLIN: See individual diseases

INVESTIGATIONS:

	"A"	"B"	"C"
• Bilirubin	: Indirect ↑	: Direct ↑	: Direct ↑
• Urobilinogen	: ↑	: Norm or ↓	: ↓
• AST, ALT	: Norm	: ↑↑	: ↑
• Alk phos	: Norm	: sl ↑	: ↑
• PT time	: Norm	: ↑	: ↑
• Albumin	: Norm	: Occ ↓	: Norm
• Reticulocytes	: ↑	: Norm	: Norm
• Coombs Test	: Occ +ve	: —	: —
• FBC	: Usually	: Usually	: Usually
	: Macro-	: Normo-	: Hypo-
	: cytic	: cytic	: chromic

- FOB + ve in: Ca ampulla, Ca head of pancreas >varices
- Viral markers: HBsAg, Paul-Bunnel, CMV; IgM Ab to HepA
- ANA, Mitochondrial & smooth muscle antibodies: PBC & CAH
- Serum Fe; Ferritin; Transferrin; Caeruloplasmin
- AXR; CXR
- Ultrasound: If no obst, no further radiology usually needed
- ERCP
- PTC
- CAT scan
- HIDA scan
- Liver biopsy

RX: See individual diseases

Indications For Liver Biopsy (LIST 27 GIT)

1. Cirrhosis
2. Portal BP ↑
3. Jaundice
4. Chr hepatitis
5. Alcoholic liver disease
6. Unexplained hepatomegaly
7. Unexplained abnormal LFT
8. Screening of relatives c FH of liver disease
9. Wilson's disease
10. Haemochromatosis
11. Systemic disease: Eg TB, Sarcoid, Brucellosis, Reticuloses
12. Liver tumours: Primary & secondary
13. Infective liver disease
14. Drug induced disease

Complications of Liver Biopsy (LIST 28 GIT)

1. Haem. Due to:
   a) Puncture of gall bladder or major bile duct
   b) Capsular tears
2. Biliary colic
3. Bile peritonitis
4. Cholangitis
5. Puncture of Pancreas: May be serious
6. Puncture of kidney or colon: Usually no sequaelae
7. Intrahepatic haematomas: Rarely symptomatic

Alcohol & the Liver

Prevalence +vely ass c̄ per capita consumption, low cost. Esp low social class; brewery workers; servicemen; doctors; publicans & company directors

AETIOLOGY: 1. NAD ↑, NADP ↑ → fatty acid accumulation & ketosis → fatty liver
2. Triglyceride ↑ → fatty liver
3. Hepatotoxicity → necrosis, hepatitis → cirrhosis

PATHOLOGY: Fatty change. Pericellular fibrosis. Mallory bodies (10%). Then micronodular cirrhosis

FATTY LIVER

CLIN: Usually asymptomatic. Liver slightly ↑. Occ Anorexia. Rarely Fat embolus, Cholestasis

RX: Reduce or stop alcohol

ACUTE HEPATITIS

CLIN: Tender liver ↑; Moderate J; Fever; Abdo pain. Occ Portal BP ↑ → varices, ascites, encephalopathy, Spider naevi; Dupuytren's contracture; Parotitis; Wernicke's syndrome. Acute attack often ppt by a binge

RX: Abstinence
In acute attack: Low salt, low protein diet; Diuretics; & Rx encephalopathy. Regular monitoring of U&E, BG, Renal function. Folate & B vits. When stable, slowly ↑ protein
Zieve's Syndrome is Alc hepatitis c̄ Haemolysis & Hyperlipidaemia & is ass c̄ pancreatitis

CHRONIC HEPATITIS

May cause both CAH & CPH

RX: Abstinence

MICRONODULAR CIRRHOSIS

May occur along c̄ acute hepatitic episodes

RX: Abstinence still useful

INVESTIGATIONS OF ALCOHOLIC LIVER DISEASE

- FBC: Macrocytosis
- Platelets ↓
- WCC ↑
- ALT/AST
- BG
- GGT ↑
- B12, Folate
- Liver biopsy
- Ultrasound
- ERCP

Viral Hepatitis

Three gps: Hep A virus, Hep B virus & Hep non-A non-B

HEPATITIS A

Esp children & young adults. Prevalent late summer to winter. F-O route. Ass c̄ poor sanitation & contaminated water. Anicteric >> icteric. 2nd attacks rare.

Alcohol Related Disease
(LIST 29 GIT)

1. Gastrointestinal:
   a) Acute gastritis, GU, Mallory-Weiss
   b) Fatty liver, Acute hepatitis, CAH, Cirrhosis, ALF
   c) Pancreatitis
   d) Malabsorption
   e) Haemosiderosis
2. Cardiac:
   a) Arrhythmias
   b) Cardiomyopathy
   c) Beri-Beri
3. Neuropsychiatric:
   a) Delirium tremens
   b) Wernicke's encephalopathy
   c) Korsakov's psychosis
   d) Cerebellar degeneration
   e) Epilepsy
   f) Psychoses
   g) Suicide
4. Metabolic:
   a) Hypoglycaemia
   b) Hyperuricaemia
   c) Ketoacidosis
   d) Hypertriglyceridaemia
   e) Porphyria cutanea tarda
   f) Nutritional deficiencies due to poor diet
5. Muscular:
   a) Acute myositis
   b) Chronic myopathy
6. Increased incidence of infections:
   Esp TB
7. Social effects:
   Eg Disordered family relationships
8. Increased incidence of road traffic accidents

MACRONODULAR CIRRHOSIS

HAEMOSIDEROSIS, HAEMOCHROMATOSIS

Quite common. Due to ↑ Fe absorption in alcoholic cirrhosis & high Fe content of some beverages

RX: Desferrioxamine

DD: Idiopathic haemochromatosis

HEPATOMA

Incub Pd 15–50 days
Infect pd lasts from 7 days pre-symptoms into icteric phase

CLIN: Mild GI upset—Abdo pain, Anorexia, Nausea; Malaise; Headache; Fever. Then may → J, dark urine, pale stools; Liver ↑. Occ Spleen ↑. When J, GIT symptoms usually clear. Often relapse ppt by alcohol

INVESTIGATIONS: • ALT, AST
- Alk phos slight ↑
- Hep A specific IgM
- WCC: Leucopenia c̄ relative lymphocytosis early

RX: Good personal hygiene, proper sewage disposal. Close contacts given human immunoglobulins. Occ barrier nurse. Vaccine being developed

PROG: Usually full recovery

HEPATITIS B

M>F. Esp in Tropics. Common infection (millions of carriers). Ass c̄ injections, Tattooing, Drug abuse, Dental procedures, Homosexuality esp M, Long stay institutions. Can be spread from carrier mother to child. ? occ spread by mosquitoes. Can have more than once. Incub Pd 15–180 days depends on size of infection, route & immunity status

CLIN: Insidious onset: Anorexia; Nausea; Abdo pain. Occ Vom. After 3/52 "Serum Sickness" c̄ Pyrexia; Skin rashes; Arthralgia (25%). Then may → J; Liver ↑. Occ Spleen ↑; Pruritus. When J, GIT symptoms usually clear. Carrier state (M>F) is particularly common in Tropics, Far E, China, Greece. Esp c̄ anicteric cases

INVESTIGATIONS: • ALT, AST
- Alk phos slight ↑
- WCC: Leucopenia c̄ relative lymphocytosis early
- HBsAg
- HBcAg: Persistence in carrier
- HBeAg: Marker of infectivity & carriage risk
- AntiHBs: Indicates protection
- AntiHBe: Carriage state
- AntiHBc: Rising titre in acute phase

RX: a) Prevention & control: Hep B Ig useful in pre- & immediate post-exposure. Screen dialysis staff; Blood & Kidney donors. Hep B vaccine to high risk gps
b) Acute episode: Bed rest, barrier nurse & care c̄ samples

HEPATITIS NON-A NON-B

Probably >2 diseases. Both F-O & parenteral route esp blood transfusion & drug abuse

CLIN: Mild GIT symptoms—N; Anorexia; Abdo pain. Then may → J; Liver ↑. Occ spleen ↑. When J, GIT symptoms usually clear

INVESTIGATIONS: • ALT, AST
- Alk phos slight ↑
- WCC: Leucopenia c̄ relative lymphocytosis early
- Viral studies eg HBsAg, HepA specific IgM, CMV: Diagnosis by exclusion

RX: Good personal hygiene. Barrier nurse

COMPLICATIONS OF VIRAL HEPATITIS

1. Post-Hepatitis syndrome
   Malaise, TATT, anorexia, abdo discomfort. LFT normal
2. Relapsing hepatitis: Hep A >Hep B, Non-A Non-B
3. Prolonged cholestatic J
4. CPH: Hep B >Non-A Non-B
   Rare
5. Cirrhosis: Hep B >Non-A Non-B
   Rare. F>M. Esp in relapsing & sub-acute cases
6. Fulminating Hepatitis (ALF): Hep B >Hep A
7. Sub-acute Hepatitis
8. Extrahepatic manifestations: Esp Hep B
   Polyarthropathy, pleurisy, nephrosis
9. CAH: Esp Hep B
10. Hepatoma: Hep B
11. Giant cell hepatitis: Esp Hep B
    Infancy. India

DD OF VIRAL HEPATITIS

1. GE
2. Glandular fever
3. Drug induced J
4. Haemolytic disease
5. Serum sickness
6. CMV
7. Other causes of cirrhosis & hepatitis

Parasitic Liver Disease

AMOEBIC LIVER ABSCESS

Esp India, Nigeria, S.Afr, Mexico. 7M:1F

CLIN: Intermittent fever; Night sweats; Wt ↓; Abdo pain & intercostal tenderness. Abdo mass. Occ Asymptomatic

INVESTIGATIONS: • FBC, ESR
- WCC ↑
- IHA test
- CFT
- Indirect IFA

- CXR
- CAT scan
- Ultrasound ± Aspiration: "Anchovy sauce" pus

RX: Metronidazole 5/7 then Diloxanide furoate 10/7 ± Needle aspiration. Rarely surgery

COMPLICATIONS: 1. Rupture of abscess: → eg:
a) Empyema
b) Lung abscess
c) Peritonitis
d) Cholangitis
2. Caval thromb
3. Portal BP ↑: Rare

KALA-AZAR (LEISHMANIASIS)

Due to *L. donovani.* Esp Sudan, E.India, S.Am, Mediterranean. Zoonosis. Spread via sand-fly to RES. Incub Pd 2/12–10yrs

CLIN: Ac & Chr forms. Intermittent fever; Cough; Anaemia; Diarrhoea; Night sweats; Wt ↓; Epistaxis; Liver ↑; Spleen ↑↑. Occ LN ↑; Rash. Often sub-clin

INVESTIGATIONS:
- FBC, WCC: Pancytopenia
- IgG ↑↑
- Leishmanin skin test
- Bone marrow culture shows parasite
- CFT
- IFA
- LFT normal

RX: Pentavalent Antimony compounds eg Na stibogluconate

COMPLICATIONS: 1. 2° infection esp pulm TB
2. Portal BP ↑
3. Amyloidosis
4. Liver fibrosis (Roger's cirrhosis)

MALARIA (INVOLVING LIVER)

CLIN: In acute attack: Liver ↑; Spleen ↑; Mild J; Fever. Occ Tropical splenomegaly syndrome develops c̄ Spleen ↑↑, Liver ↑, Portal BP ↑

INVESTIGATION: • In Tropical splenomegaly syndrome IgM ↑↑

RX: Antimalarial drugs

HELMINTHIC INFECTIONS

Helminths often cause granuloma & biliary tract obst

HYDATID DISEASE OF LIVER: (Echinococcus)
Esp N, S & E Afr, Australia, New Zealand, Wales. Host is usually dog & eggs pass in faeces to man, sheep or cattle. Liver, esp R lobe, is site of 75% of hydatid cysts. May have long latent pd

Clin: Mass in R hypochondrium; Liver ↑. Later pain

Investigations:
- FBC: Eosinophilia
- IHA (Most reliable)
- CFT
- Indirect IFA
- Casoni skin test
- AXR, CXR: Occ Ca^{2+}
- Ultrasound

Rx: Surgical excision. Mebendazole

Complications: 1. Rupture into peritoneum, GIT, pleura, Biliary tract
2. Infection
3. Obstructive J

SCHISTOSOMIASIS: Due to *S.Mansoni* (esp E.Afr & Brazil) or *S.Japonicum* (Orient)

Pathology: Periportal granulomata → fibrosis → portal vein flow ↓ → presinusoidal portal BP ↑

Clin: Liver ↑ (esp L lobe) then portal BP ↑ c̄ liver ↑, Spleen ↑↑

Investigations:
- Eggs seen in stool, rectal mucosa & liver biopsy
- LFT normal

Rx: Oxamniquine, Niridazole

CHRONIC PERSISTENT HEPATITIS

Chr inflam for >6mths

CAUSES: 1. Hep B >Non-A Non-B
2. Drugs eg Isoniazid, Paracetamol
3. Alcohol
4. Idiopathic
5. IBD
6. Post CAH

PATHOLOGY: Chr inflammation c̄ hepatocyte damage & fibrosis

CLIN: May be asymptomatic. Occ post acute hep attack. Malaise; Alcohol intolerance; Liver slightly ↑

INVESTIGATIONS: • ALT, AST ↑
• HBsAg
• IgG: Usually norm
• Liver biopsy

RX: No alcohol. Review periodically

PROG: Excellent. Very rarely → CAH

CHRONIC ACTIVE HEPATITIS

Inflam c̄ piecemeal necrosis & fibrosis

CAUSES:
1. Hep B >Non-A Non-B
2. "Lupoid" (Idiopathic)
3. Alcohol
4. Wilson's Disease
5. Drugs eg Isoniazid
6. α_1-antitrypsin def

Hep B +ve CAH

Due to Hep B. Esp in immunosuppressed; Hep B carrier. M>F

CLIN: May be asymptomatic. Occ Preceded by liver disease. Later J & ascites

INVESTIGATIONS: • Bilirubin ↑
• ALT ↑
• IgG ↑
• HBsAg, HBeAg, HBcAg present
• Liver biopsy
• Smooth muscle Ab: Usually -ve

RX: Steroids (c/i TB) ± Azathioprine

PROG: Some improve. Usually liver function ↓. Occ Hepatoma

"Lupoid" CAH

? Autoimmune aetiology. F>M esp puberty, menopause. Ass c̄ Rh Arth Ulc Colitis; Thyroid disease; Sjorgen's; RTbA

CLIN: May be asymptomatic. May follow acute hep episode. Spleen ↑; J. Occ Rashes; Arthropathy; Pleurisy; Nephritis; Amenorrhoea. Later signs of liver failure; Cirrhosis

INVESTIGATIONS: • Bilirubin ↑
• ALT ↑
• IgG ↑ ↑
• LE cells
• ANA
• Anti-smooth mucle Ab
• Anti-mitochondrial Ab
• Anti-thyroid Ab
• Liver biopsy
• Serum Cu & Ceruloplasmin to exclude Wilson's

RX: Steroids for at least 2yrs, withdrawn when biopsy shows inactivity. Cyclophosphamide if lupus nephritis

PROG: Usually good response to steroids unless Cirrhosis

CIRRHOSIS

Incidence well correlated c̄ per capita alcohol consumption. M>F. A late result of hepatic cell necrosis c̄ fibrosis, disruption of lobules, linking of portal & systemic veins, nodular regeneration & vascular derangement

Causes of Cirrhosis (LIST 30 GIT)

1. Infection:
   a) Viral hepatitis: B & Non-A Non-B
   b) Syphilis (Cong)
2. Alcohol
3. Metabolic:
   a) Haemochromatosis
   b) Wilson's disease
   c) α-1-antitrypsin def
   d) Galactosaemia
   e) Fructosaemia
   f) Glycogen storage disease
   g) Tyrosinaemia
   h) Porphyria
   i) Cystic fibrosis
   j) Thalassaemia
   k) Sickle cell disease
4. Prolonged cholestasis (2° biliary cirrhosis):
   a) Stones
   b) Strictures
   c) Tumours
   d) Biliary atresia
5. Vascular:
   a) Budd-Chiari syndrome
   b) CCF
   c) Osler-Weber-Rendu
6. Immunological:
   a) CAH
   b) PBC
7. Drugs: Eg Methyldopa, Methotrexate
8. Cryptogenic
9. Indian childhood cirrhosis

CLIN: May be asymptomatic early.
Liver ↑ then ↓; Spleen ↑; Haem; Ascites; Fever; J; TATT; Wt ↓; Dyspepsia; Oedema; Diarrhoea; Spider naevi; Clubbing; Gynaecomastia; Gonadal atrophy; White nails; Sparse body hair; Bruising; BP ↑; 2° infections. Hepatic encephalopathy → lethargy, slurring, dementia, flap, precoma → coma. Portal BP ↑ → Varices

INVESTIGATIONS:
- FBC
- Platelets ↓
- WCC ↑
- U&E
- ALT, AST ↑
- Bilirubin ↑
- Albumin ↓
- Ig ↑
- GGT
- PT time ↑
- Serum Fe, Ferritin
- Blood & urine Cu, ceruloplasmin
- Liver biopsy
- Ultrasound
- Isotope scan
- ERCP
- Splenoportogram
- Angiography

RX: If possible remove causative factor eg Stop alcohol, Penicillamine for Wilson's disease, Venesection & Desferrioxamine for Fe overload. Care in drug prescribing. High protein diet. Regular surveillance c̄ early Rx of complications (qv)

COMPLICATIONS:
1. Portal BP ↑
2. Encephalopathy
3. Ascites
4. Varices, Vit K ↓, Platelets ↓ → Bleeding
5. Infections
6. RF
7. Pruritus
8. Hepatoma

PROG: Irreversible when established
Poor risk factors:
a) Small liver
b) Hepatoma
c) Variceal bleed
d) Progressive J
e) Resistent ascites
f) RF

DD of Cirrhosis (LIST 31 GIT)

1. Infections:
   a) Viral hepatitis
   b) Schistosomiasis
   c) TB
2. Vascular:
   a) CCF
   b) Portal vein thromb
3. Malignancy:
   a) Hepatoma
   b) Leukaemia
   c) Metastases
   d) Biliary tract tumours
4. Glycogen storage disease
5. Drug cholestasis
6. CAH

Causes of Hepatomegaly (LIST 32 GIT)

1. Infections:
   a) Bacterial eg TB, Liver abscess, Weil's disease
   b) Viral eg Viral hepatitis, Infectious mononucleosis, CMV
   c) Protozoal eg Malaria, Kala-azar, Amoebiasis, Toxoplasma
   d) Helminthic eg Hydatid disease
   e) Fungal eg Histoplasmosis
2. Malignancy:
   a) Metastases
   b) Reticuloses
   c) Primary liver tumours eg Hepatoma
3. Physiological: Riedel's lobe
4. Cystic disease
   Eg Adult polycystic disease of the liver
5. Vascular:
   a) CCF
   b) Tricuspid Stenosis (Pulsatile)
   c) Budd-Chiari syndrome
   d) Veno-occlusive disease
   e) Constrictive pericarditis
6. Myeloproliferative disorders:
   Eg Myelofibrosis
7. Fatty liver:
   a) Alcohol
   b) Obesity
   c) Pregnancy
   d) Drugs eg Tetracycline
   e) Diabetes
   f) Reye's syndrome
8. Metabolic:
   a) Glycogen storage disease
   b) Mucopolysaccharidoses
   c) Wilson's disease
   d) Haemochromatosis
   e) Amyloidosis
   f) Histiocytosis X
9. Early cirrhosis (later liver ↑)
10. Chronic hepatitis
11. Biliary tract obst:
    a) Stones
    b) Strictures
    c) Tumours

Portal Hypertension

Gradient between portal venous P & IVC P is normally 2–5mmHg. If gradient is >5–15mmHg: latent portal BP ↑; if >15mmHg: symptomatic portal BP ↑. Due to obst in portahepatic circulation. 90% of adult portal BP ↑ due to cirrhosis Portal BP ↑ may be due to
a) Periportal fibrosis (Pre sinusoidal)
b) Perisinusoidal fibrosis (sinusoidal)
c) Nodular compression (Post-sinusoidal)

Causes of Portal Hypertension (LIST 33 GIT)

A. PRE-SINUSOIDAL
1. Extrahepatic portal vein obst:
   a) Sepsis
   b) Malignancy
   c) Trauma
   d) Pancreatitis
2. Intrahepatic portal vein obst:
   a) Schistosomiasis
   b) Sarcoidosis
   c) Cong
   d) Vinyl chloride monomer
   e) Arsenic & Cu
   f) Reticuloses infiltration
3. Increased portal blood flow:
   a) A-V fistula
   b) Massive splenomegaly

B. SINUSOIDAL
1. Cirrhosis

C. POST-SINUSOIDAL
1. Budd-Chiari syndrome
2. Veno-occlusive disease
3. Constrictive pericarditis
4. PBC

CONSEQUENCES OF PORTAL BP ↑:
1. Spleen ↑ ± hypersplenism
2. Spontaneous porto-caval anastomosis:
   a) via umbilical vein
   b) via inf mesenteric vein (→ Ano-rectal varices)
   c) via R gastric vein (→ Oesophageal varices)
   d) via post gastric vein
3. Ascites: Seen particularly c̄ concurrent liver cell failure
4. Portal-portal anastomosis eg cavernoma, in extrahepatic obst

CLIN: Spleen ↑; GI bleeding from oesophageal or gastric varices (In cirrhosis may ppt encephalopathy, ascites, J); TATT; Anaemia; Epistaxis, ecchymoses & purpura; L upper abdo pain due to splenic size & infarcts. Distended abdo wall veins. Occ Ascites

INVESTIGATIONS: • Identify underlying cause
- LFT: Best shunt prog if Bilirubin <25μmol/l, Albumin >40g/l
- Liver biopsy
- Endoscopy
- Splenoportogram ± Portal P measurement
- Ultrasound
- α-FP

RX OF VARICEAL BLEEDING:

1. Resus: Bed rest; Fresh blood, plasma c̄ CVP line; Enema; Catheter; Neomycin; Low protein diet

2. Find bleeding site c̄ Endoscopy: N.B. May be haem from non-variceal cause eg erosion

3. Secure Haemostasis:

A. Medical: a) Vasopressin SE Colic, Diarrhoea c/i heart disease
b) Sengstaken tube SE Airway obst, Aspiration, Ruptured Oesophagus
c) Sclerosant via L coronary vein or at endoscopy

B. Surgical: If bleeding continues Pre-op splenic venogram to assess portal vein patency. Various ops:
a) Trans-oesphageal ligation: Short term Rx
b) Porta-caval shunt: *Complications:* Encephalopathy, J, GU, Haemochromatosis
c) Distal spleno-renal shunt (c̄ splenectomy if portal vein not patent). Low rate of post-op encephalopathy but technically difficult
d) Oesophageal transection: Short term Rx
Later, Elective op esp spleno-renal shunt as rebleeds common

PROG: 25–50% mort. Better if young, no ascites, no precoma, good nutritional state

Ascites in Liver Disease

Causes of Ascites (LIST 34 GIT)

1. Carcinoma:
   Eg GIT, Ovarian, Metastases
2. Cirrhosis
3. CCF
4. CAH
5. IVC obst
6. Hypoalbuminaemia:
   Esp Nephrotic syndrome
7. Portal vein thromb
8. Hepatic vein thromb
9. Rarely:
   a) Constrictive pericarditis
   b) Pancreatitis
   c) Chylous ascites due to lymphatic obst
   d) Hypothyroidism

PATHOGENESIS: Damaged liver cells → Albumin ↓ → plasma colloid osmotic P ↓. In Cirrhosis, ascites is also due to portal vein P ↑. In Budd–Chiari syndrome, ascites is ass c̄ hepatic vein obst
Compensatory mechanisms:
a) Renal blood flow ↑
b) GFR ↑
c) Aldosterone ↑
d) Urinary Na^+ ↑

CLIN: Insidious or rapid onset. Often ass signs of liver disease eg dilated abdo wall veins, oedema. Abdo ↑ (need 2 litres for shifting dullness); Flatulence; Anorexia; Wt ↑. Occ hernias esp hiatal, umbilical, inguinal; SOB; Pulmonary atelectasis; R Pleural effusion

INVESTIGATIONS: • U&E
- Albumin
- FBC
- WCC
- Ultrasound
- LFT
- Paracentesis: Protein, WCC, C&S, Amylase, ZN stain, Cytology

RX: A Medical: Treat underlying liver disease eg abstinence, remove IVC obst in Budd-Chiari syndrome. Bed rest; Low salt diet c̄ diuretic eg Frusemide & Spironolactone (SE: Na^+ ↓, K^+ ↓, Urea ↑, Encephalopathy); Daily wt & U&E. Occ use Ethacrynic acid; Salt free albumin; Cautious aspiration; Ascitic fluid ultrafiltration

B. Surgical: Side-to-side portocaval anastomosis: Controls ascites but high op mort esp risk of encephalopathy. Rx of choice in young c̄ normal LFTs & severe Portal BP ↑

Wilson's Disease

Aut recessive. Esp 5–40 yrs. Esp Arabs, Orient

CLIN: May be acute or insidious onset. May have no neurological signs. If liver disease: Malaise; J; Fever; Bleeding varices; Ascites; Spleen ↑; Bruising. Kayser–Fleischer ring on Descemets membrane near pupils, always present if neurological signs. Poor gait; Tremor; Parkinson-like symptoms; Cataracts. Occ Haemolytic anaemia; Aminoaciduria; Osteomalacia

INVESTIGATIONS: • FBC: Occ anaemia or pancytopenia
- Serum Ceruloplasmin ↓
- Liver biopsy: Cu ↑ ↑ ± cirrhosis, CAH
- 24hr urine: Cu ↑ ↑, PO_4 ↑, Aminoaciduria, Glycosuria

RX: Penicillamine (SE: Nephrotic syndrome, Thrombocytopenia) ± low Cu diet. Standard Rx of Liver failure. Screen relatives

PROG: Good if early Rx. Fatal if no Rx

Haemochromatosis

May be 1° or 2°. Due to chr excessive Fe absorption c̄ liver overload

Causes of Haemochromatosis (LIST 35 GIT)

1. Primary (Idiopathic) Haemochromatosis
2. Secondary haemochromatosis:
   a) Erythropoetic esp Thalassaemia, Sickle cell anaemia
   b) Alcoholic liver disease
   c) Porto-caval shunt
   d) Prolonged use of iron containing drugs
   e) Repeated transfusions
   f) Porphyria cutanea tarda
   g) High dietary iron esp in Bantus from "Kaffir" beer & iron cooking utensils

PRIMARY (IDIOPATHIC) HAEMOCHROMATOSIS

10M:1F. Aut Dom. Ass c̄ HLA-A3

CLIN: "Bronzed Diabetics". Lethargy; Malaise; Wt ↓; Liver ↑; Testicular atrophy; Skin pigmentation; Arthropathy; CCF; Periph neuritis

INVESTIGATIONS:
- Serum Fe
- Serum ferritin
- TIBC: Saturated
- Liver biopsy: Tissue Fe ↑ ↑
- Desferrioxamine test

RX: Weekly venesection of 500ml blood (250mg Fe) until Hb <11g/100ml. Then venesect when necessary. May use desferrioxamine. Screen relatives

COMPLICATIONS:
1. Chondrocalcinosis
2. Cardiomyopathy
3. Hepatoma

PROG: Rx does not aid arthritis, hypogonadism

Primary Biliary Cirrhosis

F>M. Esp 40–60yrs. Progressive liver disease → cholestasis & eventual cirrhosis. Strongly ass c̄ connective tissue disease inc Sjorgen's syndrome, Scleroderma, RTbA, Hashimoto's thyroiditis, Coeliac disease, Pancreatic hyposecretion & Rh Arth

AETIOLOGY: Immunologically mediated, ? cause

CLIN: Pruritus (commonest presentation). J; Liver ↑; Spleen ↑; Clubbing; Steatorrhoea; Xanthomas; Osteoporosis. Later Ascites; Encephalopathy; Variceal haem; Osteomalacia

INVESTIGATIONS:
- AST: sl ↑
- Bilirubin: usually sl ↑
- Alk Phos ↑ ↑
- Cholesterol
- IgM ↑
- AMAb +ve 95%
- Liver biopsy: Cu ↑
- ERCP

RX: Add Vit A, D & K, Ca^{2+} & PO_4, MCT to diet. Cholestyramine for pruritus. ? Penicillamine in advanced stages. ? Liver transplant

PROG: Poor prog indicated by bilirubin ↑ ↑, cholesterol ↓ & albumin ↓. Good prog if asymptomatic. Usually survive 5–10 yrs after symptom onset

Budd-Chiari Syndrome

A venous obst between R Atrium & liver

CAUSES:
1. Ca
2. PRV
3. "Pill"
4. Ulc colitis

CLIN: Tender liver ↑; Ascites; Portal BP ↑

INVESTIGATIONS:
- Liver scan: Liver uptake↓ except for spared caudate lobe
- Venography
- Angiography
- Liver biopsy

RX: Remove IVC or hepatic vein web if present. Generally need shunt but prog poor

Veno-Occlusive Disease

Esp India, S.Afr & Caribbean due to alkaloid ingestion eg Senecio
Due to compression of the central veins followed by non-portal cirrhosis

Liver Failure

AETIOLOGY:
1. Fulminant hepatic failure (ALF) arising in previously normal liver: Symptoms within 8/52 of onset. Uncommon
   Due to:
   a) Viral hep >Herpes simplex
   b) Drugs eg Paracetamol, Halothane, Tetracycline, Methyldopa
   c) Fatty liver eg Pregnancy & Reye's syndrome
2. 2° to Chr liver disease esp cirrhosis

CLIN: J; Ascites; Bleeding; Encephalopathy; RF; Diabetes; Osteomalacia. Fever; Vom; Hepatic fetor. Late BP ↑
Encephalopathy: Due to retention of toxic metabolites. 4 grades closely related to prog:
Grade I: Slurring of speech, Confusion, Insomnia
Grade II: Drowsy, Ataxia, Asterixis
Grade III: Drowsy++, Delirium, Reflexes++; Rigidity
Grade IV: Coma, Ep, Flaccid

INVESTIGATIONS:
- HBsAg
- WCC ↑
- BG
- PT time
- U&E

- FBC
- LFT
- Tests for underlying disease if acute phase controlled

RX: Look for & treat ppt cause eg infection, diuretics. Occ need barrier nursing
For Encephalopathy: Low protein, high chd diet; No sedatives; Enema; Neomycin; ± Lactulose. ? may do liver transplant. Charcoal haemoperfusion & Prostacyclin may be useful

COMPLICATIONS:

1. **Bleeding:** Esp GIT & Skin
   Due Esp To: a) Clotting factors synthesis ↓
   b) DIC
   c) Thrombocytopenia
   d) Varices
   e) PU

Hepatic Complications of Drugs

METABOLITE RELATED HEPATOTOXICITY

PARACETAMOL: Ppt by phenobarbitone inhibited by glutathione. When glutathione used up → liver necrosis, ALF

Clin: Anorexia, N&V. Occ LOC due to BG ↓ at 24–48hrs. Liver signs not present until 48hrs, then J, Liver ↑, Encephalopathy. Occ Ht & Kidney damage

Rx: Admit all patients with an o/d of >5g. If Paracetamol level raised, give N-acetylcysteine or Methionine (depending on level & time since ingestion)

ISONIAZID: Hepatitis in 0.1% esp >35yrs.

Causes of Drug Induced Liver Disease (LIST 36 GIT)

A. DOSE RELATED HEPATOTOXICITY
   1. Paracetamol
   2. Tetracycline
   3. Salicylates
   4. Methotrexate
   5. Azathioprine

B. DOSE INDEPENDENT HEPATOTOXICITY
   1. Acute or Chr Hepatitis:
      a) Antibiotics eg Sulphonamides, PAS, Isoniazid
      b) Methyldopa
      c) Halothane
      d) Phenytoin
      e) Dantrolene
      f) Propylthiouracil
   2. Cholestasis:
      a) Chlorpromazine
      b) Chlorpropamide
      c) Erythromycin
      d) Carbimazole
      e) Methyltestosterone
      f) "Pill"
      g) Anabolic steroids
      h) Rifampicin

C. HEPATIC FIBROSIS & TUMOURS
   1. Vinyl chloride monomer
   2. Thorotrast (No longer used)
   3. Arsenicals
   4. Rarely:
      a) "Pill"
      b) Anabolic steroids

   Rx: Vit K; FFP; Blood; Cimetidine

2. **ARF:**
   Rx: Occ dialysis
3. **Cerebral oedema:**
   Rx: Dexamethasone
4. **Hypoglycaemia & Diabetes:**
   Rx: IV Dextrose. Monitor BG c̄ care
5. **Fluid retention:** → ascites, oedema, pulmonary oedema
6. **Others:** a) Acute resp failure
   b). Pancreatitis

PROG: If coma 80% mort. Haemodialysis aids RF & oedema but ? not prog. Worse prog if in deep coma; Old; Bleed++ c̄ PT time ↑; Complications

ISONIAZID: Hepatitis in 0.1% esp >35yrs.
Rapid acetylators (50% pop). Ppt by enzyme inducers eg Rifampacin, Alcohol. Usually develops within 3mths. Not dose dependent

METHYLDOPA: Occ → hepatitis. J at 3–6wks. Rarely → CAH. Very rarely → cirrhosis. May also cause J by Coombs +ve haemolysis. Not dose dependent

METHOTREXATE: Fibrosis >hepatitis >cirrhosis due to toxic metabolite

Rx: Withdraw drug

HALOTHANE: Very rare. Seen on re-exposure to drug. ? hypersensitivity

Clin: Fever 8–13/7, malaise, J 10–28/7. Eosinophilia. Hepatitis → ALF. Poor prog if ALF

CCl_4: If ppt by phenobarb, alcohol: J, PT time ↑ → haem esp gastric, ARF

DIRECT HEPATOTOXICITY

TETRACYCLINE:
Clin: Fatty liver; Protein synthesis ↓. Rarely ALF. Absolute c/i 3rd trimester of preg

HYPERSENSITIVITY

GENERAL CLIN: Unrelated to dose. Fever, Rash; Arthralgia; Eosinophilia

CHLORPROMAZINE: Occurs in 0.5%. Onset 0–4/52. Prodromal stage 4–5/7. Then Cholestatic J; Eosinophilia; Rash; Fever; Pruritus
Prog: Good

OTHERS: a) Chlorpropamide
b) Azathioprine
c) Erythromycin
d) Carbimazole
e) Phenytoin

PURE CANNALICULAR CHOLESTASIS

CLIN: No hypersensitivity. Dose related. ? genetic factor
a) Methyltestosterone
b) "Pill"
c) Anabolic steroids

PROG: Good

DRUG INDUCED HEPATIC FIBROSIS & ANGIOSARCOMA

a) Thorotrast (Obsolete contrast agent)
b) Fowler's solution (Arsenical)
c) Vinyl chloride monomer

SEX HORMONES & HEPATIC NEOPLASIA

↑ Adenoma c̄ "Pill". ↑ Ca c̄ "Pill", Anabolic steroids. Very rare

Miscellaneous Conditions

LIVER TRAUMA

Ass c̄ rib #s, penetrating wounds

CLIN: Abdo pain & tenderness. Shock due to haem. Occ delayed presentation due to haematoma formation & rupture

RX: Laparotomy & transfusion. Secure haemostasis eg sutures, IVC balloon occlusion. Resect non-viable liver. If large resection, T-Tube CBD drain

PORTAL PYAEMIA

Esp 2° to acute appendicitis, diverticulitis, umbilical sepsis

CLIN: Rigors; High swinging temp; Tender liver ↑; J

INVESTIGATIONS: • Blood culture: Often +ve
• WCC

RX: Antibiotics. Occ drain abscess

POLYCYSTIC DISEASE OF THE LIVER

Ass c̄ polycystic disease of the kidney & pancreas. Infantile Aut Rec & Adult Aut Dom types

CLIN: Occ Portal BP ↑; Spleen ↑; Varices; Abdo pain. Also signs of kidney disease

INVESTIGATIONS: • Ultrasound scan
• LFT usually norm or sl ↑

Tumours of the Liver

A. BENIGN

HEPATOCELLULAR ADENOMA: Ass c̄ "Pill" esp in F >30yrs & c̄ long term use
Clin: Often asymptomatic. Occ Abdo pain; Liver ↑; Haem
Investigations: • αFP: Norm
• Liver scan
• Angiography
Rx: Stop "Pill". Resect tumour
Prog: Good

HAEMANGIOMA: Commonest benign tumour. F>M
Clin: Usually asymptomatic. Occ Abdo pain; Haem; Purpura
Investigations: • FBC: Occ Thrombocytopenia
• Angiography
Rx: Resect if symptomatic

B. MALIGNANT

HEPATOCELLULAR Ca: Esp N.Africa, Far E c̄ peak incidence 20–40yrs. Rare in UK. M>F. Ass c̄ Cirrhosis; Aflatoxins; Chr Hep B infection; Androgen Rx; Haemochromatosis; ? "Pill"
Clin: Abdo pain; Wt ↓; Liver ↑. Occ Vom; J; Haem. Later Ascites; Spleen ↑; Fever; Bone pain. Rarely Hypoglycaemia; HyperCa^{2+}; Sexual precocity; Clubbing; Carcinoid syndrome; Porphyria cutanea lata
Investigations: • αFP ↑
• CXR
• Ultrasound
• Liver Scan
• CAT Scan

- Angiography ± Cyt.T
- Liver Biopsy
- Ca^{2+}: Occ ↑

DD of ↑ Alpha feto-protein: (If very high virtually diagnostic of Hepatoma)

1. Germinal cell tumours of testis, ovary
2. Endometrial Ca
3. Viral hepatitis
4. Cirrhosis
5. Liver trauma

Rx: Surgical resection, Cyt.T, Liver transplants & Hepatic vein ligation all show poor results

Prog: Very poor

CHOLANGIOCARCINOMA: Esp Orient. Rare in UK. Ass c̄ flukes (Clonorchis), Ulc colitis, Crohn's, Thorotrast

Clin: Liver ↑; Obst J; Abdo pain; Wt ↓; Malaise

Investigations: • αFP: Normal
- CXR
- Ultrasound
- Liver Scan
- CAT Scan
- ERCP
- Angiography

Rx: Resection, Cyt.T or X-Rad. Palliative drainage of CBD via stent placed transhepatically or via ERCP

Prog: Poor

HAEMANGIOSARCOMA: Arise from Kupfer cells. Rare. Ass c̄ Thorotrast; Arsenicals; Vinyl chloride monomer

Clin: Upper abdo pain; Wt ↓; N; Liver ↑; Malaise. Occ J; Spleen ↑; Ascites; Haem. Later ALF, Mets

Investigations: • AXR: Occ Ca^{2+}
- Liver Scan
- Ultrasound
- Angiography
- CAT Scan

Rx: Resection, Cyt.T or X-Rad

Prog: Poor

C. METASTASES

Very common

RX:
1. Wedge removal: Rarely indicated
2. Hepatic artery ligation
3. Cyt.T esp by direct infusion into artery

PROG: Poor

MISCELLANEOUS SURGICAL TOPICS

Post Operative Complications

General Post Operative Complications (LIST 37 GIT)

1. Vascular:
   a) Haemorrhage
   b) DVT
   c) MI
   d) CVA
2. Urinary:
   a) Urinary retention
   b) ARF
   c) UTI
3. Respiratory:
   a) Obst of airway
   b) Inhaled vomit
   c) Pulm collapse
   d) Bronchopneumonia
   e) Tracheobronchitis
   f) PE
4. Bed sores
5. Parotitis
6. Constipation
7. Septicaemia
8. Anaesthetic related:
   Eg Drug reaction
10. Iatrogenic:
    Eg Poor post-op management of fluid balance

Local Post Op Complications of Abdominal Surgery (LIST 38 GIT)

1. Haemorrhage:
   a) Reactionary
   b) Secondary
2. Infection:
   a) Wound infection
   b) Subphrenic abscess
   c) Pelvic abscess
   d) Residual abscess
3. Burst abdomen
4. PI
5. Adhesions → obst
6. Incisional hernia
7. Anastomotic breakdown & fistula:
   Eg Faecal, Biliary
8. Persistent sinus
9. Peritonitis
10. Pseudo-membranous enterocolitis
11. Abdo distension (may → resp distress)

WOUND INFECTIONS

Common. Esp Large bowel surgery, Elderly, Obese, Prolonged surgery. Esp Staph; Coliforms, Haemolytic Streps. Anaerobic organisms are less common but may → gas gangene, tetanus. Predisposing factors can be considered in three gps:

1. Pre-op: Infection at or near the intended site of surgical wound & any drainage site eg skin infection esp Staph from nose or hand; Peritonitis from perf viscus; Immunodef eg malnourished, steroid Rx, Ca
2. Operative: Failures in theatre technique eg poor sterilisation of instruments/dressings; Poor staff hygiene; Infection from staff esp Staph carriers; Poor surgical technique eg soiling of wound by bowel contents
3. Post-op: Self-infection of wound; Cross infection by air-borne & contact routes

CLIN: Onset usually a few days post-op. Fever; Malaise; Anorexia; Vom. Wound becomes painful, red, swollen & tender & may discharge or form abscess. May → burst wound; Incisional hernia

INVESTIGATIONS: • Swab for C&S
• WCC ↑

PREVENTION: Pre-op correction of any general disability. Ensure cleanliness of equipment & environs. Pre-op skin disinfection. Good staff hygiene. Antibiotic prophylaxis for major surgery eg single dose of Cephalosporin for cholecystectomy at time of op, Metronidazole & Cephalosporin for colorectal surgery

RX: Analgesia. If pus present, drain. Antibiotics if cellulitis or septicaemia. Allow wound to heal by 2° intention

GAS GANGRENE

An acute infection due to a mixture of clostridial organisms esp *Cl.welchii, Cl.septicum, Cl.sporogenes.* Esp deep penetrating wounds. Was common in World War 1. Incub Pd 1–3 days

PATHOGENESIS: Clostridia are Gm −ve anaerobes which produce exotoxin. Some are saccharolytic, others are proteolytic → liberation of gas by protein destruction

CLIN: Shock; Vom; PR ↑; Fever. Wound becomes red & swollen & then gangrenous. Infection spreads to involve other muscles. Occ may → Septicaemia; ARF

INVESTIGATION: • X-R: Gas in soft tissues

PREVENTION: Wound debridement. Antibiotics for gas gangrene prone wounds eg patients c̄ atheroma requiring amputation

RX: Wide debridement removing all dead & doubtfully viable tissue. If extensive gangrene amputate. Antibiotics. Analgesia. Hyperbaric O_2 may be helpful. Correction of any shock. Correct any anaemia c̄ blood transfusion

BURST ABDOMEN

Occurs in about 1% of abdo ops. Predisposing factors can be considered in 3 gps:

1. Pre-op: Cachexia c̄ Protein def; Uraemia; Vit C def; Ca; Prolonged Steroid Rx; Obesity; Chr cough; Constipation; ↑ Intra-abdo P eg bladder neck obst
2. Op: Wrong or faulty suture material; Poor technique in closing wound; Failure to decompress grossly distended bowel
3. Post-op: Wound infection; Wound haematoma; Persistence of pre-op factors; Premature suture removal

CLIN: 3 major types:
Complete & revealed: This occurs about 10th day c̄ protrusion of bowel &/or discharge through wound. Occ Preceding serous effusion (pink fluid sign)
Superficial & revealed: Noted when skin sutures removed. Separation of skin & sc layers only. Usually 2° to wound haematoma or infection
Deep & concealed: All layers separate except skin. → incisional hernia

RX: Treat any wound infection; Reassure; Analgesia. If supf, evacuate any clot & allow to heal by 2° intention. If revealed, cover protruding viscus c̄ sterile towels & perform urgent op, resuturing wound c̄ interrupted sutures passing through all layers of abdo wall

PROG: Usually good

PULM COLLAPSE

Very common esp c̄ abdo or thoracic

procedures. Predisposing factors are: Pre-existing lung disease inc smoking; Conditions making coughing difficult eg Ank Sp; Anaesthetics → ↓ bronchial ciliary action; Pain of op → disinclination to cough; Heavy sedation

PATHOGENESIS: Mucus retained in bronchial tree → blockage of small airways → absorption of alveolar air → collapse of lung segments esp basal. Occ 2° infection

CLIN: Occurs in first two days post-op. Variable severity. SOB; Fever; Painful cough; ↓ air entry over affected area. Occ Cyanosis; Rhonchi; 2° Infection

INVESTIGATIONS:
- CXR
- Sputum C&S

PREVENTION: Stop smoking. Pre- & Post-op physio

RX: Physio; Antibiotics if infection

HAEMORRHAGE

1° haem occurs at time of op. Reactionary haem occurs within a few hrs of op due to eg slipped vessel ligature. 2° haem occurs a few days post-op due to infection or clot dissolution.

CLIN: Haem may be revealed eg blood via wound or drain, or concealed eg boggy mass in pelvis. Pallor; PR ↑; BP ↓. May be peritonism

PREVENTION: Good surgical technique

RX: Control any shock. Revealed haem may be controlled by pressure dressing. If no improvement, re-op & secure haemostasis

Causes of Post-op Pyrexia (LIST 39 GIT)

1. Infection:
   Eg Wound infection, Septicaemia, Abscess, Pneumonia, UTI, Enterocolitis
2. Haematoma
3. DVT
4. PE
5. Pulmonary collapse
6. Drug reaction
5. MI

RESIDUAL ABSCESS

The persistence or reforming of an abscess following a procedure to remove it. Predisposed to by infection, inadequate drainage, haematoma formation. Esp coliforms

CLIN: Continuation of malaise & fever following procedure. Local tenderness ± mass

RX: Incision, establish free drainage. Antibiotic

SUBPHRENIC ABSCESS

The potential subphrenic spaces become distended by pus forming subphrenic abscesses. Can occur in various sites eg R or L ant & R or L post space. R sided >L. Usually 2° to peritonitis but may occur 2° to abdo ops esp stomach & biliary tree

CLIN: Variable presentation. May be acute or gradual onset. Often Anorexia; N; Hiccoughs; PR ↑; Malaise. Occ Lower chest or shoulder tip pain; Swinging temperature; Liver sl ↑; Signs of consolidation &/or pleural effusion. Rarely Palpable mass; Local redness. Classical chest signs are resonance (norm lung), dullness (pleural effusion), dullness (gas above abscess), resonance (abscess). Rarely → Empyema; Pyopneumothorax; Pericarditis; Bronchopleural fistula; Mediastinal abscess

INVESTIGATIONS:
- WCC: Usually ↑
- FBC
- ESR: Usually ↑
- CXR
- Ultrasound
- Rarely CAT scan, Isotope scan

RX: Antibiotics, Analgesics, Good diet. Drain abscess under ultrasound or occ CAT scan control, leaving tube in situ. If no resolution require op

PELVIC ABSCESS

Usually 2° to peritonitis esp PU, Perf appendicitis, Perf diverticula. May follow Gynae infections. In F abscess lies between uterus & post vagina anteriorly & rectum posteriorly (Pouch of Douglas). In M abscess lies between bladder & rectum. Predisposing factors inc poor peritoneal toilet & an infected pelvic haematoma

CLIN: Tender boggy mass on rectal or vaginal examination; Diarrhoea; Mucus or blood stained stools; Fever; Malaise; Wt ↓; Anorexia

INVESTIGATIONS: • WCC ↑
• Ultrasound

RX: If abscess not pointing, give antibiotics & observe. If abscess pointing, drain abscess

FAECAL FISTULA

A fistula is an abnormal communication between 2 int organs or an int organ & the body surface. A faecal fistula discharges faeces & may occur post-op due to eg inadequate anastomosis, perf of bowel by drain, bowel disease esp Crohn's, obst distal to an anastomosis

RX: Many post-op fistulas close spontaneously & simply require dressings. Occ require dissecting out of track & closure of bowel. Hemicolectomy may be required esp for Crohn's

PROPHYLAXIS: Empty stomach before emergency op. Starve patient for 6hrs before elective op. If possible correct metabolic disturbances pre-op. Can give anti-emetic c̄ pre-med. Can use less emetic anaesthetic agents. Avoid rough handling of abdo viscera. Good op technique

RX: Anti-emetics eg Cyclizine. Correct fluid & electrolyte balance. Treat PI, peritonitis, mechanical obst, gastric surgery complications in standard manner

RUPTURED SPLEEN

Not uncommon inj following closed abdo trauma. Occ iatrogenic due to surgery

Causes of Post-op Vomiting
(LIST 40 GIT)

1. Psychogenic:
   Esp Response to noxious stimuli eg smell
2. Drugs:
   Esp Anaesthetic agents, Analgesics
3. Metabolic:
   Eg Uraemia, Diabetic ketosis
4. PI
5. Peritonitis
6. Gastric:
   a) Gastric atony esp Post Vag
   b) Pyloric obst esp post pyloroplasty
   c) Stomal ulceration esp post gastrectomy
7. Mechanical Obst:
   Eg Adhesions
8. ↑ ICP
9. CVA

ADHESIONS

Common sequelae to op esp abdo but only occ give rise to symptoms

CLIN: May cause early or late abdo obst

PREVENTION: Careful op technique

RX: Operate to relieve obst

PERSISTENT DISCHARGING SINUS

Due to persisting infection. May occur 2° to foreign material eg swab or stitch, partially drained abscess, chr underlying disease eg Crohn's, TB

RX: Probe sinus & remove any foreign material. If persists may require exploration

POST-OP VOMITING

Commonest causes are Drugs & PI

CLIN: Vom. May → Aspiration pneumonia inc Mendelsohn's syndrome; Burst abdomen; Dehydration

CLIN: Pallor; PR ↑; Tachypnoea; BP ↓; Abdo pain esp L upper quadrant; Abdo rigidity & distension; BS ↓. Occ Bruising over splenic area

INVESTIGATIONS: • FBC
• Group & XM
• AXR
• Occ Ultrasound, Isotope scan

RX: Treat shock pre-op. Urgent laparotomy & splenectomy

PRESSURE SORES

Esp elderly, immobile, drowsy or unconscious or the very ill. Pressure sores are often an important factor in a patient's progress. Two types, supf & deep

SUPERFICIAL PRESSURE SORES: Usually due to abrasion of the skin eg by dragging patient along bed esp if skin is inflammed or soggy eg as in the urinary incontinent

Rx: Avoid incorrect handling & unsuitable positioning. Good skin care inc careful drying, cleanliness, avoidance of irritants. When supf sores have occured, clean c̄ non-irritant lotion eg Eusol & where possible left dry

DEEP PRESSURE SORES: More serious than supf sores. Occ due to compression of tissues overlying bony structure → ↓ blood flow & ischaemic necrosis esp of sc tissues & muscle. Common sites are the ext malleoli of the ankles, heels, sacrum & femoral trochanters. Uncommon in healthy as ischaemia → discomfort & hence relieving mvt

Rx: Prevention involves the avoidance of unrelieved pressure on vulnerable areas in at-risk patients. Regular 2hrly turning will virtually abolish bed sores. Ripple mattresses are a useful adjunct to turning regimes. Care over patient's position in bed is of importance. Debride established deep sores & apply non-irritant eg Eusol. Good diet. Antibiotics for any 2° infection. Occ surgery eg skin grafts may be of benefit

PROG: Deep pressure sores usually heal slowly & may delay rehabilitation. On occasion the sore is a factor in the death of the patient

Peritonitis

Widespread infection within peritoneal cavity. Usually 2° to perf, leakage or gangrene of an abdominal viscus. Occ due to Septicaemia eg due to Strep, Staph, TB; Spread of infection from F genital tract eg Pneumococcus; Penetrating wounds; Infection introduced at op

CLIN: Symptoms & signs of ppt lesion. Then severe pain ppt by mvt; Vom; Fever (Occ temperature subnorm); Pallor; PR ↑; BP ↓; Tachypnoea. Initially abdo tenderness may be localised, later generalised tenderness, rigidity & rebound tenderness; Absent BS. Later increasing malaise; Faecal vom; Distended abdo; Cold clammy skin

INVESTIGATIONS: • WCC ↑
• CXR: Occ gas under diaphragm

RX: Analgesia; Drip & suck. Antibiotics eg for large bowel surgery, Gentamycin & Metronidazole; For PU, Cefuroxime. Surgery if source of infection can be removed or closed. Drain any local collections of pus. Conservative Rx if patient is moribund, primary focus is irremovable eg pancreatitis or when infection is localised eg appendix mass

BILIARY PERITONITIS

Bile is an irritant & the extent of inflam depends on amount of intraperitoneal leakage & degree of any ass infection. May occur due to Surgery iatrogenically; Perf or gangrenous gall bladder; Trauma. Rarely idiopathic

CLIN: Variable presentation. In major leak → abdo pain; Vom; Shock. Then PI; Abdo distension. Occ No abdo rigidity

RX: Laparotomy, correct leakage

PROG: 50% mort

TB PERITONITIS

Occurs 2° to TB elsewhere. May be part of generalised miliary TB

CLIN: Classically 3 forms, the acute, ascitic & plastic. Acute form mimics general peritonitis. The ascitic type presents more gradually c̄ abdo distension & ascites. The plastic type is characterised by gross adhesions → intestinal obst

RX: Standard anti-TB chemotherapy. Op to relieve any intestinal obst

Parenteral Nutrition

Parenteral nutrition is indicated when the enteral route can't supply sufficient nutrition to the malnourished patient. It attempts to satisfy the patient's full nutritional requirements & provide a +ve nitrogen balance

Indications for Total Parenteral Nutrition (LIST 41 GIT)

1. Intra-abdominal or other major sepsis
2. Major burns
3. Intestinal fistulas c̄ no distal obst
4. Short bowel syndrome
5. Multiple visceral injuries
6. Pancreatic conditions:
   a) Trauma
   b) Fistula
   c) Abscess
   d) Pseudocyst
   e) ?Acute pancreatitis
7. Possible benefit:
   a) Major surgery complications
   b) Pre-op to raise wt nearer to ideal
   c) IBD

Complications of Parenteral Nutrition (LIST 42 GIT)

1. Complications of Catheter insertion:
   Eg Pneumothorax, Air embolism, Venous thromb, Haematoma, Nerve injury, Sepsis
2. Metabolic complications:
   a) Hypoglycaemia
   b) Rebound BG ↓
   c) Def of electrolytes, Trace elements, Vitamins
   d) Osteomalacia
   e) Metabolic acidosis
   f) Hyperammonaemia
   g) Jaundice
   h) Intrahepatic cholestasis
   i) Fatty liver

Haematology

THE ANAEMIAS

If Hb <13.5g/dl in adult male; <11.5g/dl in adult female; <11g/dl from 3mths to puberty & <15g/dl from 0–3mths then anaemia is present Note that anaemia may be masked if plasma vol ↓ eg dehydration or if blood & circulating vol ↓ eg acute bleed. Spurious anaemia is caused by ↑ circulating vol eg infusion

NON-SPECIFIC CLIN: Pallor; Lassitude; Weakness; Fatigue

Iron Deficiency Anaemia

Causes of IDA (LIST 1 HAEM)

1. Excess physiological demand:
   a) Menstruation
   b) Pregnancy
   c) Childhood growth
2. Haemorrhage:
   Eg Ulcerative colitis, PU, Menorrhagia, Haematuria
3. Low dietary iron
4. Malabsorption:
   Eg Post gastrectomy, Coeliac disease, Hookworm

Children & menstruating & pregnant women heavily dependant on dietary iron. Requirement for adult men & postmenopausal is 1mg Fe/day, for growing children 1.5–2mg Fe/day, for menstruating women 1.5–2.5mg Fe/day, for women in 3rd trimester 4–5mg Fe/day

FACTORS ENHANCING Fe ABSORPTION:
1. Vit C
2. Meat, Fish
3. Acid
4. Fe^{2+} salts
5. Erythropoietin
6. Anaemia per se
7. Inorganic Fe

FACTORS REDUCING Fe ABSORPTION:
1. Phytates
2. Phosphates
3. Eggs, Tea
4. Alkalis
5. Organic Fe^{3+} salts
6. Tetracycline

STAGES OF Fe DEF: 1. Latent: Marrow stores ↓. No anaemia
2. Early: No marrow Fe. TIBC ↑. Anaemia—normochromic/cytic
3. Late: Serum Fe low. Anaemia—microcytic hypochromic
4. Tissue: Clinically apparent

CLIN: Occ Koilonychia; Glossitis; Angular stomatitis; Pigmentation; SOB; Achlorhydria & Atrophic gastritis; Spleen ↑. Retinal oedema & haem. Ass c̄ Plummer-Vinson Syndrome

INVESTIGATIONS: • FBC: Hb ↓, MCH ↓,

MCV ↓
- Blood film: Microcytic, Hypochromic. Occ hypersegmentation. Target cells. Anisocytosis. Poikilocytosis
- FOB
- Bone marrow: Erythroid hyperplasia if due to haem
- Underlying condition eg Endoscopy; Ba studies

RX: Oral iron eg Ferrous sulphate. Reticulocytosis seen after 4 days on Fe. Treat underlying cause. Rarely parenteral Fe

Indications for Parenteral Iron Therapy:

1. Oral iron intolarence
2. 3rd Trimester of pregnancy c̄ patient unwilling to take Fe
3. Hereditary telangiectasia
4. Inoperable GI bleeding eg Ca
5. Intestinal malabsorption eg Crohn's & Ulc Colitis

Parenteral Fe is c/i in Rh. Arth & in allergic may cause anaphylaxis

DD:
1. β Thalassemia
2. 1° Sideroblastic anaemia
3. Rarely: Infection, Uraemia, Cancer, Rh Arth

Sideroblastic Anaemia

Disordered Hb synthesis. The bone marrow erythroblasts contain ring of granules around nucleus

Causes of Sideroblastic Anaemia (LIST 2 HAEM)

1. Cong (1°)
2. Primary acquired sideroblastic anaemia
3. Vit B6 def
4. Lead poisoning
5. Alcoholism
6. Drugs:
   Eg Isoniazid, Chloramphenicol
7. Rarely:
   Ca, Leukaemia, Rh Arth, Myxoedema

INVESTIGATIONS:
- Blood film: In 1° — Hypochromic microcytic. In 2° — Dimorphic RBCs & usually macrocytosis
- Bone marrow: Fe ↑, Ring sideroblasts
- Liver biopsy: Fe ↑
- TIBC: Sat ↑
- Folate: Usually ↓

RX: Pyridoxine & Folic acid. Transfuse. Treat underlying cause

Causes of Dimorphic Blood Picture (LIST 3 HAEM)

1. Partially treated IDA
2. Sideroblastic aneamia
3. Mixed IDA & megaloblastic anaemia:
   Eg Poor diet, Malabsorption, Liver disease
4. Recent transfusion

Megaloblastic Anaemia

Megaloblasts in marrow due to defective DNA synthesis

Causes of Megaloblastic Anaemia (LIST 4 HAEM)

A. VIT B12 DEFICIENCY
1. Inadequate intake (rare):
   a) Poor diet
   b) Vegans
2. Malabsorption:
   a) Gastric causes eg Pernicious anemia, Partial or total gastrectomy
   b) Intestinal causes (inc B12 use by bacteria or parasites) eg Ileal resection, TB, Crohn's disease, Ileocaecal fistula, Jejunal diverticulosis, Blind loop syndrome, Tapeworm
3. Cong (rare):
   a) Intrinsic factor def
   b) Cong Vit B12 malabsorption c proteinuria
4. Drugs:
   Eg Metformin, PAS acid, Neomycin

B. FOLATE DEFICIENCY
1. Inadequate intake:
   Esp Alcoholics, Poor, Elderly, Mentally ill
2. Malabsorption:
   Eg Coeliac disease, Tropical sprue,
   Dermatitis herpetiformis
3. Excess physiological demand:
   a) Pregnancy
   b) Lactation
   c) Growth esp prematurity

➤

4. Excess pathological demand:
   a) Haemolytic anaemias
   b) Malignancy
   c) Myeloma
   d) Chr inflammatory disease eg Rh Arth, Psoriasis, TB
5. Excess losses:
   a) CCF
   b) Chronic dialysis
   c) Active liver disease
6. Drugs:
   Eg Anticonvulsants, Barbiturates, Methotrexate, Alcohol,Trimethoprim, Cholestyramine, The "Pill"
7. Homocystinuria
8. Inborn error of folate metabolism:
   Eg Dihydrofolate reductase deficiency

C. NORMAL FOLATE & B12:
1. Aplastic anaemia
2. Liver disease
3. Hereditary orotic aciduria
4. Lesch–Nyhan syndrome
5. Cytotoxic drugs:
   Eg 6-Mercaptopurine, Hydroxurea

Dietary requirements: 2–5μg of B12/day. 200μg Folate/day

CLIN: Anaemia; Sore mouth & tongue. PA signs (qv)

INVESTIGATIONS: • FBC: Hb ↓; MCV ↑; WCC ↓; Platelets ↓
- Blood film: Neutrophil hypersegmentation ↑
- Bone marrow
- Assay B12 & Folate
- Red cell folate
- Schilling test (B12)
- Urinary methylmalonic acid excretion (B12)
- FIGLU test
- Deoxyuridine supression test

RX: Parenteral Vit B12. Oral or occ parenteral Folate

Causes of Macrocytic Anemia c̄ Normoblastic Marrow (LIST 5 HAEM)

1. Blood regeneration (Reticulocytosis):
   a) Haemolysis
   b) Haemorrhage
2. Anaemias:
   a) Aplastic
   b) Leucoerythroblastic
   c) 2° sideroblastic
3. Alcoholism
4. Liver disease
5. Hypothyroidism
6. Myeloma
7. Cytotoxic drugs
8. Scurvy

Pernicious Anaemia

Esp middle & old age, N.Europe. A megaloblastic anaemia due to B12 def caused by severe atrophic gastritis. Ass c̄ auto-immune disease & long standing Fe def

CLIN: Insidious onset of anaemia. Occ Glossitis; Diarrhoea; SOB; Liver ↑; Spleen ↑; Mild J; Retinal Haem; CNS signs eg periph neuritis, optic atrophy; Dorsolat column involvement

INVESTIGATIONS: • Bone marrow
- Intrinsic factor ↓ (IF)
- Vit B12 ↓
- Pentagastrin test—Achlorhydria
- Ab's: 85% Parietal cell Ab (5–10% norm); >50% IF Ab
- Endoscopy ± biopsy to exclude Ca

RX: Hydroxycobalamin IM every 2/12

COMPLICATION: PA is pre-malignant

Vit B12 Def in Childhood

1. Cong intrinsic factor def: Aut rec
2. Cong Vit B12 malabsorption c̄ proteinuria (Imerslund–Grasbeck Syndrome): Aut Rec
3. Foetal deprivation

Aplastic Anaemia

A pancytopenia due to bone marrow aplasia
Esp young adults. Far East >Europe, USA

Causes of Aplastic Anaemia (LIST 6 HAEM)

1. Congenital (Fanconi's anaemia)
2. Idiopathic
3. Infections:
   Eg Hepatitis, Glandular fever
4. Drugs:
   a) Cyt.T (dose dependent) esp Busulphan
   b) Antibiotics eg eg Chloramphenicol, Sulphonamides
   c) Anti-inflammatory eg Phenylbutazone
5. Chemicals:
   Esp Benzene
6. Irradiation (dose dependent)
7. SLE (rare)

CLIN: Anaemia; Haem; Purpura; Infections ↑; Bruising ↑; No LN ↑; Usually no Spleen ↑

INVESTIGATIONS:
- FBC: Pancytopenia
- MCV: Occ ↑
- Bone marrow (trephine)
- Isotope study

RX: Treat infections eg Amphotericin & Septrin. Anabolic steroids. Antithymocytic globulin. Bone marrow transplantation

PROG: 50% mortality in 6mths. Occ spontaneous remissions

DD:
1. Paroxysmal nocturnal haemoglobinuria
2. Leukaemia

Fanconi's Anaemia

Aut Rec. Pre-malignant

CLIN: Occ patchy skin pigmentation; Bony abnormalities eg Syndactyly; Microcephaly; Short stature; Squint

INVESTIGATIONS:
- FBC
- Bone marrow
- Chromosomal studies

RX: Oxymethalone & Prednisolone

Failure of Red Cell Production

INHERITED RED CELL APLASIA (DIAMOND–BLACKFAN SYNDROME)

Presents in 1st yr c̄ anaemia. Reticulocytosis ↓↓. 25% have other cong abnormalities

ACQUIRED RED CELL APLASIA

ACUTE FORM:

Causes:
1. Hereditary Spherocytosis
2. AIHA
3. Sickle cell anaemia
4. Infections
5. Drugs eg Chloramphenicol
6. Riboflavin def

Rx: Oxymethalone, Steroids. Occ transfuse

CHRONIC FORM:

Causes:
1. Idiopathic
2. Immune ass c̄ thymoma

Rx: Thymectomy. Cyclophosphamide

Failure of Granulocyte Production

Neutropenia = $<2.5 \times 10^9$/l. Agranulocytosis is a syndrome of severe infection & pronounced neutropenia, often drug induced

Causes of Neutropenia (LIST 7 HAEM)

1. Drugs:
   Eg Cyt.T; Phenothiazines; Phenylbutazone
2. Infections:
   a) Viral eg Flu, Glandular fever, Infectious hepatitis
   b) Bacterial eg Typhoid, Brucellosis, Septicaemia
3. Hypersplenism:
   Eg Rh Arth (Felty's syndrome)
4. Aplastic anaemia
5. Cyclical Neutropenia
6. Collagen vascular diseases:
   Eg SLE
7. Chronic idiopathic
8. Severe megaloblastic & IDA
9. PNH
10. Endocrine:
    a) Hypo or Hyper thyroidism
    b) Hypopituitarism
11. Inherited:
    a) Kostman's syndrome: Fatal
    b) Familial benign chr neutropenia

CLIN: Severe infections

RX: Treat underlying condition, stop possible causative drugs. Antibiotics

Leuco–erythroblastic Anaemia

Erythroblasts together c̄ primitive white cells in the periph blood

Causes of Leuco–erythroblastic Anaemia (LIST 8 HAEM)

1. Carcinoma esp marrow mets
2. Myelosclerosis
3. Myeloma
4. Myeloid leukaemias
5. Hodgkin's disease
6. Severe haemolysis
7. Miliary TB
8. Osteopetrosis
9. Lipidoses
10. Thrombotic Thrombocytopenic purpura

Commonest causes are myelosclerosis & myeloma

Anaemias 2° to Non-haematological Disorders (LIST 9 HAEM)

1. Malignancy
2. Cirrhosis
3. CRF
4. Pregnancy
5. Collagen vascular diseases
6. Infection
7. Hypothyroidism
8. Hypopituitarism
9. Addison's disease

The Haemolytic Anaemias

Haemolysis is the reduction of RBC lifespan. Bone marrow compensation until breakdown 8X norm, then Haemolytic anaemia

MECHANISMS OF HAEMOLYSIS:

1. Abnormalities of RBC structure or function
2. Unusual RBC rigidity 2° to abnormal Hb or precipitation
3. ↑ Physical trauma

Causes of Haemolytic Anaemia (LIST 10 HAEM)

A. INHERITED:
 1. Abnormal Hb:
  a) Sickle cell Anaemia (Hb S)
  b) Thalassemia
  c) Hb C; Hb D; Hb E
 2. Abnormal RBC membrane:
  a) Hereditary Spherocytosis
  b) Hereditary Elliptocytosis
  c) Acanthocytosis
  d) Stomatocytosis
 3. Metabolic Defect:
  a) G6PD def
  b) Pyruvate kinase def

B. ACQUIRED:
 1. Auto-immune:
  a) Warm Ab (IgG): Eg SLE, CLL, Idiopathic, Lymphoma, Aldomet, CAH, Hashimoto's disease, Myeloproliferative disorders
  b) Cold agglutinin (IgM): Eg Lymphoma, Mycoplasma, Idiopathic, Infectious mononucleosis
  c) Paroxysmal cold haemoglobinuria (IgG)
 2. Haemolytic disease of the newborn
 3. Haemolytic transfusion reaction
 4. Infections: Eg Gram -ve septicaemia, Malaria, TB, Cl.welchii, Typhoid
 5. CRF
 6. Cirrhosis
 7. Haemolytic uraemic syndrome
 8. Drugs & Chemicals: Eg Phenacetin, PAS acid, Snake venom, Lead, Arsenic
 9. Hypersplenism (qv)
 10. Radiation
 11. Burns
 12. Rh Arth
 13. Cardiac surgery
 14. PNH
 15. Thrombotic thrombocytopenic purpura

GENERAL INVESTIGATIONS: • Bone marrow
- Urobilinogen ↑
- Unconjugated bilirubin ↑
- Stercobilinogen ↑
- Haptoglobins ↓↓
- Reticulocytosis
- LDH ↑
- Coombs' test
- Osmotic fragility
- Red cell morphology eg Sickle cells, Target cells
- Tests for intravascular haemolysis eg Schumm test
- Chromium-51 labelling of RBC

G6PD DEF

Very common although often asymptomatic enzyme def. X-Linked. Enzyme activity ↓. Esp Blacks, Orientals & Mediterranean. Commonest cause of oxidative haemolysis

PRECIPITATING FACTORS: 1. Drugs: eg Primaquine, Nitrofurantoin, Sulphonamides
2. Hepatitis
3. Diabetic Ketoacidosis
4. Pneumonia
5. Favism

CLIN: Intravascular haemolysis ie Fever; Malaise; Prostration; Dark urine occurs 2° to the ppt factors. Neonatal J. Occ Cong non-spherocytic haemolytic anaemia

INVESTIGATIONS: • Fluorescent spot test
- G6PD assay
- Methaemoglobinaemia
- Sulphaemoglobinaemia
- Blood film: Bite cells or Heinz bodies (c̄ splenectomy)

RX: Avoid ppt factors

PYRUVATE-KINASE DEFICIENCY

A cong non-spherocytic haemolytic anaemia. Aut Rec. Esp children

CLIN: Anaemia; J; Spleen ↑. Occ neonatal J. Ass c̄ gallstones

INVESTIGATIONS: • Autohaemolysis test
- Enzyme assay

RX: Splenectomy

HAEMOGLOBINOPATHIES

TYPES: 1. Abnormal Hb configuration or stability eg Sickle cell
2. Abnormal O_2 carriage eg Hb Chesapeake
3. Slow production → globin chain imbalance eg Thalassaemia

SICKLING DISORDERS: In HbS, Valine substituted in β-chain → ↑ blood viscosity & ↓ RBC life. Sickling disorders include Sickle cell trait (the carrier state HbA-HbS), Sickle cell anaemia HbS-HbS & others eg HbS-HbC. Esp central Africa. Severity depends on amount of HbS in RBC

Clin: Sickle cell trait usually asymptomatic
Sickle cell anaemia—Painful swelling of hands & feet. J; Spleen ↑; Dorsal kyphosis; Frontal bossing. Later splenic infarct
Periodic sickle cell crises ppt by Folic acid def, infection, pregnancy, acidosis, dehydration, cold & hypoxia characterised by severe limb & back pain, fever & malaise

Investigations: • Hb electrophoresis
- Dithionite test
- Blood film: Elongated "holly leaf" RBC

Rx: Check all Blacks for HbS pre-op. Genetic counselling. Vaccinate. Avoid ppt causes. Folic acid; Transfusions

Rx of Crises: Rest, Hydration, Analgesia, Antibiotics, O_2. Occ exchange transfusions

Complications: 1. Anaemia
2. Crises
3. Chr leg ulcers
4. Infection eg Salmonella osteomeyelitis
5. Aseptic necrosis of femoral & humeral head
6. Ht ↑
7. Pulmonary fibrosis occ → pulmonary BP ↑
8. Hepatic necrosis
9. Nephrotic syndrome
10. Intra-uterine death
11. Retinal haem

Prog of Sickle Cell Anaemia: High mort

OTHER ABNORMAL HAEMOGLOBINS

1. SICKLE CELL HbC DISEASE:
Clin: Anaemia; Spleen ↑; Sudden infarctive crises; High incidence of retinal & hip disease

2. HbC; HbD & HbE:
Clin: Spleen ↑; Chr anaemia

3. UNSTABLE HAEMOGLOBINS:
Ass c̄ Heinz bodies

THALASSEMIAS

Imbalanced synthesis of globin chains due to abnormality or loss of globin gene. Esp Africa, S.Europe, Middle & Far East

Excess globin chains → RBC inclusion bodies → ↑ RBC fragility

Two main Types:

1. α-thalassemia: αchains ↓
   4 subtypes: α-thalassemia 2; α-thalassemia 1; HbH; Hb Barts
2. β-thalassemia: βchains ↓
   4 subtypes: Minima; Minor (Heterozygous); Intermedia; Major

GENERAL INVESTIGATIONS: • FBC & film
- Hb electrophoresis
- HbA2 & HbF measurement
- Serum Fe & %Transferrin sat
- Genetic counselling

α THALASSEMIA 2: The silent carrier state. Single gene deletion. Very common in Greece, Italy, S.E.Asia, China

DD: IDA

α THALASSEMIA 1: Two α gene deletion

Clin: Mild (Microcytic) anaemia

Hb H: Three α genes lost. 5–30% of adult persons Hb is HbH

Clin: Mod severe anaemia; Spleen ↑

Hb BARTS (HYDROPS FOETALIS SYNDROME): Four α genes lost → No α chains

Clin: Stillbirth due to hydrops foetalis

Hb CONSTANT SPRING: A unique α chain variant. Esp S.E.Asia

β-THALASSEMIA MINOR: Esp Italy & Greece

Clin: Mild Anaemia. Usually asymptomatic

Investigations: • FBC: MCH ↓; MCV ↓
- Blood film: Basophilic stippling, Target cells
- Electrophoresis: HbA2 ↑, Usually HbF ↑

β-THALASSEMIA INTERMEDIA: A condition intermediate between the major & minor forms not usually requiring transfusions. Usually survive into adulthood

β-THALASSEMIA MAJOR (COOLEY'S ANAEMIA): Presents in infancy

Clin: Severe anaemia; Growth ↓; Liver ↑; Spleen ↑; Bone deformities eg frontal bossing; Fever. Later infections; Haemosiderosis

Investigations: • FBC: MCH ↓, MCV ↓↓
- Blood film: Microcytic, hypochromic, target cells, reticulocytosis
- Bone marrow: Erythroid hyperplasia
- Electrophoresis: HbF ↑, HbA2 ↑ but no HbA

Rx: Blood transfusions. Splenectomy if hypersplenism. Intensive iron chelation Rx c̄ desferrioxamine. Folate. BMT

HbS β-THALASSEMIA: African form less severe than both β-Thalassemia & sickle cell anaemia. Mediterranean form more severe

Clin: Mild anaemia; Spleen ↑; Episodes of pain

Investigation: • Electrophoresis: HbS, HbA2 ↑

DISORDERS OF RED CELL MEMBRANE

HEREDITARY SPHEROCYTOSIS: Aut Dom. Onset in childhood

Clin: Anaemia; Intermittent J & splenomegaly

Investigations: • Osmotic fragility ↑
- Blood film
- Coombs' test +ve

Rx: Splenectomy after age 10yrs to ↓ risk of pneumococcal sepsis

Complications: 1. Crises
2. Gallstone formation
3. Haemochromatosis
4. Chr leg ulcers

ELLIPTOCYTOSIS: Aut Dom. Not rare

Clin: May be symptomless. Occ Symptoms of haemolysis & ↑ spleen

Rx: Splenectomy if symptomatic

ACANTHOCYTOSIS: Rare. Ass c̄ β lipoprotein absence, malabsorption, retinitis pigmentosa, CNS involvement. RBCs have spiky excrescences

STOMATOCYTOSIS: Rare. Hereditary. Reversed RBC K^+/Na^+ ratio & overhydration

DD: 1. Alcoholism
2. Liver disease
3. Lead poisoning
4. Malignancy

AUTO IMMUNE HAEMOLYTIC ANAEMIA

A. WARM ANTIBODY HAEMOLYTIC ANAEMIA (IgG):

Causes: 1. Idiopathic 50%
2. SLE
3. CLL
4. Lymphoma
5. Drug induced eg Aldomet
6. Ovarian teratoma

Clin: Anaemia. Occ J; Spleen ↑

Investigations: • Coombs test +ve
- Blood film: Spherocytosis

- Test for underlying disease eg ANA, Bone marrow

Rx: Steroids. Occ Splenectomy

B. COLD AGGLUTININ HAEMOLYTIC ANAEMIA (IgM):

Causes: 1. Idiopathic
2. Mycoplasma
3. Lymphoma
4. Infectious mononucleosis

Clin: Occ Raynaud's phenomenon; Haemoglobinuria; Spleen ↑; LN ↑

Investigations: • Autoagglutination at low temperature
- Coombs' test +ve
- PPE: IgM band
- For underlying disease

Rx: Keep warm. Folic acid

C. PAROXYSMAL COLD HAEMOGLOBINURIA: Intermittent intravascular haemolysis & Hburia caused by Donath–Landsteiner auto-Ab which is cold dependant. Caused by viral infection or syphilis. Very rare

INTRAVASCULAR HAEMOLYSIS

Rare causes of haemolytic anaemia where RBC destroyed in vascular space

Causes of Intravascular Haemolysis (LIST 11 HAEM)

1. PNH
2. Paroxysmal cold haemoglobinuria
3. Prosthetic heart valves
4. March haemoglobinuria
5. Microangiopathic haemolytic anaemia
6. Favism
7. Malaria (Blackwater fever)
8. Cl.welchii septicaemia

INVESTIGATIONS: • Haemoglobinuria
- Urine haemosiderin
- Methaemalbuminaemia (Schumm's Test)

PAROXYSMAL NOCTURNAL HAEMOGLOBINURIA (PNH)

PATHOGENESIS: RBC membrane sensitive to lysis by complement esp if pH ↓. Esp 30–50yr old

CLIN: Early morning haemoglobinuria. Abdo pain due to thromb or infarct. Headaches. Ass c̄ aplastic or hypoplastic anaemia, acute leukaemia

INVESTIGATIONS: • Ham's test: +ve acid lysis
- Sucrose water test
- Cold Ab lysis test: +ve Anti-I

RX: Transfusion of washed RBCs. Occ Oxymethalone

PROSTHETIC HEART VALVE ANAEMIA

Artificial or diseased valve esp aortic → red cell trauma

CLIN: Often asymptomatic. Occ Symptoms of intravascular haemolysis

RX: Prophylactic anti-coagulation. Occ replace valve

MARCH HAEMOGLOBINURIA

Hburia following heavy physical excercise

MICROANGIOPATHIC HAEMOLYTIC ANAEMIA

Disease of small vessels → fragmented RBC & intravascular haemolysis

CAUSES: 1. Haemolytic uraemic syndrome
2. Malignancy
3. Thrombotic Thrombocytopenic purpura
4. Septicaemia
5. Collagen–vascular diseases
6. Eclampsia
7. Cavernous haemangiomata
8. Malignant BP ↑

1. HAEMOLYTIC URAEMIC SYNDROME: Esp childhood. Ass c̄ RF

Clin: Often preceded by URTI or GE. Oliguria; Anaemia; Nephritis; Fever; Purpura. Occ Abdo pain; J; Hburia; D&V; BP ↑; Coma

Investigations: • Blood film: RBC fragmentation; Spherocytes; Polychromasia
- WCC ↑, Platelets ↓
- Urea ↑
- Urinalysis
- Coagulation tests: Occ evidence of DIC

Rx: Standard Rx for RF. Occ Heparin used

Prog: Fair

2. MALIGNANCY: Esp found in disseminated mucus secreting Ca esp stomach

3. THROMBOTIC THROMBOCYTOPENIC PURPURA: Esp 10–40yrs. F>M. Often 2° to infection

Clin: Sudden onset. Fever; Purpura; Anaemia; Hburia; Paralysis; Psychosis;

Coma. Occ Spleen ↑; Uraemia; DIC

Rx: Plasmapheresis. FFP. Occ Steroids, Dipyrimadole

OTHER ACQUIRED RED CELL MEMBRANE DEFECTS

CHRONIC LIVER DISEASE: A severe haemolytic anaemia c̄ spur cells is occ seen

RENAL FAILURE: Burr cells are ass c̄ uraemia

LYMPHOPROLIFERATIVE DISEASE

Acute Lymphoblastic Leukaemia (ALL)

85% of childhood Leukaemia is ALL. In UK annual incidence = 0.3/million children <15yrs of age. Esp 3–5yrs of age

Aetiology usually unknown but viruses suspected. Rarely due to X-Rad, Chemicals eg Benzene. Ass c̄ Down's, Bloom's Syndromes; Fanconi's Anaemia

CLIN: Anaemia; Malaise; Fever; Infection; Purpura. Occ Gum or GI haem; Spleen ↑; LN ↑; Bone & jt pain. Mediastinal mass (Sternberg presentation). Later spread to CNS; Skin; Testes; Ovaries; Kidneys; GIT; Peritoneum; Bones

INVESTIGATIONS:
- WCC
- Platelets ↓
- Blood film: Occ lymphoblasts
- Bone marrow: Hypercellular c̄ blast cells
- Type for T, B, or null cell

RX: Induction of remission: >90% success c̄ Cyt.T eg Vincristine, Asparginase & Prednisolone preceded by hydration, alkalinisation of urine & Allopurinol. Transfuse, Antibiotics

CNS prophylaxis: Cranial X-Rad & Intrathecal Methotrexate

Maintenance chemotherapy for 2–3yrs eg Mercaptopurine & Methotrexate. Regular monitoring inc bilat testicular biopsy

SE of Rx:
1. Hazards of immunosuppression eg Measles, Chicken pox, Pneumocystis infection
2. Drug SE eg Periph neuropathy
3. Methotrexate-radiation toxicity: Ep & dementia

CLIN OF CNS LEUKAEMIA: Headache; Vom; Papilloedema

Adverse prognostic factors:
1. Male sex
2. Age <2 or >12yrs
3. High WCC
4. Organomegaly
5. CNS disease
6. Mediastinal mass
7. T-cell >B-cell ALL

DD:
1. ITP
2. Infectious mononucleosis
3. Aplastic anaemia

Chronic Lymphocytic Leukaemia

2M:1F. At diagnosis 80% aged 40–70yrs. Esp the West

Aetiology unknown, not due to radiation. 1% is T-cell CLL

CLIN: Many presentations, occ an incidental finding. LN ↑; Anaemia; Malaise; Spleen ↑; Lassitude; Purpura; Infections. Occ Haemolytic anaemia; Organ infiltration eg L'homme rouge (skin); Pleural effusion; Ascites; Mikulicz's syndrome. Gradual or fast progression c̄ ↑ susceptibility to infections

Ass c̄ ↑ in other Ca, but no progression to Acute Leukaemia

INVESTIGATIONS:
- FBC: Lymphocytosis occ Anaemia
- Platelets ↓
- Hypogammaglobulinaemia (60%)
- Coombs Test: Occ +ve
- Bone marrow

RX: Observe if asymptomatic. Cyclophosphamide & Chlorambucil. Steroids for AIHA, Thrombocytopenia, Marrow failure but ↑ risk of infection. X-Rad for local LN ↑. Transfusions

PROG: Median survival about 5yrs

Sezary Syndrome

Probably a leukaemic variant of mycosis fungoides. Abnormal mononuclear cells of T-cell origin in blood

CLIN: Severe pruritis; LN ↑ & oedematous exfoliative erythroderma

RX: Alkylating agents

Hairy Cell Leukaemia

Uncommon. Chr leukaemia characterised by mononuclear cell c̄ "Hairs" in marrow, spleen & blood. M>F esp middle age

CLIN: Spleen ↑; Infections esp TB

RX: Splenectomy. Chlorambucil. Interferon may help

PROG: Fair

Prolymphocytic Leukaemia

Rare variant of CLL. M>F esp elderly

CLIN: Spleen ↑↑

INVESTIGATION: • Promyelocytes in blood & marrow. WCC ↑↑↑

RX: Cyt.T & X-Rad

PROG: Poor

Causes of Lymphocytosis (LIST 12 HAEM)

1. Infections:
   a) Viral eg Exanthemata, Infectious mononucleosis
   b) Bacterial eg TB, Brucella, Pertusis, Typhoid
   c) Protozoal eg Toxoplasmosis
2. Physiological in early childhood
3. ALL, CLL
4. Malignancy
5. Post splenectomy

Acute Myelogenous Leukaemia

All ages but ↑ incidence >50yrs. M>F. Ass c̄ X-Rad & ?viruses
Variants:
80% Myeloblastic or myelomonoblastic;
5% Promyelocytic;
10% Erythroleukaemia (DiGuglienos); 1–2% Monoblastic

CLIN: Various presentations. Anaemia; Haem eg SAH or intracerebral; Infection esp Herpes, CMV; Tissue infiltration esp skin & kidneys → RF; Hyperuricaemia; LN ↑; Spleen ↑; Bone pain; J; Mouth ulcers c̄ candida. Gingivitis c̄ Gum hyperplasia. Focal CNS involvement eg cranial nerve palsy

CLIN OF ACUTE PROMYELOCYTIC FORM: Purpura; Epistaxis; Haemoptysis; Haematemesis; Malaena; Retinal haem. DIC

INVESTIGATIONS:
- Blood film: Blast cells. Auer rods. ↓ Mature granulocytes. WCC ↓ (aleukaemic leukaemia) or ↑
- Bone marrow: Blast cells
- Careful search for infection (Difficult to detect)

RX: Induction of remission ie <5% bone marrow blasts & normal FBC c̄ combination chemotherapy ± Immunotherapy
Red cell transfusion; Granulocyte transfusions; Platelet transfusion. Antibiotics. Reverse barrier nursing. Maintenance Cyt.T. Occ BMT esp in young (Cyclosporin A to help prevent GVHD)

PROG: Poor

Chronic Myeloid Leukaemia (CML)

All ages but esp middle aged. M sl>F. Ass c̄ radiation
Variants: CGL; Atypical CGL; Juvenile CML; Chr myelomonocytic Leukaemia; Chr neutophilic Leukaemia; Eosinophilic Leukaemia

CHRONIC GRANULOCYTIC LEUKAEMIA (CGL)

CLIN: Weakness; Fatigue; Malaise; Wt ↓; Pallor; SOB; Sweating; Liver ↑; Spleen ↑ → abdo discomfort, dyspepsia. Occ Haem into gums, skin, retina. Rarely Osteolysis; Gout. Later further spleen ↑; Blastic crisis ie fever, sweating, haem, bone pain

INVESTIGATIONS:
- FBC: Hb ↓
- WCC ↑↑
- Blood film: Myelocytes, Metamyelocytes & blast cells; Eosinophilia; Basophilia

- Platelets: Usually ↑, Occ ↓
- NAP ↓
- B12 & B12 binding protein ↑↑
- Bone marrow: Hypercellular; Usually ↑ blast cells
- Philadelphia chromosome: in 80%

N.B In blast crisis: Hb ↓; WCC ↑↑; Blast cells ↑

RX: Busulphan ± 6-Thioguanine. Occ Splenectomy; X-Rad. Rarely BMT. In blast crisis combination chemotherapy

PROG: >90% initial remission. Median survival 3yrs

PHILADELPHIA NEGATIVE CGL (ATYPICAL CGL)

No Philadelphia chromosome. Respond less well to Cyt.T

PROG: Poor

JUVENILE CHRONIC MYELOID LEUKAEMIA

Uncommon. Infants & young children. No Philadelphia chromosome

CLIN: LN ↑; Liver ↑; Spleen ↑; Skin lesions; Bruising

PROG: Poor

CHRONIC MYELOMONOCYTIC LEUKAEMIA

Esp elderly. Uncommon. No Philadelphia chromosome

CLIN: Spleen ↑↑

INVESTIGATIONS:
- Bone marrow: Usually blast cells
- Blood film: Mixed monocytosis & granulocytosis
- Serum lysozyme ↑

Causes of Monocytosis (LIST 13 HAEM)

1. Leukaemia:
   a) Chr monocytic
   b) Chr myelomonocytic
2. Hodgkins disease
3. Infections:
   a) Viral eg Infectious mononucleosis
   b) Bacterial eg TB; Brucellosis; Typhoid; Listeria
   c) Protozoal eg Malaria; Kala–Azar; Trypanosomiasis

CHRONIC NEUTROPHILIC LEUKAEMIA

Rare. Marked peripheral blood neutrophilia c̄ no immature forms. No Philadelphia chromosome

CLIN: Spleen ↑

DD: 2° Leukaemoid reactions

EOSINOPHILIC LEUKAEMIA

Rare. Immature cells in blood & marrow

CLIN: Liver ↑; Spleen ↑; LN ↑. Visceral infiltration esp Heart

RX: Cyt.T & Steroids

PROG: Poor

Causes of Eosinophilia (LIST 14 HAEM)

1. Parasites:
   Eg Ascaris; Hookworm; Tapeworm; Filaria; Hydatid; Bilharzia; Strongyloides; Toxocara
2. Skin disease:
   a) Scabies
   b) Eczema
   c) Urticaria
   d) Dermatitis herpetiformis
   e) Erythema neonatorum
3. Allergy:
   a) Food
   b) Drugs
   c) Asthma
   d) Hay fever
4. Malignancy:
   Eg Hodgkin's Disease; Eosinophilic leukaemia
5. Pulmonary Eosinophilia:
   a) Aspergillosis
   b) Tropical Eosinophilia
   c) PAN
   d) Loeffler's
6. Hypereosinophilic syndrome
7. Post splenectomy
8. Eosinophilic granuloma
9. Irradiation

THE LYMPHOMAS

Conventionally divided into Hodgkin's & Non-Hodgkin's lymphoma

STAGING: Stage I: Single LN region or single extralymphatic organ or site affected
Stage II: 2 or more LN on same side of diaphragm or involvement of extralymphatic organ & LN on same side of diaphragm
Stage III: LNs involve both sides of diaphragm ± involvement of spleen &/or extralymphatic organ
Stage IV: Diffuse involvement of extralymphatic organs ± LNs

Hodgkin's Disease

Malignant Lymphoma. M>F. Bimodal age distribution c̄ peaks at 25 & 70yrs
Four pathological types c̄ prognostic significance:
1. Lymphocyte predominant (best prog)
2. Nodular sclerosing
3. Mixed cellularity
4. Lymphocyte depleted (worst prog)

Characteristic Reed–Sternberg multinucleated cell

CLIN: Usually arises in LN. Painless rubbery LN ↑ (Pain c̄ alcohol); Spleen ↑; Liver ↑; Fever (Occ periodic "Pel–Ebstein"); Anaemia; Wt ↓; Weakness; Malaise; Pruritis. Occ Osteosclerosis (ivory vertebra) → extradural compression; Gout; Peripheral neuropathy; Pulmonary infiltration; 2° infection esp TB, Herpes, Cryptococcus; Pleural effusion; Skin nodules & pigmentation. Later J; Ascites
"B" symptoms ie 10% body Wt ↓ in 6/12, Fever >38° C, Night sweats are poor prognostic signs

INVESTIGATIONS:
- LN biopsy
- ESR ↑
- CXR
- FBC: Occ Lymphopenia; Leucocytosis; Eosinophilia
- Platelets occ ↓
- Bone marrow
- LFT
- Liver scan
- CAT scan
- Lymphangiography
- Laparotomy c̄ Splenectomy for staging

RX: Stage I & II: Mantle X-Rad & Adjuvent Cyt.T
Stage IIIA: Combination chemotherapy eg MVPP & nodal X-Rad
Stage IIIB & IV: Combination chemotherapy

PROG: 5yr survival: Stage I, IIA 90% Stage IIB, III 75% Stage IV 50%

Non-Hodgkin's Lymphoma

Esp middle aged & elderly. Commoner than Hodgkin's disease
Classification is difficult. The Lukes–Collins classification is based on immunohistochemical techniques. Other classifications inc Kiel & Modified Rappaport's classification

Modified Rappaport's Classification:
A. Nodular forms:
- Poorly differentiated nodular lymphocytic lymphoma
- Mixed nodular histiocytic lymphocytic lymphoma
- Nodular histiocytic lymphoma
- Nodular (follicular) lymphoma

B. Diffuse forms:
- Well differentiated diffuse lymphocytic lymphoma
- Poorly differentiated diffuse lymphocytic lymphoma
- Mixed diffuse histiocytic lymphocytic lymphoma
- Diffuse histiocytic lymphoma
- Lymphoblastic Lymphoma (Sternberg presentation)
- Undifferentiated diffuse lymphoma (Inc Burkitt's)

Generally best prog is c̄ small cells & nodular forms

CLIN: Often presents in stage IV. LN ↑; Spleen ↑; Liver ↑. Often infiltration of GIT, CNS, Bone marrow. Wt ↓; Fever; Sweating. Occ AIHA. Later Marrow failure; Hypersplenism. In Diffuse histiocytic lymphoma often infiltration of thyroid, testes & bone. Occ Well differentiated diffuse lymphoma becomes a CLL

INVESTIGATIONS:
- FBC
- ESR ↑
- LFT
- Liver biopsy
- Bone marrow

- LN biopsy (N.B Inflam changes in axillary & groin LN often make them poor choice for biopsy)
- CXR
- IVU
- Bone scan
- CAT
- PPE: Hypogammaglobulinaemia >IgM ↑ >Polyclonal gammopathy
- Rarely: Ba meal & follow through, Lymphography

RX: X-Rad for Stage I, II & palliation. Cyt.T (more intensively if poor prog) & Steroids

PROG: Good prog gp: Median survival 5yrs
Diffuse histiocytic lymphoma: Good if remission achieved
Poor prog gp: 5yr survival 20%

Burkitt's Lymphoma

Esp E.Africa. Esp children. Due to E-B herpes virus
Characteristic biopsy picture

CLIN: Multifocal tumour esp Jaw; Abdominal viscera; Ovaries; Retroperitoneum; Spinal cord; Thyroid. Rarely affects lymphoid tissue

RX: CyT.T

PROG: Very good

Mycosis Fungoides

A chronic skin lymphoma (T-cell)

CLIN: Chr psoriasiform lesion over many years → skin tumour c̄ LN & RES involvement

RX: PUVA. Local X-Rad or topical chemotherapy

Sternberg's Sarcoma

A thymic lymphoma (T-cell). Esp young males

CLIN: Bone marrow infiltration. Symptoms of ALL

RX: As for ALL

Causes of Lymphadenopathy (LIST 15 HAEM)

1. Infection
2. Malignancy
3. Hodgkin's disease
4. Non-Hodgkin's Lymphomas
5. ALL, CLL
6. Sarcoidosis
7. Collagen vascular disease
8. Histiocytosis X
9. Drugs:
   Eg Phenytoin

GRAFT VERSUS HOST DISEASE

Due to the transference of competent lymphoid cells from a donor to a recipient which is incapaple of rejecting them, the grafted cells subsequently reacting against the foreign host. May occur in immunologically anergic receiving transplants eg BMT for severe combined immunodef

CLIN: In acute GVHD macular pruritic rash esp mucous membranes, palms & soles develops about 10–14days post transplant. Fever; Anaemia; Diarrhoea; Wt ↓; Spleen ↑
Chr GVHD is sometimes preceded by acute GVHD & occurs >3mths post transplant. Mottling of skin → sclerosis. Occ Alopecia; Loss of nails

RX: Cyclosporin A

MYELOPROLIFERATIVE DISORDERS

Polycythaemia Rubra Vera

Idiopathic condition. M>F. Esp Elderly
RBC marrow production ↑ – RBC mass ↑; PCV ↑; Red cell count ↑

Causes of Polycythaemia (LIST 16 HAEM)

A. RELATIVE
  1. Dehydration
  2. Erythrocytosis (Stress polycythaemia)

B. ABSOLUTE
  1. PRV
  2. Secondary
    i) Tumours
      a) Renal Ca
      b) Hepatoma
      c) Phaeochromocytoma
      d) Uterine myomata
      e) Androgen secreting Ca
      f) Cerebellar Haemangioblastoma
    ii) Respiratory
      a) COAD
      b) Pulmonary fibrosis
      c) Pickwickian Syndrome
    iii) High altitude (Hypoxia)
    iv) R–L shunt eg Cyanotic CHD
    v) Renal cysts & hydronephrosis
    vi) Abnormal haemoglobins eg Methaemoglobinaemia
    vii) Benign familial

CLIN: Plethoric appearance; Pruritis; Headache; Dizzyness; Haem; Dyspepsia; Thrombosis eg Cerebral, Coronary, Lower limbs; Spleen ↑. Occ DU; BP ↑; Liver ↑; Myelofibrosis & bone marrow failure; Leukaemia

INVESTIGATIONS:
- FBC: Hb ↑; PCV ↑; WCC ↑
- Platelets ↑
- Serum B12 & B12 binding protein ↑
- NAP ↑
- Uric acid ↑
- CXR
- IVU
- Isotope assay for red cell mass
- Lysozyme ↑
- Bone marrow
- LDH ↑

RX: Busulphan or repeat venesection until PCV <0.5 then radioactive phosphorus

PROG: Median survival 15yrs. Small risk of leukaemia after prolonged Rx c̄ radioactive phosphorus

Myelofibrosis

Fibrous tissue deposited in bone marrow. Primary form late middle age

Causes of Myelofibrosis (LIST 17 HAEM)

1. Primary (Idiopathic)
2. Other myeloproliferative diseases
3. Malignancy: Esp Mets
4. Chr infection: Eg TB
5. Irradiation
6. Benzene
7. Fluorosis
8. Mastocytosis
9. Hodgkin's Disease
10. SLE
11. Osteopetrosis (Marble bone disease)
12. Renal osteodystrophy

CLIN: Insidious onset. Weakness; Fatigue; Pallor; Night sweats; Wt ↓; Spleen ↑. Occ Bruising; Haem eg GI bleed, epistaxis; PU; Gout; Obst uropathy. Liver ↑ occ → portal BP ↑, varices. 2° infections. Later Spleen ↑↑

INVESTIGATIONS:
- WCC: ↑, norm or ↓
- NAP: Norm or ↑
- Blood film: Tear drop poikilocytes; Anisocytosis; Nucleated RBC. Leucoerythroblastic anaemia
- X-R bone: Occ osteosclerosis
- Bone marrow trephine

RX: Blood transfusions. Allopurinol. Folic acid. Pyridoxine. Oxymethalone. Occ Busulphan. Splenectomy if symptoms from spleen ↑↑, or severe thrombocytopenia

PROG: Median survival 4yrs

MALIGNANT MYELOFIBROSIS

Rare

CLIN: Rapid downhill course. Anaemia; Haem; No spleen ↑; 2° infections

INVESTIGATIONS:
- WCC ↓↓
- Platelets ↓
- Hb ↓
- Blood film: Myeloblasts; Reticulocytes ↓
- Bone marrow trephine
- Bone biopsy

RX: As above but usually refractory to Rx

PROG: Few months

Essential Haemorrhagic Thrombocythaemia

Thrombocythaemia may complicate any of the myeloproliferative diseases but may be an isolated abnormality

CLIN: Haemorrhage tendency ↑ eg epistaxis; GI bleed; ↑ menstrual bleeding. Spleen ↑; Anaemia; Thromboses

INVESTIGATIONS: • Bone marrow: ↑ in size & number of megakaryocytes
- Platelets ↑↑ but abnormal function
- WCC ↑
- NAP ↑

RX: Periodic radioactive phosphorus or Busulphan
N.B Risk of severe haem or thromb c̄ surgery

Causes of Splenomegaly (LIST 18 HAEM)

A. CAUSES OF MASSIVELY ENLARGED SPLEEN
1. Infections & Infestations:
   a) Malaria
   b) Kala–Azar
2. CML
3. Myelofibrosis

B. CAUSES OF MODERATELY ENLARGED SPLEEN
1. Causes of A
2. Leukaemias
3. Haemolytic Anaemias
4. Portal BP ↑
5. Lipid Storage Disorders
6. Lymphomas

C. CAUSES OF SLIGHTLY ENLARGED SPLEEN
1. Causes of A & B
2. Myeloproliferative disease
3. Infections:
   Eg Typhus; Typhoid; TB; Brucellosis; SABE; Septicaemia; Hep B; Infectious mononucleosis; Hydatid cyst
4. Malignant lymphomas
5. Benign tumours & cysts
6. Collagen vascular diseases:
   Eg Rh Arth, SLE
7. Megaloblastic anaemia
8. ITP
9. Myeloma
10. Amyloidosis
11. Sarcoidosis

HYPERSPLENISM

The ass of splenomegaly c̄ a reduction of one or more blood elements

Causes of Hypersplenism (LIST 19 HAEM)

1. Portal BP ↑
2. Myelofibrosis
3. Malignant lymphomas
4. CML, CGL
5. Chronic infections eg TB; Brucella; Malaria
6. Felty's Syndrome (Rh Arth)
7. Sarcoidosis
8. Gaucher's & Nieman Pick's disease
9. Tropical splenomegaly syndrome
10. Idiopathic

PLASMA CELL NEOPLASMS

Plasma cell neoplasms arise from an uncontrolled proliferation of β-lymphocytes to form a large monoclonal population

Causes of Monoclonal Gammopathy (LIST 20 HAEM)

A. BENIGN
1. Benign monoclonal gammopathy
2. Transient 2° to infection
3. Chronic cold agglutinin disease
4. Rarely α heavy chain disease

B. NEOPLASTIC
1. Myeloma
2. Macroglobulinaemia
3. Amyloidosis
4. Heavy chain diseases
5. Plasma cell neoplasms of skin
6. CLL & Diffuse lymphomas (rare)

Myeloma

Esp 50–70yrs. Characterised by bone lesions, paraprotein in serum/urine & infiltration of marrow c̄ plasma cells

CLIN: Bone pain; Infections eg Herpes, bacterial; Haem; Fever; Purpura; Anaemia. Later renal involvement c̄ signs of ARF or CRF; Wt ↓. Occ Amyloidosis → Nephrotic syndrome, carpal tunnel syndrome, macroglossia, neuropathy

INVESTIGATIONS:
- Blood film: Rouleaux. Occ plasma cells or leuco-erythroblastic anaemia
- ESR ↑
- Bone marrow: Plasma cells usually >10%
- PPE: Monoclonal gammopathy IgG >IgA >Light chains
- Proteinuria
- Platelets: ↑ or ↓
- Urine electrophoresis: Often light chains (Bence–Jones protein)
- X-R: Usually osteoporosis &/or osteolytic areas. Rarely Osteosclerosis
- Serum Ca^{2+}: Often ↑
- Urea, Creatinine
- Uric acid
- Alk phos
- Occ Myelogram, Rectal Biopsy

RX: Relieve pain c̄ X-Rad, Analgesia, Spinal support. Push fluids. Steroids for hyperCa. Allopurinol. Antibiotics. Local X-Rad for bony lesions. Cyt.T (Melphalan & Prednisolone) esp if platelets ↑. Regular follow up

COMPLICATIONS:
1. Hypercalcaemia
2. Renal failure
3. Infections
4. Amyloidosis
5. Acute leukaemia

PROG: Median survival 30mths. Poorer prog if Uraemia

Waldenstrom's Macroglobulinaemia

Malignant disease of IgM plasma cells

CLIN: Anaemia. Hyperviscosity → Haem eg Epistaxis, CCF, purpura, retinopathy, lethargy, headache, vertigo, nystagmus, coma, Pulmonary BP ↑. Cold sensitivity eg Raynaud's, AIHA. LN ↑; Spleen ↑. No bone destruction. Occ 2° infections; Amyloidosis. Rarely RF

INVESTIGATIONS:
- PPE: Monoclonal IgM ↑
- Immunoelectrophoresis
- Blood film: Rouleaux
- ESR ↑
- Bone marrow

RX: Plasmapheresis, Chlorambucil & Prednisolone

Heavy Chain Disease

Rare. Esp middle aged. M>F

CLIN: Rapid course. LN ↑; Spleen ↑; Weakness; Wt ↓; GI involvement

RX: Cyt.T

PROG: Poor

Benign Monoclonal Gammopathy

Higher prevalence than myeloma

CLIN: Usually asymptomatic. No bone lesions, anaemia or wt ↓

INVESTIGATIONS:
- PPE: Usually monoclonal IgG ↑
- Serum Ig <0.3g/l
- Bone marrow: 5–15% plasma cells

PROG: Very good but 20% develop myeloma within 10yrs

Amyloidosis

Syndromes c̄ deposition of amyloid. Amyloid is an Ig related protein/chd aggregate

CLASSIFICATION: 1. Primary Familial: Occ ass c̄ Familial Mediterranean fever
2. Primary Atypical
3. Secondary: Due to
   a) Chr suppurative disorders
   b) Malignancy
   c) Myeloma
   d) Reticuloses
   e) Rh Arth
   f) Leprosy
   g) Ulc colitis
   h) Chr pyelonephritis
4. Para-amyloid
5. Localised

CLIN: Primary Atypical: Malabsorption; Diarrhoea; Neuropathy; Myopathy; Skin lesions. Occ Bence–Jones protein
Primary Familial: Neuropathy; Nephrotic syndrome; Cardiomyopathy
Secondary: Spleen ↑; Liver ↑; Nephrotic syndrome; Renal vein thromb; Renal failure. Occ Bence–Jones protein. 10% of myeloma → amyloidosis

INVESTIGATIONS: • Rectal biopsy
• Renal biopsy

RX: ?Melphalan

HAEMORRHAGIC DISORDERS

Blood coagulation is mediated via an extrinsic pathway involving tissue thromboplastin & factors VII, X, V & an intrinsic pathway involving factors XII, XI, IX, VIII, X, V, II. The final common pathway is for thrombin to convert fibrinogen to fibrin
It is convenient to discuss haemorrhagic disorders under three headings: Coagulation, Platelet & Vascular abnormalities

CLIN OF COAGULATION DEFECT:
Large bruises; Haemarthrosis; Haematuria; Late post-op bleeding

CLIN OF PLATELET/CAPILLARY DEFECT:
Bleeding++ from cuts controlled by pressure; Epistaxis; GI bleed. Early post-op bleed

GENERAL INVESTIGATIONS FOR HAEMOSTASIS: • Platelets
• Prothrombin time
• Thrombin clotting time
• Activated partial thromboplastin time
• Bleeding time

Vascular Abnormalities

HEREDITARY TELANGIECTASIA

Familial. Esp childhood. Aut Dom. Lack of muscle & elastic coats of vessels

CLIN: Skin & mucous membrane lesions. Epistaxis; GI haem; Haemoptysis. Ass c̄ A-V fistulae in lung, liver & spleen

RX: Local pressure; Transfusions; Oestrogens

Causes of Vessel Defects
(LIST 21 HAEM)

A. CONGENITAL
1. Hereditary Telangiectasia (Osler–Weber–Rendu)
2. Connective tissue disorders: Eg Ehlers–Danlos syndrome
3. Haemangiomatosis

B. ACQUIRED
1. Vasculitis
2. Infections: Eg Meningococcal septicaemia
3. Senile pupura
4. Drugs: Eg Steroids
5. Simple bruising
6. Dermatoses: Eg Eczema
7. Systemic diseases: Eg Cushing's, Scurvy, BP ↑, Diabetes, Ca, Uraemia
8. Fat embolism

EHLERS–DANLOS SYNDROME

Rare. Hereditary. Connective tissue disorder

CLIN: Elasticity & fragility of skin ↑; Jt laxity & hyperextensibility; Large bruises; Painful bleed into muscles; Epistaxis; GI bleeding; Haematuria

SCURVY

Vit C def

CLIN: Ecchymoses in calves, thighs, buttocks → bruising; Haem; Subperiosteal bleeding (esp young)

RX: Vit C

Platelet Defects

Causes of Thrombocytopenia (LIST 22 HAEM)

A. DECREASED PRODUCTION
1. Drugs & Chemicals
2. Marrow infiltrations: Eg Myelofibrosis, Leukaemia, Myeloma
3. Aplastic anaemia
4. Congenital:
   a) Fanconi's anaemia
   b) Wiskott–Aldrich Syndrome
   c) Thrombocytopenia with absent radii
5. Uraemia
6. Megaloblastic anaemia

B. DECREASED SURVIVAL
1. Immunological:
   a) ITP
   b) Drugs eg Thiazides, Rifampicin
   c) SLE
   d) CLL, Lymphomas
   e) AIHA c ITP (Evans' Syndrome)
   f) Neonatal infections eg CMV, Rubella syndrome
   g) Incompatible blood transfusions
2. Hypersplenism
3. DIC
4. Thrombotic Thrombocytopenic purpura
7. Infections: Eg SABE, Meningococcal septicaemia, Typhus, Rocky Mountain Spotted fever

C. DILUTION
Massive transfusion of stored blood

D. LOSS
Massive haemorrhage

Causes of Platelet Dysfunction in Absence of Thrombocytopenia (LIST 23 HAEM)

1. Hereditary Haemorrhagic Thromboasthenia
2. Von Willebrand's Disease
3. Platelet factor def
4. Uraemia
5. Drugs: Eg Aspirin, Sulphinpyrazone, Indomethacin
6. Chronic liver disease
7. Scurvy
8. Thrombocytosis:
   a) Post splenectomy
   b) Haemorrhage
   c) Trauma
   d) Malignancy
   e) Inflam bowel disease
   f) Myeloproliferative disorders Eg Essential haemorrhagic thrombocythemia, PRV, Myelofibrosis

TESTS OF PLATELET ABNORMALITIES:
1. Bleeding time ↑
2. Tourniquet test
3. Platelet aggregation tests
4. Impaired clot retraction
5. Impaired thromboplastin generation

ITP

Esp children & young adults. Usually post viral infection

CLIN: Petechiae on arms, legs, chest, neck; Epistaxis; Menorrhagia; Anaemia. Usually feels well. Occ Spleen ↑. Usually self limiting but occ → chr ITP

INVESTIGATIONS: ● FBC
- Platelets ↓
- WCC occ ↑
- Bone marrow Megakaryocytes ↑
- Bleeding time ↑
- Coagulation tests normal

RX: May recover spontaneously. Azathioprine &/or Steroids. If steroids fail, Splenectomy

HEREDITARY THROMBASTHENIA (GLANZMAN'S DISEASE)

Aut Rec

CLIN: Bleeding; Purpura; Bruising; Epistaxis; Menorrhagia

INVESTIGATIONS: ● Platelets norm number but abnorm function

- Bleeding time ↑
- +ve tourniquet test
- Defective clot retraction
- No aggregation c̄ ADP & thrombin

RX: Platelet concentrates

Coagulation Defects

Acquired coagulation defects are occ ass c̄ thrombocytopenia

Causes of Coagulation Disorders (LIST 24 HAEM)

A. CONGENITAL
1. Haemophilia
2. Christmas Disease
3. Von Willebrand's Disease
4. Other cong factor defs

B. ACQUIRED
1. Vit K def
2. Anticoagulant drugs
3. Chr liver disease
4. DIC
5. Massive transfusion of stored blood
6. SLE
7. Advanced renal failure

GENERAL TESTS FOR COAGULATION DISORDERS: 1. PT time
2. Thrombin clotting time: ↑ in fibrinolysis
3. Activated partial thromboplastin time: ↑ in intrinsic pathway defect
4. Specific factor assays
5. FDPs

HAEMOPHILIA

Sex-linked recessive. Lack of Factor VIII

CLIN: Spontaneous or post traumatic haem. Haemarthrosis → jt deformity esp knee, chr synovitis; Haematuria; Haematomas. Rarely GIT or Brain haem

INVESTIGATIONS: • Activated partial thromboplastin time ↑
- Factor VIIIC ↓
- Assay factor VIII

RX: Genetic counselling

RX OF HAEMARTHROSES: Prompt factor replacement. Arthroscopy. Occ synovectomy or osteotomy. Physio. Avoid Aspirin

RX OF HAEMATURIA: Bed rest. Push fluids. Factor replacement
Surgical preparation: Ensure sufficient factor replacement available. Give factor VIII pre-op & periodically thereafter till 10days post-op. In minor op can use DDAVP instead of factor VIII

RX IN GENERAL: Factor dosage depends on patient's plasma vol, baseline level & desired factor elevation. Factor VIII is available as a lyophilized factor concentrate, cryoprecipitate or FFP. Anti-fibrinolytic agents eg Tranexamic acid are useful post dental extraction. Train suitable persons for home therapy

Complications of Rx: 1. 5–10% have Ab to factor VIII
2. HepB
3. Allergic reactions
4. AIDS

CHRISTMAS DISEASE (HAEMOPHILIA B)

Sex-linked recessive. Factor IX def

CLIN: Identical to haemophilia. Haemarthrosis etc

RX: As for haemophilia except use factor IX concentrate or FFP

VON WILLEBRAND'S DISEASE

Aut Dom. Abnormality of factor VIII & platelet function

CLIN: Bruising; Bleeding; Menorrhagia. Rarely Haemarthroses

INVESTIGATIONS: • Bleeding time ↑
- Platelet numbers normal
- Activated partial thromboplastin time ↑
- Factor VIIIC, VIIIRAg, VIIIWF all ↓
- Platelet aggregation c̄ ristocetin ↓
- Factor IX norm

RX: Factor VIII concentrate, Cryoppt

FACTOR V DEF

Aut Rec. Rare

CLIN: Epistaxis; Bruising; Menorrhagia

FACTOR II, VII, X DEF

All Aut Rec & rare. Not improved by Vit K

FACTOR XI DEF

Aut Rec. Rare. Esp Jews. Mild disorder

RX: FFP

FACTOR XIII DEF

Aut Rec. Presents early c̄ bleeding from umbilical stump

RX: FFP

ACQUIRED CLOTTING FACTOR DEF

VIT K DEF: Factor II, VII, IX, X produced in liver & require Vit K

Causes of Vit K Def: 1. Prematurity
2. Liver disease
3. Anticoagulants eg Coumarin
4. Extrahepatic biliary obst
5. Malabsorption

Clin: Ecchymoses; GI bleeding; Mucosal membrane bleeding; Haematuria. Bruising

Rx: Vit K. Occ FFP, Cryoppt

URAEMIA: Disorder of coagulation & thrombocytopenia. Platelet factor 3 low therefore inhibiting prothrombin conversion to thrombin

Rx: Dialysis

DISSEMINATED INTRAVASCULAR COAGULATION (DIC)

DIC is an intermediary mechanism of disease c̄ simultaneous thromb & haem of variable severity. In severe DIC there is uncompensated consumption of coagulation factors & fibrinolysis → haem

Causes of DIC (LIST 25 HAEM)

1. Obstetric:
   a) Abruptio placenta
   b) Retained dead foetus
   c) Retained placenta
   d) Amniotic fluid embolus
   e) Eclampsia
2. Trauma & surgery esp Burns, Cardiopulmonary surgery
3. Incompatible blood transfusion
4. Hypoxia
5. PE
5. Infection:
   a) Septicaemia esp Gm -ve & meningococcal
   b) Malaria
   c) Staph aureus
   d) Purpura fulminans
6. Liver disease:
   a) Cirrhosis
   b) Fulminant liver failure
7. Malignancy:
   a) Mucin secreting Ca
   b) Ca prostate
   c) Metastatic Ca
   d) Ac promyelocytic leukaemia
8. Anaphylaxis
9. Venoms
10. Haemangioma
11. Hypothermia

CLIN: In severe cases haem esp skin, GIT. Occ Thrombophlebitis; Periph gangrene; Renal failure; J; CCF; Resp failure

INVESTIGATIONS:
- Thrombin clotting time ↑
- Platelets ↓
- FDPs ↑
- Fibrinogen level ↓
- PT time ↑
- Activated partial thromboplastin time
- Blood film: Fragmented RBC

RX: Treat underlying condition. Restore fluid balance. Treat hypoxia, acidosis & shock. FFP & platelet concentrates. Heparin indicated in purpura fulminans. Tranexamic acid to inhibit excess fibrinolysis c̄ heparin to prevent thrombosis

PROG: Poor in severe DIC

BLOOD TRANSFUSIONS

There are at least 100 blood gp antigens which are all inherited independently. The most important system is ABO, others include Rhesus, Kell, Lewis. It is therefore important to cross match blood prior to transfusion

Complications of Blood Transfusions (LIST 26 HAEM)

A. EARLY
1. Haemolytic reaction:
   a) Mismatched transfusion
   b) Poor storage of blood
2. Circulatory overload
3. Febrile allergic reaction: Eg to HLA Ab, Plasma hypersensitivity
4. Clotting abnormalities eg after multiple transfusions
5. Air embolism
6. Hyperkalaemia esp in CRF
7. Excess citrate → bleeding (Rx Ca^{2+} gluconate)
8. Thrombocytopenia after massive transfusion
9. Excess ammonia (in stored blood) → precoma in cirrhosis

B. LATE
1. Sensitisation eg to rhesus antigen
2. Disease transmission:
   a) HepB
   b) Syphilis
   c) CMV
   d) Malaria
   e) AIDS
3. Transfusion siderosis
4. Development of circulating anticoagulants

Endocrinology, Metabolic Disorders & The Breast

DIABETES MELLITUS

A state of chr hyperglycaemia ass c̄ arterial, retinal, renal & neurological complications. Occ may be 2° eg 2° to Acromegaly, Cushing's syndrome; Pancreatitis; Phaeochromocytoma

INVESTIGATIONS: • Random BG
- Fasting BG: >8mmol/l
- Occ GTT: BG >12mmol/l 2hrs after 75g load

TYPES: Insulin dependent (juvenile); Non-insulin dependent (maturity onset); Impaired glucose tolerance (2–4% p.a become diabetic); Gestational (present during pregnancy, remitting afterwards)

Insulin Dependent Diabetes (IDDM)

Esp 15–30yrs

AETIOLOGY: Genetic & environmental factors. Ass c̄ HLA-A8, HLA-BW15 & viral infection eg Coxsackie B4, Rubella

CLIN: Usually rapid onset c̄ thirst, polyuria, Wt ↓. ↑ incidence of infection may ppt coma. Occ present c̄ complications eg poor vision, impotence, paraesthesiae

CONTROL of IDDM: Inject insulin according to lifestyle requirements eg Degree of activity; Type, amount & timing of meals; State of health. Generally use b.d monocomponent insulin

Dietary advice:
a) Recognise importance of cultural, economic & personal preference factors.
b) Usually advise ↓ sat fats, ↑ high fibre foods & ↓ rapidly absorbed sugars

Artificial endocrine pancreas: Continuous monitoring by machine of BG c̄ appropriate infusion of insulin. Experimental

Non-insulin Dependent Diabetes (NIDDM)

Esp middle aged & elderly, but NIDDM in youth well recognised

AETIOLOGY: 1. Genetic susceptibility
2. Obesity
3. Ageing

CLIN: Usually slow onset of symptoms. Occ Asymptomatic. Obese

RX OF UNCOMPLICATED NIDDM:
1. Diet: Wt, chd, fats all ↓. If BG not controlled try drugs
2. Oral Anti-diabetic drugs:
   a) Sulphonylureas eg Chlorpropamide, Tolbutamide, Glibenclamide
   b) Biguanides eg Metformin (SE: Lactic acidosis esp Phenformin)

Diabetic Comas

TYPES: Ketoacidotic Hyperglycaemic; Hypoglycaemic; Hyperosmolar Hyperglycaemic; Lactic Acidosis; Uraemic acidotic; Non-metabolic coma

KETOACIDOTIC HYPERGLYCAEMIA COMA

Due to insulin def. Often ppt by infection, inadequate insulin dose or disease eg MI

CLIN: Tiredness; Thirst; Polyuria; Vom; Abdo pain. Then usually >1wk later Dehydration; Hyperventilation; Acetone on breath; BP ↓; PR ↑; Warm skin

INVESTIGATIONS:
- BG ↑↑
- Urea ↑
- HCO_3↓
- Astrup: pH ↓, pO_2 ↓
- FBC: PCV ↑
- Ketone bodies in blood & urine
- ECG
- Look for infection

RX:
a) Rapid fluid replacement c̄ Norm saline (if [Na]>155mmol/l use N/2 saline), when BG<14mmol/l use 5% dextrose
b) Rapid acting insulin i-m or continuous IV eg 20Units i-m initially then 5Units/hr. Monitor BG
c) Initially use 20mmolK /hr. If [K]>5mmol/l ↓ rate; If [K]<4mmol/l ↑ rate
d) If pH<7 give 100mmol $NaHCO_3$ & 20mmol KCl over 1hr. Repeat if Astrup pH remains <7
e) Ancillary measures: Gastric aspiration; Antibiotics. Occ Heparin; Catheterisation; use CVP line; O_2 if pO_2 <11kPa
f) When BG is <15mmol/l give IV Glucose c̄ KCL IV & 2hrly 6 Units Insulin i-m. Continue until patient eating

HYPOGLYCAEMIC COMA

Commonest

CLIN: Can often be recognised & dealt with by patient in early stages. Dizzy; Sweat++; LOC. Occ Occurs during sleep

INVESTIGATION:
- BG

RX: If BG ↓ suspected give immediate trial of Rx. If conscious, oral glucose, otherwise IV. Glucagon IV/IM

HYPEROSMOLAR HYPERGLYCAEMIC NON-KETOTIC COMA

Esp Elderly; Black; New diabetics. About 5% of BG ↑ comas. Pathogenesis unknown

CLIN: Dehydrated++; Consciousness ↓. No ketosis; No acidosis; No hyperventilation

INVESTIGATIONS:
- BG >50mmol/l
- Urea >20mmol/l
- Osmolality >350mmol/l
- Na^+: Often >150mmol/l
- Astrup

RX: If Na^+ >150mmol/l use N/2 saline c̄ CVP. If Na^+ <150 use norm saline. Insulin Rx as for ketoacidotic coma. Heparin as risk of DIC & thromb is high

LACTIC ACIDOSIS

Now rare c̄ ↓ use of phenformin. Esp seen if taking biguanides c̄ coexisting renal & liver impairment

CLIN: Malaise; Consciousness ↓; Acidosis

INVESTIGATIONS:
- BG: ↓ to ↑↑
- Some ketone bodies
- pH ↓↓

RX: Stop biguanide. Large amounts of HCO_3. Peritoneal or haemodialysis. Control BG c̄ Insulin & Glucose

PROG: 50% mort

OTHER COMAS

Esp 2° to renal failure

Neurological Complications

Nerve conduction study abnormalities very common. Clinically apparent forms often mild. M>F

SYMMETRICAL SENSORY POLYNEUROPATHY

CLIN: Glove & stocking distribution, feet >>hands. Numbness. Occ Pain; Paraesthesiae. Rarely Motor weakness; Pressure ulcers; Charcot's jts

MOTOR POLYNEUROPATHY

Often asymmetrical

CLIN: Rapid onset usually painful muscle weakness in legs. Esp quads (Amyotrophy of Garland). Occ ass c̄

Sensory symptoms; Charcot's jts

MONONEUROPATHIES

a) Cranial nerve palsies eg IIIn, VIn, Vn, VIIn, VIIIn. Rapid onset, usually recover
b) Pressure palsies esp Carpal tunnel syndrome; Ulnar nerve compression; Foot drop

AUTONOMIC NEUROPATHY

Ass c̄ periph neuropathy

CLIN SYNDROMES INC: Postural BP ↓; Abnormal valsalva; PR ↑; Sweating; Diarrhoea; Atonic bladder; Impotence; Sudden cardiac death

Diabetic Nephropathy

M sl>F. Esp if diabetic for >30yrs

PATHOGENESIS: Thickened more permeable basement membrane, initially reversible by good BG control. Later damage to glomerular capillaries & arterioles c̄ ↑ fibrin deposition → renal ischaemia & therefore ↓ glomerular & tubular function. Often ass c̄ infection & pyelonephritis
Types of glomerular lesion (Diabetic glomerulosclerosis): Diffuse; Exudative; Hyaline; Kimmelstiel–Wilson (nodular)Tubular lesions inc glycogen laden vacuoles (Armani–Ebstein) Interstitial lesions inc UTIs & renal papillary necrosis

CLIN: Initially asymptomatic proteinuria. Then oedema. After variable time → RF c̄ anaemia; BP ↑ & arterial disease very common

RX: Often need less insulin. Diuretics. Strict control of BP ↑. Antibiotics for UTIs. Low protein, high chd diet if uraemic. CAPD. Transplant if ESRF

PROG: 75% are in ESRF after 10yrs continuous proteinuria

Diabetic Retinopathy

Commonest cause of blindness in UK between ages 30–64yrs. 80% c̄ IDDM develop retinopathy after 15–20yrs

4 CLIN STAGES: Mild background retinopathy; Background retinopathy c̄ maculopathy; Proliferative retinopathy; Advanced eye disease

Mild Background Retinopathy: Potentially reversible
Clin: Asymptomatic. Microaneurysms; Haem. Occ Hard exudates; Cotton wool spots
Rx: Good diabetic control. 6mthly review. Fluorescein angiogram useful for monitoring esp if ↓ acuity

Background Retinopathy c̄ Macular Oedema: Esp NIDDM, middle-aged & elderly
Clin: Visual loss due to macular oedema or foveal exudate
Rx: Photocoagulation

Proliferative Retinopathy:
Clin: New vessel formation in underperfused retina. Multiple cotton wool spots & large blot haem. Venous beeding, loops & reduplications. If untreated many develop blindness due to advanced eye disease
Rx: See below

Advanced Eye Disease:
Clin: Vitreous haem; Fibrous tissue formation ass c̄ new vessels (Retinitis proliferans) & thrombotic glaucoma c̄ Rubeosis Iridis. Blindness
Rx: Photocoagulation to destroy abnormal leaking vessels & abnormal nonperfused retina. Occ vitrectomy to remove vitreous haem & fibrous tissue
Prog: Best if treated early. Photocoagulation often improves sight in those c̄ new vessels arising from disc

Diabetic Foot

CAUSES: 1. Sepsis
2. Neuropathy
3. Ischaemia
4. Combination of 1 to 3

CLIN: Neuropathy → callus formation esp 1st metatarsal & painless skin ulceration occ followed by osteomyelitis &/or gangrene. Rarely Charcot's jt. Ischaemia → claudication, rest pain & gangrene

PREVENTION: Prophylactic cleanliness, inspect feet daily, cut nails transversely, stop smoking. Appropriate shoes

RX: Medical Rx: Rest; Antiseptics. Systemic antibiotics if severe infection
Surgical Rx: Indicated if: Gangrene; Osteomyelitis; To release pus

Arterial Disease

Ass c̄ ↑ risk of coronary, cerebral &

periph arterial disease. Risk partially mediated by BP ↑ & lipids ↑

CORONARY HEART DISEASE

MI more likely to be fatal in diabetics

RX: Prevention by treating BP ↑ eg non-thiazide diuretics. Treat hyperlipidaemia with low fat, high fibre diet. Stop cigs. If established, treat as for IHD
N.B Non-selective β blockers can mask hypoglycaemia

PERIPHERAL ARTERIAL DISEASE

Esp arteries below the knee. Often ass c̄ sensory neuropathy

RX: Surgery is difficult if small arteries affected. Drugs & sympathectomy for IC of little value

CARDIOMYOPATHY

Rare. Ass c̄ IDDM. ↑ risk of congestive cardiomyopathy

Necrobiosis Lipoidica

Uncommon complication. May precede diabetes. Esp 20–40yrs. Can occur in non-diabetics

CLIN: Oval or irregular indurated slowly enlarging plaques c̄ central atrophy or sclerosis esp front of lower legs. Occ Ulceration

RX: Ulcerated lesions may require excision grafting

Care of The Surgical Diabetic

ON DIET ALONE

Nil by mouth pre-op. BG post-op

ON ORAL DRUGS

Nil by mouth pre-op. If minor surgery BG post-op. If major surgery b.d insulin

ON INSULIN

STABLE: Convert to b.d soluble regime pre-op & maintain till eating again

UNSTABLE: Give insulin & glucose at op, then sliding-scale or continuous infusion. When oral foods tolerated revert to b.d

HYPOGLYCAEMIA

Two types: Reactive postprandial & fasting. Fasting BG ↓ indicates an underlying disease. Post prandial BG ↓ usually occurs without organic disease

GENERAL CLIN: Sweating; Palps; PR ↑; Pallor; Slurred speech; Inco-ordination; Poor concentration. Later Ep; Transient CVA; Diplopia; Coma. If BG drops rapidly, adrenergic features predominate; If BG drops slowly CNS signs dominate

CAUSES: See LIST 24 GIT

Idiopathic Reactive Hypoglycaemia

Quite common

CLIN: Sweating; Palps; Lightheadedness 1–3hrs after meal

INVESTIGATION: • GTT: Low BG 1.5–2.5hrs after load

DD: Anxiety

HYPERLIPIDAEMIA

An ↑ level of Cholesterol &/or Triglyceride. There are 4 main lipoprotein classes : HDL, LDL, VLDL & Chylomicrons. HDL is Cholesterol-rich, VLDL & Chylomicrons are Triglyceride-rich. Chylomicrons transport dietary fat; VLDL transport endogenous triglyceride; LDL transport cholesterol to periph cells; HDL transport cholesterol from periph cells. Most 1° causes are familial, 2° causes include Obesity; Alcohol; Hypothyroidism; Uraemia; Diabetes. Frederickson's classification gives 5 types: Type I: Familial Hyperchylomicronaemia; Type IIa: Familial hypercholesterolaemia; Type IIb: 2° hyperβlipoproteinaemia of normal density; Type III: Dysβlipoproteinaemia; Type IV: Hyperpreβlipoproteinaemia; Type V: Mixed hyperlipoproteinaemia. A high level of HDL appears to be cardioprotective

GENERAL INVESTIGATIONS OF HYPERLIPIDAEMIAS: • Fasting lipids (×2)
- BG
- MCV
- GGT
- U&E
- PPE
- TFT

N.B Fasting lipids raised post MI

Hypertriglyceridaemia

The Aut Dom familial combined hyperlipidaemia & 2° causes of hypertriglyceridaemia are ass c̄ ↑ risk of CVS disease

Causes of Hypertriglyceridaemia (LIST 1 ENDO)

A. OVERPRODUCTION
1. Primary:
   a) Familial combined hyperlipidaemia
   b) Hypertriglyceridaemia
2. Secondary:
   a) Obesity
   b) Alcohol
   c) Acromegaly
   d) Cushing's syndrome
   e) Oestrogen excess

B. IMPAIRED REMOVAL
1. Primary:
   a) 1° lipoprotein lipase def
   b) Lipoprotein lipase activator def
2. Secondary:
   a) Diabetes
   b) Hypothyroidism
   c) Uraemia

CLIN OF SEVERE HYPERTRIGLYCERIDAEMIA: Eruptive xanthomas; Lipaemia retinalis; Pancreatitis; Abdo pain

RX: Advise stop cigs, restrict alcohol, high chd low sat fat diet if obese. Occ drugs eg Clofibrate, Nicotinic acid, esp young 1° cases c̄ FH of IHD & all c̄ severe hypertriglyceridaemia (ie >15mmol/l). Treat underlying cause

Remnant Removal Disease (Dysβlipoproteinaemia)

Rare. Impaired conversion of remnants to LDL

CLIN: Planar (palmar) xanthomas

INVESTIGATIONS: • Fasting blood lipids: Triglyceride ↑, Cholesterol ↑
- Ultracentrifugation
- Apoprotein assay: E apoprotein ↓
- PPE

RX: Low sat fat diet. Occ Clofibrate

Hypercholesterolaemia

Ass c̄ premature CVS disease

Causes of Hypercholesterolaemia (LIST 2 ENDO)

1. Familial combined hyperlipidaemia
2. Familial hypercholesterolaemia
3. Common hypercholesterolaemia
4. Hypothyroidism
5. Nephrotic syndrome
6. Renal transplant patients
7. Glucocorticoid Rx

FAMILIAL HYPERCHOLESTEROLAEMIA

Esp S.Afr

CLIN: Tendon xanthomas esp hands, Achilles tendon; Xanthelasma. Homozygous form causes earlier more severe IHD

INVESTIGATION: • Cholesterol ↑; LDL ↑; Triglyceride norm

FAMILIAL COMBINED HYPERLIPIDAEMIA

FH

CLIN: Presents in adulthood. No xanthomas. Premature IHD

INVESTIGATION: • Cholesterol ↑; Triglyceride ↑; LDL & VLDL ↑↑

COMMON HYPERCHOLESTEROLAEMIA

Polygenic inheritance. Diet of aetiological importance. Common. Risk of IHD increases c̄ ↑ cholesterol level but risk not as high as for familial form

GENERAL RX: Stop cigs. High chd low sat fat diet if obese. Occ drug Rx esp for young 1° cases c̄ FH of CVS disease ie Cholestyramine (SE: Diarrhoea, Poor absorption of fat soluble vits. Therefore use multivit supplements nocte) & nicotinic acid

THYROID DISORDERS

Goitre

A goitre is an enlargement of the thyroid. Esp premenopausal F. F>M. Commonest cause worldwide is iodine def. Goitres & thyroid nodules are only occasionally toxic

Causes of Goitre (LIST 3 ENDO)

1. Iodine Def
2. Physiological:
   a) Puberty
   b) Pregnancy
3. Graves disease
4. Goitrogens:
   Eg Anti-thyroid drugs, Iodine containing drugs, Li, Cassava
5. Thyroiditis:
   a) Hashimoto's
   b) De Quervain's
   c) Riedel's
   d) Septic
6. Dyshormonogenesis:
   Eg Pendred's syndrome
7. Tumours:
   a) Adenoma
   b) Carcinoma
   c) Lymphoma
8. Sarcoid
9. TB
10. Syphilis

GENERAL INVESTIGATIONS: • TSH
- Serum T3
- Serum T4
- Thyroid Ab
- Isotope scan
- Ultrasound scan
- Biopsy
- TRH (Not if low TSH or basal TSH ↑)
- Rarely: Resin uptake test (derive FTI); TBG

Simple Euthyroid Goitre

Usually idiopathic or due to I_2 def. I_2 def is very common worldwide. Occ physiological or due to Dyshormonogenesis or goitrogens. Pendred's syndrome is goitre & cong deafness

CLIN: Diffuse goitres are usually asymptomatic. Multinodular goitres very rarely cause pressure symptoms, haem or become malignant. May → hypothyroidism

INVESTIGATIONS: • As above.
- I_2 uptake ↓ in iodide trapping defects
- K^+ perchlorate Test: Abnormal in Pendred's syndrome
- Clearance of I_2: Increased in coupling & dehalogenase defects

RX: Occ cosmetic surgery. Thyroxine Rx may reduce size of goitre esp if diffuse & TSH ↑. If P symptoms, partial thyroidectomy

Acute/Subacute (de Quervain's) Thyroiditis

May be viral cause eg Mumps, Coxsackie. F>M

CLIN: Usually tender goitre. Early transient hyperthyroidism which may be followed by transient hypothyroidism. Pyrexia; URTI; Malaise; Dysphagia

INVESTIGATIONS: • T4 ↑
- Radio-active I_2 uptake ↓
- ESR ↑

RX: Analgesics; NSAID; Steroids

PROG: Usually recovery by 4–6mths

Riedel's Thyroiditis

Rare. Akin to retroperitoneal or mediastinal fibrosis

CLIN: Woody hard gland c̄ fibrosis extending into surrounding tissue. Occ P symptoms eg stridor; Hypothyroidism

RX: Thyroxine if hypothyroid. Surgery to relieve P symptoms

DD: Anaplastic Ca

Hypothyroidism

F>M. Esp 40–60yrs. Cong & juvenile forms well recognised. Due to def of circulating thyroid hormone

Causes of Hypothyroidism (LIST 4 ENDO)

A. 1° THYROID CAUSES
1. Autoimmune Thyroiditis
2. Iodine Def
3. Goitrogens
4. Irradiation
5. Surgery
6. Acute/Subacute thyroiditis
7. Dyshormonogenesis
8. Cong absence or maldevelopment
9. Replacement of Thyroid by Ca or Other disease

B. 2° TO PITUITARY/ HYPOTHALAMIC DISEASE

CLIN: Many presentations. Onset usually insidious. Often Fatigue; Lethargy; Physical & mental sluggishness; Cold intolerance; Constipation; Wt ↑; Gruff voice; Dry thickened scaly skin; Typical facies c̄ periorbital puffiness, thickened sc tissue; Halitosis; Coarse brittle hair; PR ↓; Reflexes ↓; Goitre. Occ Anaemia; Alopecia; Psychosis (Myxoedema madness); Carpal tunnel syndrome; Polyneuritis; Cerebellar syndrome; Myopathy; Arthralgia; Menorrhagia; Angina; CCF; Deafness
N.B Clin of Juvenile & cong forms see Paediatrics

INVESTIGATIONS:
- Serum T4 ↓
- T3 resin uptake
- FTI (= Serum T4 × T3 resin uptake) ↓
- TSH: ↑ in 1° thyroid disease
- Serum T3: Often ↓
- Occ TRH-TSH test: Exaggerated prolonged TSH ↑ in thyroid disease & slow response in pituitary disease

RX: L-Thyroxine; In elderly or if IHD introduce thyroxine in small dose & gradually increase to maintenance level

COMPLICATION:

Myxoedema Coma: May present c̄ coma but usually a gradual increase in somnolence precedes coma. Esp winter. Esp elderly. May be ppt by drugs or infection. Usually ass c̄ hypothermia
Rx: IV thyroxine; IV fluids; O_2; Nurse in warm room. Occ Cortisol; Assisted ventilation
Prog: 50% mort

Hashimoto's Thyroiditis

Common cause of goitrous hypothyroidism. Occ FH. F>M. Esp 10–20yrs. Ass c̄ other auto-immune diseases eg PA; Vitiligo; RTbA

PATH: Ashkenazi cells in thyroid histology

CLIN: Hypothyroidism >Euthyroidism. Rarely LN ↑. Occ Transient hyperthyroidism

RX: Thyroxine

Hyperthyroidism

Due to an excess of circulating T3 &/or T4. Commonest causes are Graves' disease & toxic uni- & multi-nodular goitres. Other causes are rare. F>M

Causes of Hyperthyroidism (LIST 5 ENDO)

1. Graves disease
2. Toxic multinodular goitre
3. Toxic adenoma
4. Extraneous Thyroid Hormone:
   a) Excess thyroxine Rx
   b) Thyroid Ca c mets
   c) Struma ovarii
4. Excess TSH or TSH like substance:
   a) Pituitary tumour
   b) Choriocarcinoma
   c) Hydatidiform mole
   d) Embryonal testicular Ca
5. Jod–Basedow phenomenon (excess I_2)
6. Thyroiditis (Transient): Eg Hashimoto's, de Quervain's, Silent subacute, X-Rad
7. Neonatal hyperthyroidism (Transient): Usually due to maternal Graves disease

GENERAL CLIN: Usually gradual onset. Many presentations. Often Wt ↓ despite good appetite; Sweating; Heat intolerance; Warm skin; Tremor; Nervousness; Palps; PR ↑; D&V; Prominent eyes; Lid lag; Lid retraction; Proptosis; Goitre; Reflexes ↑. Occ SOB; Angina; AF; CCF; Psychosis; Proximal myopathy; Palmar erythema; Spider naevi; Oligo- or amenorrhoea; Loss of libido; Gynaecomastia (M); Ophthalmoplegia; Conjunctivitis; Bone pain (2° to osteoporosis). Rarely Pretibial myxoedema; Thyroid acropachy; Vitiligo; Spleen ↑; Myasthenia gravis; Steatorrhoea. In elderly often "apathetic" hyperthyroidism c̄ predominant CVS &/or CNS symptoms A thyroid crisis c̄ Fever; Stupor; CCF; Abdo pain; J; Diarrhoea → coma may be ppt by infection or thyroidectomy in poorly prepared patient

GENERAL INVESTIGATIONS: • Tests directed towards determining free T4 & T3. Serum T4 is mainly protein bound to TBG. [TBG] is ↑ or ↓ by many factors without affecting free T4 eg ↑ by oestrogens, pregnancy, Hep & ↓ by salicylates, steroids, hypoalbuminaemia

- Serum T4
- Serum T3: In T3 toxicosis, T3 ↑ T4 norm
- T3 resin uptake
- FTI (= Serum T4 × T3 resin uptake) ↑
- [TBG]
- T4:TBG ratio ↑
- TSH ↓↓
- TRH test: No response of TSH
- Thyroid uptake tests (seldom used): Usually ↑ but ↓ in thyroiditis
- Ca^{2+}: Sl ↑
- Usually T4 determination is sufficient for diagnosis

GRAVES DISEASE

F>M esp 20–40yrs. Diffuse hyperplasia & hypertrophy of thyroid occ ass c̄ ocular involvement. Eye signs may occur in absence of hyperthyroidism or after successful Rx of systemic disease

PATHOGENESIS: IgG antibodies against TSH receptor of thyroid follicular cell (Thyroid stimulating Igs). Also thyroid growth Igs. Different proportions of these Igs probably account for variable clinical picture

CLIN: Diffuse goitre; Hyperthyroidism. Ocular involvement may be mild eg lid lag & retraction or severe c̄ chemosis, proptosis, ophthalmoplegia & periorbital oedema which may → papilloedema, blindness. Usually both eyes involved

DD: Anxiety

MULTINODULAR GOITRE & TOXIC ADENOMA

F>M. Esp 40–70yrs

CLIN: Nodular goitre; Hyperthyroidism. CVS symptoms common. Eye signs infrequent

RX OF HYPERTHYROIDISM: 3 forms of Rx. All require careful follow up:

1) **Anti-thyroid Drugs:** Often first choice in pregnant, children & small goitres. Choice of 2 gps of drugs, Carbimazole & Thiouracil derivatives. Similar SE: Transient skin rash; J; LN ↑; N&V; Fever; Arthralgia; Agranulocytosis (Often preceded by sore throat when need FBC & stop drug). Drugs may be used c̄ β blocker to prepare for surgery or to control illness until Radio I_2 Rx has taken effect. Long term Rx aims to maintain patient in euthyroid state for at least 12–18mths when Rx is discontinued. Relapse is common esp c̄ toxic nodule or multinodular goitre
2) **Surgery:** Often first choice in large goitre, pressure symptoms, severe disease, recurrences, failed medical Rx, middle aged, cosmetic need. Patient must be euthyroid before surgery eg by anti-thyroid drugs for 1–2mths & I_2 for 7–10days then partial thyroidectomy. In 5–10% hyperthyroidism recurs, in 20–30% hypothyroidism develops over next 10yrs. Rarely post-op hypoPT or recurrent laryngeal nerve damage, occ transient hyperCa^{2+}
3) **Radio I_2:** Often first choice in post-op recurrent disease, >45yrs & when surgery c/i. Acts by destroying effective function of thyroid cells. Dose of I_2 is related to size of goitre. Takes 6–10wks for clinical response during which time anti-thyroid drugs & Propranolol may be used for control. Further doses may be given if still toxic at 4mths. After 2yrs about 10–15% are hypothyroid, rising to about 50% at 20yrs. Some deliberately give large dose to induce hypothyroidism & then give Thyroxine replacement Rx

RX THYROID CRISIS: Large doses of anti-thyroid drugs. Oral I_2 at least 1hr after start of anti-thyroid drug Rx. IV Propranolol, Dexamethasone (inhibits T3 & T4 tissue effects), IV fluids. Antipyretics & ice packs; Antibiotics. If CCF: Dig, Diuretics & O_2. Occ require plasmapheresis

Silent Subacute Thyroiditis

Not infrequent in USA

CLIN: Hyperthyroidism for 1–2mths; Non-tender goitre

INVESTIGATIONS:
- T4 ↑
- Radio I_2 uptake ↓

RX: β blocker

Thyroid Cancer

Types inc Papillary Ca, a common slow growing form; Follicular Ca & Anaplastic tumours. F>M. Well differentiated Ca are commoner in young adults; Anaplastic Ca commoner in elderly

CLIN OF WELL DIFFERENTIATED Ca: May present as solitary nodule or occ Cv LN ↑. Usually late spread to other organs

CLIN OF ANAPLASTIC Ca: Hard irregular fixed goitre which spreads rapidly to lungs, bone & brain. Usually local P symptoms

INVESTIGATIONS:
- Isotope scan: Cold nodule indicates area of ↓ uptake which may be due to Ca
- Needle biopsy

RX: All solitary cold nodules should be surgically explored & excised to exclude Ca (most will be benign adenomas). If Ca found do total thyroidectomy. Then T3 to suppress TSH for 6–8wks, discontinue for a wk & do whole body isotope scan to look for mets. If +ve give larger dose of Radio I_2 & start replacement Rx. Then review regularly c̄ scan. If anaplastic Ca found surgery only of palliative value & Radio I_2 ineffective

PROG: Papillary & Follicular Ca approx 50% 10yr survival. Very poor if anaplastic

Medullary Ca of Thyroid

Arise from parafollicular cells. May be uni- or bilat. Ass c̄ Phaeochromocytoma, HPT & Mucocutaneous neuromas (MEA type II). Often FH. Produce calcitonin

CLIN: Usually present c̄ a thyroid swelling. Occ Multiple small neuromas on eyelids, tongue & lips

INVESTIGATIONS:
- Plasma calcitonin
- Isotope scan
- Biopsy
- Tests for parathyroid adenoma & phaeochromocytoma

RX: If phaeochromocytoma present, treat before thyroid surgery to avoid a BP ↑ crisis. Total thyroidectomy c̄ excision of any involved LNs ± X-Rad. Then Thyroxine replacement Rx

PROG: Approx 50% 5yr survival

PARATHYROIDS & CALCIUM METABOLISM

1° Hyperparathyroidism

F>M esp post-menopausal. Usually due to parathyroid adenoma but occ due to parathyroid hyperplasia or malignant parathyroid tumour. Hyperplasia is ass c FH of HPT & MEA type I

PATHOGENESIS: Excess PTH secretion → ↑ renal reabsorption of Ca^{2+}, ↑ GIT absorption of Ca^{2+}, ↑ bone turnover, ↑ VitD synthesis, ↑ PO_4 excretion → ↑ serum Ca^{2+}, ↓ serum PO_4

CLIN: Many presentations. Commonest is renal stone. Occ Nephrocalcinosis;

BP ↑; Polyuria; Thirst; Bone disease eg pain, #; PU; N&V; Constipation; Pancreatitis; Psychiatric (may be subtle changes or frank psychosis); Proximal myopathy; Arthropathy inc pseudogout, chondrocalcinosis; Corneal calcification. May be asymptomatic. A parathyroid Ca is often palpable

INVESTIGATIONS: • Serum Ca^{2+} ↑
- Serum PO_4 ↓
- PTH usually ↑
- Cl^- ↑ (usually mild hyperchloraemic acidosis)
- Serum albumin
- U&E
- Alk Phos: Occ ↑
- AXR
- Bone X-R esp hands: Occ Subperiosteal erosions; Pepper-pot skull; Path #; Jaw/Long bone cysts (Brown tumours)
- ECG: Occ ˆQT↓ˆ
- Rarely Hydrocortisone suppression test: Usually no suppression of Ca^{2+} (in other causes of HyperCa^{2+}, Ca^{2+} often falls)

RX: Surgery to remove adenoma or 7/8ths of parathyroid tissue if hyperplasia. Occ more exact localisation required before op—achieved by multiple PTH samples obtained by neck vein catheterisation, CAT scan or isotope subtraction studies. Occ post-op hypoCa^{2+} & hypoMg → tetany Rx Ca^{2+}. As post-op Ca^{2+} ↓ is very common in severe bone disease, prophylactically given Vit D 3days pre-op to 1–2wks post-op

2° HPT

In chr diseases where serum Ca^{2+} is low eg CRF & Malabsorption, prolonged stimulation of PTH → parathyroid hyperplasia → metabolic bone disease

INVESTIGATIONS: • Serum Ca: Norm or ↓
- Alk phos ↑

RX: Vit D analogues (↑ GIT Ca^{2+} absorption). Treat underlying cause

3° HPT

When parathyroid tissue mass becomes very large a state of relative parathyroid autonomy may occur (3° HPT). The serum Ca^{2+} rises

RX: Subtotal parathyroidectomy

Causes of Hypercalcaemia (LIST 6 ENDO)

1. 1° & 3° HPT
2. Malignancy:
   a) Bony Mets
   b) Multiple myeloma
   c) Ectopic PTH secreting tumour
3. Drugs:
   Eg Vit D intoxication, Thiazides, Lithium
4. Sarcoidosis
5. Milk alkali syndrome
6. ARF (Polyuric recovery phase)
7. Hyperthyroidism
8. Idiopathic infantile hyperCa^{2+}
9. Addison's disease
10. Immobilisation
11. Familial hypocalciuric hyperCa^{2+}

GENERAL RX OF SEVERE HYPERCALCAEMIA: Rehydrate. Brisk saline diuresis c̄ Frusemide; PO_4 if no renal impairment; Steroids. Occ Peritoneal or haemodialysis. Occ sc Calcitonin. Mithramycin is effective but SE of bleeding diathesis & nephrotoxicity

Malignant Hypercalcaemia

Common cause of symptomatic Ca^{2+} ↑. Bony mets from Ca breast often cause Ca^{2+} ↑. Ectopic PTH secreting tumours have usually been described c̄ squamous cell lung Ca & Ca kidney & are ass c̄ mild hypoK^+ alkalosis

Milk–Alkali Syndrome

Usually due to excess use of proprietary alkalis containing Ca^{2+} → HyperCa^{2+}, renal stones

INVESTIGATIONS: • Ca^{2+} ↑
- PO_4: Norm or ↑
- Urinary Ca^{2+} norm
- KUB

RX: Low Ca^{2+} diet; Withdraw Ca^{2+} containing drugs

Familial Hypocalciuric Hypercalcaemia

Aut Dom. Rare

CLIN: Often few symptoms. Rarely pancreatitis

INVESTIGATION: • Urinary Ca^{2+}: Usually <3mmol/day

RX: Often discovered when removal of parathyroid glands does not relieve hyperCa^{2+}

Vit D Intoxication

May occur in any patient using Vit D. Actions of 1,25 DHCC → Alk Phos ↑; ↑ Ca^{2+} binding protein; ↑ Ca^{2+} active transport in GIT; Control of bone resorption

CLIN: HyperCa^{2+}. Later RF

RX: Stop Vit D (HyperCa^{2+} may last for many months); Steroids

Hypoparathyroidism

Results from failure of PTH secretion. Commonest cause is post surgery but also idiopathic form (children >adults). Idiopathic form occ ass c̄ DiGeorge syndrome, Addison's disease, Systemic candidiasis. Severe Mg^{+} ↓ also → hypoPT

CLIN: Often Tetany → carpopedal spasm, stridor, abdo pain; Paraesthesiae; Ep (esp children); Psychiatric symptoms; +ve Trousseau & Chvostek signs. Occ Cataracts

INVESTIGATIONS:
- Ca^{2+} ↓
- PTH ↓↓
- PO_4 ↑
- 1,25 DHCC ↓
- PTH provocation test: ↑ in urinary cyclic AMP excretion

RX: 1,25 DHCC is preferred to other Vit D analogues as any Ca^{2+} ↑ responds quickly to stoppage of drug. Treat tetany c̄ Ca^{2+}

Pseudohypoparathyroidism

Due to defective PTH tissue receptors. Rare. Occ FH

CLIN: Present in childhood. Short stature; Short 4th metacarpal; Obesity; IQ ↓; Tetany; Ep. Occ Cataracts

INVESTIGATIONS:
- Ca^{2+} ↓
- PTH ↑
- PTH provocation test: No ↑ in urinary cyclic AMP

Pseudopseudohypoparathyroidism

A term to describe people c̄ morphological signs similar to those of pseudohypoPT but c̄ no biochemical abnormality

Causes of Hypocalcaemia (LIST 7 ENDO)

1. HypoPT
2. PseudohypoPT
3. CRF
4. Hypoalbuminaemia
5. Acute Pancreatitis
6. Vit D def
7. Neonatal Hypocalcaemia
8. Thyroid Medullary Ca

METABOLIC BONE DISEASE

Osteoporosis

A reduction of bone mass per unit volume c̄ norm mineral & chemical composition. Very common in elderly, F>M

Causes of Osteoporosis (LIST 8 ENDO)

A. PRIMARY
1. Senile
2. Post menopausal
3. Juvenile
4. Adult

B. SECONDARY
1. Cushing's syndrome
2. Steroid Rx
3. Hyperthyroidism
4. HPT
5. Alcoholism
6. Immobilisation
7. Hypogonadism
8. CRF
9. Myeloma
10. Scurvy
11. Acromegaly
12. Rarely: a) Osteogenesis imperfecta
    b) Werner–Rothmund syndrome
    c) Childhood cirrhosis
    d) Glycogen storage disease
    e) Systemic mastocytosis

AETIOLOGY: Bone mass normally decreases c̄ age accounting for most senile cases. Oestrogen levels fall post menopausally → ↑ bone resorption relative to bone formation. Glucocorticoids are the other common cause → ↑ rate of bone loss

CLIN: Often asymptomatic. Occ # esp Femoral neck, Vertebral bodies, Colles'. May → Kyphosis, ↓ Hgh, root symptoms

INVESTIGATIONS: • Ca^{2+} norm
- PO_4 norm
- Alk Phos norm
- FBC
- ESR
- U&E
- Appropriate X-R: Loss of bony density. Occ vertebral wedging, "cod-fish" vertebrae
- Tests for underlying disease: Eg Cortisol

RX: Good diet. Encourage exercise. Oestrogens ± progestogen for early menopausal & ?established osteoporosis (SE: ↑ risk of endometrial Ca, Thromboembolism). High Ca^{2+} diet may be helpful

Osteomalacia

A reduction in bone mineral content per unit volume. Usually due to vit D def. In childhood causes rickets

Causes of Osteomalacia
(LIST 9 ENDO)

1. Deficient Synthesis & Supply of Vit D:
   a) Poor diet
   b) Inadequate sunlight exposure
   c) Post-gastrectomy
2. Impaired Vit D Absorption:
   Malabsorption
3. Impaired 25-Hydroxylation of Vit D:
   Chr liver disease
4. Impaired 1-Hydroxylation of Vit D:
   a) CRF
   b) Vit D dependent rickets
5. Hypophosphataemic rickets:
   a) Familial
   b) Adult onset
   c) Tumour associated
6. Epileptics on anticonvulsants
7. RTbA

PATHOGENESIS: Vit D enters body via food (Commonest cause of Osteomalacia is a diet lacking Vit D esp seen in elderly, housebound, infants, Asian immigrants in UK) or due to skin synthesis in sunlight (Poor skin synthesis of vit D is not usually a major aetiological factor except in housebound elderly). Vit D is converted in the liver to 25(OH)D, a process interfered c̄ by anticonvulsants. In the kidney 25(OH)D is converted to 1,25 DHCC

CLIN OF ADULT OSTEOMALACIA: Variable presentation. Occ Bone pain; Proximal myopathy. Rarely signs of hypoCa^{2+} eg Tetany

INVESTIGATIONS: • Serum Ca^{2+}, PO_4: CaxPO_4 product ↓ (except in CRF)
- Alk Phos ↑
- X-R: Often loss of bone density, "cod-fish" vertebrae, Looser's zones (pseudo#s) esp long bone shafts, scapulae, pubic rami
- Bone biopsy: Excess osteoid, disrupted calcification front
- Serum 25(OH)D: ↓ if 2° to dietary, malabsorptive or hepatic cause
- Tests for underlying disease eg U&Es, LFTs

RX: Nutritional osteomalacia use 1000–2000IU/day Vit D2. For malabsorptive osteomalacia require about 50,000IU/day Vit D2. Hypophosphataemic rickets require high dose Vit D c̄ PO_4 supplements. Monitor Rx, risk of HyperCa^{2+} if excess Vit D given

Osteopetrosis

Severe Aut Rec & mild Aut Dom forms

CLIN: Severe form presents in infancy c̄ Anaemia, Purpura, #s. Milder form presents later c̄ #s

INVESTIGATION: • X-R: Dense thickened cortical bone

RX: BMT

PORPHYRIA

Inborn errors of metabolism occurring at different enzymic sites at haem biosynthetic pathway. F>M

CLASSIFICATION: A. Acute Porphyrias
1. Acute Intermittent Porphyria
2. Hereditary Coprophyria
3. Variegate Porphyria
4. Plumboporphyria

B. Cutaneous Porphyrias
1. Cutaneous Hepatic Porphyria
2. Erythropoetic Protoporphyria
3. Cong porphyria

Acute Porphyrias

General ppts of acute attack: Many drugs eg Barbiturates, Sulphonamides, Steroids, Anticonvulsants. Occ pregnancy & pre-menstrual period provoke attack

ACUTE INTERMITTENT PORPHYRIA

F>M. Aut Dom. Esp young adults. Uncommon

CLIN: Acute episode often c̄ Colicky abdo pain; Vom; Muscular aches; BP ↑; PR ↑. Often motor neuropathy esp symmetrical. Occ Anxiety or frank psychosis; Ep. No frank photosensitivity. Rarely Resp paralysis

INVESTIGATION: • Urinary ALA, PBG & Uroporphyrin ↑↑

HEREDITARY COPROPORPHYRIA

Aut Dom. Rare

CLIN: Features of acute & cutaneous porphyria. Photosensitivity

INVESTIGATIONS: • Urinary ALA, PBG, Coproporphyrin ↑↑
• Faecal coproporphyrin ↑

VARIEGATE PORPHYRIA

Aut Dom

CLIN: Severe skin lesions eg bullous eruptions, scarring. Photosensitivity. Occ Hypertrichosis; Pigmentation; Skin fragility

INVESTIGATIONS: • Urinary ALA, PBG ↑↑
• Faecal X, porphyrin, protoporphyrin ↑↑

PLUMBOPORPHYRIA

Aut Dom. Rare. ALA dehydratase activity also depressed in Pb poisoning

CLIN: Resembles acute intermittent porphyria

INVESTIGATION: • Urinary ALA, uroporphyrin ↑↑

GENERAL TREATMENT OF ACUTE PORPHYRIAS

Avoid c/i drugs; Stringent dieting. In acute attack maintain good chd intake, IV laevulose, IV haematin to reduce overproduction of porphyrin. Symptomatic Rx may inc Analgesics, Antiemetics, Anti BP ↑ eg Propranolol, Neostigmine for severe constipation, Anticonvulsants eg Clonazepam, Anxiolytics eg Lorazepam. If resp paralysis, tracheostomy & IPPV. β-carotene may help photosensitivity

Cutaneous Porphyrias

All deposit photosensitising porphyrins in upper epidermal layer

CUTANEOUS HEPATIC PORPHYRIA

Aut Dom & acquired form eg 2° to Oestrogenic steroids, Polyhalogenated hydrocarbons, Liver tumours

CLIN: Usually ppt by alcohol. Erythema → vesicles → bullae which may haem & scar. Pruritis; ↑ skin fragility; Pigmentation; Hirsutism. Liver ↑; Hepatic siderosis

INVESTIGATIONS: • Urinary uroporphyrin ↑↑
• Faecal X, porphyrin & coproporphyrin ↑↑

RX: Avoid ppt agents. Venesect until Hb <12g/dl. Chloroquine

ERYTHROPOETIC PROTOPORPHYRIA

Aut Dom. Rare

CLIN: Pruritis; Photosensitivity; Urticaria; Burning pains. Later chr liver disease → ALF

INVESTIGATIONS: • RBC protoporphyrin ↑↑
• Faecal protoporphyrin ↑↑

RX: β-carotene for photosensitivity. Cholestyramine may delay onset of liver disease

CONG PORPHYRIA

Aut Rec. Very rare

CLIN: Presents in childhood. Severe skin lesions eg scarring c̄ deformity of hand. Occ Nail dystrophy; Scarring of lens → blindness; Brown–pink teeth; Spleen ↑ Anaemia

INVESTIGATIONS:
- RBC protoporphyrin & coproporphyrin ↑↑
- Urinary uroporphyrin & coproporphyrin ↑↑

RX: Splenectomy; Chloroquine

PROG: Short life expectancy

THE PITUITARY & HYPOTHALAMUS

The ant pituitary releases ACTH, TSH, LH, FSH, GH & Prolactin. These hormones are regulated by a feedback loop c̄ Hypothalamus via Corticotropin releasing factor, TRH, LH-RH, GHRH & PIF respectively. In most cases a feedback loop between the target gland & the pituitary is also recognised
The post pituitary releases Oxytocin & ADH

Pituitary Tumours

Usually adenomas but occ craniopharyngioma, carcinoma, meningioma, chondroma, chordoma

GENERAL CLIN: 3 main presentations: Local SOL effects; Hypopituitarism; Hypersecretion of pituitary hormone
SOL effects: Bitemporal hemianopia or other field defects → ↓ vision. Occ Papilloedema; Diplopia; Ep; Focal CNS signs. Acute enlargement may → haem infarct & pituitary apoplexy c̄ vision ↓, ↓ consciousness, focal CNS signs, meningism
Hypopituitarism: Usually develops sequentially c̄ functional loss of GH then LH, FSH, TSH & ACTH. If PIF cannot act on pituitary, hyperprolactinaemia occurs. DI is rare

GENERAL INVESTIGATIONS:
- SXR: Occ enlarged fossa, double floor
- CAT scan
- Pituitary function tests ie Plasma cortisol at 9am, T4, T3, Prolactin, Testosterone (M), Oestradiol (F). If cortisol norm do combined pituitary stimulation test c̄ Insulin, GnRH, TRH injection & measurement of BG, Cortisol, GH half hrly for 2hrs & LH, FSH, TSH measurement half hrly for 1hr (c/i h/o IHD, Ep)

ACROMEGALY & GIGANTISM

Due to excessive secretion of GH → gigantism if starting before epiphyseal fusion & acromegaly after fusion. Esp middle aged. Usually due to pituitary tumour rarely due to ectopic hormone production eg from pancreatic tumour. Uncommon. Part of MEA type I syndrome

CLIN OF ACROMEGALY: Enlarged extremities; Large tongue; Hyperhydrosis; Prognathism; Greasy thick skin; BP ↑; Ht ↑; Visceromegaly; Headache; Visual field defects. Occ Diabetes; Cranial nerve palsies; Kyphosis; Carpal tunnel syndrome; Psychiatric symptoms; Goitre; Hirsutism; Loss of libido & sexual potency; Arthropathy. Rarely HyperCa^{2+}; Hyperthyroidism; Galactorrhoea

INVESTIGATIONS:
- ↑ GH levels not suppressed after oral glucose load (diagnostic)
- Often inappropriate stimulation of GH by TRH or LH-RH
- SXR: Large sella
- ↑ heel pad thickness
- Other hormones: Prolactin occ ↑; GnRH, TSH, ACTH occ ↓

RX: Trans-sphenoidal surgery c̄ X-Rad unless GH concentration <5mU/l. Trans-frontal surgery for large tumours. Bromocriptine may reduce GH levels & be an adjunct to Rx. Replacement hormone therapy as necessary

PROLACTINOMA

Prolactinomas are commoner than GH or ACTH producing tumours. Non functioning pituitary tumours may prevent PIF (ie dopamine) from acting thereby causing prolactin excess

CLIN: Headache; Visual field defects; Cranial nerve palsies. In F: Infertility; Amenorrhoea; Oligomenorrhoea; Galactorrhoea; Hirsutism; Acne. In M: Impotence; Loss of libido; Gynaecomastia; Hypogonadism; Rarely Galactorrhoea. F usually present earlier, pregnancy may exacerbate

INVESTIGATIONS: • Prolactin ↑↑
• No LH surge c̄ oestrogens

RX: Bromocriptine in slowly increasing dose. Monitor c̄ serial CAT scans. Withdrawal of drug may → recurrence & therefore X-Rad & trans-sphenoidal surgery remain alternatives

PROG: Bromocriptine usually shrinks tumour & allows norm gonadal function if gonadotrophin secretion is intact

TSH SECRETING TUMOURS

Rare. May → hyperthyroidism

GONADOTROPHIN SECRETING TUMOURS

Rare. Do not usually cause clinical syndrome

CUSHING'S SYNDROME

Cushing's syndrome (qv) may be caused by an ACTH secreting tumour arising from basophil or chromophobe cells

NELSON'S SYNDROME

The Rx of Cushing's disease by bilat adrenalectomy may later → formation of locally invasive pituitary tumour c̄ hyperpigmentation (Nelson's syndrome). High levels of ACTH & β-lipotrophin which stimulates melanocytes are found. Nelson's syndrome is usually prevented by pituitary irradiation at time of adrenalectomy

NON FUNCTIONING PITUITARY TUMOURS

About 30% of pituitary tumours are not hormonally active

CLIN: SOL effects; Progressive hypopituitarism. Occ Pituitary apoplexy; Cranial nerve palsies due to lat tumour extension

GENERAL RX OF PITUITARY TUMOURS

Trans-sphenoidal surgery often c̄ microsurgical technique is very safe & effective in relieving microadenomas without loss of pituitary function. Larger tumours may require trans-cranial approach. X-rad is routine after large adenoma removal. It is useful in reducing recurrence risk but late development of hypopituitarism is not uncommon. Occ Stereotactic Yttrium implantation; Drugs eg Bromocriptine

Hypopituitarism

Causes of Hypopituitarism (LIST 10 ENDO)

1. Tumours:
   a) Non-hormone producing adenoma
   b) Suprasellar tumours
2. Trauma
3. Surgical removal
4. Post X-Rad
5. Granulomas: Eg TB, Sarcoid
6. PPH (Sheehan's syndrome)

Rare. Commonest cause is a chromophobe adenoma

CLIN: Presentation depends on cause eg slow progression c̄ Pituitary tumour. Hypogonadism; Dwarfism & infantilism in children; Hypothyroidism; Hypoadrenalism. Occ DI; Hyperprolactinaemia

INVESTIGATIONS: • Basal level of Cortisol (at 9am), T4, T3, Prolactin, Testosterone (in M), Oestradiol (in F). Then inject Insulin, GnRH, TRH & measure BG, Cortisol, GH, LH, FSH, TSH over following 90mins
• Rarely Clomiphene test (To test hypothalamic/pituitary axis)

RX: Remove pituitary tumour by surgery ± X-Rad; Replacement Rx c̄ GH in children, Oestrogens & Progestogens in F, Testosterone in M, Thyroxine, Hydrocortisone. If fertility desired, Gonadotropins

Post Pituitary Disorders

ADH (Arginine vasopressin) is synthesised in hypothalamus & passes to the post pituitary. Secretion of ADH is mainly determined by plasma osmolality. ADH principally acts on kidney collecting ducts to allow concentration of urine

DIABETES INSIPIDUS

May result from ADH def (Cranial DI) or renal resistance to ADH (Nephrogenic DI)

Causes of Diabetes Insipidus (LIST 11 ENDO)

A. CRANIAL DI
1. Idiopathic
2. Trauma
3. Surgery
4. Tumours:
   Eg Pituitary tumour, Craniopharyngioma, Mets
5. Granuloma:
   Eg Sarcoid, TB, Histiocytosis
6. Post Infectious:
   Esp Basal meningitis
7. Vascular insult:
   Eg Sheehan's syndrome, Sickle cell anaemia
8. Familial

B. NEPHROGENIC
1. Familial
2. HypoK^+
3. HyperCa^{2+}
4. Chr renal disease:
   Eg Polycystic kidneys, Amyloidosis
5. Post obst uropathy
6. Pyelonephritis
7. Lithium

CRANIAL DI

Mainly acquired causes but rarely familial c̄ Aut Dom or Aut Rec inheritance

CLIN: Polyuria; Thirst; Polydypsia

INVESTIGATIONS:
- Urine osmolality
- Plasma osmolality
- Serum ADH
- Water deprivation test ie record urine & plasma osmolality during 8hr fluid fast & following ADH injection: Cranial DI is indicated by hypotonic urine following dehydration but ability to concentrate c̄ ADH; Nephrogenic DI is indicated by hypotonic urine even c̄ ADH; 1° polydipsia → hypertonic urine on dehydration
- Hypertonic saline infusion: ↓ response of ADH to osmotic stimulation in cranial DI

RX: DI may be transient after surgery or head injury. ADH replacement therapy. Chlorpropamide is rarely used
N.B DI can be masked by ACTH def which ↓ water excretion

DD: 1° polydipsia

INAPPROPRIATE SECRETION OF ADH

A syndrome of dilutional hyponatraemia due to inappropriate ADH secretion

Causes of Inappropriate ADH Secretion (LIST 12 ENDO)

1. Tumours:
   Eg Ca lung, Ca pancreas, Leukaemia, Thymoma
2. Chest disease:
   Eg Pneumonia, TB, CF, Emphysema
3. CNS disorders:
   Eg Meningitis, Encephalitis, Head inj, Brain abscess, Brain tumour, Guillain–Barre, Hydrocephalus, Porphyria
4. Drugs:
   Eg Chlorpropamide, Clofibrate, Thiazides
5. Hypothyroidism
6. Idiopathic
7. IPPV

CLIN: Excessive water retention without oedema. Severe hyponatraemia → drowsiness, nausea, confusion & later Ep & coma

INVESTIGATIONS:
- Urine Na^+ ↑
- Serum Na^+ ↓
- Serum & urine osmolality: Low serum osmolality c̄ inappropriately high urine osmolality
- ADH assay

RX: Treat underlying cause. Restrict fluid intake. Occ require Demeclocycline or Li^+ to inhibit ADH

Hypothalamic Disorders

The hypothalamus produces a series of factors to control pituitary ie Corticotropin releasing factor, GnRH, GRF, GHRIH, TRH, PIF & ADH. In addition hypothalamus is concerned c̄ sexual activity, body temperature, sleep,

water & appetite regulation
Deficient production of hypothalamic hormones can result from any hypothalamic disease esp Tumours eg craniopharyngioma, chromophobe adenoma, pinealoma, mets; Granulomas eg TB, sarcoid, Hand–Schuller–Christian; Trauma

GENERAL CLIN: Most present c̄ DI & variable def of ant pituitary lobe hormones. Rarely alterations in calorie balance, temperature or sleep control. Precocious puberty is occ due to a pinealoma or Albright's polyostotic fibrous dysplasia of bone
N.B Frohlich's syndrome of obesity & hypogonadism usually merely represents normal obese boys c̄ late puberty

LAURENCE–MOON–BIEDL SYNDROME

Aut Rec. Syndrome of obesity; Hypogonadism; IQ ↓; Retinitis pigmentosa; Polydactylism. Probably due to hypothalamic disease → isolated GnRH def

CUSHING'S SYNDROME

A syndrome caused by inappropriately raised levels of glucocorticoid steroids

Causes of Cushing's Syndrome (LIST 13 ENDO)

1. Pituitary/Hypothalamic disease (Cushing's Disease)
2. Ectopic ACTH secreting tumours
3. Exogenous glucocorticoid or ACTH
4. Adrenal Adenoma
5. Adrenal Carcinoma
6. Micronodular adrenal dysplasia

Commonest cause is corticosteroid Rx. Pituitary tumours occur esp in middle aged F

PATHOGENESIS: Cushing's disease is due to overproduction of corticotropin releasing factor or ACTH secreting pituitary tumours. Adrenal adenomas & Ca are non-ACTH dependent

CLIN: Obesity esp truncal; Moon face; Striae; Thin skin; BP ↑; Oedema; Muscle weakness. Occ Bruising; Amenorrhoea; Impotence; Diabetes; Pigmentation; Poor wound healing; Infections; Acne;Psychiatric disturbances.
In children growth ↓. Less often Hirsutism; #. If cause is an ectopic ACTH syndrome the clinical course is rapid & weight loss common

INVESTIGATIONS:
- U&E: K^+ ↓ in ectopic ACTH syndrome
- FBC: WCC ↑, Eosinophils ↓
- Cortisol at 12pm & 9am: Loss of diurnal rhythm
- Low dose Dexamethasone suppression test: No suppression of plasma cortisol
- Urinary 11-OHCS ↑
- ACTH at 9am & 12pm: ↑ in Cushing's disease & ectopic ACTH syndrome & ↓ in adrenal adenoma or Ca
- CAT scan
- High dose Dexamethasone suppression test: Steroid suppression in Cushing's disease but not ectopic ACTH syndrome or adrenal lesions
- Seleno–cholesterol isotope adrenal scan
- CXR
- Occ X-R bones: Occ #, Osteoporosis, Kyphosis, Aseptic necrosis
- Rarely:
  a) Metyrapone test: Marked response in Cushing's disease ie ↑ 17-oxogenic steroids; No response in ectopic ACTH syndrome
  b) GTT
  c) Angiography

RX ADRENAL TUMOURS: Resect as fully as possible. Cyt.T; Metyarpone can curb cortisol excess

RX ECTOPIC ACTH SYNDROME: Small cell lung Ca may respond to Cyt.T; Metyrapone can curb cortisol excess

RX CUSHING'S DISEASE: Trans-sphenoidal pituitary surgery usually preferred to X-Rad or Yttrium implant. X-Rad virtually eliminates risk of Nelson's syndrome. Metyrapone (c̄ Dexamethasone to prevent dramatic drop in cortisol level) is used pre-surgery to produce remission

ADDISON'S DISEASE

1° hypoadrenalism due to destruction of adrenal cortex. Uncommon. Autoimmune adrenalitis is commoner in F in adults & in M in childhood

Causes of Primary Hypoadrenalism (LIST 14 ENDO)

1. Autoimmune adrenalitis
2. TB
3. Bilat adrenalectomy
4. Granulomas
5. Mets
6. Cong adrenal hypoplasia
7. Cong adrenal hyperplasia
8. Meningococcal septicaemia
9. AIDS
10. Drugs: Eg Rifampicin, Anticoags
11. Birth trauma $\rightarrow$ haem
12. Adrenoleukodystrophy
13. Amyloidosis
14. Haemochromatosis

Commonest causes are autoimmune adrenalitis & TB. Autoimmune adrenalitis may be ass c̄ Hashimoto's disease, Schmidt's syndrome, PA, 1° ovarian failure, IDDM & Hypoparathyroidism. 2° hypoadrenalism is usually due to pituitary/hypothalamic disease

PATHOGENESIS: Aldosterone def $\rightarrow$ Na^+ & water loss, K^+ retention $\rightarrow$ $\downarrow$ plasma vol $\rightarrow$ $\uparrow$ renin & $\uparrow$ ADH secretion $\rightarrow$ water retention. Cortisol def $\rightarrow$ inability to excrete water load, mild acidosis & $\downarrow$ GFR; $\downarrow$ liver glycogen & $\downarrow$ gluconeogenesis $\rightarrow$ BG $\downarrow$

CLIN: May present acutely c̄ weakness, dehydration, malaise, postural BP $\downarrow$, or chronically. Lassitude; Muscle weakness; Anorexia; Wt $\downarrow$; Nausea; Vom; Dizziness (postural BP $\downarrow$); Pigmentation of skin & buccal mucosa; Loss of body hair (F). Occ Vitiligo; Depression; Nocturia; Abdo pain; Dyspepsia; Impotence; Hypoglycaemia; Diarrhoea

INVESTIGATIONS:
- Plasma cortisol $\downarrow$
- U&E: Often Urea & K^+ $\uparrow$; Na^+ & Cl^- $\downarrow$
- AXR: Occ calcified adrenals
- Short Tetracosactrin (Synacthen) test: Do cortisol level then give Synacthen & take cortisol levels at 30 & 60mins. In Addison's disease cortisol level remains low
- Depot Synacthen test: In 1° hypoadrenalism, cortisol level rise is impaired whereas in 2° hypoadrenalism or post long term steroid Rx a delayed rise is seen
- Autoimmune antibodies
- BG
- Ca^{2+}: Occ $\uparrow$

RX OF ACUTE ADRENAL CRISIS: Take blood for U&E, cortisol & BG & start IV glucocorticoids & fluids immediately. If high doses of Hydrocortisone are given a mineralocorticoid is not required. Oral Rx can usually be started after 1–2 days

RX OF CHR HYPOADRENALISM: Hydrocortisone replacement therapy. Usually also require mineralocorticoids eg Fludrocortisone. Dose needs to be increased in illness, surgery & prior to labour but care c̄ Rx needed to prevent iatrogenic Cushing's syndrome

DD:
1. TB
2. Malignancy
3. CRF

CONN'S SYNDROME
(1° HYPERALDOSTERONISM)

Usually due to adrenal adenoma or adrenal hyperplasia. Very rarely due to adrenal Ca. F>M. Esp 30–50yrs. causes about 1% of all cases of BP $\uparrow$

CLIN: Polydipsia; Polyuria; Nocturia; Muscle weakness; BP $\uparrow$. Occ Tetany; Paraesthesiae. Rarely oedema

INVESTIGATIONS:
- U&E: K^+ $\downarrow$, HCO_3 $\uparrow$, Na^+ >140mmol/l
- Plasma renin: $\downarrow$ in 1° & $\uparrow$ in 2°

hyperaldosteronism
- CAT scan
- Occ adrenal vein sampling of aldosterone for localisation

RX: Spironolactone whilst awaiting diagnosis & for bilat hyperplasia (SE: Gynaecomastia). Surgery for adenoma

2° HYPERALDOSTERONISM

Overproduction of aldosterone due to excessive stimulation of norm adrenals due to extra-adrenal disease. Commonly due to conditions which decrease blood vol eg nephrotic syndrome → ↑ renin & compensatory ↑ aldosterone to maintain blood vol

Causes of 2° Hyperaldosteronism (LIST 15 ENDO)

A. WITH FLUID RETENTION
1. Cardiac oedema
2. Cirrhosis
3. Nephrotic syndrome
4. Persistent idiopathic oedema

B. WITHOUT FLUID RETENTION
1. Renal ischaemia (Usually renal artery sten)
2. Accelerated BP ↑
3. Na^+ losing nephritis

C. MISCELLANEOUS
1. Drugs: Eg Carbenoxolone, Mineralocorticoids
2. Juxtaglomerular hyperplasia
3. Renin secreting tumour

Juxtaglomerular Hyperplasia (Bartter's Syndrome)

Rare. Aut Rec. Esp children

CLIN: Short stature; No BP ↑; Failure to thrive; Polyuria; Polydipsia

INVESTIGATIONS:
- U&E: Metabolic acidosis, K^+ ↓
- Renin ↑
- Aldosterone ↑
- Angiotensin ↑
- Renal biopsy: Juxtaglomerular hyperplasia

RX: Spironolactone, Na^+ restriction. May try prostaglandin inhibitor eg Indomethacin

PHAEOCHROMOCYTOMA

A tumour of neural crest tissue origin. 90% originate in adrenal medulla & 10% are extra-adrenal esp in para-aortic bodies of Zuckerkandl. Often multiple. About 10% malignant. Esp 25–55yrs. May be part of MEA type II syndrome

CLIN: Symptoms due to persistent or intermittent catecholamine production. Intermittent or persistent BP ↑; Headaches; N&V; Palps; Pallor & sweating. Paroxysms may last minutes or hours. Occ → Renal damage; BG ↑

INVESTIGATIONS:
- 24hr urine metadrenaline or VMA ↑
- Plasma Adrenaline &/or noradrenaline: Often ↑
- BG
- CAT scan
- Rarely Phentolamine suppression test

RX: α & β blockade to control BP ↑ eg Nitroprusside or Phentolamine & Propranolol. Then surgery

MULTIPLE ENDOCRINE ADENOMATOSIS SYNDROMES

It is postulated that these syndromes may represent neoplasia of APUD cells (Amine precursor uptake & decarboxylation). APUD cells migrate from neural crest to ectoderm during embryogenesis & secrete protein hormones

MEA type I (Werner's Syndrome)

Aut Dom. Commonest MEA. Most have HPT & Pancreatic islet adenomas eg → ZE or WDHA syndromes. Occ Pituitary adenoma & adrenocortical adenomas eg → Acromegaly, Cushing's syndrome, Prolactinoma, Hypogonadism

MEA type IIa

Aut Dom. Thyroid medullary Ca ass c̄ Phaeochromocytoma. Occ HPT

MEA type IIb

Thyroid medullary Ca, Phaeochromocytoma, neurological abnormalities eg Marfanoid habitus, mucosal neuromas, ganglioneuromatosis of the bowel

OBESITY

Acceptable wt ranges for M & F according to height have been determined. A wt 10–20% above the upper limit of acceptable range is termed overweight whilst obesity describes a wt >20% above. The cause of obesity is usually unknown but rarely due to endocrine disorders eg hypothyroidism, Cushing's disease. Obesity is ass c̄ ↑ early mort esp if grossly obese; BP ↑; Diabetes; Hernias; Gallstones; OA. Gross obesity is ass c̄ endometrial Ca

RX: ↓ energy intake c̄ adequate intake of protein, fibre, vits & electrolytes. Exercise whilst dieting may help prevent rebound wt gain on stopping diet. Occ jaw wiring or jejuno–ileal bypass are used. Surgery has a high mortality & morbidity & its use is therefore limited

THE BREAST

In F the breasts develop under the influence of oestrogens at puberty. During pregnancy the breasts enlarge & develop further in response to circulating placental hormones ie oestrogens, progestogens & HPL, & prolactin. Post-delivery levels of placental hormones fall & prolactin levels remain up esp if breast feeding

Cystic Mastitis

In each menstrual cycle, oestrogens → duct tissue stimulation & progesterone → alveolar secretory activity prior to menstruation. Common

CLIN: Slight breast tenderness; "Heavy" breasts. Occ ↑ breast nodularity. Relieved by menstruation

RX: Reassurance, well fitting bra. Occ Diuretics ± Progesterone for last few days of cycle. Rarely use Danazol or Bromocriptine

Traumatic Fat Necrosis

Trauma of breast fat cells → foreign body giant cell reaction → fibrosis & occ Ca

CLIN: h/o breast trauma. Breast lump occ c̄ skin tethering. Occ Axillary LN ↑

RX: Excision

DD: Ca breast

Acute Bacterial Mastitis

Esp Staph. Esp during lactation

CLIN: Cellulitis → abscess after several days; Breast engorgement

RX: Relieve milk engorgement eg by breast pump. Antibiotics if cellulitis. Poultice then drainage if abscess

Chronic Abscess

Rare. Due to TB; Gumma; Actinomycosis or inappropriate antibiotic Rx of acute abscess

CLIN: Bloodstained discharge; Abscess

Fibroadenosis

Esp 30–50yrs

CLIN: Painful lumpy breasts esp upper outer quadrant. Usually no LN ↑ or skin tethering

INVESTIGATIONS:
- Needle aspirate & cytology
- Biopsy to exclude Ca
- Mammography

RX: Biopsy

Fibroadenoma

Esp 25–40yrs. Common. Benign

CLIN: Rounded well defined mobile tumours

RX: Excision biopsy

Duct Papilloma

Benign

CLIN: Serous or bloody nipple discharge; Small tumour normally near nipple

RX: Excision biopsy

Mammary Duct Ectasia

Esp menopause. → stagnant secretions in duct system

CLIN: Occ green or brown thick discharge; Wormlike thickening beneath areola. May be 2° infection

DD: Ca breast

Mamillary Fistula

Rare. Usually a track between a major duct & the skin near the areola. Often h/o parareolar abscesses

Carcinoma of the Breast

Esp UK; USA; Europe. Commonest F Ca in UK. Occ FH. ↑ risk in nulliparous eg nuns & early menarche. ↓ risk if early completed pregnancy. Mastitis may predispose. M breast Ca is rare & ass c̄ Klinefelter's syndrome. Many pathological types eg Scirrhous

CLIN: Usually present c̄ hard painless lump which may be fixed to skin (In advanced cases → "Peau d'orange"). Occ Nipple retraction; Blood stained discharge. Early spread to axillary LN. Later spread esp to lung, liver, bones, brain, ovaries, adrenal. Early or late development of Ca in other breast is well recognised

INVESTIGATIONS:
- Excision biopsy c̄ frozen section or formal histology
- Mammography: MicroCa^{2+} suggests Ca
- Cytology of any aspirate/discharge
- CXR
- Skeletal survey
- Radioisotope bone scan

RX: Presymptomatic screening by palaption & mammography is probably of benefit in older women. Psychological & admin factors can prevent early reporting of symptoms

Type of Rx depends on clin stage
Rx Stage I & II ie Lump confined to breast or Mobile axillary glands: No consensus on Rx. Options inc Lumpectomy ± X-Rad; Quadrant/segment mastectomy ± X-Rad; Simple mastectomy ± axillary clearance ± X-Rad; Rarely radical mastectomy. Surgery may proceed directly following a frozen section or be carried out in two stages ie biopsy & then definitive surgery
Rx Stage III & IV ie fixed axillary LN, distant LN spread or mets: No consensus on Rx. About 30% of tumours are hormone responsive esp in F c̄ cytoplasmic oestrogen receptors & pre menopausal, respond to Tamoxifen. Occ surgical hormonal ablation performed ie Oopherectomy, Adrenalectomy, or Hypophysectomy. Simple mastectomy. Cyt.T may be of value. Local X-Rad for palliation esp bone pain. Occ toilet mastectomy to control local disease

PROG: 5yr survival stage I 70%. Poor if stage III or IV. Particularly malignant during pregnancy. Loss of breast often → psychiatric problems, hence importance of minimal disfigurement from surgery & good post-op support

Paget's Disease of the Nipple

Rare. Esp Middle-aged & elderly. Always ass c̄ breast Ca

CLIN: Unilat dry, red, bleeding, eczematous lesion round nipple

RX: Mastectomy

Causes of Nipple Discharge (LIST 16 ENDO)

1. Lactation
2. Carcinoma
3. Duct papilloma
4. Mammary duct ectasia
5. Breast abscess
6. Fibroadenosis & cysts
7. Non puerperal Galactorrhoea:
   a) Pituitary/Hypothalamic lesions
   b) Hypothyroidism
   c) Drugs eg Phenothiazines, Methyldopa

Gynaecomastia

Male breast development is usually due to an altered oestrogen/androgen balance

Causes of Gynaecomastia (LIST 17 ENDO)

1. Physiological:
   a) Neonatal
   b) Pubertal
2. 1° testicular failure
3. Hypogonadotrophic hypogonadism
4. Tumours:
   Eg Adrenal Ca, Leydig cell tumour
5. Liver disease
6. Refeeding post starvation
7. Endocrine disorders:
   Eg Pituitary tumours, Hyperthyroidism
8. Drugs:
   Eg Oestrogens, Spironalactone, Griseofulvin, Digoxin

Neonatal Gynaecomastia is due to high levels of placental oestrogens. Mild gynaecomastia is common in norm pubertal boys. ↑ oestrogen production occurs in cirrhosis, thyrotoxicosis & c̄ some tumours. ↓ androgen production eg Klinefelter's syndrome, castration or panhypopituitarism often → gynaecomastia

INVESTIGATIONS:
- Serum oestradiol
- Serum testosterone
- Serum LH & FSH
- LFTs
- CXR
- Occ require TFT, Chromosomes, CAT scan

RX: Testosterone for androgen def or Danazol & Tamoxifen. In severe disease a subcutaneous mastectomy may be required

Infectious Diseases

PUO

The following criteria are generally accepted to define PUO: Illness of >2wks duration; Temp >38.3° C on several occasions; No diagnosis after 1wk in hospital. Most causes of PUO are unusual presentations of common diseases or one of a gp of diseases which are difficult to diagnose. Infections, malignancies & collagen vascular diseases are common causes

INVESTIGATIONS: • Thorough reappraisal of history, examination & routine tests. Further tests often include serological tests for Ab to micro-organisms; General ultrasound examination of abdo & pelvis. Occ Biopsy; Isotope or CAT scan indicated. Sometimes a therapeutic trial is indicated when diagnosis not apparent eg a course of anti-TB Rx or steroids

Causes of PUO (LIST 1 INFD)

1. Infection:
   Esp TB, SABE, Brucellosis, Localised abscesses
2. Malignancy:
   Esp Hodgkin's disease, Lymphoma, Leukaemia, Renal Ca
3. Collagen vascular disease:
   Esp Still's disease, SLE
4. Drugs
5. Factitious fever
6. Sarcoidosis
7. Rarely:
   a) Familial mediterranean fever
   b) Whipple's disease
   c) Weber–Christian disease
   d) Phaeochromocytoma

INTESTINAL INFECTIONS

Enteric Fever (Typhoid)

Esp Afr, Central & S.Am, S. & E.Europe, Middle & Far East. In UK most cases are related to foreign travel.

Due to *Salmonella typhi*. Transmission is by F–O route. Often spread by asymptomatic human carrier via faecal or urinary contamination of food or water. Incub Pd 10–20 days

PATHOGENESIS: Organism flourishes in unhygienic food & water. On ingestion multiplies in ileum then spreads to mesenteric LN & via thoracic duct to bloodstream c̄ resulting clin illness. Reinvasion of GIT via bile & multiplication in RES inc → Peyer's patches. Gall bladder often reservoir of pathogen

CLIN: Insiduous onset c̄ Fever; Headache; Abdo pain; Non-productive cough; Constipation. In 2nd wk occ rose spots on trunk; Spleen ↑; Relative PR ↓; Diarrhoea. In 3rd wk often Toxic confusional state & occ GI complications. Then usually spontaneous recovery. 2nd attacks may occur (approx 10%)

INVESTIGATION:
- Blood culture
- Stool cultures (from 2nd wk): Often excrete organism for 1–3mths
- Urine culture
- Widal's test: Difficult to interpret. Often +ve from previous infection, immunisation or anamnestic reaction
- WCC: Usually ↓

PREVENTION: Clean water supply will dramatically ↓ incidence in endemic areas. Modern sewage disposal methods. General hygiene eg washing hands after lavatory, hygienic storage of food. Killed vaccines give 70–80% protection for about 5yrs. Carriers should not be employed in food or water industries

RX: Barrier nurse; Rehydrate. Chloramphenicol (SE: Aplastic anaemia) or Cotrimoxazole for 2wks. 2–5% become permanent carriers & these may respond to prolonged antibiotic Rx. Stool & urine culture required to monitor post Rx clearance. Inform Community Physician. Cholecystectomy is rarely indicated

COMPLICATIONS:
1. GIT: Haem; Perf; Cholecystitis
2. Resp: Pneumonia; Sore throat; Empyema
3. CVS: Myocarditis; Pericarditis; DIC; SABE
4. GUS: Cystitis; Orchitis
5. CNS: Meningitis; Encephalopathy; Polyneuritis; Psychosis
6. Abscesses
7. Osteomyelitis

Paratyphoid Fevers

Due to *Salmonella paratyphi A, B & C*. In UK, *S.paratyphi B* is commonest

CLIN: Clin features & complications are similar but less serious than typhoid

Salmonellosis

Common. There are more than 1700 serotypes of Salmonella. 2 main categories: Enteric fever organism ie *S.typhi* & *S.paratyphi*; Serotypes responsible for food poisoning which are parasites of animals eg *S.typhimurium*, *S.hadar*, *S.virchow*. Found in wide range of birds & animals, common sources are poultry, pigs & cattle. Food poisoning occurs through poor food preparation eg insuf cooking of frozen foods, contamination of cooked food by contact c̄ raw contaminated food. Outbreaks occur by F–O route. Esp institutions. Incub Pd 12–48hrs

CLIN: May be asymptomatic. Sudden onset of Abdo pain (usually mild); D&V. Occ Malaise; Fever. Rarely Septicaemia; Toxic dilatation of colon. Usually recovery starts after 3–4 days. May be cause of PUO

INVESTIGATIONS:
- U&E
- Stool culture

RX: Ensure good hygiene. Rehydrate. Notify Community Physician. Antibiotics eg Chloramphenicol for septicaemia. Chr carrier state rare

Shigellosis

Common. Prevalent world wide. 4 gps of organisms: *Sh.sonnei*, *Sh.dysenteriae* (*Sh.shigae*), *Sh.boydii*, *Sh.flexneri*. Man is disease reservoir. Esp overcrowding, poor hygienic conditions, institutions. In temperate countries *Sh.sonnei* is common, in tropics *Sh.flexneri* is common. Incub Pd 1–4 days. Usually F–O spread, in tropics spread by flies

CLIN: Abrupt onset. Abdo pain; Fever; Watery stools ± blood & mucus.

In tropics, dysentery c̄ Dehydration; Shock; Bloody stools may occur. Sonnei dysentery is usually mild

INVESTIGATIONS:
- Stool cultures
- U&E

RX: Good hygiene. Rehydrate; Antibiotics often required for *Sh.flexneri* & *Sh.shigae*. Food handlers should be excluded from work until 3 stool cultures are −ve

COMPLICATIONS:
1. Arthritis
2. Haemolytic–Uraemic Syndrome

Campylobacter

Common cause of GE. Most cases are sporadic. Incub Pd 3–5 days

CLIN: May be asymptomatic. Occ Diarrhoea ± blood in stools; Abdo pain; Fever; Nausea. May exacerbate existing IBD

INVESTIGATION: • Stool culture

RX: Usually no Rx needed. In severe or prolonged illness, Erythromycin

COMPLICATIONS: 1. Arthritis
2. Pancreatitis
3. Septicaemia

E.Coli

3 pathogenic forms of *E.Coli*: Enterotoxigenic; Enteroinvasive; Enteropathogenic

ENTEROTOXOGENIC E.COLI

These strains produce heat labile &/or heat stable toxins which produce diarrhoea. Important cause of traveller's diarrhoea

ENTEROINVASIVE E.COLI

Certain "O" serotypes produce invasive inflam change in large intestine. Occ cause of dysentery

ENTEROPATHOGENIC E.COLI

A cause of infantile GE

Yersinia enterocolitica

Found worldwide. Most infections are sporadic

PATHOGENESIS: Heat stable enterotoxin affecting terminal ileum

CLIN: Often Fever; Abdo pain; Diarrhoea. Occ Arthritis; Erythema nodosum; Reiter's syndrome; Uveitis; Thyroiditis

INVESTIGATIONS: • Stool culture
• Serology

RX: If severe bowel symptoms or extraintestinal disease antibiotics eg Chloramphenicol

Cholera

Due to enterotoxin of *Vibrio cholerae* esp El Tor biotype. Esp India. Causes periodic epidemics. F–O spread, transmitted via water or food. Incub Pd 0.5–5 days

CLIN: May be asymptomatic. Rapid onset of Diarrhoea++; Vom; Cramps. Occ → Shock; ARF. In children often Ep; BG ↓; Stupor

PREVENTION: Clean water supply systems; Good personal hygiene. Vaccine gives partial protection

RX: Prompt replacement of fluids & electrolytes (WHO solution for oral repletion usually obviates need for IV Rx). Antibiotics eg Tetracycline may benefit but drug resistance may occur. Carrier state is common

Vibrio parahaemolyticus

Esp Japan. Usually spread via contaminated seafood. Incub Pd 0–3 days

CLIN: Profuse watery diarrhoea

RX: Rehydrate. Occ require antibiotics eg Tetracycline

Bacillus cereus

Illness often due to inadequate reheating of cooked fried rice. 2 types c̄ Incub Pd of 1–5hrs & 8–16hrs

CLIN: Short Incub Pd illness ass c̄ Vom. Other type → diarrhoea & abdo pain

Clostridium perfringens

Usually due to inadequate reheating of cooked meat. Incub Pd 12hrs

CLIN: Diarrhoea; Abdo pain. Rarely Vom

Traveller's Diarrhoea

A general term for GIT disturbance of traveller's esp to Tropics. Usually due to Shigella, Salmonella, Campylobacter, *E.coli* or Giardia

CLIN: D&V; N; Abdo pain. Usually lasts few days

Intestinal Worms

Helminths are divided into Nematodes (Roundworms), Cestodes (Tapeworms), Trematodes (Flukes). These worms are an important cause of intestinal illness worldwide esp Tropics

NEMATODES

The 6 commonest intestinal Nematode infections can be divided into 2 gps. The infective stage is swallowed c̄ Ascaris, Enterobius & Trichuris infections & the infective stage penetrates the skin c̄ Strongyloides, Ancylostoma & Necator infections. Most are soil transmitted

ASCARIASIS (ROUNDWORM): Caused by *Ascaris lumbricoides*. Very common esp Tropics, Far E. Esp low social class

Life Cycle: Eggs passed in faeces mature in soil. If mature eggs are swallowed, larvae escape into sm intestine & burrow through wall passing via blood to liver & lungs & thence through resp airways to be swallowed, becoming adult worms in the sm intestine. Adult worms live for approx 1yr

Clin: Larval ascariasis → Liver ↑; Pneumonia; SOB; Wheeze. Occ Fever; Haemoptysis; Loeffler's syndrome; Urticaria. The adult worm (intestinal) phase may cause Colic; ↓ nutritional status. Occ intestinal obst; Appendicitis; Perf; Volvulus; Malabsorption; Cholecystitis; Pancreatitis. Symptoms related to number of worms. Rarely D&V

Investigations:
- Faeces for ova
- Sputum for larvae
- Serology: +ve early
- Eosinophilia: High early

N.B Occ worm passed in stools or vomited

Prevention: Proper faecal disposal could control disease. Endemic ascariasis can be controlled by 3–6mthly community-orientated chemotherapy

Rx: Levamisole, Mebendazole or Piperazine. Cure 80–90%

ENTEROBIASIS (PINWORM): Due to *Enterobius vermicularis*. Very common worldwide esp Tropics. Esp children

Life Cycle: Infection by ingestion of eggs via dirty hands or food. Worms develop in caecum where they survive for 4–6wks. A F worm migrates to rectum & lays many eggs which are deposited on perianal skin at night. Infective larvae develop in eggs in approx 6hrs. Chr autoinfection is common

Clin: Perianal pruritus esp nocte. Occ Appendicitis; 2° infection; Vulvovaginitis; Endometritis

Investigations:
- Eggs can be recovered from a strip of sticky tape applied to perianal skin
- Worms sometimes seen in stools

Prevention: Good personal hygiene esp washing hands after passing stools

Rx: All family members should be examined & treated if necessary. Piperazine or Mebendazole

TRICHURIASIS (WHIPWORM): Due to *Trichuris trichiura*. Common esp Tropics. Esp children

Life Cycle: Excreted eggs mature in soil. Man swallows infected eggs via dirty hands or food. Eggs hatch in small intestine & larvae attach to GIT mucosa esp caecal & develop into adult worms. Eggs passed in faeces

Clin: Most infections are mild. In severe infections Chr diarrhoea; Anaemia; GIT bleeding; Appendicitis; Intussusception; Failure to thrive; Abdo pain; 2° infections; Rectal prolapse; Clubbing

Investigations:
- Quantitative faecal examination to establish number of eggs per g of faeces
- Eosinophilia
- FBC: Hb ↓
- Occ Stools for Charcot–Leyden crystals

Rx: Treat if heavy infection or pronounced symptoms c̄ Mebendazole. Effective in 70–80% of cases

ANCYLOSTOMIASIS (HOOKWORM): Hookworm infection is caused mainly by 2 nematodes *Ancylostoma duodenale* & *Necator americanus*. *A.duodenale* is prevalent in Far E, China, S.Europe, S.Am & *N.americanus* is common in humid tropics eg Afr, S.E.Asia, Central Am

Life Cycle: Similar in both species. Eggs form rhabditiform larvae which feed on faeces & develop into infective filariform larvae which penetrate skin by direct contact c̄ infected soil. Larvae migrate via blood to liver & lungs, & via trachea to GIT. Adult worm develop in sm intestine & pass eggs in faeces. Adult worms live 3–5yrs in GIT

Clin: Itchy dermatitis esp feet. Occ Abdo pain; Protein ↓; Anaemia; Failure to thrive; Diarrhoea. Rarely Resp symptoms (Wakana disease) c̄ SOB, cough, haemoptysis

Investigations:
- Faecal egg count: May

be detected 2mths after earliest symptoms

- FBC: Often IDA
- Eosinophilia

Prevention: Wear shoes to ↓ risk of infection. Improve sanitary conditions. Community–orientated selective chemotherapy

Rx: Bephenium for *A.duodenale.* Thiabendazole for *N.americanus.* Fe ± folic acid for any anaemia

STRONGYLOIDIASIS: Due to *Strongyloides stercoralis.* Esp Tropics eg Afr, S.Am, Far E

Life Cycle: Infection may arise from outside body or within GIT (autoinfection). Free living larvae are derived from a free living cycle in soil & penetrate the skin, whilst larvae from perianal skin or intestine burrow through intestine to reach blood stream. Larvae are carried to lungs & thence to intestine via trachea. Adult worms develop in sm intestine. Eggs are passed containing rhabditiform larvae

Clin: Within a week of exposure, transitory creeping itchy red skin eruption. Then resp symptoms eg Pneumonia, Loeffler's syndrome which may be chr in autoinfection. Occ Abdo pain; Diarrhoea; Malabsorption; Cholecystitis; Anaemia. In immunosuppressed, acute dissemination may occur

Investigations:
- Stool examination usually demonstrates larvae
- Duodenal aspiration may reveal larvae
- Specific serology

Prevention: Wear shoes. Avoid damp shady places

Rx: Thiabendazole

CESTODES (TAPEWORMS)

TAENIA SAGINATA: Esp Tropical Afr, Middle E, S.E.Asia. Man is the only definite host. Larval stages develop in cattle

Life Cycle: Man is infected by eating undercooked beef c̄ larval stage. Cysticerus (larva) attaches to the sm intestine & adult worm develops. Eggs are passed in faeces. Cattle swallow eggs & embryo is liberated in GIT & migrates into muscles & tissues developing into cysticerci. Cysticerci are usually detectable by routine meat inspection

Clin: Often asymptomatic. Vague abdo pain; Diarrhoea; Change in appetite. Occ Appendicitis; Obst; Malabsorption; Perianal discomfort

Investigation: • Faecal examination for eggs. Occ worm segments

Prevention: Good hygiene. Cook meat thoroughly

Rx: Niclosamide, Diclorophen or Praziquantel

TAENIA SOLIUM: Esp Central Am, Middle E, Afr, E.Europe

Life Cycle: Man is infected by eating undercooked pig c̄ cysticerus larvae. Tapeworms live for years in sm intestine. Oncosphaera in an embryo phore is passed in faeces & ingested by pig or man. Cysticercus larvae develop in muscle or organs eg brain, eye

Clin: May be asymptomatic. Occ Abdo pain; Diarrhoea; Spread to tissues (cysticercosis). Cysticerci take about 4mths to develop & cause symptoms on dying eg Fever; Headache; Urticaria; sc nodules; Ep; Focal CNS symptoms

Investigations:
- Faecal examination for eggs (to distinguish from *T.saginatum* examine scolex)
- X-R: May show calcified cysticerci
- Brain scan will show cysts

Prevention: Good hygiene. Cook meat thoroughly

Rx: Niclosamide & Praziquantel. Care in handling faeces

DIPHYLLOBOTHRIASIS: Due to *Diphyllbothrium latum* (fish tapeworm). Esp Scandinavia, N.E.Europe, Canada, Japan

Life Cycle: Insuf cooked fish containing plerocercoids eaten by man. Adult worms develop in 3–5wks in sm intestine. Eggs are passed in human faeces & after 10–15 days in water become infective to Cyclops (a crustacean) in which a coracidium is formed which develops into a procercoid. When Cyclops are eaten by fish the procercoid penetrates the GIT & migrates to muscle where a plerocercoid is formed

Clin: May be asymptomatic. Fatigue; Abdo pain. Occ Anaemia; Malabsorption. Rarely CNS symptoms

Investigations:
- Faeces for eggs
- FBC: Occ Megaloblastic anaemia

Rx: Niclosamide. Expulsion of scolex is evidence of success

HYMENOLEPIASIS: Due to dwarf tapeworm, *Hymenolepsis nana.* Esp Tropics. Common in insanitary overcrowded conditions. Esp children. Spread by F–O route. May be chr due to autoinfection

Clin: Occ Growth ↓; Wt ↓; Anorexia; Weakness; Abdo pain; Diarrhoea; Kerato–conjunctivitis

Investigation: • Repeated faecal examinations for eggs

Rx: Niclosamide. May recur

TREMATODES (FLUKES)

Intestinal Trematodes eg Metagonimus yokagawai are uncommon

EXTRA-INTESTINAL WORM INFECTIONS

Toxocariasis

A disease due to infection c̄ larvae of the Nematodes, *Toxocara canis* & *T.cati.* Esp young children. Ass c̄ pica. Common infection but often asymptomatic. Visceral larva migrans is a general term covering syndromes where helminth larva lodge in int organs causing granuloma & eosinophilia

LIFE CYCLE: In dogs, *T.canis* lives in intestine & produces eggs in faeces. Eggs become infective after 3–4wks. Infection may spread prenatally, or by ingestion of infected rats or mice. *T.cati* lives in GIT of cats. Spread of infection to humans is by swallowing infective eggs. Eggs release larvae in intestine which are carried to viscera in blood or lymph. Larvae do not multiply in man

CLIN: Most infections are subclinical. Symptoms depend on the number of larvae ingested, sites to which they are carried & host reaction. Occ Fever; Anorexia; Wt ↓; Ocular symptoms eg blurred vision; Liver ↑; Resp symptoms eg cough, asthma; Spleen ↑; LN ↑. Rarely Ep; Myocarditis; Blindness due to retinal destruction. Illness usually lasts for wks or mths & then improves spontaneously

INVESTIGATIONS:
- Toxocaral fluorescent Ab test
- Toxocara ELISA test
- Eosionophilia: Esp in visceral larva migrans
- CXR
- Igs: IgM & IgE ↑ in visceral larva migrans

PREVENTION: Prevent contact of humans c̄ areas used by dogs for defaecation. Dog owners can have animals wormed

RX: Diethylcarbamazine. In ocular toxocariasis, steroids & Diethylcarbamazine

DD:
1. Retinoblastoma (Ocular disease)
2. Tropical eosinophilia
3. Asthma
4. Other helminth infections

Schistosomiasis

A gp of diseases caused by Trematodes. Commonest species are *S.haematobium*, *S.mansoni*, *S.japonicum*. *S.haematobium* & *S.mansoni* are endemic in Afr & Middle E. *S.japonicum* esp prevalent in Far E

LIFE CYCLE: Man is the definitive host. Contact c̄ freshwater schistosome cercariae → penetration of skin. Cerecariae become schistosonules & travel via blood & lymph to pulm vessels. Settle in portal venous system & develop into adult worms in 6–12wks. Then migrate to final habitat (*S.haematobium*—bladder & prostate; *S.mansoni*—inf mesenteric veins; *S.japonicum*—sup & inf mesenteric veins). Worm lives for years producing eggs which are deposited in terminal blood vessels of bladder or intestine & passed in urine or faeces. Eggs hatch in water & liberate miracidia which must penetrate specific snail host within one day. Sporocysts develop in snail. Daughter sporocysts develop cercariae

PATHOGENESIS: Eggs which pass into tissues cause granulomatous reaction. Severity of disease is related to intensity of infection & host reaction

GENERAL CLIN: 1° infection causes papular itchy rash at site of skin penetration. 4–6wks later, Severe toxaemia;

Fever; Eosinophilia. Later effects of complications due to granuloma

CLIN OF S.HAEMATOBIUM: Freq; Dysuria; Suprapubic pain; Haematuria. Occ later Dribbling; Incontinence; Obst uropathy; Repeated UTIs. May be premalignant → Ca bladder

CLIN OF S.MANSONI: Abdo pain; Diarrhoea ± blood & mucous. Occ later Anaemia; Ascites; Varices; Liver failure; Nephrotic syndrome; OA

CLIN OF S.JAPONICUM: Spleen ↑; Ascites; Dysentery. Occ Acute serum sickness-like illness (Katayama fever)

CLIN OF PULM SCHISTOSOMIASIS: All species may cause arterial or parenchymus lesions. May → Cor pulmonale; Bronchitis; Bronchiectasis; Emphysema; Asthma

CLIN OF CNS SCHISTOSOMIASIS: *S.japonicum* mainly affects brain while other species affect spinal cord. May → Ep; Focal CNS signs; Encephalitis; Myelitis

INVESTIGATIONS OF URINARY SCHISTOSOMIASIS:
- Urine examination for terminal spined eggs
- KUB: Occ Ca^{2+}
- Cystoscopy
- Renogram
- ELISA in non-endemic areas

INVESTIGATIONS OF INTESTINAL & ASIATIC SCHISTOSOMIASIS:
- Stools for eggs
- Rectal biopsy for eggs
- ELISA test in non-endemic areas

PREVENTION: Clean water & good sanitation facilities. Wearing of protective clothing. Snail destruction eg by molluscicides. Mass Rx c̄ Oxamniquine to ↓ egg excretion

RX: Early Rx to reduce risk of obst lesions. Niridazole, Oxamniquine esp for *S.mansoni*, or Metriphonate esp for *S.haematobium*

Filarial Infections

A gp of infections caused by filarial worms whose larval stage develop in arthropods. Man is the natural host of 8 species which are confined to the Tropics. Most important filiariases are *Wuchereria bancrofti* & *Onchocerca volvulus*. Adult worms do not multiply in man

LYMPHATIC FILARIASIS

Due to *Wuchereria bancrofti* or less commonly *Brugia malayi*. Common. Esp E.Afr, Pacific, India, S.E.Asia

LIFE CYCLE: Commonest vectors are mosquitoes. Insects ingest microfilariae c̄ blood meal which grow in thorax & then migrate to proboscis. When mosquito feeds, larvae are deposited on skin & migrate to LN. M & F worms mate to produce microfilaria which enter blood stream

CLIN: Early features include Epididymitis; Tender LN ↑; Orchitis. Later Hydrocoele. Rarely Elephantiasis esp legs c̄ lymphoedema, thickening of skin & occ 2° infection; Tropical pulm eosinophilia syndrome

INVESTIGATION:
- Midnight blood for filariae ± concentration techniques

PREVENTION: Prophylaxis against mosquitoes eg nets, larvacides

RX: Diethylcarbamazine (death of worms can → fever, lymphangitis, abscess). Surgery for hydrocoele. Elephantiasis is difficult to treat

ONCHOCERCIASIS

Due to *O.volvulus*. Common worldwide esp African savanna. Important cause of blindness

LIFE CYCLE: *O.volvulus* is spread by the vector Simulium fly, whose larval stages depend on the presence of well oxygenated river water

PATHOGENESIS: Disease severity depends on duration & intensity of worm load. Microfilariae cause major pathology due to immunotoxic reaction to their death

CLIN: Papular rash; LN ↑; Fever; Malaise. Later thickened skin c̄ depigmentation (leopard skin) & loss of elasticity. Ocular onchocerciasis initially cause opacities & photophobia.

Later a sclerosing keratitis → blindness & glaucoma. In the Yemen, Sowda (ie unilat hyperkeratosis, hyperpigmentation, tender LN ↑) is common

INVESTIGATIONS:
- Skin snips to look for microfilariae
- Mazzotti test if skin snips −ve ie Diethylcarbamazine → ↑ itching
- Fundoscopy may show microfilariae

PREVENTION: Protective clothes. DDT destroys larval stage of vector

RX: Remove any onchocerca nodules on head. Diethylcarbamazine kills microfilariae but not worms, therefore recurrence inevitable. Repeat Rx → Mazzotti reaction, which can be helped by steroids. Occ Suramin which kills worm is used (SE: Nephrotoxicity). Rx of advanced disease is disappointing

LOIASIS

Due to *Loa loa*. Esp African rain forest. Vector is Chrysops fly

CLIN: sc swellings. Occ migrating worms seen under conjunctiva

INVESTIGATIONS:
- Eosinophils ↑↑
- Blood for microfilariae

PREVENTION: Protective clothing. Prophylactic Diethylcarbamazine

RX: Diethylcarbamazine

Hydatid Disease

A zoonosis caused by Echinococcal infection. Two important species, *E.granulosus* common in Middle E, Asia, N.Afr, S.Am, Australasia c̄ man interacting c̄ dog/sheep or dog/cow cycle; & *E.multilocularis* common in Europe, Japan & N.Am c̄ a rodent host

LIFE CYCLE: Eggs shed in faeces are ingested by carrier animal eg sheep, & eggs hatch in duodenum, larvae migrating through gut to disseminate via blood esp to liver. Larvae develop into hydatid cysts. When infected sheep organs are eaten by dog, adult worms develop. Man is infected by ingestion of eggs after contact c̄ dogs & as in sheep, larvae migrate to viscera esp liver & lung to form cysts

CLIN: May be asymptomatic. Liver cysts may → Liver ↑; J; PUO; Cholangitis. Pulm cysts may → SOB; Haemoptysis; 2° infection; Coughing up of daughter cysts; Resp distress. Rarely symptoms from cysts in kidney, brain, bone or pancreas. Rupture of cyst may → anaphylactic shock or disease dissemination

INVESTIGATIONS:
- CXR: Rounded well defined opacity. Occ rupture → "water-lily" sign
- Ultrasound
- CAT scan: Esp for brain cysts
- Occ Casoni's test for serology (not very specific)
- Eosinophilia: Occ

PREVENTION: Deworm dogs regularly. Do not feed dogs uncooked meat

RX: Surgery for symptomatic cysts (care to avoid leakage which may → anaphylaxis or dissemination of disease). If surgery is c/i can use Mebendazole

Clonorchiasis

Due to trematode *Clonorchis sinensis*. Common esp Far E. Usually acquired by eating raw fish. Flukes lodge & live in bile ducts for many years

CLIN: May be symptomless. Occ Anorexia; Dyspepsia; Liver ↑; Cholangitis; Biliary cirrhosis; J; Diarrhoea. May → cholangioCa of liver

PREVENTION: Control of snail, the intermediary host. Adequate cooking of fish

RX: Praziquantel

Fascioliasis

Disease of herbivores esp sheep & cattle. Due to eating raw contaminated water plants. Due to *F.hepatica* & *F.gigantica*

CLIN: Dyspepsia; Fever; Diarrhoea

RX: Bithionol

Fasciolopsiasis

Due to F.buski esp S.E.Asia, India. Due to eating contaminated water plants

CLIN: Often asymptomatic. Occ Malabsorption; Ascites; Rashes

RX: Praziquantel

Opisthorchiasis

Due to liver fluke Opisthorchis. Common esp Far E, N.E.Europe, India. Usually acquired by eating raw fish containing larvae. Flukes lodge & live in bile ducts for many years

CLIN: Weakness; Anorexia; Diarrhoea; Loss of

taste; Abdo pain; Hot sensations esp on trunk; Cholangitis; J

INVESTIGATIONS: • PTC: Dilated biliary tree
• Duodenal fluid examination
• Faeces for eggs

RX: Praziquantel

Paragonimiasis

Due to lung fluke Paragonimus. Esp China, Thailand. Usually acquired by eating raw infected crab or crayfish

CLIN: May be asymptomatic. Early symptoms are Diarrhoea; Abdo pain. Later chest signs may include Cough; SOB; Chest pain; Night sweats; Fever; Haemoptysis; Pleural effusions. Occ sc nodules; Abscesses; CNS signs

INVESTIGATIONS: • Sputum or stools for eggs (occ – ve)
• Specific serology tests
• CXR

RX: Praziquantel

Dracontiasis (Guinea Worm Disease)

Due to nematode, *Dracunculus medinensis*. Common esp W.Afr, India. Spread by drinking fresh water containing larvae carried by Cyclops or water fleas

CLIN: Often ulcers esp lower leg. Occ Arthritis

RX: Niridazole. Dress ulcers c̄ Ca^{2+} hypochlorite. Can extract worms manually or by surgery

Trichinosis

Due to nematode *Trichinella spiralis*. Common worldwide. Usually spread by eating infected raw meat esp pork

CLIN: Most are asymptomatic. 3 stages. Initially D&V; Colic; Maculopapular rash. Then Myalgia; Fever; Orbital oedema. Later severe toxaemia. Occ Myocarditis

INVESTIGATIONS: • Serology
• Muscle biopsy for larvae
• Eosinophils ↑↑

RX: Steroids for allergy until fever ↓. Mebendazole

BACTERIAL INFECTIONS

Tetanus

A disease caused by the neurotoxin of *Clostridium tetani* characterised by muscle rigidity & spasm. Common esp developing countries. Predispositions to infection are anaerobic conditions eg necrotic tissue, pyogenic sepsis, poor blood supply to wound & delay in Rx. Neonatal sepsis may follow cultural practice of covering umbilical stump c̄ animal dung. Incub Pd usually 6–10 days but may be longer or shorter (in a minority of cases no infection site can be identified)

CLIN: Early Trismus (lockjaw); Myalgia esp neck & back. Occ Malaise; Fever; Sweating; Dysphagia; Headache; Irritability. Later muscular rigidity → abdo rigidity, lumbar lordosis & neck retraction. Muscle spasms occur periodically & may → characteristic facies eg risus sardonicus, opisthotonus, dysphagia, resp arrest. Severe tetanus → sympath overactivity c̄ arrhythmias, BP ↑ or ↓, pyrexia, sweating & salivation. Rarely tetanus remains localised around wound site. Course is unpredictable. Attacks may last 2wks to many mths

INVESTIGATION: • Tetanus is a clinical diagnosis

PREVENTION: Active immunisation c̄ tetanus toxoid esp pregnant mothers in endemic areas. Destruction of environmental spores eg by heat or chemicals such as formaldehyde, esp in high risk areas eg operating theatres. Clean & debride all wounds thoroughly. Antibiotics for wound sepsis. Active immunisation for supf wounds if patient not immune. In more severe wounds, give toxoid booster if patient known to be immune. If patient not immune

& wound is severe, give HTIG & then active immunisation

RX: HTIG im & if indicated, early intrathecally. Debride wound. Antibiotics. Sedatives & muscle relaxants eg Diazepam. Tracheostomy if dysphagia or laryngeal spasm. In severe tetanus may require curarisation, IPPV, IV rehydration, naso–jejunal feeding. Sympath overactivity may require α &/or β blockers

PROG: Bad prognostic factors are Old age; Drug addiction; Tetanus neonatorum; Puerperal tetanus; Occurrence of generalised spasms; Short Incub Pd; <2 days between 1st symptom & 1st spasm; Sympath overactivity; Resp infections; High fever. Mort varies between 10–60% in developed world, but is approx 80% elsewhere

DD:
1. Functional muscle spasm (hysteria)
2. Phenothiazine dystonia
3. Tetany

Brucellosis

A specific disease of animals which is occ transmitted to man. Caused by 3 main Brucella species: *B.melitensis*, an infection of goats & occ sheep; *B.abortus*, an infection of cattle; *B.suis*, an infection of pigs. *B.melitensis* is usually spread via raw milk whilst other species are spread by direct contact c̄ raw meat & animals. Esp Vets, meat handlers & farmers

CLIN: Several types of disease are recognised ie acute, subacute, localised & chr forms

Acute brucellosis has an Incub Pd of 1–3wks & may present c̄ High pyrexia; Rigors; Sweating; Low back pain; Sciatica; Headache; Irritability; Large jt monoarthritis; Spleen ↑; Liver ↑. Usually illness spontaneously remits after 2–3wks

Subacute brucellosis may develop insidiously or after an acute illness. Characteristic undulant fever. Occ Malaise; Tiredness; Specific organ involvement eg spondylitis, arthritis, meningitis. Between attacks patient is well. Many recover spontaneously

Localised brucellosis presents insidiously c̄ evidence of local infection. Often Osteitis; Spondylitis; Arthritis; Meningism. Occ SABE; Pneumonia; Epididymo–orchitis; Sciatica. Rarely Hepatitis; Meningo–encephalitis; Cord compression

Chr brucellosis. Occ symptoms recur for prolonged periods. Usual symptoms are Malaise; Anorexia; Wt ↓; Sweating; Cough; Headaches. Occ Liver ↑; Spleen ↑; LN ↑; Temperature slightly ↑ in evenings

INVESTIGATIONS:
- WCC: Often ↓ c̄ relative lymphocytosis
- Blood cultures ×3
- Cultures of urine, marrow, aspirates
- Serology

PREVENTION: Pasteurise or boil all milk. Protective clothing & good hygiene when handling potentially infective animals. Vaccinate young animals. Screen animals for brucella & slaughter any who are +ve

RX: Tetracycline

PROG: *B.melitensis* infections are the most severe & are likeliest to cause chr infection. Appropriate Rx results in negligible mort & morbidity

DD:
1. TB
2. Other causes of PUO

Leprosy

Very common worldwide esp Tropics, Subtropics, Middle E. Due to *Mycobacterium leprae*. Incub Pd mths to yrs

PATHOGENESIS: 3 major clin forms depending on type & extent of immune response

Tuberculoid leprosy occurs when cell mediated immunity is strong. Bacilli are rare & disease is localised. Histology shows non-caseating granulomas

Lepromatous leprosy causes a widespread infection. Cell mediated immunity is weak. Bacilli are numerous. Bacilli are shed from resp tract & inhalation is thus common method of infection

Borderline (Dimorphous) leprosy is an unstable state lying in the middle of the spectrum of leprosy types. Often divided into 3 forms ie borderline lepromatous, borderline leprosy & borderline tuberculoid

CLIN OF INDETERMINATE LEPROSY: The simplest early manifestation of leprosy. Esp children. Small hypopigmented macule which may show hypoaesthesia & ↓ sweating. Most heal spontaneously but some develop one of the spectrum of leprosy forms

CLIN OF TUBERCULOID LEPROSY: 1–4 circular large well defined anaesthetic hypopigmented hairless dry lesions. Occ lesion is numb. Often thickening of periph nerve esp ulnar nerve at elbow, median nerve at wrist, lat popliteal nerve, great auricular nerve, post tibial nerve

CLIN OF BORDERLINE TUBERCULOID LEPROSY: Common esp in Afr & Asia. Smaller more numerous skin lesions compared to tuberculoid form. Sensation usually impaired. Often thickened periph nerves. May present c̄ acute motor weakness

CLIN OF BORDERLINE LEPROSY: Unstable form. Numerous asymmetrical lesions which may be macular, papular, plaques or annular lesions c̄ broad rims & hypopigmented anaesthetic areas. Often enlarged nerves

CLIN OF BORDERLINE LEPROMATOUS LEPROSY: Common in Europe & Asia. Numerous skin lesions of variable size c̄ hypo- or hyper-pigmented macules, papules, nodules or plaques. Nerve involvement often not prominent

CLIN OF LEPROMATOUS LEPROSY: Insidious onset. Usually present c̄ widespread symmetrical hypopigmented macular rash esp on face, upper trunk & extensor surfaces of limbs. Often nasal mucosa is yellow & thickened & may produce bloody discharge. Occ Iritis. Later the initially mild periph nerve signs ↑ c̄ ↓ sensation esp at extremities, & thickening of nerves. Also later ↑ thickening & nodularity of skin esp facial; Loss of eyebrows; ↑ ear lobes; Swelling of lips, fingers & feet; Conjunctivitis; Iritis; Keratitis; LN ↑; Testicular atrophy. Occ Erythema nodosum; Saddle nose deformity; Nodular infiltrates esp palate & nose; Septicaemia; Amyloidosis; Nephritis

INVESTIGATIONS:
- Skin smears: AFBs found in Borderline & Lepromatous forms
- Lepramin test: +ve in tuberculoid leprosy but −ve in lepromatous forms
- Histology: Non-caseating granulomas & lymphocytes are seen in Tuberculoid form. In Lepromatous form AFBs, histiocytes & immune complexes are common

RX: Best carried out by experts. Care to avoid damage to anaesthetic areas. Physio for weak muscles. Tuberculoid, Boderline Tuberculoid & Indeterminate forms are treated c̄ Dapsone & Rifampicin once monthly for 6mths. Borderline forms may gain cell mediated immunity on treatment c̄ resulting subacute inflam, this reversal reaction is treated c̄ steroids. Borderline & Lepromatous forms require triple drug therapy eg Dapsone, Rifampicin & Ethionamide until AFB smear −ve. Lepromatous patients should be isolated until infectivity controlled (approx 4 days post start of drug Rx). Rx of Lepromatous leprosy should last at least 2yrs. Erythema nodosum responds to Thalidomide. Steroid & Atropine eye drops for iritis. Occ plastic surgery esp for facial deformities; Orthopaedic ops eg tendon transplants

PROG: Best if early Rx & in paucibacillary disease

Plague

Zoonosis due to *Yersinia pestis*. Esp Asia, Afr, S.Am. Infection is transmitted to animals including humans by bites of infected fleas which normally feed on rodent hosts. In Afr the rat, Mastomys natalensis is important reservoir of disease

CLIN: 3 major forms: Bubonic, Pulmonary, Septicaemic. May be asymptomatic. Often painful tender local LN ↑ (bubo) c̄ surrounding cellulitis esp inguinal or femoral. May → Fever; Malaise; Headache; Septicaemia; Periph gangrene; Pneumonia. Rarely present c̄ meningitis or cervical buboes

INVESTIGATIONS:
- Blood cultures
- Sera for *Y.pestis* Abs
- Aspiration & culture of bubo material
- WCC ↑↑
- ELISA test

PREVENTION: Treat contacts c̄ prophylactic Tetracycline. Vaccinate those in high risk occupations (gives partial protection). Control rodents eg by gassing & poisoning. Control fleas eg c̄ DDT

RX: Isolate all patients c̄ pneumonic plague. Tetracycline ± Streptomycin

PROG: Good if early Rx

Legionnaires Disease

Due to Legionella pneumophila. Infection by inhalation from environmental source eg air condition cooling towers. Incub Pd usually 2–10 days

CLIN: Occ asymptomatic. Fever; Wt ↓; Anorexia; Sweating; Headache; Myalgia. Then 2–4 days later cough, SOB. Later Pneumonia; Confusion. Occ Diarrhoea; RF; Pleural effusion

INVESTIGATIONS:
- WCC: Usually ↑, Lymphocytes ↓
- ESR ↑
- U&Es: Serum Na^+ usually ↓
- Albumin: Usually ↓
- CXR
- LFT
- Urinalysis: Occ microscopic haematuria
- Sputum C&S: No organisms shown by conventional stains
- Abs to *L.pneumophilia* rise

PREVENTION: Water sources which are warm & still eg air conditioning water towers should be regularly cleaned & treated c̄ chlorine & other bactericides

RX: Erythromycin. Advanced cases often require supportive Rx eg respirator

PROG: Mort 10%. Poor in Elderly, Immunocompromised

Pontiac Fever

Due to *Legionella pneumophilla*. Rare

CLIN: Acute onset of Malaise; Fever; Headache; Myalgia. Usually quick recovery

RX: Erythromycin

Anthrax

Principally a disease of herbivores. Man acquires anthrax by close contact c̄ infected animals (including skins) or by eating infected animals. Esp Afr, Far E, USSR, S.Am. Ass c̄ occupational exposure. Due to spores of *Bacillus anthracis*. Cutaneous anthrax is due to penetration of spores into skin, GIT anthrax is due to spore ingestion & pulm anthrax is due to spore inhalation. Pulm & GIT anthrax are rare. Incub Pd 1–5 days

CLIN OF CUTANEOUS ANTHRAX: Small itchy papule that blisters & becomes surrounded by erythematous swelling. Later 2° vesicles form which are gradually covered by an eschar (malignant pustule). LN ↑. Occ Headache; Anorexia; N; Fever; Rigors. Later may → septicaemia

CLIN OF PULM ANTHRAX (WOOL SORTER'S DISEASE): Present c̄ malaise & fever, then SOB, cough, haemoptysis. Occ Pleural effusions; Pulm oedema

CLIN OF GIT ANTHRAX: Anorexia; Vom; Abdo pain; Bloody Diarrhoea; Septicaemia

INVESTIGATIONS OF CUTANEOUS ANTHRAX:
- C&S of vesicle fluid
- Blood culture
- Serology

PREVENTION: Vaccinate all at risk animals. Avoid using unsterilised animal products. Vaccinate at-risk persons. Good attention to hygiene in at-risk occupations

RX: Benzylpenicillin (does not affect natural h/o cutaneous lesion but relieves systemic symptoms)

PROG: Poor in pulm & GIT forms. Good c̄ Rx in cutaneous form

Leptospirosis

3 main causes: *Leptospira icterohaemorrhagiae* → Weil's disease; *L.canicola* → canicola fever; *L.hebdomadis* → hebdomadis infection

WEIL'S DISEASE

Common in rats where organism is established in kidney & urine is infective. Infection spread to humans by water usually via skin abrasion. Esp at risk occupations eg sewage workers. Incub Pd 5–19 days

CLIN: Acute onset c̄ Fever; Sweating; Headache; Myalgia. Occ Oliguria → RF; Epistaxis; Petechiae; Haematuria; GI bleed; Meningitis; J after 4th day; Myocarditis. Often improve in 3rd wk c̄ Fever ↓; J ↓; Diuresis

INVESTIGATIONS: • Serial Abs: Rise in titre
- WCC ↑
- CSF: ↑ protein & lymphocytes. Sugar norm
- Blood culture: +ve in first wk

PREVENTION: Protective clothing for at-risk occupations. Control of rat population

RX: Tetracycline. Usual Rx of RF

PROG: Mort 10–15% if J

CANICOLA FEVER

Common disease of dogs & pigs. Spread to humans by contact c̄ infected water. Incub Pd 5–19 days

CLIN: Milder illness than Weil's disease. Often mild meningitis. Occ Nephritis; J

PREVENTION: Vaccination of dogs

RX: Tetracycline

Tularaemia

Due to *Francisella tularensis.* Esp N.Hemisphere (not UK). Humans are incidental hosts. *F.tularensis* may contaminate water sources & its natural cycle involves blood sucking arthropods eg Ticks & various mammals eg rabbits, birds, amphibians & fish. Two biotypes, a more virulent arthropod-borne & a milder water-borne form. Infection may be by penetration of skin, inhalation or ingestion. Incub Pd 1–14 days

CLIN: Sudden onset of Fever; Malaise; Myalgia; Chills. Cutaneous form → Ulcer; LN ↑; Septicaemia. Ingestion → Typhoid-like illness. Inhalation → Pneumonia; Pleurisy. Conjunctival infection → purulent conjunctivitis. Occ membranous pharyngotonsillitis

INVESTIGATION: • ELISA test

PREVENTION: Boil untreated water. Wear gloves while skinning animals. Live attenuated vaccine for endemic areas eg USSR

RX: Streptomycin or Gentamicin

Actinomycosis

Usually due to *A.israelii.* Ass c̄ dental caries

CLIN: 3 main forms. Cervico-facial occurs after tonsillitis & → swelling over angle of jaw, local induration, trismus. Then sinus develops & discharges thin pus. Occ direct spread to orbit, skull, jaw. Pulm actinomycosis usually follows inhalation from infected mouth. Abdominal actinomycosis usually occurs 2° to perf PU or perf appendix & → hard mass c̄ abscesses & discharging sinuses. May → portal pyaemia

RX: Penicillin. Drain any collection of pus

Melioidosis

Due to *Pseudomonas pseudomallei.* Esp S.E.Asia, Australia. Infection via soil by penetration of skin or inhalation. Incub Pd variable

CLIN: Often asymptomatic. Occ Chr skin lesions; Septicaemia

INVESTIGATIONS: • Blood culture
- CFT

RX: Tetracycline, Chloramphenicol & Kanamycin

Glanders

Disease of horses. Occ spread to man. Due to *Pseudomonas mallei*

CLIN: Skin nodules → deep ulcers & necrosis. Inflam of mucous membranes

RICKETTSIAL DISEASES

Rickettsiae are obligate intracellular parasites usually transmitted to man by arthropods & intermediate in size between bacteria & viruses

Transmission of Rickettsial Diseases (LIST 2 INFD)

1. Transmitted by Louse:
   Epidemic typhus
2. Transmitted by Flea:
   Murine typhus
3. Transmitted by Tick:
   a) Rocky Mountain Spotted fever
   b) Fievre Boutonneuse
   c) Siberian tick typhus
   d) Queensland tick typhus
4. Transmitted by Mite:
   a) Rickettsial Pox
   b) Scrub typhus

Epidemic Typhus

Due to *R.prowazekii.* Man is major disease reservoir. Spread by louse, *Pediculus humanus.* Louse feeds on infected human blood & deposits rickettsiae in its faeces around bite sites. Scratching the irritant bite site → infection. Ass c̄ wars & famine. Incub Pd 7–21 days

CLIN: Acute onset c̄ Fever; Malaise; Headache; Constipation; Chills. After 1wk, Maculopapular rash esp on trunk; Drowsiness; Fever; Torpor. In 2nd to 3rd wks, Poor mental state; BP ↓; Fever; Weakness++; Spleen ↑. Occ Gangrene; Coma. If patient recovers prolonged convalescence before full recovery
Occ there is a recrudescence of epidemic typhus (Brill–Zinsser) disease c̄ a milder version of the illness

INVESTIGATIONS:
- IFA
- CFT
- Occ Wiel–Felix reaction (non-specific)

PREVENTION: DDT dusting of lousy individuals. Vaccine

RX: Tetracycline (Prolonged course → ↓ risk of recrudescence)

DD:
1. Other rickettsial disease esp Murine typhus
2. Typhoid
3. Malaria
4. Meningococcaemia

Murine Typhus

Due to R.typhi. Natural infection of rats. Transmission to man by rat flea, *Xenopsylla cheopis.* Incub Pd 6–10 days

CLIN: Gradual onset c̄ Headache; Myalgia; Fever; Chills; Painful eye mvts; Macular rash esp trunk. Usually recover in 2wks

INVESTIGATIONS:
- IFA
- CFT
- Occ Wiel–Felix reaction

RX: Tetracycline

Rocky Mountain Spotted Fever

Due *R.rickettsii.* Man is incidental host. Tick vector. Esp USA, S.Am. Incub Pd 3–12 days

CLIN: Acute onset of Fever; Headache; Malaise; Chills; Photophobia; Myalgia; Arthralgia; Prostration. Maculopapular rash esp extremities, usually appears on 3rd–4th day. Occ fever remits in mornings. Later rash spreads to trunk & becomes petechial, occ → gangrene of extremities; Headache; Confusion; Restlessness. Occ coma. If patient recovers, slow convalescence usually starting in 3rd wk

PREVENTION: Vector control eg insecticides. Application of repellent to clothing

INVESTIGATIONS:
- IFA
- CFT
- Occ Wiel–Felix reaction

RX: Tetracycline

Fievre Boutonneuse

Due to *R.conorii.* Man is incidental host. Tick spread. Esp S.Europe, Afr, Middle E. Incub Pd 5–7 days

CLIN: Eschar; LN ↑; Headache; Fever; Malaise. Maculopapular rash occurs 3–4 days later spreading from extremities to trunk. Rarely haemorrhagic ulceration. Prolonged convalescence

INVESTIGATIONS:
- IFA
- CFT

RX: Tetracycline

Siberian Tick Typhus

Due to *R.siberica*. Tick spread. Esp Asia, Far E. Incub Pd 5–7 days

CLIN: As for Fievre Boutonneuse

INVESTIGATIONS: • IFA
• CFT

RX: Tetracycline

Queensland Tick Typhus

Due to *R.australis*. Tick spread. Esp Queensland. Incub Pd 5–7 days

CLIN: As for Fievre Boutonneuse

INVESTIGATIONS: • IFA
• CFT

RX: Tetracycline

Rickettsialpox

Due to *R.akari*. Spread by blood sucking mite. Infection of mice. Esp N.Am, USSR, Korea. Rarely reported. Incub Pd 10–24 days

CLIN: Mite bite → red papule → vesicle which may → eschar. Then sudden onset of Fever; Chills; Headache; Myalgia. 1–4 days later, maculopapular rash which becomes vesicular; LN ↑; Photophobia. Full recovery in 1–2wks

INVESTIGATIONS: • IFA
• CFT

RX: Tetracycline

Scrub Typhus

Due to *R.tsutsugamushi*. Spread by mites. ? animal reservoir is wild rodents. Esp area from Pakistan to Japan & southward to N.Australia. Incub Pd 6–18 days

CLIN: Occ eschar develops at site of larval mite feeding. LN ↑; Remitting fever; Headache; Malaise; Chills; Painful eye mvts. Occ maculopapular rash develops in 1st wk esp affecting trunk. Usually recovery starts after 2–3wks. Milder disease seen in endemic areas

INVESTIGATIONS: • WCC: Large lymphocytes ↑
• CFT

PREVENTION: Vector control eg insecticides. Chemoprophylaxis c̄ Tetracycline for those at risk

RX: Tetracycline

DD:
1. Malaria
2. Infectious mononucleosis
3. Typhoid
4. Dengue
5. Leptospirosis

VIRAL INFECTIONS

Herpes Simplex

There are two strains, HSV-1 & HSV-2. HSV-1 is spread via oral secretions & is commonly seen esp in children & low social classes. HSV-2 is spread by genital secretions (see STD section)

CLIN OF 1° INFECTION: 1° infection may be asymptomatic. Various presentations occ seen:
Gingivostomotitis c̄ Fever; Sore throat; Vesicles on pharynx, buccal mucosa, tongue & gums; Pain on eating & drinking; Cv LN ↑. Occ ulceration. Usually recover after 10–14 days
Unilat follicular conjunctivitis c̄ photophobia; Oedema; Dendritic ulcer. Occ deeper stromal involvement. Usually recover in 2–3wks
Rarely HSV-1 → herpetic whitlow (esp health workers) or anal infection (esp homosexuals)

CLIN OF RECURRENT INFECTION:
Usually occur at site of 1° infection.
Severe infection is common in immunocompromised
Herpes labialis (Cold sore) may be ppt by fever, trauma, strong emotion, menstruation. Vesicles occur on or around lips & form ulcers & crusts over following 3 days. Usually recovery in 7 days
Eye infections recur as supf keratitis → corneal ulceration. Occ uveitis → permanent visual loss

INVESTIGATIONS: • Electron microscopy or IMF of vesicle fluid

RX: Herpes labialis, use topical Idoxuridine or Acyclovir. Dendritic or amoeboid ulcers, use topical Idoxuridine or Acyclovir. Stromal disease use steroids &/or topical Acyclovir. In immunocompromised inc prophylaxis for organ transplants, use IV Acyclovir

COMPLICATIONS: 1. Herpes simplex encephalitis
2. Kaposi's varicelliform eruption: In those c̄ atopic eczema vesicles develop in large crops becoming pustular & occ haemorrhagic. Fever; 2° infections

Shingles

Due to *Herpes varicella–zoster* virus. Man is only host. 1° infection → chickenpox. Virus then remains dormant in dorsal root ganglion. Reactivation of virus → shingles. Cause of reactivation often unknown, occ due to immunosupression, malignancy, spinal cord disease. Esp elderly

CLIN: Often several days of radicular pain c̄ hyperaesthesia of affected segment. Then erythematous rash in dermatome distribution which becomes vesicular. Rash encrusts & scabs separate after 8–10 days. Commonly affected dermatomes are thoracic, lumbar nerves & ophthalmic div Vn. Occ a sparce chickenpox rash is seen. Less commonly → Ramsay–Hunt syndrome. Usually full recovery occurs but post-herpetic neuralgia c̄ prolonged burning pain in affected segment is not uncommon. Occ Meningitis; Encephalitis; Myelitis

RX: Analgesia. Acyclovir or Vidarabine early in illness in immunocompromised. Antiviral drugs do not affect frequency or severity of post-herpetic neuralgia but high dose steroids early in course of infection may be effective. Post-herpetic neuralgia is often resistent to Rx

Rabies

Due to RNA virus. Primarily an animal infection. Transmitted to man by animal bites eg dog, fox. Rabies is common in most of world, rabies-free areas being UK, Scandinavia, Australasia, Japan, Antartica. Incub Pd usually 20–90 days

CLIN: Non-specific symptoms of Fever; Myalgia; Headache; Sore throat; Pain at wound site. Then "furious" or paralytic rabies symptoms develop. Furious rabies is commoner form & → insp muscle spasms & hydrophobia which may → Generalised convulsions; Hallucinations; Autonomic disturbance; Cranial nerve lesions; Meningism. Death due to cardiac or resp arrest during spasm, or later due to coma c̄ generalised flaccid paralysis. Paralytic rabies → an ascending flaccid paralysis not usually ass c̄ hydrophobia; Death occuring in 2–3wks

INVESTIGATIONS: • IFA of brain of rabid animal
- Histology of brain of rabid animal: Negri bodies
- Viral immunoflourescence of skin, corneal or brain biopsy
- Virus isolation from secretions eg saliva

PREVENTION: Inform public about risks of rabies. Vaccinate domestic animals yrly in endemic countries. Muzzle dogs, eliminate strays. Supply health centres c̄ vaccine & antiserum. Pre-exposure vaccination to high risk occupations eg vets
If in contact c̄ possibly rabid animal clean wound thoroughly & give serum & vaccine (if possible test animal for rabies). Preferred vaccine is human diploid cell c̄ 6 doses in 3mths. Anti-rabies serum or human rabies immunoglobulin is useful during the 1st wk after initial bite. If animal remains healthy for >5 days can stop Rx (if doubt remains eg uncertainty over source of bite, give full prophylaxis)

RX: Analgesia, sedation & intensive care

PROG: Very poor

DD: 1. Tetanus
2. Cerebral malaria
3. Viral encephalitis eg Herpes virus simiae

Viral Haemorrhagic Fever

A gp of diseases c̄ similar clinical manifestations. Many are due to togaviruses (arbovirus) & arenaviruses

GENERAL RX: Good personal hygiene. Barrier nursing. Prompt Rx of shock. Convalescent plasma sometimes helpful. Correction of fluid, electrolyte & acid-base balance. Symptomatic drug Rx eg analgesics

YELLOW FEVER

Due to an arbovirus. 2 distinct cycles, urban yellow fever viz man to domestic mosquito to man & jungle yellow fever viz monkey to forest mosquito to monkey. Esp Afr. Incub Pd 3–6 days

CLIN: Acute onset of Fever; Headache; Rigor; J; Oliguria; N; Vom; Constipation; Abdo pain. Pulse rapid then falls whilst fever still high (Faget's sign). In mild cases, improvement starting on day 4 or 5 continues whilst in severe cases, relapse between 6th–12th day c̄ Fever; PR ↓; J; Haem; RF

INVESTIGATION: • Liver biopsy: Midzonal degeneration. Occ Councilman bodies, Torres bodies

PREVENTION: Vaccination c/i in infants & pregnant. Protects for 10yrs. Control vector

RX: Supportive measures

PROG: If recovery, rapid convalescence c̄ no sequelae

DENGUE FEVER

Due to an arbovirus. Mosquito vector. Esp S.E.Asia. Incub Pd 5–8 days

CLIN: Acute onset of Fever; Headache esp frontal; Myalgia; Arthralgia; Cv LN ↑; Transient rash. Then improvement on 5th or 6th day c̄ relapse between 6–10th day c̄ Fever; Vom; Malaise; Widespread itchy maculopapular rash. Prolonged convalescence. Occ, esp in children, the clin course is severe (Dengue haemorrhagic fever) c̄ additional signs of shock; Haem; Effusions; Myocarditis

INVESTIGATIONS OF SEVERE FORM:
- WCC ↓
- Platelets ↓
- CXR
- Liver biopsy

PREVENTION: Control vector

CHIKUNGUNYA

Due to an arbovirus. Esp Far E. Mosquito vector

CLIN: Acute onset. Fever; Maculopapular rash; Painful arthralgia; Haem

PREVENTION: Control vector. Vaccination

RIFT VALLEY FEVER

Due to an arbovirus. May be spread via infected animals eg sheep or by infected mosquito. Esp N.Afr. Incub Pd 3–12 days

CLIN: Fever; Headache; Malaise; Rigors; Haem; Arthralgia; Myalgia. Occ Retinitis; Encephalitis

PREVENTION: Control vector. Vaccination

OMSK HAEMORRHAGIC FEVER

Due to arbovirus. Tick vector. Esp summer. Esp E.USSR. Incub Pd 3–8 days

CLIN: Fever; Headache; N; Vom; Prostration; LN ↑; Rash. Occ Haem. If recovery, prolonged convalescence

PROG: 1–10% mort

KYANASUR FOREST HAEMORRHAGIC FEVER

Due to arbovirus. Tick vector. Esp India

CLIN: As for Omsk haem fever

PROG: 25% mort

CRIMEAN HAEMORRHAGIC–CONGO–HAZARA FEVER

Due to arbovirus. Tick vector. Esp E.Europe, USSR, Central Afr Esp summer. Incub Pd 7–12 days

CLIN: Sudden onset Fever; Headache; N; Vom; Pain; Diarrhoea; Widespread rash; Haem. Occ Pneumonia. If recovery, prolonged convalescence

LASSA FEVER

Due to an arenavirus. The rat *Mastomys natalensis* is both vector & reservoir. Incub Pd is 5–17 days. Esp W.Afr

CLIN: Insidious onset. Malaise; Headache; Fever; Conjunctivitis; Generalised pains; LN ↑; N; Vom; Oropharyngeal papules & ulcers. Occ Haem; RF; Effusions; CCF; Encephalopathy. In convalescence, occ deafness & alopecia develop. May be asymptomatic

INVESTIGATION: IFA on biopsy

RX: Supportive Rx. Barrier nursing. ?antiviral drugs & convalescent plasma

ARGENTINIAN HAEMORRHAGIC FEVER

Due to an arenavirus. Reservoir & vector is infected rodent. Esp summer. Esp Argentina. Incub Pd 10–14 days

CLIN: Gradual onset. Fever; Headache; Malaise; Haem; Rash; Oropharyngeal petechiae. Occ Encephalitis; RF; BP ↓; Tremors; Shock

PROG: 10% mort

MARBURG–EBOLA VIRUS FEVER

Probably a zoonosis. Esp Central Afr. Incub Pd 3–10 days

CLIN: Sudden onset. Fever; PR ↓; Generalised pains; Conjunctivitis; Haem; LN ↑; Orchitis; Encephalitis; Oropharyngeal eruptions. Later maculopapular rash

INVESTIGATIONS:
- Viral studies
- WCC ↓
- Platelets ↓

RX: Supportive Rx. Barrier nursing

KOREAN HAEMORRHAGIC FEVER

Transmitted via mites from rodent reservoir. Esp N.Europe, Asia. Incub Pd usually 12–16 days

CLIN: Fever; Prostration; Vom; Body pains. Then Haem; RF; Shock

PROG: 6% mort

HAEMORRHAGIC FEVER WITH RENAL FAILURE SYNDROME

Due to Hantaan virus. Esp Asia. Rodent reservoir

CLIN: Fever; Abdo pain; RF. Occ Haem

Other Arbovirus Infections

GENERAL RX: Supportive Rx

SANDFLY FEVER

Sandfly (Phlobotomus) vector. Man is reservoir. Esp tropics & subtropics in summer & autumn. Incub Pd 3–7 days

CLIN: Sudden onest. Fever; Sweating; Photophobia; Headache; Orbital pain; Anorexia; N; Vom; Body pains. Occ PR ↓; Bronchitis. No rash or LN ↑. Recover in 3–4 days c̄ slow convalescence

RX: Supportive Rx

O'NYONG NYONG

Mosquito vector esp Central & E.Afr

CLIN: Sudden onset. Fever; Prostration; Arthralgia; LN ↑. Later morbilliform rash. On recovery, slow convalescence

JAPANESE B, St LOUIS, MURRAY RIVER ENCEPHALITIS

These 3 diseases all have a bird reservoir & a mosquito vector. The Japanese B form is most severe

CLIN: May be asymptomatic. Headache; Meningoencephalitis

RUSSIAN SPRING/SUMMER ENCEPHALITIS

Tick vector. Rodent or duck reservoir. Esp Central Europe, USSR. Incub Pd 8–14 days

CLIN: Sudden onset. Fever; Headache; Photophobia; N; Vom; Body aches. Occ Paralysis of shoulder girdle

PREVENTION: Vaccinate at-risk

VENEZUELAN EQUINE ENCEPHALITIS

Disease of horses. Esp Central Am. Incub Pd 2–5 days

CLIN: Fever; Headache; Myalgia. Occ CNS symptoms. Usually full recovery

PREVENTION: Vaccinate at risk

CALIFORNIAN ENCEPHALITIS

Mosquito vector. Esp USA. Esp children

CLIN: Acute onset. Fever; Headache; Meningoencephalitis

PROG: 10% mort. 20% have sequelae

COLORADO TICK FEVER

Wild rodent reservoir. Tick vector. Esp N.Am

CLIN: Acute onset. Fever; Malaise; Headache; Prostration; Photophobia; Myalagia; Arthralgia; N; Vom. Occ Maculopapular rash; Meningoencephalitis; Haem; Myocarditis; Orchitis; Chorioretinitis; Pleurisy

PREVENTION: Vaccinate at risk

DD: 1. Rocky mountain spotted fever

2. Tularaemia

ROSS RIVER FEVER

Mosquito vector. Incub Pd 10 days

CLIN: Acute onset. Fever; Rash; LN ↑; Arthralgia. Usually full recovery

Miscellaneous Viral Diseases

HAND, FOOT & MOUTH DISEASE

Due to Coxsackie virus. May occur as small epidemics

CLIN: Vesicles on mouth & pharynx. Maculopapular rash which becomes vesicular on hands & feet

DD: Herpangina: Due to Coxsackie. Clin of sudden fever c̄ vesicles on fauces & soft palate

BORNHOLM DISEASE

Due to Coxsackie virus. Incub Pd 2–14 days

CLIN: Sudden onset of Headache; Fever; Paroxysmal muscular pains esp lower chest or upper abdo ppt by mvt, coughing & deep breathing. Occ Myalgia; Cutaneous hyperaesthaesia; Pericarditis; Meningitis; Orchitis. Generally recover in 1wk

INVESTIGATIONS:
- Viral studies
- CXR
- ECG

RX: Supportive therapy

CAT SCRATCH FEVER

?Due to small bacillus

CLIN: Small pustule develops at site of injury eg Cat scratch. 2–6wks later, area becomes inflammed c̄ pain, swelling, LN ↑. Occ systemic signs eg fever, headache, conjunctivitis, spleen ↑, meningoencephalitis

INVESTIGATION:
- Intradermal injection of heated pus from proven case → +ve skin reaction

RX: Supportive Rx. Occ surgical drainage of suppurating nodes

ACQUIRED CMV INFECTION

Esp children in tropics. In UK, commonest in young adults. Spread is probably via close contact c̄ asymptomatic excretors. Rarely spread by transfusion

CLIN: Many cases are asymptomatic or mild. Occ Liver ↑. Less often LN ↑; Spleen ↑; J; Pharyngitis; Tonsillitis. Rarely Polyneuritis; AIHA; Pneumonia; Arthritis; Pericarditis. An influenza-like illness may persist for some weeks. In immunosuppressed, a more severe illness is recognised c̄ Fever; Rashes; Purpura; Pneumonia; Arthralgia; Hepatitis; Choroidoretinitis

INVESTIGATIONS:
- WCC: Atypical lymphocytosis
- Paul–Bunnell test –ve
- LFTs
- Serial viral studies
- Liver biopsy

RX: Symptomatic Rx. Screen blood donors for graft recipients for CMV Abs

DD:
1. Glandular fever
2. Toxoplasmosis

PROTOZOAL INFECTIONS

Malaria

Due to 4 species of the parasite Plasmodium ie *P.vivax*, *P.falciparum*, *P.malariae*, *P.ovale*. Malaria is very common in Afr, S.Am, S.E.Asia, N.India, Central Am, Middle E. Imported cases to non-endemic areas are not infrequent. Vector is *Anopheline mosquito*. Infection is more severe in non-immune & pregnant. Incub Pd is usually 12–28 days, the shortest pd is for *P.falciparum* & longest for *P.malariae*

LIFE CYCLE: The infected mosquito passes sporozoites into man's bloodstream whilst feeding. Sporozoites pass to liver & by 6–11 days develop into schizonts which release merozoites into the blood which invade RBCs. The merozoites develop into trophozoites which mature into schizonts that burst RBCs & release more trophozoites. This asexual cycle lasts 48hrs in RBCs infected c̄ *P.vivax* & *P.ovale* (→ tertian fever) & 72hrs in RBCs infected c̄ *P.malariae* (→ quartan fever). In *P.falciparum*, parasites in the liver die out after erythrocytic phase, whilst in other forms there is a persistent liver phase (Exo–erythrocytic cycle). The schizonts also may liberate M & F gametocytes rather than trophozoites. Following mosquito bite, gametocytes within RBCs mate inside mosquito's body forming zygote which develops into an oocyst in mosquito's stomach. The oocyte liberates sporozoite which migrate to the salivary gland in preparation for transference to human bloodstream

CLIN OF FALCIPARUM MALARIA (MALIGNANT TERTIAN MALARIA): Many manifestations. Commonly swinging temperature; Headache; Malaise; N; Vom; Arthralgia. Then may develop severe manifestation eg Cerebral malaria (often preceded by confusion) c̄ Ep, Coma, Fever, CNS signs; ARF; Liver failure → J; Severe anaemia → Ht failure, Hburia; Watery diarrhoea. In semi-immune people, mild or asymptomatic course is usual

CLIN OF VIVAX MALARIA (BENIGN TERTIAN MALARIA): Classically an intermittent fever occuring every other day c̄ cold, hot & sweating stages. General symptoms usually milder than in falciparum malaria. Often Spleen ↑; Anaemia. Severe manifestations rare

CLIN OF MALARIAE MALARIA (QUARTAN MALARIA): Usually a mild illness. In children may → quartan malaria nephrosis

CLIN OF OVALE MALARIA (BENIGN TERTIAN MALARIA): Clin picture resembles that of vivax malaria

INVESTIGATION: • Periph blood film: Parasitaemia confirms infection

PREVENTION: Control of vector eg insecticides, mosquito nets. Chemoprophylaxis for travellers: In areas of Chloroquine–resistant falciparum malaria (increasingly common esp S.Am, S.E.Asia) give Pyrimethamine & Sulphadoxine (Fansidar) or Pyrimethamine & Dapsone (Maloprim), & either Chloroquine or Proguanil as prophylaxis against P.vivax; In Chloroquine–sensitive areas give Chloroquine, Proguanil, Pyrimethamine or Amodiaquine. Start chemoprophylaxis 1wk before travelling & continue 4wks after return

RX OF VIVAX, OVALE, MALARIAE MALARIA: Chloroquine (SE: GIT disturbances, Pruritus. If Rx for >1yr may → retinopathy) for 3 days then Primaquine for 14–21 days

RX OF UNCOMPLICATED ATTACKS OF FALCIPARUM MALARIA: Chloroquine in Chloroquine–sensitive areas, or Quinine for 3 days then Sulphadoxine & Pyrimethamine in Chloroquine–resistant areas

RX OF COMPLICATED ATTACKS OF FALCIPARUM MALARIA: IV Quinine bd until oral Rx feasible. Then oral Chloroquine or Quinine depending on Chloroquine status of area. Supportive Rx is very important eg careful monitoring of fluid balance. Cerebral malaria use steroids ± Mannitol. If Ep, use Diazepam or Paraldehyde

Acquired Toxoplasmosis

Due to obligatory intracellular parasite *Toxoplasma gondii.* Common worldwide. Spread by eating undercooked or raw contaminated meat or by ingestion of mature oocytes derived from cat species. Sexual phase of life cycle occurs in cat's GIT

CLIN: Most infections are subclinical. Often only symptom is painless LN ↑ esp cervical. Occ Malaise; Fever; Spleen ↑; Weakness. Rarely affects other organs esp CNS, unless immunosuppressed. Usually complete recovery within mths

INVESTIGATIONS: • Blood film: Occ Atypical lymphocytosis
• Paul–Bunnell test –ve
• Sabin–Feldman dye test +ve

RX: Usually no Rx required. If systemic symptoms give Spiramycin. If other organs involved, use Pyrimethamine & Sulphadiazine

Giardiasis

Due to *Giardia lamblia* infection of duodenum & jejunum. Esp Tropics. Esp children. Man is major animal reservoir. The trophozoite lives in upper small intestine where it gives rise to cysts which can survive in moist conditions. Infection is by F–O route esp via contaminated water. Occ outbreaks in families & institutions. Transmission amongst homosexuals is well recognised. Incub Pd usually 8 days but occ >2wks

CLIN: Most are asymptomatic. Often slight change in bowel habit. Occ outbreaks of severe diarrhoea lasting 1–2wks c̄ abdo pain, N, Vom esp in institutions & in travellers. Occ children c̄ chr infection fail to thrive. Chr giardia contributes to malabsorption

INVESTIGATIONS:
- Stool examination: May find trophozoites or cysts esp in diarrhoeal stools & in 2nd wk of illness
- Jejunal aspirate: May find trophozoite

RX: Metronidazole

Amoebiasis

Due to *Entamoeba histolytica*. Man is major disease reservoir. Infection is by swallowing of cysts passed in stools. Water-borne spread is rare. Esp poor environmental conditions

LIFE CYCLE: Amoeba in large bowel grow & divide by binary fission. Some amoebae are passed to rectum where absorption of water from bowel causes amoeba to encyst & become infective. Gut wall invasion occ occurs esp in immunosuppressed & → bowel wall damage & ingestion of RBCs by amoeba

N.B Any cause of diarrhoea → passage of amoeboid form (trophozoites) as there is insufficient time to encyst

CLIN: May be asymptomatic. Invasive intestinal amoebiasis → amoebic dysentery. Amoebic dysentery does not cause constitutional upset but → bloody diarrhoea & occ pain on defaecation. In endemic areas, an occ finding is a chr inflam lesion usually in caecum (Amoeboma) which may → fever, abdo tenderness, intestinal obst. Rarely fulminating infection → gangrene of colon. Commonest extraintestinal manifestation is a liver abscess

INVESTIGATIONS:
- Stools, biopsy or ulcer scrapings: May show trophozoites esp if examined quickly in warm (special stains available)
- Stools: Cysts may be found (do not of course demonstrate invasive disease)
- Serology: Occ false – ves

RX: Metronidazole ± Diloxanide furoatė. In severe cases can use Emetine & Tetracycline. Carriers may require Rx c̄ Diloxanide or Metronidazole

Trypanosomiasis

There are two main African types, W.African & E.African. Chagas' disease occurs in Central & S.Am

WEST AFRICAN TRYPANOSOMIASIS

Due to *T.brucei gambiense*. Vector is Tsetse fly. Esp river valleys. ↑ occupational risk c̄ eg fisherman, road & railway construction workers

CLIN: Usually acute onset. Chancre may occur at site of infective bite. Then irregular fever gradually increasing in severity. Often Malaise; Headache; Wt ↓; Arthralgia; LN ↑ esp post Cv; Blotchy irregular large macular rash esp on trunk. Personality changes; Insomnia. Following a variable period of indifferent health, onset of more severe symptoms c̄ CCF; Anaemia; CNS signs esp cerebellar. Later Negativism; Antisocial behaviour; Chorioathetosis; 2° infections; Irresistible sleep (hence "sleeping sickness"). Course of disease often very protracted esp in natives

EAST AFRICAN TRYPANOSOMIASIS

Due to *T.brucei rhodesiense*. Vector is Tsetse fly. Esp woodlands. Animal reservoir of ungulates. More virulent than W.African form

CLIN: Acute onset of paroxysms of intense fever. Swelling of face & extremities; Wt ↓; Weakness; Myocarditis; LN ↑. Rapid deterioration rarely allows development of pronounced CNS signs, thus tremor & personality changes are seen in later mths but pathological sleeping is rare. Untreated usually die in <1yr

GENERAL INVESTIGATIONS OF AFRICAN FORMS:
- Thick blood film usually shows trypanosomes
- LN aspirates often show trypanosomes
- CSF examination: If parasites not demonstrated by other tests

- Serological tests

RX OF AFRICAN FORMS: Hospitalise except in early cases. Analgesia. Antibiotics for 2° infection. May need dietary supplements. Suramin (SE: Idiosyncracy, Nephrotoxicity) is useful before CNS involvement (can't pass blood brain barrier). Pentamidine (SE: BP ↓) is useful for W.African form c̄ no CNS involvement. Melarsoprol IV (SE: Diarrhoea; J; Encephalopathy) is used if CNS involvement. Examine CSF 6mths post Rx to assess effectiveness of Rx

PROG: If no CNS involvement, Rx gives good results. Poor results if CNS involvement. Can relapse after Rx

Chagas' Disease

Due to *T.cruzi*. Transmitted to man by Triatomid bugs. Many mammals are disease reservoir

CLIN: Occ at site of bite a painless indurated nodule (Chagoma) develops c̄ regional LN ↑. If infection via conjunctiva, eyelids are swollen & reddish–violet in colour. In about 5%, an acute phase occurs 14–28 days post infection. Symptoms inc Paroxysms of fever; PR ↑; LN ↑; Liver ↑; Spleen ↑. Occ Arrhythmias; BP ↓; Diarrhoea; Anaemia; Meningoencephalitis. Acute phase lasts 1–3mths. Many years later about half develop symptoms of the chr stage eg Ht ↑; Arrhythmias inc Ht block; Dilatation of oesophagus & colon; IQ ↓

INVESTIGATIONS:
- Periph blood film: Trypanosomes occ seen
- Xenodiagnosis ie clean bugs fed on suspected patient & after 2wks contents of bug's gut examined for organisms
- CFT

RX: Rx is unsatisfactory. Nifurtinox may be helpful

Leishmaniasis

Due to protozoan Lieshmania. 4 species cause infection in man ie *L.donovani* → Kala–azar, *L.tropica* → Oriental sore, *L.mexicana* → Chicle ulcer & *L.braziliensis* → Espundia. Many animal reservoirs inc man. Rarely transmission by blood or cong

LIFE CYCLE: Amastigote form lives intracellularly in man & other mammals. When F sandfly has a blood meal the protozoa develop into promastigote in pharynx & migrate to salivary glands over following 10 days in preparation for infection of next victim

KALA–AZAR

Esp Central Afr, Mediterranean, S.Am, E.India. In Mediterranean esp children aged 2–4yrs. Main disease reservoirs are man, dogs, & rodents. Wide variety of manifestations depending on immune status of individual. Incub Pd is usually 4–6mths but may be many yrs

CLIN: Most infections are subclinical. Common presentations are Cough; Diarrhoea; Epistaxis; Pain from spleen ↑. Then Fever esp biphasic rise during day; Spleen ↑↑; Liver ↑; Anaemia. Occ J, LN ↑. Few constitutional symptoms. Rarely Granulomatous tumours of nasopharynx & nose esp Afr; Generalised LN ↑ esp Mediterranean; Tonsil ↑ c̄ Cv LN ↑. Skin lesion c̄ macular depigmented rash & papular eruption on face & upper trunk is usually sign of recovery

INVESTIGATIONS:
- WCC ↓
- Platelets ↓
- Hb ↓
- IgG ↑↑
- Urinalysis: Often proteinuria
- Parasite may be cultured from marrow, spleen or LN smear
- Leishmanin test
- CFT
- IFA

RX: Sodium stibogluconate or N-methylglucamine antimonate. Spleen usually of norm size by end of 30 day course. Persistence of fever usually indicates inactivated drug, pulm BP ↑ or concurrent pulm TB. Rarely splenectomy required

PROG: Good c̄ drug Rx. May relapse but respond to further drug Rx

ESPUNDIA

Due to *L.braziliensis*. Esp S.Am. Esp seen in road construction workers

CLIN: Skin nodule at bite site which ulcerates

leaving scar. Mths later fungating ulcers occur on the nose, mouth, tongue & buccal cavity → destruction of nose, larynx & pharynx. Often 2° infection; Regional LN ↑

INVESTIGATIONS: • Leishmanin tests +ve • IFA

RX: Pentavalent Antimony or Amphotericin B

DD:
1. Blastomycosis
2. Syphilis
3. Yaws
4. Leprosy

CHICLE ULCER

Due to *L.mexicana*. Esp Central Am. Main reservoir are forest rodents. Esp rain forest

CLIN: Skin lesions esp pinna of ear. Lesions heal within 6mths except on ear where infections may be chr. Ear infection may → destruction of pinna

RX: As *L.mexicana* cannot be distinguished from skin lesion of *L.braziliensis*, give Antimony compound

ORIENTAL SORE

Due to *L.tropica*. Esp N.India, Central Afr, Middle E. L.Tropica major is a rural disease c̄ a disease reservoir of rodents. L.tropica minor is an urban disease c̄ a disease reservoir of dogs. In endemic areas most children contract disease

CLIN: Urban infection is usually more chr. Small itchy papule becomes scaly & then forms a brown raised indurated nodule which crusts. When crust is removed a shallow ulcer remains. May be multiple ulcers (esp c̄ L.tropica major) or single. Common sites are face & limbs. Heal c̄ scarring in 6mths. In middle E occ have a chr cutaneous leishmaniasis (Leishmaniasis recidiva) c̄ a slowly growing facial lesion → "apple jelly" nodules. In Ethiopia & Kenya, a chr non-ulcerative lesion occurs on face esp nose & spreads to involve the body over many yrs (Diffuse cutaneous leishmaniasis)

INVESTIGATIONS: • Demonstrate parasites from biopsy
• Lieshmanin skin test: +ve at 2–3mths (−ve in diffuse cutaneous leishmaniasis)

RX: Pentavalent antimony. Grenz rays may help Leishmaniasis recidiva. Diffuse cutaneous leishmaniasis is difficult to treat, can try Pentamidine

Babesiosis

Protozoal infection c̄ tick vector. Rare. Esp immunocompromised

Balantidiasis

Due to protozoan *B.coli*. Rare. Common infection of pigs

CLIN: Severe diarrhoea

RX: Tetracycline

Cryptosporidiosis

Protozoan infection affecting immunocompromised esp in AIDS

CLIN: Severe diarrhoea

INVESTIGATION: • Parasite in faeces or biopsy

RX: None known

FUNGAL INFECTIONS

Fungal Infections (LIST 3 INFD)

1. Superficial Mycoses:
   a) Pityriasis versicolor
   b) Ringworm
   c) Superficial candidosis
   d) Black or white piedra
   e) Tinea ñigra
2. Subcutaneous mycoses:
   a) Mycetoma
   b) Chromomycosis
   c) Sporotrichosis
   d) Phaeohyphomycosis
   e) Lobo's disease
   f) Subcutaneous zygomycosis
3. Systemic mycoses:
   a) Cryptococcosis
   b) Blastomycosis
   c) Histoplasmosis
   d) Coccidioidomycosis
   e) Paracoccidioidomycosis
   f) Aspergillosis
   g) Systemic candidosis
   h) Mucormycosis

Blastomycosis

Due to *B.dermatitidis*. Esp N.Am

CLIN: Usually → chr resp illness c̄ Fever; Malaise; Cough. Occ extrapulm infiltrations → Bone pain; Epididymitis; Nodular or warty skin lesion

INVESTIGATIONS: • Histology & culture • Serology

RX: Amphotericin B

Paracoccidioidomycosis (South American Blastomycosis)

Due to *P.brasiliensis*. Esp Central & S.Am. M>F

CLIN: Present c̄ chr pulm disease or disseminated granulomas. Disseminated disease may → LN ↑; Mucosal ulceration; Pulm infiltrates

RX: Ketoconazole

Cryptococcosis

Due to *C.neoformans*. Usually an opportunistic infection in Hodgkin's, Sarcoidosis, SLE or if Rx c̄ systemic steroids

CLIN: Commonest presentation is meningitis which may → obst hydrocephalus. Occ → resp, skin or bone lesions

INVESTIGATION: • Indian ink stain eg of CSF

RX: Amphotericin B & Flucytosine

DD: TB meningitis

Systemic Candidosis

An opportunistic infection due to candidal yeasts in immunodepressed esp due to malignancy, diabetes

CLIN: Many different manifestations. May cause blood infection (candidaemia) esp in ass c̄ IV lines. Deep focal candidosis usually occurs by direct spread from infected area which may → dysphagia, meningitis, peritonitis, UTI. Rarely Endocarditis. Occ disseminated candidosis → Fever; Myalgia; Abscesses; Retinal opacities

INVESTIGATIONS: • Blood cultures • Serology (often false – ves)

RX: Remove any ppt cause eg IV line, urinary catheter. Amphotericin B

Mucormycosis

Due to Zygomycete fungi. Rare. Esp seen in immunocompromised

CLIN: May → orbital cellulitis

RX: Amphotericin B

Chromomycoses

A chr skin infection due to pigmented fungi. Esp Central & S.Am, Far E, S.Afr

CLIN: Large warty growth esp extremities which slowly spread

INVESTIGATION: • Skin scraping or biopsy histology

RX: Flucytosine

Sporotrichosis

Due to *S.schenckii*. Esp Americas, Afr, Australia

CLIN: Nodules which ulcerate esp along lymph channels. Rarely causes systemic infection

INVESTIGATION: • Culture of scrapings or biopsy

RX: Potassium iodide

DD: 1. Cutaneous leishmaniasis
2. Mycobacterium marinum

INFECTIONS IN IMMUNOCOMPROMISED

Many factors can → ↓ immunocompetence including neutropenia, malnutrition, extremes of age, drugs eg steroids,

AIDS. 1° immunodef diseases are rare

Causes of Fever in the Immunocompromised Patient (LIST 4 INFD)
A. INFECTIVE
1. Fungal: Eg Candida, Cryptococcus, Aspergillus, Mucormycosis
2. Viral: Eg CMV, Herpes simplex
3. Bacterial: Eg TB, Legionella, Mycoplasma, Nocardia, Pseudomonas, Salmonella
4. Protozoal: Eg Pneumocystis, Toxoplasmosis, Cryptosporidiosis
B. NON-INFECTIVE
Eg PE, Pulm oedema, Radiation, Drugs, Haemorrhage

GENERAL RX: Try to treat c̄ least toxic & most specific agents but urgency of starting therapy often → empirical choice. Generally choose combination of 2 of the following 3 classes of antibiotics: Penicillins, Aminoglycosides, Cephalosporins. If neutropenic & no response to antibiotics after 5 days add antifungal agent eg Amphotericin B. Acyclovir is effective against *Herpes simplex* & *varicella–zoster. Pneumocystis carinii* responds to high dose Cotrimoxazole or Pentamidine. Granulocyte transfusions may be helpful

SEXUALLY TRANSMITTED DISEASES

Important worldwide. Increasing in prevalence. Esp seen in young adults. High risk gps include prostitutes, entertainment industry, travellers, seamen

Gonorrhoea

Due to *Neisseria gonorrhoeae.* Almost always transmitted by sexual contact. Incub Pd for urethral gonorrhoea in M 1–10 days

CLIN: In M urethritis usually → dysuria & urethral discharge. The F may be asymptomatic or complain of dysuria & vaginal discharge. Rectal & pharyngeal gonorrhoea are commoner in homosexuals & may be asymptomatic or → rectal discharge, sore throat. Later complications occur esp in F. These include: In F, bartholinitis &/or pelvic infection, occ → infertility; In M, epididymitis (uni- or bilat), rarely prostatitis. Occ GC causes complications outside the GUS esp arthritis, rash, fever. In prepubertal girls, GC vulvovaginitis may occur

INVESTIGATIONS:
- Urethral discharge C&S (easier to diagnose in M)
- Vaginal or cervical C&S
- Rectal & pharyngeal swabs C&S

PREVENTION: Sheath & diaphragm offer partial protection. Contact tracing of sexual partners

RX: Single dose of Penicillin. Follow up to ensure Rx success. If penicillin resistance use Spectinomycin

PROG: Very good if early Rx. Penicillin resistance is increasing

Syphilis

Due to *Treponema pallidum.* May be cong or acquired. Traditionally divided into early & late forms; early form covering first 2yrs of illness when supf lesions are infectious

1. PRIMARY ACQUIRED SYPHILIS

CLIN: Incub Pd 9–90 days (median 23 days). Small pink macule on genitalia, in M usually on coronal sinus of penis becoming papular & then developing into a painless ulcer c̄ well defined edges (1° chancre); Regional LN ↑. In F commonest site is vulva, whilst homosexuals may develop anal or rectal chancres. Chancre heals in 3–8wks

INVESTIGATIONS: • Examine ulcer serous transudate for *T.pallidum*
• Serum Ab tests become +ve after appearance of ulcer

RX: IM Procaine Penicillin for 10–12 days. Long follow up to ensure satisfactory result

2. SECONDARY ACQUIRED SYPHILIS

CLIN: 2° signs occur 6–8wks after appearance of 1° chancre. Often Symmetrical maculopapular rash which spreads to involve face, palms & soles, limbs esp flexor surfaces; Fever; Headache; Malaise; Myalgia. In warm moist areas eg perianal region skin lesions become large (condylomata lata). Occ Discrete rubbery LN ↑; Mucosal ulcers which may join to produce a snail track ulcer. Rarely involvement of bones, CNS, eyes, viscera

INVESTIGATIONS: • Examine ulcer serous transudate for *T.Pallidum*
• Serum Ab tests +ve

RX: Procaine Penicillin for 15 days. Long follow up to ensure satisfactory result

3. LATENT SYPHILIS

The outward signs & symptoms of 2° Sy gradually resolve & a latent period lasting some yrs is entered. Latent Sy cases are divided into early or late depending on whether time since initial exposure is < or > 2yrs. Many do not appear to progress to tertiary Sy

INVESTIGATION: • Serum Ab tests

4. TERTIARY ACQUIRED SYPHILIS

CLIN: Usually develops 3–10yrs after 1° stage. Gummas occur esp on: Skin (nodules healing leaving shiny scars); Mucous membranes → punched-out ulcers & occ bony destruction; Bone which may → osteoperiostitis

INVESTIGATIONS: • Biopsy
• X-R
• Serum Ab tests

RX: Procaine Penicillin for 15 days. Lifelong follow up

5. QUATERNARY SYPHILIS

CLIN: Usually develops 5–20yrs after 1° stage. CVS & CNS problems predominate inc AI; Aortic aneurysm esp ascending; Coronary osteal stenosis which may → angina, MI; Mengiovascular Sy which may → meningitis, cranial nerve lesions, pupillary abnormalities; Tabes dorsalis; GPI → change in personality, dementia

INVESTIGATIONS: • CXR
• Echocardiography
• Serum Ab tests
• CSF: In NeuroSy usually cells ↑, protein ↑, +ve Ab tests

RX: Procaine Penicillin for 21 days. Give steroids at start of course to reduce any Jarisch–Herxheimer reaction. Control any cardiac failure c̄ diuretics ± Dig

PROG: Good for GPI, fair for CVS Sy, poor for Tabes

GENERAL PREVENTION

Screen serologically all pregnant women (even late Rx in pregnancy should prevent Cong Sy). Contact tracing esp early cases

SEROLOGICAL TESTS FOR SYPHILIS

Two main gps, the non-specific (lipoidal) tests & the specific tests
Non-specific tests do not detect specific anti-treponemal Ab & are prone to false +ve results. They become +ve in 1° Sy & usually remain so until 4° stage. In treated disease, test becomes −ve in early Sy but remains +ve in late form. Examples of these tests are the WR, Kahn, VDRL, & RPR. VDRL & RPR are the preferred non-specific tests
Specific tests detect anti-treponemal Ab. They become +ve in 1° Sy & remain so throughout disease even after Rx. Examples of specific tests are FTA, TPHA, TPI, RPCFT

DD OF SYPHILIS

1. YAWS: A treponemal infection indistinguishable serologically from Sy. Not a STD. Esp Central & S.Am, N. & Central Afr, S.E.Asia, India. Esp rural areas. Incub Pd 3–6wks

Clin: Nodular erythematous macule which heals in 2–8wks. Then 2 or more crops of painless itchy skin lesions esp face & genital areas & occ palms & soles. Occ 2° infection → LN ↑; Ulceration; Bone lesions eg → dactylitis. After a latent period of yrs may develop 3° lesions occuring in skin c̄ ulcers, nodules, scarring & contractions, in bone c̄ severe periostitis → bony destruction

Rx: Penicillin

2. PINTA: A treponemal infection indistinguishable serologically from Sy. Not a STD. Esp Central & S.Am

Clin: sc red or bluish black granuloma c̄ satellite lesions which slowly grows → depigmented atrophic skin. Similar painless lesions (pintids) occur in crops after 6–12mths. Occ LN ↑. No visceral lesions

Rx: Penicillin

> **Causes of False Positive WR (LIST 5 INFD)**
>
> 1. Acute infections: Esp Malaria, Leptospirosis, Viral pneumonia
> 2. Subacute & Chr infections: Esp TB, Connective tissue disease eg SLE
> 3. Vaccinations

Acquired Immune Deficiency Syndrome

A STD esp in homosexuals, rapidly increasing in incidence esp in USA. Due to Human T-cell Lymphotropic Virus III. Milder form of disease seen in Haiti, Central Afr. Esp 20–50yrs of age. M>>F. Spread to F partners is rare in USA. Can be spread by blood transfusion & blood products, thus ↑ risk to Haemophiliacs & IV drug abusers. Incub Pd variable

CLIN: Variable presentation. 4 major patterns: Febrile prodrome followed by opportunistic infection; Abrupt onset of opportunistic infection; Presentation c̄ Kaposi's sarcoma; AIDS-related complex

Febrile prodrome followed by opportunistic infection: Fever; Sweating esp nocte; Wt ↓. Occ Diarrhoea; Seborrhoeic dermatitis; Generalised LN ↑, usually slight but occ very large nodes. Then 1–6mths later, develop symptoms of opportunistic infection eg cough & SOB due to pneumocystitis

Abrupt onset of opportunistic infection: Less common than presentation c̄ febrile prodrome

Presentation c̄ Kaposi's sarcoma: Usually M homosexuals c̄ no systemic infections. Insidious onset of red plaques of sarcoma esp hard palate, conjunctiva

AIDS-related complex: May present c̄ LN ↑; Wt ↓; Fever; Diarrhoea; Night sweats; Malaise. May later develop opportunistic infections or Kaposi's sarcoma. Some cases do not progress to develop AIDS

Later: ↑ susceptibility to infections (Opportunistic infections are common eg CMV, Candida, Toxoplasma, Cryptosporidium, Atypical mycobacteria); LN ↑. Occ CNS signs eg Personality changes, Ep, Hemiplegia, Depression; Malignancies eg lymphoma

INVESTIGATIONS:
- WCC
- LFTs
- Blood cultures
- CXR
- HTLV III Ab test

PREVENTION: Screen blood products. Health education. Contact tracing

RX: Supportive Rx. Specific Rx for identified infections. Advise patients to avoid situations c̄ a high risk of contact c̄ infection

PROG: Kaposi's sarcoma & Pneumocystis pneumonia have a high mort. In US, about 80% die within 3yrs of diagnosis

Nonspecific Urethritis

Commonest causative organism is *Chlamydia trachomatis* (TRIC agent). Symptoms more marked in M. Incub Pd usually 2–3wks

CLIN: May be asymptomatic. Dysuria; Mucoid or mucopurulent urethral discharge. In M may → Prostatitis; Epididymitis; Reiter's syndrome. In F may → pelvic infection

INVESTIGATION: • Urethral discharge culture

N.B Exclude Gonorrhoea

RX: Tetracycline or Erythromycin for 2–3wks. Follow up as relapse may occur. Test & treat sexual partner

PROG: 80–90% respond to drug

Genital Herpes

Principally caused by HSV-2. Esp seen in promiscuous. May be pre-malignant for Ca cervix. Incub Pd 4–5 days

CLIN: A few vesicles appear on genitals which rupture to leave painful tender irregular erosions which bleed on minor trauma. Common sites are the vulva & cervix in F & the glans, prepuce & shaft of penis. Usually heal in 10 days unless 2° infection but often recurrent episodes. Rarely ass c̄ meningoencephalitis, herpetic whitlow. Infection may be spread during parturition

INVESTIGATIONS: • Serological tests (Only useful for 1° infections)
• Virus culture
N.B Exclude syphilis

RX: Clean genitals to reduce risk of 2° infection. If 2° infection use a non-treponemicidal antibiotic eg Sulphonamide

Genital Warts (Condylomata Acuminata)

Due to Papova virus. Increasing incidence in UK. Incub Pd 1–6mths. May be spread by intercourse or via skin warts on hand

CLIN: On warm moist genital areas develop large filiform warts esp coronal sulcus, glans, vulva, perianally, whilst on cold dry genital areas develop small flat warts

RX: Good genital hygiene eg keep affected parts clean, cool & dry. Local applications of Podophyllin. Occ cautery or cryotherapy of warts is required. Contact tracing. Sheath must be worn during intercourse to prevent spread

PROG: Most warts remit after prolonged Rx. Malignant change very rarely occurs

Balanitis

An inflam of the glans penis

Causes of Balanitis (LIST 6 INFD)

1. Candidiasis esp in diabetics
2. Trichomoniasis
3. Reiter's Syndrome (Circinate balanitis)
4. Behcet syndrome
5. Stevens–Johnson syndrome
6. Erythroplasia of Queyrat
7. Syphilis
8. Chancroid
9. Gonorrhoea

Chancroid

Due to *Haemophilus ducreyi.* Esp S.Am, Tropical Africa, Far E. Incub Pd 1–8 days

CLIN: Multiple, painful, tender papules → pustules → ulcers; Firm, tender inguinal LN ↑ (buboes). Occ Phimosis; Paraphimosis; LN suppuration; Destruction of penile tissue (phagedena)

INVESTIGATIONS: • Gram stain
• Culture
• Biopsy & histology
• Tests to exclude Sy

RX: Good genital hygiene. Sulphadimidine or Cotrimoxazole

Granuloma Inguinale

Due to Donovania granulomatis. Esp Tropics & Sub-tropics. Esp Blacks. Incub Pd <3mths

CLIN: Painless papules → granulomatous ulcers c̄ rolled edges. Lesions may spread from ext genitalia to surrounding skin. Occ 2° infection c̄ inguinal LN ↑; Fibrosis → elephantiasis. Rarely Malignant change; Extra-genital lesions

INVESTIGATIONS: • Biopsy c̄ Giemsa's stain: Donovan bodies
• Test to exclude Sy

RX: Streptomycin or Oxytetracycline

Dermatology

ECZEMA

Common conditions characterised by erythema, oedema, vesicles, itching & lichenification (ie thickened epidermis c̄ ↑ skin markings) of skin. Classified into endogenous & exogenous forms. The endogenous forms are termed atopic, varicose, discoid, pompholyx, seborrhoeic & asteatotic. The exogenous are termed allergic contact, irritant contact, infective & photo-allergic

Varicose Eczema (Stasis Eczema)

Usually occurs 2° to long standing varicose veins & venous stasis

CLIN: Eczema around ankle esp medially. Occ Eczema of leg, trunk or arms. Often 2° stasis ulceration

RX: Topical steroid. Protect area by bandage or support stocking. Often useful to remove VVs. If ulceration rest leg. Use topical antibiotics for infection (but risk of sensitisation or development of resistance)

Discoid Eczema (Nummular Eczema)

Common. Coin shaped areas of chr eczema on trunk & limbs. Two main types affecting the limbs of M >40yrs or the hands of young F. Relapsing & remitting course

RX: Moderately potent topical steroids

DD:
1. Psoriasis
2. Ringworm
3. Atopic eczema

Pompholyx

Characterised by large blisters on palms & soles. Unknown aetiology

CLIN: Sudden development of crops of blisters on palms &/or soles which become confluent, subside & then desquamate after 2–3wks

RX: Lead & Zn soaks or K^+ permanganate. Large blisters may need deroofing. Often require local steroids

Adult Seborrhoeic Eczema

Common. Esp young adults c̄ greasy skin

CLIN: Scalp commonly involved, may also affect face, flexures, trunk. Facial form often → blepharitis. Truncal form involves infrascapular regions & hairy areas, lesions may be petaloid or diffuse. Intertrigo may occur where two skin surfaces are in contact esp groins, axilla, submammary areas in F

RX: Use medicated shampoo & steroid scalp application for seborrhoeic eczema of scalp. Use weak steroids & antiseptics in other areas

DD: 1. Atopic eczema
2. Psoriasis

Asteatotic Eczema

Esp elderly c̄ dry skin. May occur in hypothyroidism

CLIN: Dry scaly erythematous skin c̄ crazy paving pattern

RX: Moderately potent topical steroid ointment. Avoid degreasing agents such as soap (replace by emollients)

Contact Dermatitis

Caused by agents which come into contact c̄ skin. Often occupational. Irritants & allergens can penetrate epidermis → irritant & allergic contact dermatitis respectively

IRRITANT CONTACT DERMATITIS

Esp if very fair or dry skin. Occ ass c̄ atopic dermatitis. Most irritants appear to directly damage cells. Common irritants are oils, alkalis, detergents & organic solvents

ALLERGIC CONTACT DERMATITIS

Contact allergens combine c̄ proteins at epidermal/dermal junction & set up a cell-mediated type IV reaction. Substances vary in their sensitising potential, most contact allergens have a molecular wt <1000. Sensitisation may occur at first contact or after prolonged contact. Common sensitisers are perfumes, Nickel, Chromate, plastic monomers, Lanolin, epoxy resins & Neomycin

CLIN: When sensitised skin comes into contact c̄ allergen, dermatitis will occur at site of contact. Often characteristic distribution patterns. Occ 2° spread to other body sites; Swelling of eyelids

INVESTIGATION: • Patch test

GENERAL RX: Prevent contact c̄ allergen or irritant eg by use of gloves. Compresses give symptomatic relief. Persistent contact dermatitis may require topical fluorinated steroids. Occ a change in occupation is unavoidable

DD: 1. Atopic dermatitis
2. Discoid eczema
3. Seborrhoeic dermatitis
4. Tinea
5. Psoriasis
6. Lichen Planus
N.B It is often difficult to distinguish irritant & allergic contact dermatoses

PSORIASIS

An inflam skin disease characterised by well defined papules or salmon pink plaques of varying size covered c̄ silvery scales. Common. Often FH. Onset esp in young adult—mean age 28yrs. About 5–10% have a sero -ve arthropathy

PATHOGENESIS: Cause of rash is unknown. Large increase in number of proliferating epidermal cells in the lesions

CLIN: Rash c̄ natural h/o relapses & remissions. Relapses are occ triggered by skin trauma (Koebner's phenomenon) or *Strep pyogenes* infection (→ guttate psoriasis). Sharply defined erythematous, scaly lesions c̄ silvery covering. Lesions may be arranged in plaques or be discoid, guttate or papular (chr plaque form is commonest). Esp affects scalp & extensor surfaces. Scalp psoriasis may → hair loss c̄ regrowth in remission. Psoriasis of nails may → onycholysis, pits, thickening or loss. No scarring. Occ pustules occur in discoid or plaque psoriasis but pustular psoriasis of palms & soles can occur without psoriasis elsewhere. Rarely the whole skin is erythematous c̄ multiple sterile pustules (generalised pustular psoriasis). Occ a red scaly rash develops all over body in a person c̄ h/o classical psoriasis (erythrodermic psoriasis) which is indistinguishable from other erythrodermas. The arthropathy may mimic Ank Sp

RX: A. Clearing Lesions: Choice is between tar or Dithranol topically & photochemotherapy (PUVA). Traditionally Dithranol is applied in Lassar's paste (ZnO & Salicylic acid) to each lesion, covered c̄ dressings & renewed every 24hrs. Included in regime are tar baths & ultraviolet light irradiation after removal of paste. PUVA is suspected of being carcinogenic & therefore is used in the elderly & more severe cases. PUVA works because furocoumarins eg 8-methoxypsoralen in presence of UVA combine in skin c̄ pyrimadines to ↓ epidermal proliferation. PUVA Rx is much cleaner than Dithranol but probably takes longer to act & requires careful monitoring. Eyes must be shielded from UVA during Rx & eyes & skin must be shielded from extraneous UVA for 12hrs post Rx ie period of photosensitivity. Topical corticosteroids are often used for psoriasis of face, palms & soles, & scalp. Systemic steroids may be needed in erythrodermic or generalised pustular psoriasis c̄ antimitotics eg Methotrexate, when acute phase is over. Social factors often influence choice of Rx

B. Preventing Recurrence: PUVA given weekly reduces recurrence rate. Tar baths & UVB are generally ineffective

DD:
1. Eczema
2. DLE
3. Fungal infections

LICHEN PLANUS

An acute or chr inflam disease characterised by polygonal violaceous papules esp on flexor surfaces. Esp adults. F>M. Cause unknown

CLIN: Sudden or gradual onset. Papules are initially tiny increasing to pea size & occ coalescing. Lesions are flat topped, polygonal, shiny, violaceous, scaly papules esp on flexor surfaces; Pruritus. Papules often have fine light coloured streaks & dots (Wickham's striae). Often mucous membranes affected c̄ milky white papules or lattice of thin streaks. Occ non specific nail changes. Koebner's phenomenon is common. Rarely lesions are thicker (lichen planus hypertrophicus) or bullous (lichen planus bullosus)

RX: Topical steroids may help esp oral lesions

PROG: Often spontaneous remission after 6–24mths. May recur

PRURITUS

Pruritus is an unpleasant cutaneous sensation which evokes desire to scratch. May be localised or diffuse.

Causes of more severe pruritus are given in LIST 1

Causes of Pruritus (LIST 1 DERM)

A. DUE TO SKIN DISEASE
1. Eczema
2. Scabies
3. Insect bites
4. Lichen planus
5. Pediculosis
6. Urticaria
7. Drug rashes
8. Dermatitis herpetiformis
9. Prurigo
10. Prickly heat (Miliaria rubra)

B. DUE TO SYSTEMIC DISEASE
1. Liver disease (due to bile acids)
2. CRF
3. Malignancies & Myeloproliferative disorders: Esp Lymphomas, PRV
4. Pregnancy
5. Psychogenic
6. IDA
7. Hypothyroidism
8. Diabetes
9. Parasites: Eg Onchocerciasis, Trichiniasis
10. Drugs: Eg Opiate addiction

If skin disease is not readily manifest, systemic disease should be suspected. However some dermatological causes of pruritus can have minimal skin changes eg scabies, atopic eczema, lichen planus, drugs

GENERAL RX: Topical Rx to skin lesions may be helpful eg c̄ emollients, Calamine or weak steroids. Promethazine is often used for systemic cases

THE PHOTODERMATOSES

A group of conditions with abnormal reactions to UVR. Four gps:

1. Idiopathic inc prickly heat, actinic prurigo, chr actinic dermatitis & solar urticaria;
2. Metabolic inc porphyrias & xeroderma pigmentosa;
3. Chemical & drug photosensitivity
4. UVR exacerbated dermatoses inc psoriasis, SLE, Erythema multiforme

Causes of Photosensitivity (LIST 2 DERM)

1. Prickly heat
2. Metabolic:
   Eg Porphyrias; Pellagra
3. Drugs:
   Eg Phenothiazines, Tetracyclines; Thiazides
4. Contact photosensitisers:
   Eg Furocoumarins, Tar
5. Lack of protection from UVR:
   Eg Albinism, Vitiligo, PKU, Hypopituitarism
6. Chr actinic dermatitis
7. Actinic prurigo
8. Solar urticaria
9. Hydroa vacciniforme
10. Xeroderma pigmentosa
11. Exacerbation of pre-existing dermatoses:
    Eg SLE, Herpes simplex, Rosacea, Psoriasis

Prickly Heat

Common. Esp young adults. Probably due to UVB exposure

CLIN: On exposure to sun, symmetrical rash develops. Usually pruritic papular erythematous eruption but occ vesicles or plaques. Healing occurs if exposure is avoided

RX: Avoid UVB. Sunscreens eg β-carotene may help. In severe cases PUVA given before summer

DD: Other photodermatoses

Actinic Prurigo

Uncommon. F>M. Induced by UVB. Worse in summer

CLIN: Excoriated papules esp on exposed areas. Often mild scarring on face. May remit at puberty

RX: Avoid UVB. Use sunscreens. Thalidomide (SE Cong malformations) is effective after 1–3mths

DD:
1. Atopic Eczema
2. Insect bites
3. Prurigo nodularis

Chr Actinic Dermatitis

Rare. M>F. Esp elderly. Worse in summer. Induced by UVR & visible light

CLIN: Widespread eczematous lesions on exposed skin c̄ later lichenification. Often Erythroderma; Loss of eyebrows & eyelashes; Hypo- & Hyper-pigmentation; Petechiae. Occ Covered skin involved

INVESTIGATIONS:
- Histology
- Irradiation skin tests

RX: Avoid UVR. Sunscreens. Steroids & Azathioprine may help

DD:
1. Mycosis fungoides
2. Airborne contact dermatitis

Sunburn (Acute Actinic Damage)

Due to overexposure of skin to UVR. Esp fair skinned

CLIN: Prolonged exposure to sun → erythema. In severe case Oedema; Blistering; Tenderness; Collapse. On recovery, peeling of skin & pruritus

RX: Prevent by gradual introduction to sunbathing & use of sunscreens. Cooling preparations & fluids. If severe burns use steroids

Chr Benign Actinic Damage

Due to prolonged exposure to UVR. Esp fair skinned in hot dry countries

CLIN: Premature ageing of skin ie thick atrophic skin, "crow's feet". Later Telangiectasia; Hyper- & Hypo-pigmentation; Yellowish thickened neck furrows (cutis rhomboidalis); Yellowish papules & plaques. Occ Actinic chelitis due to sunlight & wind

RX: No specific Rx

Solar Keratoses

Pre-malignant. Induced by chr sunlight exposure

CLIN: Small scaling lesions c̄ hypo- or hyper-pigmentation. Enlargement, ulceration or bleeding suggest malignancy

INVESTIGATION: • Skin biopsy

RX: Supf cryotherapy or topical Cyt.T

Bowens Disease (Carcinoma-in-Situ)

Pre-malignant. Induced by chr sunlight exposure. Esp >40yrs. Lesions may occur on non-exposed areas

CLIN: Slowly enlarging, discrete, erythematous, scaly lesions

INVESTIGATION: • Skin biopsy

RX: Supf cryotherapy or topical Cyt.T or excision

Hutchinson's Melanotic Freckle

Pre-malignant. Induced by chr sunlight exposure. Esp elderly

CLIN: Macular pigmented slow growing freckles esp facial

RX: Careful follow up. Occ surgical excision

DISORDERS OF PIGMENTATION

Vitiligo

Common. Esp Asians. Occ FH. Ass c̄ autoimmune disease eg PA, Addison's disease, Thyroid disease

CLIN: Symmetrical depigmented areas of skin esp hands, feet, axilla, groins, genitalia & around eyes & mouth. Koebner's phenomenon is common

RX: Cosmetic masking occ indicated. PUVA can be effective

Partial Albinism

Aut Dom

CLIN: White forelock c̄ triangular depigmented area on forehead. Circumscribed symmetrical areas of depigmented areas on trunk or limbs

Oculocutaneous Albinism

Rare. Many types, mainly Aut Rec

CLIN: ↓ pigmentation of iris, hair & skin. Photosensitivity. ↑ risk of skin Ca

Causes of Hypomelanosis (LIST 3 DERM)

1. Vitiligo
2. Partial albinism
3. Oculocutaneous albinism
4. PKU
5. Tuberous sclerosis
6. Hypopituitarism
7. Chemicals:
   Eg Hydroquinone
8. Post inflam depigmentation:
   Eg Post eczema esp pityriasis alba; Post psoriasis
9. Leprosy
10. Sy
11. Pityriasis versicolor

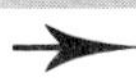

12. Kwashiorkor
13. Vit B12 def
14. Solar keratosis
15. Chr actinic dermatitis
16. Benign chr actinic damage

Causes of Hypermelanosis (LIST 4 DERM)

1. Cong/Genetic:
   a) Neurofibromatosis
   b) Peutz–Jegher syndrome
   c) Freckles
   d) Albright's syndrome
   e) Xeroderma pigmentosum
   f) Mongolian blue spot
   g) Pigmented naevi
   h) Multiple lentigines syndrome
   i) Incontinentia pigmenti
2. Endocrine:
   a) Cushing's syndrome
   b) Nelson's syndrome
   c) Addison's disease
   d) Pregnancy
3. Metabolic:
   Eg Haemochromatosis; PBC; Porphyria; CRF
4. Post inflam:
   Eg Resolving lichen planus, eczema
5. Idiopathic
6. Drugs:
   Eg Phenothiazines, The "Pill", Psoralens, Chloroquine, Phenolphthalein, Arsenic
7. Acanthosis nigricans (usually underlying Ca)

BULLOUS DISORDERS

Bullae are accumulations of serous fluid within or under the epidermis c̄ a diameter >0.5cm

Causes of Bullae (LIST 5 DERM)

1. Inherited:
   a) Epidermolysis bullosa
   b) Benign familial pemphigus
2. Pemphigus vulgaris
3. Bullous pemphigoid
4. Dermatitis herpetiformis
5. Herpes Gestationis
6. Porphyria
7. Benign chr bullous dermatosis
8. Toxic epidermal necrolysis
9. Drugs:
   Eg a) Photosensitivity reaction —Psoralens
   b) Fixed drug eruptions—Barbiturates
   c) Pemphigus—Rifampicin
   d) Pemphigoid—PUVA
   e) Erythema multiforme—Phenytoin
10. Trauma:
    Esp Frostbite, Friction, Sunlight, Pressure, Burns
11. Infection:
    Eg Impetigo, Herpes simplex (usually vesicular)
12. Pompholyx
13. Dermatitis artefacta
14. Subcorneal pustular dermatosis
15. Epidermolysis bullosis acquisita
16. Malignancy

Epidermolysis Bullosa

Rare. Bulla develop 2° to trauma. Aut Dom & Rec forms. Most present in infancy

Benign Familial Pemphigus (Hailey-Hailey Disease)

Rare. Not related to true pemphigus. FH

CLIN: Present at 10–30yrs c̄ erosions, vesicles & bullae in axillae, groins & neck. Occ 2° infection

DD: Intertrigo

Pemphigus Vulgaris

Rare. Esp 40–60yrs. Esp Jews

CLIN: Easily ruptured thin roofed bullae (thus Nikolsky's sign +ve) which crust & heal without scarring. Often presents in mouth c̄ painful ulceration. Occ Flexural hypertrophic lesions (Pemphigus vegetans)

INVESTIGATIONS:
- Direct IMF of peribullous skin: IgG between epidermal cells
- Indirect IMF: Circulating intercellular IgG

RX: Steroids in high dose in acute episode. Maintenance Rx c̄ steroid & Azathioprine

PROG: Spontaneous remission may occur after several years

VARIANTS OF PEMPHIGUS

Pemphigus may present as supf erosions (Pemphigus foliaceus) ± LE like rash on face (Pemphigus erythematosus)

Bullous Pemphigoid

Esp elderly

CLIN: Red itchy plaques c̄ weals & tense bullae esp abdo & limb flexures. Rarely affects mouth

INVESTIGATIONS:
- Direct IMF: Deposit of IgG & C3 on basement membrane
- Indirect IMF: Anti-basement membrane IgG Ab

RX: Steroids ± Azathioprine

PROG: Usually spontaneous remission within 2yrs

Cicatricial Pemphigoid

CLIN: Bullae & erosions of mucous membranes c̄ 2° scarring → ocular pterygium & occ blindness

INVESTIGATION: • IMF

RX: Dapsone

Dermatitis Herpetiformis

M>F. Often HLA-A8 +ve. Often ass c̄ gluten sensitive enteropathy

CLIN: Vesiculo-bullous eruption easily ruptured by scratching; Pruritus; Erythematous papules esp shoulders, elbows, knees, scalp, sacrum; Lesions are grouped. ↑ incidence of Ca eg Lymphoma

INVESTIGATIONS:
- Histology
- Direct IMF: IgA in tips of dermal papillae of normal skin
- Jejunal biopsy
- WCC: Occ eosinophils ↑

RX: Dapsone (SE: Haemolysis, Periph neuropathy). Gluten free diet (Helpful even if jejunal biopsy norm)

PROG: Response to Dapsone is dramatic but Rx usually required for 2–3yrs to prevent relapse

Herpes Gestationis

Very rare. Occurs in pregnancy. Not due to Herpes virus. Histology similar to bullous pemphigus

CLIN: Bullous rash resolving in puerperium but recurring in subsequent pregnancies

Benign Chr Bullous Dermatosis

Esp young children

CLIN: Groups of tense bullae on genitalia, inner thighs & face. Condition clears by puberty

RX: Dapsone

Toxic Epidermal Necrolysis

Due to *Staph aureus* phage type 71 or drug reaction

CLIN: Widespread supf stripping of necrotic epidermis

RX: Antibiotics

Other Infections

Impetigo is a common cause of bullae in children. Many viral infections occ produce bullae although vesicles are commoner eg *Herpes simplex*

Subcorneal Pustular Dermatosis (Sneddon–Wilkinson Disease)

May be variant of pustular psoriasis

CLIN: Pustules & bullae esp axilla & groin. Rarely → myeloma

RX: Dapsone

PROG: Usually spontaneous remission at 5–10yrs

Epidermolysis Bullosa Acquisita

Ass c̄ IBD, Amyloidosis & Ca

CLIN: Bullae 2° to trauma esp limbs

Erythema Multiforme

An acute inflam c̄ symmetrical macules, papules, vesicles & occ bullae. It may be caused by drugs eg Sulphonamides, Systemic diseases eg Nephritis, Serum sickness, Viral infection eg Glandular fever, Pregnancy

CLIN: Malaise, then sudden onset of maculopapular rash. Round lesions c̄ dark centres esp hands, forearms, mucous membranes, face, legs, genitalia. Usually remits in 3–4wks. In Stevens–Johnson syndrome illness is more severe c̄ high fever, pain, arthralgia, involvement of mucous membranes

RX: Bed rest; Remove cause if possible. Steroids may be needed in Stevens–Johnson syndrome. Antibiotics for 2° infection

SKIN INFECTIONS

Folliculitis

Esp seen in beard area of adult M. May be due to curling beard hairs growing back into skin → irritation & 2° infection. Occ a boil (furuncle) develops, esp back of neck

RX: Treat any seborrhoeic eczema. Growing beard will cure. Occ antibiotics required

Cellulitis

An acute or chr skin inflam. Usually 2° to wound or ulcer. Esp Strep

CLIN: Swelling; Redness; Tenderness. Often Fever; Malaise

RX: Treat underlying disease. Antibiotics

Pseudomonas aeruginosa

Ass c̄ use of heated whirlpools

CLIN: Pruritic erythematous pustular rash affecting submerged areas except palms & soles. Occ Mastitis; Fever; Malaise; LN ↑

INVESTIGATION: • Swab

TB of the Skin

Clinical features depend on immune status of the patient. Lupus vulgaris & TB verrucosa cutis occur if strong immunity. Incidence of TB skin is similar to that of TB in general

LUPUS VULGARIS

CLIN: Red-brown nodules or plaques esp head & neck. May scar. Often TB elsewhere

TB VERRUCOSA CUTIS

Warts due to direct inoculation. Occ occupational history

GENERAL RX

Standard anti-TB drug regime

Molluscum Contagiosum

Esp childhood

CLIN: Shiny umbilicated papules. Resolve usually within mths

RX: Prick papules c̄ stick dipped in liquid phenol

Orf

Viral disease of sheep & goats. Spread by direct contact. Esp farmers

CLIN: Maculopapule becomes multiloculated hard vesicle & crusts over within 2 wks. Occ Fever; LN ↑; Erythema multiforme

INVESTIGATION: • Viral studies on vesicular fluid

RX: Keep lesion dry. Healing occurs in 3–4wks

PROG: Recurrences rare

Viral Warts

Many viruses have been identified in the aetiology of warts. Esp immunosuppressed

RX: For most cases adhesive plaster occlusion or salicylic acid preparations. Cryotherapy or cautery occ used. Podophyllin for genital warts (c/i pregnancy)

Pityriasis Versicolor

Due to yeast *Malassezia furfur*. Esp hot climates

CLIN: Pale brown scaly patches esp trunk

RX: Topical preparations eg Whitfield's ointment or Miconazole. Rarely oral Ketoconazole indicated

Mycetoma (Madura Foot)

A chr granulomatous skin infection characterised by swelling, draining sinuses & grains (fungus balls). Can be caused by many fungi. Esp barefoot outdoor workers. Incub Pd variable—may be yrs

CLIN: Often presents as painless nodule which later becomes fistulous discharging grains. Later invasion of deeper tissues

RX: Depends on causative organism eg Dermatophytes Rx Griseofulvin; *Actinomyces israeli* Rx Penicillin. Often surgical incision & drainage of abscesses needed. Eradication of infection is often difficult

Tinea Nigra

Esp Afr, Asia, S.Am. Due to *Exophiala. werneckii*

CLIN: Dark macules esp palms

RX: Whitfield's ointment

DD: Malignant melanoma

Hendersonula toruloidea

Due to *Hendersonula toruloidea.* Esp immigrants in UK

DD: *Tinea pedis*

Piedra

Caused by *Piedraia hortai* (Black piedra) in S.Am & S.E. Asia or *Trichosporon beigellii* (White piedra) in S.Am & Europe

CLIN: Fungus infection of hairy areas

RX: Shave affected areas

Chromoblastomycosis

Due to Phialophora or Cladosporium fungi. Esp barefoot outdoor workers in tropics

CLIN: Subcutaneous nodules which ulcerate & heal c̄ scarring & keloid formation, esp legs

RX: Amphotericin

URTICARIA

Urticaria consists of transient weals ass c̄ itching & pricking which clear completely leaving no scaling. The process in sc tissues → angiooedema. F>M. Cause usually unknown but occ due to food allergy, cold, pressure, drugs & parasites. Many chr cases have a psychogenic element

PATHOGENESIS: Rash mediated by histamine, SRS-A, 5-HT & kinins → dermal vessel dilatation → serous fluid production & epidermal vesicle formation

CLIN: Sudden onset; Weals of variable size, site & number; Pruritus. Weals usually last few hrs. Occ Bullae. Course may be acute or chr. Occ Scratching trauma → weals (dermographism)

RX: Antihistamines. In chr cases look for ppt factors & if possible remove

Hereditary Angiooedema

Aut Dom. Due to a def of C1 esterase inhibitor

CLIN: Acute swellings ppt by trauma or tiredness may be preceded by rash. Swelling esp mouth & larynx may threaten life. Occ Abdo colic; Vom

INVESTIGATION: • C1 esterase inhibitor def

RX: In emergency transfuse c̄ FFP. Maintainance Rx c̄ anabolic steroids eg Stanozolol

Urticarial Vasculitis

CLIN: Urticaria ass c̄ Arthralgia; Abdo pain; Fever; LN ↑. Weals often longer lasting than in other forms of urticaria

INVESTIGATIONS: • ESR ↑
• Serum complement: Occ ↓

RX: Steroids

ROSACEA

Chr inflam disorder. F>M. Ppt by persistent reflex flushing of face. Esp outdoor workers

CLIN: Gradual onset c̄ bouts of facial flushing. Erythematous eruption esp nose, chin, cheeks & forehead. Often ass telangiectasia & acne. No blackheads. Occ Papules; Pustules. Occ Gross hypertrophy & reddening of nose (Rhinophyma) esp M alcoholics; Iritis; Conjunctivitis

RX: Avoid predisposing factors. Occ long term Tetracycline Rx indicated

DISORDERS OF KERATINISATION

The Ichthyoses

A gp of cong disorders c̄ persistent non inflam generalised scaling. N.B The name is occ used for localised disorders c̄ inflam

ICHTHYOSIS VULGARIS

Commonest type of ichthyosis

CLIN: Dry scaling skin esp shins, outer upper arms & back. Occ Eczema develops in scaly areas

SEX-LINKED ICHTHYOSIS

X-linked inheritence. Affected have prolonged labour

CLIN: Severe ichthyosis esp neck & face. Occ Fissures & eczema occur in involved areas

INVESTIGATION: • Skin histochemistry: Def of steroid sulphatase

BULLOUS ICHTHYOSIFORM ERYTHRODERMA (EPIDERMOLYTIC HYPERKERATOSIS)

Rare. Aut Dom. Presents at birth

CLIN: Shiny brittle skin (Collodion babies) is shed after 2wks leaving severe scaling redness & blisters. Trauma → further bullae. Normally improves c̄ age. Adults usually affected less but may have marked hyperkeratosis. Occ Localised to palms & soles; Ectropion; Ear deformities

NON BULLOUS ICHTHYOSIFORM ERYTHRODERMA

Rare. Aut Rec

CLIN: Severe generalised scaling & redness. Occ Ectropion

LAMELLAR ICHTHYOSIS

Rare. Probably Aut Rec

CLIN: Born c̄ shiny brittle skin (Collodion babies). Severe scaling & hyperkeratosis (Lizard skin)

REFSUM'S DISEASE

Rare. Aut Rec. Defect of OHlation of branch chain fatty acids eg phytanic acid

CLIN: Present in late childhood c̄ skin scaling. Ass c̄ Deafness; Ataxia; Retinitis pigmentosa; Polyneuritis

RX: Diet excluding green vegatables

SJOGREN–LARSSON SYNDROME

Aut Rec. Ichthyosis, spastic diplegia & IQ ↓

ACQUIRED ICHTHYOSIS

May occur 2° to malignancy, lepromatous leprosy, drugs eg Nicotinic acid, abnormalities of fat metabolism

CLIN: Resembles ichthyosis vulgaris

GENERAL RX OF ICHTHYOSIS

Emollients & keralytic agents eg Salicylic acid. Etretinate (a vit A derivative. c/i pregnancy) for severe scaling & hyperkeratosis. Avoid frequent hot water baths & low humidity eg central heating

DISORDERS OF HAIR

Alopecia

Causes of Diffuse Hair Loss (LIST 6 DERM)

1. Common baldness
2. Acute physical or mental stress (Telogen effluvium): Eg Bereavement, Fever, Malnutrition
3. Alopecia areata
4. Cong alopecia
5. Post partum
6. Drugs: Eg Lithium, Anticoags, Cyt.T
7. Endocrine disorders: Eg Hypothyroidism, Hypopituitarism
8. Trauma
9. DLE
10. Lichen planus
11. Psoriasis
12. Menke's kinky hair disease

CONG ALOPECIA

Hair may be completely absent or less dense. May be ass c̄ other ectodermal abnormalities

COMMON BALDNESS

CLIN: In M post pubertal hair loss is not a disease & occurs c̄ a characteristic pattern eg receding frontal hair line. In post menauposal F occ diffuse alopecia occurs

RX: Occ False hair is required for psychological reasons

ALOPECIA AREATA

Occ FH. Ass c̄ Down's syndrome & autoimmune disease eg vitiligo, PA, Hypothyroidism. Esp 10–30yrs

CLIN: Rapid loss of discrete areas of hair usually scalp. May lose all scalp hair (alopecia totalis) or all body hair (alopecia universalis). Occ Nail pitting

RX: Steroids may help

PROG: Most regrow new hair within 6–9mths. The longer alopecia lasts the worse the prog

SCARRING ALOPECIA

Patchy alopecia c̄ loss of follicles & scarring. Rare. May be due to Lichen planus, DLE, Pseudopelade

Hirsutism

The growth in a F of adult M hair pattern

Causes of Hirsutism (LIST 7 DERM)

1. Racial
2. Endocrine:
   a) Cushing's syndrome
   b) Acromegaly
   c) Virilising ovarian tumours
   d) Adrenogenital syndrome
   e) Precocious puberty
   f) Adrenal tumours
3. Drugs:
   Eg Minoxidil, Steroids, Anticonvulsants
4. Anorexia nervosa
5. Idiopathic
6. Stein–Leventhal syndrome

GENERAL INVESTIGATIONS: • Plasma androgens
• Urinary 17 oxosteroids

Dandruff

Excess production of the norm process of the formation of dead squamous scalp cells

CLIN: Dandruff; Itching. Occ Slight hair loss

RX: Regular shampooing. Severe cases may require topical steroids

DISORDERS OF THE NAILS

Paronychia

Infection of nail fold. May be acute or chr. Finger >Toenail

CLIN: Red, swollen, tender nail. May have 2° infection eg c̄ candida

RX: Keep digit dry. Treat any infection eg c̄ Miconazole

Onycholysis

Localised separation of the nail from nail bed. Usually idiopathic, occ seen in thyroid diseases or 2° to obsessive handwashing. Risk of 2° infection

RX: Keep nails short. Miconazole

Yellow Nail Syndrome

Syndrome ass c̄ pleural effusions, LRTI, lymphoedema, hypothyroidism

CLIN: Yellow curved nails

Ingrowing Toenails

Pressure necrosis of nail wall & sulcus due to contact c̄ nail plate. Predisposed to by Short toe nail; Soft, lax pulp; Crowded foot; Hypercurved nail; Subungual exostosis

CLIN: Ingrowing toenail. May → ulcer, inflam & suppuration → nail wall & sulcus swelling

RX: Conservative Rx is by Correct trimming of nail; Prevention of excess sweating; Placing cotton wall under nail plate edge; Well fitting shoes. If pain or discomfort persist, surgery eg nail avulsion or wedge resection of nail bed

Onychogryphosis

Excessive growth of nail plate

CLIN: Thick, long piled up toenail ("ram's horn")

RX: Repeated trimming of toenail. Occ excision of nail root

Subungual Haematoma

CLIN: Crush inj → tense, painful haematoma

RX: Evacuate haematoma through a trephine hole

Subungual Exostosis

Small overgrowth of bone on dorsal distal phalanx

CLIN: Hard nodules deforming nails

RX: Surgical excision

DD: Subungual wart

Glomus Tumour

CLIN: Very painful tiny tumours. Occ seen through nail as dark spot

RX: Surgical excision relieves pain

Transverse Ridging

Due to self-inflicted interference of the cuticle & nail of one thumb by nail of adajacent finger causing transverse ridges

DRUG REACTIONS

The appearance of rashes due to drugs is extremely common

Causes of Cutaneous Drug Reactions (LIST 8 DERM)

1. Urticaria:
   Eg Aspirin, Penicillin, Sulphonamides, Morphine
2. Exanthematic eruptions:
   Eg PAS acid, Phenylbutazone, Barbiturates
3. Erythroderma:
   Eg Oxyphenbutazone, Gold, Barbiturates, Allopurinol
4. Lichenoid eruptions:
   Eg Chloroquine, Chlorpropamide, Propranolol, Gold
5. Bullous eruptions:
   Eg Barbiturates, Sulphonamides, Bromides, Iodides
6. Purpura:
   Eg Phenylbutazone, Indomethacin, Cyt.T
7. Eczema:
   Eg Tolbutamide, Thiazides, Sulphonamides
8. Drug induced LE:
   Eg Hydrallazine, Procainamide, Methyldopa
9. Erythema multiforme:
   Eg Phenylbutazone, Sulphonamides, Barbiturates
10. Toxic epidermal necrolysis:
    Eg Gold, Allopurinol, Sulphonamides
11. Pigmentation:
    Eg Phenothiazines, Arsenic, PUVA, Oral contraceptives
12. Erythema nodosum:
    Eg Sulphonamides, Penicillin, Barbiturates
13. Alopecia:
    Eg Cyt.T, Oral contraceptives
14. Hypertrichosis:
    Eg Steroids, Minoxidil, Diazoxide
15. Acneiform eruptions:
    Eg Isoniazid, ACTH, Iodides, Androgens
16. Skin necrosis:
    Eg Warfarin
17. Fixed drug eruptions:
    Eg Barbiturates, Tetracyclines, Dapsone, Sulphonamides
18. Ichthyosis:
    Eg Nicotinic acid

PSYCHOLOGICAL FACTORS IN SKIN DISORDERS

Psychological factors are very important in skin disease. A few diseases are a direct result of psychological disorder but many others are triggered by emotional upset

Dermatitis Artefacta

Self induced skin disease. F>M. Esp young F. Many possible ppt events eg sexual, family or marital problems

CLIN: Many possible lesions; Often bizarre c̄ well defined edges

RX: Psychiatric Rx often indicated

Acne Excoriée

F>M. Esp 15–30yrs

CLIN: Excoriated lesions esp face, shoulders, neck, upper chest. Initially ass c̄ acne but may persist after all trace of acne has gone. Occ Evidence of phobic state

RX: Resistent to Rx. May try psychotherapy

Dysmorphophobia

A state in which the patient believes that there is a noticeable physical defect but there are no objective examination findings. F>M

CLIN: In F common worries are breasts, genitalia, face & hair. Common complaints are burning, itching, too much or too little hair. Often ass c̄ depression. Facial complaints esp re nose in F are ass c̄ ↑ risk of suicide & psychosis. Complaints of excess hair loss are ass c̄ marital problems & depression

RX: Difficult to manage. Psychotherapy may help. Amitriptyline occ benefits

Trichotillomania

Uncontrollable desire to pull out one's hair. Children >Adults

CLIN: Patches of relative baldness. Emotional problems. May → Trichobezoar

CYSTIC LESIONS

Sebaceous Cyst

A retention cyst due to obst to mouth of sebaceous gland

CLIN: Fluctuant cyst often c̄ central punctum esp face, ear lobe, scalp, scrotum & vulva. Contents are malodourous & "cheesy". Occ Infection; Ulceration (Cock's peculiar tumour); Horn formation; Ca^{2+}. Very rarely → Ca

RX: Incise, evacute & avulse cyst. If infected drain & later excise

Ganglion

Common. Tense, cystic swelling related to jt synovial membrane or tendon sheath esp dorsum wrist or foot

CLIN: Occ pain & discomfort or cosmetic problem

RX: Occ excise. Often recur

Implantation Dermoid

Cystic sc swelling esp on fingers. ? due to traumatic implantation of epithelial cells. Cyst contains white greasy material

RX: Excise

Dermoid Cyst

Occur at sites of embryonic fissure closure eg Inner or outer angle of orbit; Midline of neck, abdo, or scalp. Unilocular cyst containing hair, follicles, sweat & sebaceous glands

RX: Excise

GRANULOMA ANNULARE

Unknown cause. Esp Children, Young adults. F>M. A necrobiotic disorder

CLIN: A ring of small, smooth, firm, non-pruritic papules esp back of hand. Lesions may be single or multiple & disappear without scarring in mths or yrs

RX: Reassurance

BURNS

Burns may be partial (part or whole of germinal epithelium intact) or full thickness. Full thickness burns destroy skin

CLIN: Pain, esp supf burns; Shock. Occ Anaemia; 2° infection. Partial thickness burns blister & form a slough which falls off after 7–14 days leaving pink new skin beneath. Full thickness burns blister & slough; when slough separates 3–4wks later granulation tissue remains which heals c̄ scarring & contractures

RX: A. Partial thickness burns: Clean wound & apply sterile dressing. Analgesia
B. Full thickness burns: Analgesia; Plasma replacement usually c̄ CVP control (a rough guide is 1l of fluid per 9% of body affected—head & neck; & each arm = 9%; Each leg; front of trunk; & back of trunk = 18%; Perineum = 1%). Antibiotics. Wound may be nursed open c̄ limb elevated to ↓ oedema or closed when burn is cleaned & sterile dressings applied. When slough separates full thickness burns are excised & covered c̄ skin grafts. Skin grafts are done early if burn is small or if eyelid burnt to prevent ectropion & corneal ulceration

PROG: Depends on surface area of burn

TUMOURS

Lipoma

Common benign tumour of fat esp sc tissue of trunk & limbs. Esp adults

CLIN: Soft lobulated fluctuant tumous c̄ well defined edges. Occ calcify

RX: Excise if large or unsightly

Kerato-acanthoma (Molluscum Sebaceum)

Esp >50yrs. Occurs on hair bearing areas exposed to sun esp face, neck, hands

CLIN: Rapidly growing nodule c̄ elevated dome, umbilication & a keratotic plug. Disappears over 4–9mths to leave faint white scar

RX: Excise

DD: Epithelioma

Papilloma

Common benign sessile or pedunculated tumour eg Common wart (verruca vulgaris)

RX: Excise. Plantar warts may require $AgNO_3$, curettage or excision

Seborrhoeic Wart

Esp elderly. Common benign

CLIN: Dark brown papules on face, limbs or trunk

RX: Curettage or cauterisation

DD: Melanoma

Pigmented Naevi

JUNCTIONAL NAEVI

Commonest

CLIN: Smooth, flat or elevated brown naevi esp palms, soles, digits, genitalia. Suspect malignant change if: ↑ size; ↑ pigment; Ulcerate; Crusting; Haem; Satellite pigment

INVESTIGATION: Excision biopsy of all suspicious lesions

INTRADERMAL NAEVUS

Esp elderly

CLIN: Papillary, flat or warty naevi. Often hairy. Not pre-malignant

SPITZ NAEVUS (JUVENILE MELANOMA)

Rare. Benign. Esp children

CLIN: Pigmented, hairless, warty lesions. No dermal invasion

Keloid

Firm irregular shaped tumour, usually occuring at site of scar or previous inj. Esp Blacks

CLIN: Gradual onset. Initially small red lesion which increases in size & lightens in colour

RX: Intralesion Hydrocortisone early can help

Granuloma Pyogenicum

A single soft raspberry-like tumour sometimes caused by minor trauma

CLIN: Sudden onset. Smooth nodular bright red lesion esp finger, back or leg. Occ bleeds

RX: Excision & cautery of bleeding surfaces. May recur

Squamous Cell Carcinoma

Malignant. Esp elderly. M>F. Esp fair skinned, outdoor workers. Predispositions inc solar keratosis, Bowen's disease, Lupus vulgaris, Xeroderma pigmentosum, X-Rad, leukoplakia, varicose ulcer, Marjolin's ulcer, pitch, tar, & soot

CLIN: Rapidly growing raised nodule esp face & hands. Surrounding skin may be leathery, scaly & hyperpigmented. Later ulcer c̄ raised everted edges. Mets not uncommon

INVESTIGATION: Biopsy

RX: X-Rad or surgery

PROG: Good if early Rx

Basal Cell Carcinoma

Commonest cutaneous malignancy. Esp elderly but occurs earlier in sunnier climates. M>F

CLIN: Slow growing nodular lesion esp on line joining angle of mouth to ear lobe. Later central necrotic ulcer c̄ raised, rolled, pearly edge (Rodent ulcer). Fine blood vessels around ulcer. Direct slow spread. Mets rare

INVESTIGATION: Biopsy

RX: X-Rad or surgery. If cosmetic result important can use Mohn's chemosurgery c̄ removal of malignant cells layer by layer

PROG: Very good

Malignant Melanoma

Rare. Esp 40–60yrs. In UK F>M. Esp Australia. Often h/o pre-existing pigmented naevus

CLIN: Pigmented lesion esp on exposed skin (although in Japan commonest on soles of feet). Locally invasive & mets

INVESTIGATION: Excision biopsy

RX: Wide excision biopsy & grafting. Occ Cyt.T

PROG: Poor if mets. Better if on foot & excised early. Occ spontaneous regression

Kaposi's Sarcoma

Esp equatorial Afr. M>F. Esp homosexuals. May occur 2° to AIDS

CLIN: Painless bluish or brown nodules on hands &/or feet. Later oedema & ulceration of extremities; LN ↑; Spread to viscera eg GIT, Liver, Lungs

RX: X-Rad for local lesions. If disseminated, Cyt.T eg Vincristine & extended field X-Rad

PROG: Poor if 2° to AIDS. A variety seen esp in Poles is less aggressive

Rheumatology

RHEUMATOID ARTHRITIS

Rh Arth is a systemic connective tissue disorder predominantly affecting synovial jts
F>M. Esp "developed" countries. Onset esp 25–55yrs. Occ FH. Ass c̄ HLA DR4. >60% c̄ disease have +ve Rh F cf 5% in general pop. Ass c̄ auto immune disease eg PA

AETIOLOGY: Cause unknown but ?virus stimulates autoimmune Rh F (IgM) → immune complexes c̄ complement activation → tissue damage

CLIN: Variable presentations: Acute polyarthritis; Early morning stiffness, malaise & pain; Myalgia; Monoarthritis; Effusions esp knee; Tenosynovitis; Bursitis eg Baker's cyst; Acute rupture of synovial sack eg knee (DD:DVT); Systemic eg pericarditis. Usually later develop a characteristic bilat symmetrical arthritis esp small jts of hands & feet, morning stiffness & often non-articular signs eg nodules
Jts involved: MCP, PIP, Wrist, MTP, Knees >Elbows, hips, neck. Acutely jts are swollen, painful & warm. Later Jt effusions; Flexion deformities; Jt instability eg subluxation → ulnar deviation; Tendon rupture eg → Boutonniere' deformity. Eventual jt destruction; Occ ankylosis esp children. Characteristic late signs are: Spindling of PIPs; Swan neck deformity of fingers; Ulnar deviation at MCP jts. Rarely Atlanto–axial subluxation; Septic arthritis; Hoarseness due to crico–arytenoid arthritis; Deafness due to arthritis of auditory ossicles
Commonest non-articular manifestations are: Malaise; Anaemia; Wt ↓; Pleural effusions esp M; Firm non-tender mobile subcutaneous nodules esp extensor surfaces; Muscle weakness; Vasculitis esp digital; Supf ulcers. Less common are Pericarditis; Myocarditis; Valvulitis; Vertebral collapse; Rheumatic nodules in other sites eg lung & pleura; Fibrosing alveolitis; LN ↑; Carpal tunnel syndrome; Periph neuropathy; Cv cord or root compression; Felty's syndrome; Sjogren's syndrome; Amyloidosis; Depression; Kerato–conjunctivitis sicca; Scleritis occ → scleromalacia perforans or uveitis

SPECIFIC CLIN:

1. **Felty's Syndrome:** Splenomegaly, Leucopenia & Rh Arth. Ass c̄ ↑ risk of infection; LN ↑; Leg ulcers
2. **Sjogren's Syndrome:** Xerostomia, Kerato–conjunctivitis sicca & connective tissue disease esp Rh Arth. Ass c̄ Skin vasculitis; LN ↑; Raynauds; Other auto-immune diseases
3. **Caplan's Syndrome:** Massive fibrosis around rheumatoid nodules in pneumoconiotic lung. Esp coal miners

INVESTIGATIONS: • FBC: Often normocytic normochromic anaemia
- ESR ↑
- WCC: ↑ in infection, steroid Rx. ↓ in Felty's
- Serum Fe: Occ ↓
- TIBC: Occ ↑
- Platelets: ↓ in Felty's
- ANA: Occ +ve
- DAT, SCAT, Latex (Rh Factors): Often +ve
- Alk phos: Occ ↑
- X-R: Early sign juxta-articular porosis. Then bony marginal erosions esp MCP, MTP, PIP jts. Later subluxations, bony destruction etc. Do Cv spine X-Ray pre-op
- U&E, Creatinine: Rarely RF c̄ amyloidosis
- Jt fluid analysis: Occ Latex +ve
- Arthroscopy
- Albumin: Occ ↓
- PPE: Diffuse gammopathy
- Rarely: HLA, Synovial biopsy, Renal biopsy, Pleural & lung biopsy

RX: A. Medical: 1.General: Bed rest for acute episode. Splint in position of function to rest swollen jts. Physio. Discuss c̄ patient changes in life style. Provide home aids

2. Drugs for symptomatic relief eg NSAID such as Propionic acid, Aspirin & Indomethacin (SE:GIT disturbances). If non-effective use potentially disease modifying drugs eg Gold, Penicillamine, Chloroquine. Rarely the transiently effective drugs eg steroids are required

Gold: Disease modifying drug of choice. Slow clin effect: onset 4–8wks maximal 4–8mths. May reduce X-Ray progression

SE: Rashes; GN → nephrotic syndrome; Marrow depression

Penicillamine: Slow clin effect maximal 4–6wks. Can improve both jt & extra-articular features. May reduce X-Ray progression

SE: Rashes; Mouth ulcers; Bitter mouth taste or loss of taste; Nausea & anorexia; Nephrotic syndrome; Thrombocytopenia; Marrow depression; SLE. Can cause polyarthritis. Rarely Myasthenia

Chloroquine: Less effective than Gold or Penicillamine. No evidence of reduction of X-Ray progression. Use is limited by ocular toxicity which occurs if therapy is continued for >1yr. Monitor blood levels. Slow clin effect

SE: Nausea; Flatulence; Retinopathy. c/i Pregnancy

Azathioprine: Can retard X-Ray progression

SE: Neutropenia; GIT disturbances

Levamisole: Can induce remission. SE common

SE: Neutropenia; Vascultic rashes

Steroids: Fast clin effect. Potent anti-inflammatory effect can suppress symptoms but no alteration of disease course. Local injections may be useful but systemic use should be avoided because of the SE which are increasingly likely as dosage has to be increased to achieve same symptomatic response

SE: As for Cushing's syndrome inc vertebral collapse

B. Surgical: Indications: Nerve & tendon compression; Tendon rupture; Severe persistent pain unrelieved by medical Rx; Marked jt instability; Major loss of jt function

Four major types of op: Synovectomy, arthroplasty, osteotomy & arthrodesis

Synovectomy: Rarely used as jt lavage is a less invasive alternative

Arthroplasty (any op which reconstitutes a jt): Good for pain relief & mobility. Usually prefered to arthrodesis. Excision of metatarsal heads (Fowler's op) is useful Rx for metatarsalgia

Osteotomy (division of a bone near to a jt but outside jt capsule). Occ used for small jts of feet & knee jt

Arthrodesis (Fusion of jt surfaces): Good for jt stability but loses jt mobility

PROG: About 10% progress to severe disability. Poor prog factors at presentation : Nodules; Vasculitis or other systemic lesions; +ve DNA binding; Early bony erosions; High Rh F titre; HLA-DR4 &/or DR3

SLE

9F:1M. Esp black Americans, W.Indies, Chinese. Esp 20–40yrs. Occ FH. Ass c̄ HLA-B8/DR3

PATH: Formation of immune complexes containing ANA → tissue damage eg GN

CLIN: Relapsing & remitting disease. A variety of symptoms may be present. Skin signs eg classical butterfly rash, vasculitic rashes, non pruritic urticaria, palmar erythema, DLE (may occur in isolation), alopecia, photosensitivity; Fever; Malaise; Wt ↓; Anaemia; Arthralgia; Symmetrical polyarthritis (usually non-deforming, pain may be out of proportion to signs); Pleuritic chest pain; ↓ lung function; CNS signs eg depression, psychoses, Ep, cranial nerve palsies, chorea, periph neuropathy; BP ↑; LN ↑; Liver ↑; Spleen ↑; GN; Nephrotic syndrome; Endocarditis, myocarditis, pericarditis; Raynaud's; Shrinking lung syndrome. SLE may worsen in pregnancy (converse of Rh Arth)

INVESTIGATIONS:
- FBC: Usually normocytic, normochromic anaemia. Occ haemolytic anaemia
- Platelets ↓
- WCC: Occ ↓
- U&E & creatinine
- Urinalysis
- ANA
- Anti DNA Ab level reflects disease activity
- LE cells
- Complement ↓
- CXR, X-R Jts as necessary
- False +ve WR
- Rarely Arthroscopy, Synovial biopsy, EEG, Renal biopsy etc

RX:
1. Mild disease: NSAID &/or Chloroquine
2. More severe disease: Azathioprine. Steroids are usually also required

PROG: Excellent for mild disease. Death usually due to renal disease or infections 2° to immunosuppression. Many develop CNS disease eventually

Drug Induced SLE

A number of drugs can induce ANA production eg Hydrallazine, Procainamide. Can mimic SLE except that cerebral & renal disease less common, M=F, no anti-DNA Ab's

RX: Stop drug

DLE

F>M. Esp 30–40yrs old. Esp ass c̄ HLA B7. About 5% develop SLE

CLIN: Various clin forms. Lesions may start spontaneously or be ppt by UVR, stress & trauma
In chr form lesions on the head & neck are often well defined erythematous scaly discoid patches. Characteristically some follicles are plugged by scales. Heal c̄ scarring, local atrophy & depigmentation. If scalp involved may → alopecia. Occ similar lesions are found elsewhere on body. Occ Chilblains; Raynaud's
In LE profundus well defined nodules occur singly or in gps esp on face & buttocks. Healing c̄ atrophy & scarring
Cutaneous LE usually occurs in subacute form either as annular lesions esp extensor aspects of limbs & chest or papulosquamous lesions esp back of hands. Annular lesions do not scar on healing although central depigmentation occurs. Rarely ulceration

INVESTIGATIONS:
- ANA: +ve in approx 35%
- FBC
- WCC
- ESR
- Rh F

RX: Topical steroids. If steroids unhelpful try Chloroquine (SE: Eye problems on prolonged Rx) for 6wks. Often systemic steroids are required

PROG: Remission occurs in about 40%. SLE is likely to occur if lesions are widely disseminated. Chilblains, scalp involvement & Raynaud's are often resistant to Rx

SCLERODERMA

F>M. Esp Blacks. Ass c̄ PBC

CLIN: Two stages, the pre-fibrotic c̄ puffy fingers & Raynaud's & then the fibrotic c̄ thickened inelastic skin. Skin changes are initially Raynaud's & swollen shiny sausage shaped fingers. Later Skin elasticity lost & Skin creases disappear except round mouth; Tethering; Contractures; Loss of hair & sweating in affected areas. Occ CRST syndrome (Calcinosis, Raynaud's, Sclerodactyly, Telangiectasia). Oesophageal & other GI hypomotility is very common → oesophagitis, strictures, malabsorption, wide mouthed diverticula. Less commonly Pulmonary fibrosis; Pulmonary BP ↑; Arthralgia; Myopathy; Anaemia; Pericarditis. Late Kidney involvement → malignant BP ↑. Rarely Cardiomyopathy
If only skin involved termed Morphoea. White plaque lesions c̄ violaceous borders persisting for yrs. Linear lesions occur on limbs & may interfere c̄ growth. Lesions usually eventually remit

INVESTIGATIONS:
- FBC: Occ Anaemia
- ESR: ESR ↑ or norm
- ANA: +ve in 40–60%
- Appropriate X-Rays

RX: Avoid cold. Treat BP ↑. Antibiotics to prevent steatorrhoea. Physio

POLYMYOSITIS & DERMATOMYOSITIS

F>M. Usually idiopathic but occ ass c̄ Scleroderma, SLE & Rh Arth. In adults underlying Ca found in 5–10% cases

CLIN: Slowly progressive limb-girdle weakness; Muscle pain & tenderness; Violaceous rash on upper eyelids, shoulders, elbows, knees, chest.
Occ Photosensitivity; Skin ulcers; Raynaud's; Bluish-red plaques esp fingers; Transient arthritis; Dysphagia; Resp failure. In children Occ Ca^{2+} in skin, subcutaneous tissues & muscles

INVESTIGATIONS:
- CPK ↑
- EMG
- Muscle biopsy
- ESR: ↑ or norm
- ANA, Rh F occ +ve
- For occult Ca

RX: Steroids ± Azathioprine. Physio

MIXED CONNECTIVE TISSUE DISEASE (MCTD)

There is much overlap between connective tissue diseases but a fairly distinct group have been defined as having MCTD. Patients have elements of SLE, polymyositis & scleroderma

CLIN: Raynaud's; Sausage shaped fingers c̄ scleroderma like skin; Arthritis; Myositis. Rarely renal or CNS disease

INVESTIGATIONS:
- Ab's to Ribonucleoprotein ↑↑
- ANA ↑

RX: Steroids

EOSINOPHILIC FASCIITIS (SCHULMAN'S SYNDROME)

Rare. M>F. Can be confused c̄ scleroderma

CLIN: Sudden painful induration & swelling of subcutaneous tissues & deep fascia of limbs & trunks. No Raynauds or visceral involvement

INVESTIGATIONS:
- Periph blood eosinophilia
- Hypergammaglobulinaemia

RX: Steroids

LICHEN SCLEROSUS ET ATROPHICUS

Rare. Unknown aetiology. Ass c Morphoea & Vitiligo & other auto-immune conditions

CLIN: Small ivory macule or papule c̄ prominent sweat duct or pilosebaceous orifices on the surface. Esp anogenital area, trunk, flexor surface of wrist. Lesions may occur in gps. In girls, vulval lesions usually appear at 3–6yrs & remit at the menarche. Anogenital lesions in older F are pre-malignant → squamous cell Ca, & can cause soreness, pruritus, purpura & dyspareunia. In M, lichen sclerosus can → phimosis, meatal stenosis & recurrent balanitis (Balanitis xerotica obliterans)

RX: Non-genital lesions do not require Rx. Vulval lesions may be helped by topical oestrogen or steroid preparations. Regular review as risk of Ca. In M, balanitis may be helped by testosterone ointment, intralesional steroid injection or potent topical steroids

POLYARTERITIS NODOSA (PAN)

An inflam multisystem disorder chiefly affecting medium sized arteries causing infarction. An ill defined disorder or gp of disorders. 25–50% have HepB Ag. M>F. Esp elderly. Ass c̄ Leukaemias. May follow use of drugs eg Sulphonamides

CLIN: Diverse manifestations. Usually Fever; Malaise; PR ↑; Wt ↓; Anaemia. Occ Proteinuria; Haematuria; BP ↑; Skin lesions eg Nodules, necrosis, ulceration & livido reticularis. Myalgia; Arthralgia; Periph neuropathy; Abdo pain eg 2° to PU, organ infarcts, mesenteric ischaemia; Retinal haem & exudates; Later RF. Acute vascular episodes can occur in other sites eg Testes, Heart → CCF, Pancreas, Brain
Some classify PAN type disorders c̄ lung involvement as a variant of PAN. These have resp illness ie bronchitis, asthma or pneumonia which precedes the systemic disease. Other features are Blood eosinophilia; Necrotising lesions or polyarteritis in lungs & Granulomas

INVESTIGATIONS:
- FBC
- WCC ↑
- Alk phos ↑
- Arteriography
- HBsAg

RX: Prednisolone ± Azathioprine. Treat BP ↑. Rarely plasma exchange therapy

PROG: 70% 5yr survival

WEGENER'S GRANULOMATOSIS

Very similar to PAN. Rare

CLIN: Sinusitis; Rhinitis; Nasal ulceration; Skin lesions eg nodules, purpura; GN; URT & LRT granulomata. Rarely BP ↑. Later RF

RX: Prednisolone & Cyclophosphamide

POLYMYALGIA RHEUMATICA

Closely related to temporal arteritis. Esp >55yrs. F>M. Rarely due to occult Ca or chr infection

CLIN: Acute or insidious onset. Wt ↓; Malaise; Fever; Pain & stiffness in shoulders, neck, pelvic girdle; Synovitis in shoulders hips & knees; Proximal muscle tenderness

INVESTIGATIONS:
- FBC
- ESR ↑
- Biopsy temporal artery if signs of temporal arteritis

RX: Steroids

SERONEGATIVE ARTHRITIS

The term seronegative arthritis (or more accurately seronegative spondarthritis) is applied to a group characterised by sacro-iliitis, absence of Rh F & an ass c̄ Ank Sp. The gp comprises: Psoriatic arthritis, Ank Sp, Reiter's Syndrome, Enteropathic arthritis ass c̄ Ulc colitis, Crohn's & Whipple's, Behcet's Syndrome

Causes of Sacroiliitis (LIST 1 RHEUM)

1. Seronegative spondarthritis
2. Still's disease
3. TB, Brucellosis

Psoriatic Arthritis

Occurs in approx 10% of patients c̄ psoriasis. F=M. 1/3 FH. Ass c̄ HLA B27

CLIN: Psoriasis usually precedes arthritis. 5 types of arthritis recognised: DIP jt involvement; Arthritis mutilans; Rh Arth-like (Sero -ve); Monoarthritis; Ank Sp alone or in conjunction c̄ other types. Often Psoriatic nails & occ skin lesions. Rarely Iritis; Conjunctivitis; Keratoconjunctivitis sicca; Aortitis; Koebner phenomenon

INVESTIGATIONS:
- FBC
- ESR ↑
- Jt fluid analysis
- X-R: No juxta-articular porosis, Sacroiliitis

RX: NSAID. Physio. Local steroid injections. If ineffective, Gold or Penicillamine. Chloroquine c/i as it can → exfoliative dermatitis

PROG: Good except for arthritis mutilans

Causes of Arthritis Mutilans (LIST 2 RHEUM)

1. Rh Arth
2. Still's Disease
3. Psoriasis
4. Reticulohistiocytosis

Ankylosing Spondylitis

M>F. Onset 15–30yrs. Often FH. Esp Caucasians. Often HLA B27 +ve, eg in UK 95%

PATHOLOGY: Principally affects the attachments of ligaments & tendons to bone. Inflammation & bony erosion → fibrosis & new bone formation.

Esp affects ant & post spinal ligs → "bamboo spine", In.v discs → syndesmophytes, SIJs

CLIN: Intermittent gradually worsening episodes of lumbosacral morning pain often c̄ sciatic radiation which is improved by exercise. Later Chest expansion ↓; Bilat chest pain; Stooped position, Kyphosis. Occ presents as Monoarthritis esp Knee; Asymmetrical periph arthritis of large jts. Fever; Wt ↓. Occ Plantar fasciitis; Buttock tenderness

INVESTIGATIONS: • FBC
- ESR ↑
- Immunoglobulins ↑
- X-R spine & SIJ: eg Bilat sacro-iliitis, "squaring" of vertebral bodies, Romanos lesion
- CXR
- Rarely HLA

RX: NSAID. Exercise. Physio, teach patients to do exercises. Occ local X-Rad

COMPLICATIONS: 1. 2° Amyloidosis
2. Iritis
3. Aortic incompetence
4. Upper lobe lung fibrosis
5. Rare: Atlanto-axial subluxation → tetraplegia; Pericarditis; Cardiomyopathy; Aortic aneurysm

Reiter's Syndrome

A triad of NSU, conjunctivitis & sero -ve arthritis. May be Post-dysenteric or sexually transmitted. M>>F. Onset 20–30yrs. Ass c̄ HLA B27 (75%). Often FH

CLIN: 4–6wks after exposure, acute arthritis esp knee, conjunctivitis & urethritis. Occ a chr polyarthritis ensues. Occ Sacro-iliitis; Plantar fasciitis; Tendinitis; Circinate balanitis; Keratoderma blenorrhagica; Nail dystrophy; Buccal or lingual ulcers. Rarely Periph neuropathy; Amyloidosis; Aortitis

INVESTIGATIONS: • MSU
- Urethral swab
- ESR
- Immunoglobulins: Occ ↑
- X-R: Occ chr erosive jt disease

RX: Tetracycline for NSU. NSAID ± local steroid injections

PROG: Most recover in 2-4wks. A few develop chr arthritis or have recurrence

Ulcerative Colitis & Crohn's Disease

2 ass types of arthritis. M=F

a) Enteropathic arthritis (12% Ulc colitis, 20% Crohn's): Acute monoarthritis. Large jt >small. Esp Knee. The arthritis is related to activity of bowel disease
b) Ankylosing spondylitis: May precede gut disease

RX: NSAID. Local steroid injections. Treat bowel disease—total colectomy for Ulc colitis cures monoarthritis, bowel resection in Crohn's usually helpful. Ank Sp is not influenced by bowel Rx

Whipple's Disease

Rare. M>F. Often develop a migratory polyarthritis & Arthralgia. Occ sacroiliitis & Ank Sp

RX: Tetracycline

PROG: Good

Behcet's Syndrome

Esp S.E. Europe, Japan

CLIN: Oral & genital ulcers; Conjunctivitis; Uveitis; Recurrent non deforming arthritis esp Knee; Erythema nodosum; Cutaneous pustules & nodules; Thrombophlebitis; Meningoencephalitis; Sacroilitis; Colitis

RX: NSAID. Occ steroids

GOUT

M>F. Hyperuricaemia is a necessary prerequisite. Esp Elderly, developed countries. Occ FH

N.B Most people c̄ hyperuricaemia are asymptomatic

PATH: Caused by deposition of urate or uric acid crystals

Causes of Hyperuricaemia (LIST 3 RHEUM)

A. INCREASED URIC ACID PRODUCTION
1. Increased cell turnover:
   a) Myeloproliferative diseases & reticuloses
   b) Ca
   c) Chr haemolysis
   d) Psoriasis
   e) 2° polycythaemia
   f) Gaucher's disease
2. Increased purine synthesis:
   a) Idiopathic
   b) Lesch–Nyhan syndrome
   c) Type 1 glycogen storage disease (Von Gierke's)

B. DECREASED RENAL EXCRETION OF URIC ACID
1. Primary idiopathic gout
2. CRF
3. Ketoacidosis
4. Drugs:
   Eg Thiazides, Frusemide, Salicylates (Low dose)
5. Endocrine:
   a) Hyperparathyroidism
   b) Hypothyroidism
6. Nephrogenic diabetes insipidus
7. BP ↑
8. Down's syndrome
9. Alcoholism
10. Starvation
11. Idiopathic hypercalcuria
12. Lead poisoning

C. DEMOGRAPHIC FACTORS
1. High protein diet
2. Increased age
3. Urban dwelling
4. Increased weight
5. High social class

Acute Gouty Arthritis

PRECIPITATING FACTORS: 1. Surgery
2. Exercise
3. Trauma
4. Starvation
5. High purine diet
6. Alcohol
7. Drugs
8. Systemic illness

CLIN: Ac synovitis. Mono- or poly-articular presentation. Esp 1st MTP >Ankle, Knee >Hands & feet. Severe throbbing in jt c̄ erythematous shiny overlying skin. Occ Pyrexia; Rigors; Tenosynovitis; Bursitis; Cellulitis. Untreated, subsides in days to wks occ → pruritis & desquamation. Frequency of episodes is very variable. Recurrent acute attacks can → bony erosion, tophi, OA & disability

INVESTIGATIONS: • FBC
- U&E
- Serum urate
- WCC ↑
- –ve birefringent needle crystals from jt aspirate
- Appropriate X-R: Normal in early stages
- For underlying cause

RX: NSAID eg Indomethacin or Colchicine. Avoid ppt drugs inc Allopurinol (Xanthine oxidase inhibitor)

DD:
1. Ac septic arthritis
2. Other crystal arthopathies
3. 1st MTP bursitis
4. Traumatic arthritis
5. Rh Arth
6. Haemarthrosis
7. Spondarthritides c̄ periph jt involvement

Chronic Tophaceous Gout

The result of recurrent acute attacks

CLIN: Bone destruction; 2° OA; Asymmetric polyarthritis; Tophi (local urate deposits) esp Pinna, tendon sheaths, near jts eg olecranon bursa cause nobbly swellings. Often ass c̄ renal disease

INVESTIGATION: • As for acute gout. X-R shows "punched out" erosions, jt destruction, tophi, soft tissue swelling

RX: Between attacks life-long Allopurinol (interrupts purine synthesis thus uric acid production ↓) c̄ initial (for 3mths) Colchicine cover to prevent Allopurinol-induced acute attack. Alternatives are Probenecid & Sulphinpyrazone (uricosuric drugs) Regular review of BP, Wt, renal function

COMPLICATIONS: 1. Urolithiasis: Esp hot climates. Stones may be radiolucent (urate) or radio-opaque (Ca^{2+} salt). Not inevitably ass c̄ hyperuricaemia or hyperuricosuria

2. **Renal failure**
3. **Acute Urate Nephropathy:** Usually follows Rx of myeloproliferative disease c̄ ppt of uric acid in collecting ducts
   Rx: Allopurinol or high fluid intake & urine alkalinisation
4. **Chr Urate Nephropathy:** Rare
   N.B IHD & Diabetes are ass c̄ gout & hyperuricaemia but the latter are not risk factors

DD: 1. Nodular Rh Arth
2. OA
3. Xanthomatosis

Lesch–Nyhan Syndrome

X-linked inheritance. Rare. Due to enzyme defect

CLIN: Gout. Compulsive self-mutilation, choreoathetosis, IQ ↓. Occ Neonatal muscular hypotonia; Nephropathy

INVESTIGATIONS: • FBC: Occ megaloblastic anaemia
• Specfic enzyme assay: HG-PRTase ↓

RX: Can demonstrate by amniocentesis

OTHER METABOLIC ARTHROPATHIES

Pseudogout

An acute inflammatory synovitis due to deposition of Ca^{2+} pyrophosphate dihydrate crystals. Sporadic cases esp in elderly, younger cases often have FH. Ass c̄: Diabetes; Gout; HPT; Haemochromatosis

PRECIPITATING FACTORS: 1. Trauma
2. Surgery
3. Acute illness

CLIN: Recurrent acute arthritis esp Knees; Jt is painful, warm, swollen & tender c̄ redness of overlying skin. 1st MTP rarely involved. Rarely mimics Rh Arth & OA rather than gout. Later OA develops

INVESTIGATIONS: • Weakly +ve birefringent crystals in aspirate
• X-R: Chondrocalcinosis esp Knee, pelvis, wrist
• Arthroscopy

RX: Jt aspiration. NSAID. Occ Colchicine

Causes of Chondrocalcinosis (LIST 4 RHEUM)

1. OA
2. Pseudogout
3. Gout
4. HPT
5. Haemochromatosis
6. Acromegaly
7. Diabetes
8. Rarely:
   Wilson's disease,
   Hypothyroidism

Ochronosis

Aut Rec. Esp young adults. M>F. Def of homogentisic acid oxidase

CLIN: Alkaptonuria (urine turns black on standing). Spondylosis; Athritis esp Knees >Shoulder >In.v disc. Blue-brown pigmentation of cornea, ear cartilage, skin. Occ deafness

INVESTIGATIONS: • Alkaptonuria
• X-R: Loss of jt space, osteophytes, chondrocalcinosis

Haemochromatosis

Occ present c̄ painful arthropathy. Can affect small & large jts
Ass c̄ pseudogout

INVESTIGATION: • X-R: Chondrocalcinosis, cystic changes, destructive change

Wilson's Disease

Rheumatological problems not common. Occ Bone fragmentation; Osteochondritis dissecans; Chondrocalcinosis; Small jt arthropathy (similar to Rh Arth)

Hyperlipidaemias

Type II is ass c̄ a migratory polyarthritis & type IV is ass c̄ arthralgia & arthritis

Fabry's Disease

Rare. Due to α-galactosidase def → widespread deposition of glycolipid. X-linked Rec. Onset post-puberty

CLIN: Severe jt pain. Fever; Vascular skin lesions. Renal & CNS involvement

PROG: Invariably fatal

Reticulohistiocytosis

Rare. F>M

CLIN: Multiple small skin nodules. Mutilating synovitis

INVESTIGATION: • X-R: Arthritis mutilans

RX: Nil known

ENDOCRINE ARTHROPATHIES

Acromegaly

Six types of rheumatic complaints: Low back ache; Limb arthropathy esp Knees, shoulders & hips c̄ creps throughout range of mvt; Compression neuropathies esp carpal tunnel syndrome & occ spinal cord compression; Raynaud's Phenomenon; Premature OA; Mild myopathy

INVESTIGATIONS: • X-R: Dorsal kyphosis; Osteophytes; Tufting & "spade like" terminal phalanges; Chondrocalcinosis; ↑ in heel pad thickness; At first widening of periph jt spaces, later features of degenerative jt disease

Hypothyroidism

Occ ass c̄ Carpal tunnel syndrome; Myopathy; Knee effusions; Gout. In cong form have epiphyseal dysgenesis

RX: Respond to thyroid replacement

Thyroid Acropachy

Rare syndrome of hyperthyroidism often following Rx

CLIN: Swelling of fingers & toes. Clubbing; Pre-tibial myxoedema

Hyperparathyroidism

CLIN: Bone pain; #s; Waddling gait; Erosive symmetrical arthritis esp knees, hands, feet; Osteoporosis; 2° gout; Pseudogout; Traumatic synovitis. Symptoms due to HyperCa^{2+} are commoner

INVESTIGATIONS:
- Ca^{2+}
- Urinary Ca^{2+}
- Alk phos ↑
- HPT
- X-R: Digital subperiosteal erosions; Chondrocalcinosis; Rugger jersey spine

Vertebral Ankylosing Hyperostosis

Forestier's disease. Ass c̄ diabetes & obesity. Esp elderly

CLIN: Rarely symptomatic. If in Cv spine can cause dysphagia

INVESTIGATION: • X-R large bony overgrowths esp dorsal spine

INFECTIVE ARTHROPATHIES

Viral

Most viral infections can be ass c̄ a transient arthritis eg Mumps, Glandular fever, Varicella. Arthritis is usually a late feature

RUBELLA

CLIN: A joint synovitis occ occurs after rash settles. Same condition can occur 2–3wks post-vaccination. Occ → carpal tunnel syndrome. Recovery in <3wks

HEPATITIS B

CLIN: Arthralgia, Fever & Urticaria occur in prodrome. Chr infection can be ass c̄ PAN

ARBOVIRUSES

Common in malarial regions. Usually transmitted by mosquitoes

CLIN: Marked arthralgia & arthritis

Bacterial

Septic arthritis is now uncommon due to introduction of antibiotics for systemic infection

GENERAL CLIN: Acute onset. Rigors; Fever; Arthritis usually monoarthritis c̄ hot red tender jt

GENERAL INVESTIGATIONS:

- Blood culture
- Synovial fluid: WCC ↑, Sugar ↓, culture
- X-R
- ESR

GENERAL RX: Splint in optimal position. Antibiotics. Jt aspirations

LYME ARTHRITIS

Esp E & W coast USA. Tick borne spirochete

CLIN: Erythema chronicum migrans; Asymmetric large jt synovitis which can last years. Occ Pericarditis

RX: Penicillin

BACILLARY DYSENTERY

CLIN: Polyarteritis esp knees, elbows, wrists & fingers. 2–3wks post-infection. Occ → Reiter's syndrome

SALMONELLA

Esp children

CLIN: Usually monoarticular esp knees. Occ Osteomyelitis esp if ass c̄ sickle cell anaemia

BRUCELLA

CLIN: Recurrent fever; Sweating; Vom; Myalgia; Arthralgia. Occ Monoarthritis esp hip

GONOCOCCAL ARTHRITIS

F>M. Adequate Rx of gonorrhoea prevents arthritis

CLIN: Fever; Rigors; Migratory polyarthritis esp knees, ankles, wrists, MTP jts >Monoarthritis. Occ Skin lesions eg erythema, vesicles which may → pustules c̄ central necrosis; Tenosynovitis of fingers. Onset 3wks after infection. Can → jt destruction

INVESTIGATION: • Culture of synovial fluid & blood

RX: Penicillin. Rest jt. Occ aspirate jt

SABE

Immune complex deposition → synovitis. Ass c̄ +ve Rh Factor

MENINGOCCOCAL ARTHRITIS

CLIN: Arthritis may occur at onset of illness but usually occurs >5days after onset, affecting 2 or 3 large jts. Chr meningococcaemia → rigors, fever, jt pain, purpura

YERSINIA ENTEROCOLITICA ARTHRITIS

Ass c̄ HLA B27

CLIN: Mild GI illness followed 3wks later by a polyarthritis esp knees & ankles. Occ Sacroiliitis. Self limiting

INVESTIGATION: • Rising agglutination titre

MISCELLANEOUS ARTHROPATHIES

Hypertrophic Pulmonary Osteoarthropathy (HPOA)

Usually acquired esp 2° to Ca lung. Rarely cong

CLIN: Clubbing. Occ Bone pain; Synovial effusions

INVESTIGATION: • X-R: Symmetrical periosteal reactions esp distal radius & ulna

Leukaemia

Bone & jt symptoms are quite common

CLIN: Arthralgia; Bone pain; Migratory asymmetric polyarthritis. May be presenting feature of acute leukaemia

Sarcoidosis

CLIN: Erythema nodosum. Arthritis esp ankles & knees

Relapsing Polychondritis

Cause unknown. Repeated episodes of inflam of hyaline & fibrocartilaginous structures → destruction

CLIN: Swelling, redness & tenderness esp external ear, trachea, larynx, nose, sclera, articular cartilage. Swollen tender jts

RX: Analgesics. Occ steroids

Familial Mediterranean Fever

CLIN: Recurrent episodes of fever, arthritis. Usually a painful large jt arthropathy. Later amyloidosis

RX: Colchicine prophylaxis

OSTEOARTHROSIS

F>M. Esp elderly. Major cause of sickness absence

PREDISPOSING FACTORS (2° OA):

1. Aseptic necrosis:
   a) Idiopathic
   b) Occupational
   c) Kashin–Beck disease
   d) Hbopathies
   e) Thiemann's disease
   e) Gaucher's
2. Articular deformity:
   Eg Multiple epiphyseal dysplasia; Slipped femoral epiphysis; Malunited #; Menisectomy; Mucopolysaccharidoses
3. Inflammatory articular disease
4. Articular abuse:
   a) Occupation eg Footballers; Drillers
   b) Charcot's jts eg Diabetics
   c) Jt laxity eg Acromegaly, Ehlers–Danlos syndrome, Marfan's syndrome
5. Metabolic:
   a) Gout
   b) Pseudogout
   c) Chondrocalcinosis
   d) Ochronosis
   e) Haemochromatosis
   f) Acromegaly
   g) Wilson's disease
6. Haemophilia & Christmas disease

Most cases have no predisposing factor & are said to be primary

Obesity is not directly related to OA

PATHOGENESIS: Loss of surface matrix of articular cartilage → cleft → enzyme infiltration → cartilage degeneration → replacement by eburnated bone & osteophytes (proliferation of new skeletal material at margins). Occ subchondral bone cysts

CLIN: Esp effects DIP (Heberden's nodes), PIP (Bouchard's nodes), CMC of thumb, knee, hip, Cv spine, lumbar spine & 1st MTP jt. Dull aching pain esp on jt use; ↓ jt mvts; Stiffness. Occ Soft tissue swelling; Effusion; Crepitus. Later jt deformity but jt function often preserved

INVESTIGATION: • X-R: Loss of jt space; Osteophytes; Juxta-articular sclerosis (eburnation) & cysts. Changes do not correlate c̄ symptoms & signs

RX: A. Medical: Diet if obese. Physio & OT. Analgesics

B. Surgical:

Indications: 1. Pain++
2. Valgus, varus deformities
3. Severe ↓ functional capacity
4. Impending or actual instability
5. Gross bone destruction

Osteotomy to hip or knee is sometimes used for the younger patient. Arthrodesis is often used for wrist, MCP jt & ankle; Also used if one knee is immobile. Arthroplasty is usually op of choice for OA hip

SOFT TISSUE LESIONS

Tendinitis

If a true sheath involved = tenosynovitis

CLIN: Pain & tenderness on use. Occ crepitus

RX: Rest. Reduce tendon excursion eg wrist strapping. NSAID

Enthesopathy

Injuries at tendo-periosteal junctions due to overuse eg Tennis elbow, plantar fasciitis

RX: Rest. Local protection. NSAID. Occ Local steroids, Physio

Muscle Injuries

May be due to extrinsic trauma or sudden activity eg torn hamstring

RX: Ice compression & elevation. Ultrasound. Careful mobilisation

Bursitis

Due to overuse & trauma. Often related to occupations

COMMON FORMS:

1. **Bunions:** Due to rubbing foot wear. Over 1st metatarsal head
2. **Baker's Cyst:** Semimembranous bursa of knee. Ass c̄ OA & Rh Arth
3. **Housemaid's Knee:** Pre-patellar bursitis

GENERAL CLIN: Swelling & pain

GENERAL RX: Local aspiration & culture; Rest; Physio; NSAID. Occ steroid injections

Fibrositis

CLIN: Widespread aching for at least 3mths; Multiple tender points; Stiffness. Occ Fibrotic nodules; Sleep disturbance

INVESTIGATION: • No rheumatological abnormality

THE PAINFUL SHOULDER

Causes of Painful Shoulder (LIST 5 RHEUM)

1. Tendinitis:
   Esp Supraspinatus, Infraspinatus, Bicipital
2. Sub-Acromial bursitis
3. Trauma
4. Arthritis of shoulder:
   Eg Rh Arth, OA, Polymyalgia Rheumatica
5. Frozen shoulder
6. Shoulder–hand syndrome
7. Fibrositis (Periscapular myalgia)
8. Rarely:
   a) Neuralgic amyotrophy
   b) Aseptic necrosis
   c) Vth Cv root pain

Frozen Shoulder

Imprecise diagnosis. Usually applied to a painful stiff shoulder not caused by trauma. May occur spontaneously or 2° to immobilisation of arm eg c̄ CVA, MI, herpes of Cv root

Garrods diathesis = frozen shoulder, Dupuytren's & spongy gums

CLIN: 1st phase increasing pain esp nocte for 3–6mths; 2nd static phase for 3–6mths; Recovery in 3rd phase. No muscle loss

Shoulder–hand Syndrome

A frozen shoulder syndrome ass c̄ sympath overactivity. Occ FH

CLIN: Phase 1 swollen hand, pain on jt mvts except DIP; Frozen shoulder; Sweating; Usually unilat. In phase 2 the hand is cold c̄ atrophic skin & contractures

INVESTIGATION: • X-R: Sudeck's disuse osteoporosis, no erosions

RX: Phase 1: Ice; Indomethacin for pain; Exercise esp hand
Phase 2: Active shoulder stretching

SJOGREN'S SYNDROME

A syndrome of keratoconjunctivitis sicca & xerostomia. Often ass c̄ connective tissue diseases esp Rh Arth. Esp middle aged F

RAYNAUD'S PHENOMENON

Intermittent pallor or cyanosis of the hands & feet ppt by cold c̄ return to normal between attacks. Due to excessive vasoconstriction of digital arteries in response to cold

CLIN: Fingers are white during attack occ c̄ cyanosis. On recovery fingers pinken & then go bright red & tingle. Occ supf ulcers

RX: Avoid cold

Causes of Raynaud's Phenomenon (LIST 6 RHEUM)

1. Idiopathic
2. Cold injury
3. Vibration
4. Cervical spondylosis
5. Collagen vascular diseases:
   Eg Rh Arth, SLE, Systemic sclerosis, PAN, Takayashu's
6. Haematological:
   a) Dysproteinaemias
   b) Polycythaemia
   c) Leukaemia
   d) Cold agglutinins
7. Drugs & toxins:
   Eg Ergot, Heavy metals
8. Arterial occlusion:
   Eg Thoracic inlet syndromes, Buerger's disease

TRANSIENT MIGRATORY ARTHRITIS

Causes of Transient Migratory Arthritis (LIST 7 RHEUM)

1. Rheumatic fever
2. SLE
3. Reiter's disease
4. Infections:
   Eg Rubella, Gonnococcal, Meningococcal, HepB, Mycoplasma
5. Henoch–Schonlein purpura
6. Serum sickness
7. Whipple's disease
8. Leukaemia

Orthopaedics

BONE INJURY

Mechanisms of Bone Healing

After #, blood is lost ± damage to nerves, blood vessels. Max swelling 2–3 days. Osteoblasts migrate to haematoma to form temporary callus. Primitive bone cells migrate to the bone around and between the # to form permanent or hard callus. Then remodelling occurs
In summary: Haematoma → granulation → callus → remodelling of bone

Signs of Fracture (LIST 1 ORTH)

1. Tenderness
2. Swelling
3. Deformity
4. Abnormal mvt
5. Crepitus

Greenstick

Only in children, due to ↑ bone flexibility. Under P, bone bends and springs back. Small # on convex side of bend. Stable

Compound Fractures

A fracture that communicates with skin via wound. Potential for infection.

MANAGEMENT: 1. Scene of accident: Local P dressing, elevate limb, keep warm, splint

2. A&E Assessment:
   a) Correct shock: Blood transfusion. Analgesics cautiously (mask symptoms)
   b) Prevent infection: Debridement, antibiotics, tetanus ± gas, gangrene prophylaxis
   c) Assess extent of local and assess inj: Skin loss, nerve and arterial damage. X-R of #
3. Operation: Sterile conditions impt
   Muscle: Divide fascia. Remove necrotic foreign material
   Vessels: Repair major vessels. Tie small
   Nerves: Mark ends c̄ suture
   Tendons: Appose if little infection
   Bone: Remove fragments, clean ends, reduce
   If unstable # can:
   a) Int fixation—if little infection; <6hrs post inj; or major vessel damage
   OR
   b) Ext Splintage ± Steinmann pins
   Skin: Remove as little as poss. Aim is 1° skin closure unless infection++. May need graft. If infection++ pack
4. Plaster: Include joints above and below #. Pad well. Split from end

to end to allow for oedema. X-R control

5. Post-op:
   a) i-v fluids; Analgesia; Physio esp Leg & Chest exercises
   b) Elevate limb → Venous return ↑; Swelling ↓
   c) Plaster care:
      1. Mark limits of blood staining
      2. Smell plaster. Bad smell may indicate infection
      3. If too tight → swollen discoloured digits
      Rx: Remove plaster
   d) Continue antibiotics for 5/7
   e) Wound: Don't disturb
   f) Immobilise eg 3/12 for # femur or tibia
      Signs of union:
      1) Tenderness
      2) Pain on springing
      3) X-R: Callus, no # line
   g) Rehabilitate: Physio & OT

COMPLICATIONS:

Complications of Fracture (LIST 2 ORTH)

1. Infection
2. Delayed or non-union
3. Malunion
4. Joint stiffness
5. Arterial damage
6. Nerve inj
7. Delayed wound healing
8. Sudeck's atrophy

1. Infection: Tetanus, Gas gangrene, Aerobic infection

2. Delayed or non-union:

Causes of Delayed or Non-union (LIST 3 ORTH)

1. Wide separation of fragments
2. Infection
3. Interposition of soft tissue
4. Inadequate immobilisation
5. Poor blood supply: Eg Avascular necrosis

Rx: Bone graft if no signs of union

3. Joint Stiffness: Due to adhesions. Capsular and ligamentous fibrosis
Rx: Active exercises

4. Arterial Damage: Leads to Volkmann's contracture
Rx: Remove plaster, if no improvement within 1hr re-op

5. Delayed Wound Healing:
Rx: Provide free drainage of infected wound. remove sequestra. Continue immobilisation

6. Nerve Injury:
Rx: Resuture after bony union

7. Sudeck's Atrophy:
Clin: 2/12 post inj pain, swelling and marked jt stiffness
Rx: Physio

FRACTURES AND DISLOCATIONS (UPPER LIMB)

Clavicle

Occurs in mid-shaft

RX: Children: If no displacement sling for 1/52
Older: splint for 3–4/52 c̄ 2 circular slings. By 6/52 full mvts

Neck of Humerus

Aged. Lower fragment displaced medially

CLIN: Bruising of arm; Danger of stiff shoulder

RX: In the young immobilise for 2–3/52

Supracondylar # Humerus

May or may not be displaced

CLIN: Tender swelling. Occ Deformity or crepitus. Lower fragment backwards.

Risk to circulation and nerves esp Brachial artery; Median nerve → claw hand; Volkmann's contracture. Occ Myositis ossificans

RX: Keep elbow at 90° flexion. Reduce by rotation c̄ slight pressure on olecranon

Signs of Volkmann's Contracture

EARLY: 1. Pain, pallor of hand
2. No radial pulse
3. Weak forearm
4. Pain on moving fingers

LATE: 1. Immobile painless hand
2. Nerve palsies

RX: RUA, collar & cuff sling. Splintage

or Separation of Medial Condyle

Med condyle pulled off by flexor muscles attached. Form hole on medial side of elbow jt. Occ displaced condyle migrates via the hole into the elbow jt

RX: Manipulation of elbow in valgus. Op and resite fragment but risk of ulnar nerve damage. Rest for 5/52

Capitellum

of lat condyle. May never unite

RX: Surgically replace and fix with screw

COMPLICATION: Occ never unite. Risk OA

Forearm

Esp middle 1/3 of shaft of radius and ulna. Ass c̄ Sudeck's atrophy

RX: Usually RUA c̄ elbow at 90° in PoP. Occ internal fixation plating & screw
Movement from 10th day. Bony union about 10/52
Galleazi Fracture: # radial shaft c̄ dislocation inf radio–ulnar jt
Monteggia Fracture: # radial shaft c̄ dislocation of radial head (Mont = head)

Colles Fracture

lower end radius. Often 4cm from distal end. Change of bone structure at this point, less cortex. Often comminuted. Ass c̄ # ulnar styloid or rupture ulnar collateral ligament

CAUSE: Fall over outstretched hand. Lower end displaced backwards and radially. (If displaced forwards = Smith's #)

CLIN: Pain over ulnar styloid >over radius

RX: RUA Plaster 4/52. Place hand in ulnar deviation & slight flexion. Make sure fingers move. Exercises. In 2/12 check that wrist mvts are good

COMPLICATIONS: 1) General (see LIST 2 ORTH)
2) Disuse atrophy
3) Rupture Ext Pollicis Longus
4) Shoulder hand syndrome
5) Carpal tunnel syndrome (rare)

Scaphoid

Fall on outstretched hand or sudden dorsiflexion. Usually across waist of scaphoid.

CLIN: Painful wrist mvts; Poor grip. Poor blood supply therefore often non-union (except polar # often good union), avascular necrosis in 1/3. Sometimes no X-R signs for 10/7

RX: Immobilise wrist for 7/52. Put hand in flexion. May exercise radial styloid to assist mvt of wrist.
If ass perilunar dislocation → median nerve palsy. Occ OA

Triquetral

Best seen on lateral X-R

Bennett's

Base of 1st metacarpal. Easy to reduce, difficult to maintain, need pins

Phalanges of Fingers

Immobilise for 3/52. Plaster splint in flexion. Can → mallet finger

Dislocation of Shoulder

Ant >Post. Usually caused by fall on outstretched arm. Head of humerus comes out in front of shoulder and lies beneath coracoid process. Cannot abduct

RX: Closed reduction (Kocher maneouvre).

Hippocratic method. The older the person the less the shoulder should be immobilised. Don't allow elevation as it may tear a hole in the capsule esp in the young. In young, splint in int rotation for 3/52

COMPLICATION: Occ get damage to circumflex nerve or axillary artery

Dislocation of Acromioclavicular Joint

Fall on shoulder tip. Outer end of clavicle elevated

RX: No special Rx. Rest in sling 1/52 or screw. Rest does not relocate but allows full mvt. Screw often results in ↓ mvt

Dislocation of Elbow

Forearm is dislocated back on upper arm

RX: Reduction by traction 4–5/52 rest

COMPLICATIONS: Post traumatic ossification (Myositis Ossificans). Brachial artery damage. Ulnar nerve damage

Dislocation of Lunate

Through middle of carpus between two rows of carpal bones. Lunate bone usually displaced forward in carpal tunnel. The contents of canal are flexor tendons of wrist and fingers and the median nerve. Results in wasting of muscles supplied by median nerve
X-R findings: Lat X-R shows ant displacement c̄ loss of normal "3" cup sign

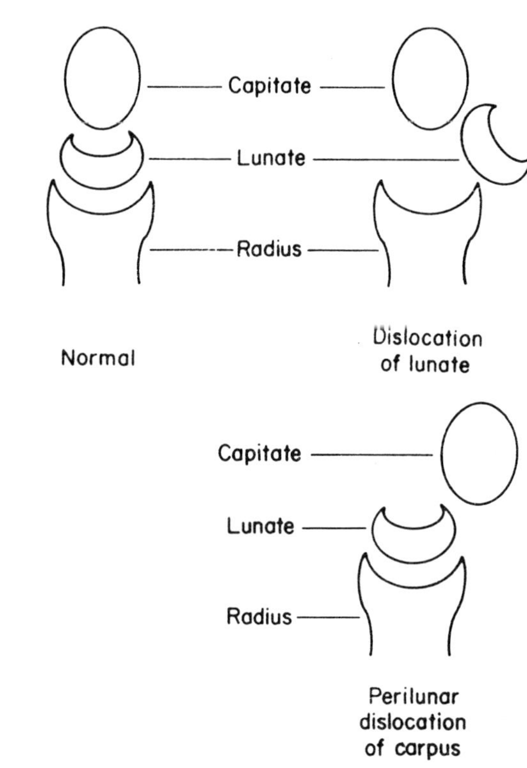

Figure 1 X Ray appearances of dislocation lunate.

RX: Replace or remove lunate within first 2 days

OTHER DISLOCATIONS

a) Perilunar dislocation of carpus
b) Dislocation of lunate & 1/2 scaphoid
c) Trans-scapho-perilunar dislocation of carpus
d) Dislocation of lunate & scaphoid
e) Peri-scapho-lunar dislocation of carpus

HAND INJURIES

Assessment & Rx

HISTORY: Mechanism & circumstances of injury. ? previous tetanus prophylaxis. Time from accident. Occupation

EXAMINATION: a) Skin loss: Decide if skin loss irrecoverable
b) ?#: X-R
c) Nerve injury:
Median nerve test—no thumb abduction
Ulnar nerve test—pass extended thumb across palm c̄ no flexion at PIP. Adduct little finger
d) Tendon inj: Posture of digit indicates eg c̄ Ext digitorum
Distal division → "mallet finger", no distal ext; Central division → "boutonniere", no PIP ext
e) Ligamentous inj: Esp c̄ dislocations

TREATMENT: If clean injury—repair. If untidy—debridement, then repair

Anaesthesia: use digital block for digit, brachial block for palm
Use avascular field c̄ pneumatic cuff. Skin closure c̄ no tension. Put PoP in position of function eg MCP jts flexed, thumb palmar abducted. Then put in sling & elevate hand. Tetanus prophylaxis & antibiotics

Special Types of Injury

SLICE OFF INJURIES TO TIP

RX: Thick split skin graft

LONGITUDINAL BURSTING INJURY

RX: Debridement. Bandage. Oedema slowly ↓

FINGER AMPUTATION

RX: If thumb or index finger try to preserve length. Occ microsurgery or replantation

SUBUNGUAL HAEMATOMA

RX: Drill through nail plate then bandage

COMPOUND # DISTAL PHALANX

RX: Remove wedge of contused necrotic tissue

TENDON REPAIR

RX: If tidy, 1° repair, good as no muscle contractures. Use avascular field & mattress suture. Immobilise for 2–3/52. put in PoP for 3/52. If finger flexors damaged, retain profundus not sublimis tendons

NERVE INJURIES

RX: Avascular fields. Trim ends. Immobilise for 3/52

FINGER

RX: Reduce finger precisely

2° Reconstructive Procedures

1. Neurovascular Island Flap transfer
   Eg to restore sensation to thumb
2. Replantation
   Eg use toe to reconstruct thumb

OTHER CONDITIONS OF UPPER LIMB

Driller's Disease

Cystic change in hand & wrist due to prolonged exposure to vibration of frequency 2500hz

Stenosing Tenosynovitis (De Quervain's Disease)

Ass c̄ tennis elbow. Inflam of ext pollicis longus or abductor pollicis over radial styloid. ? cause

CLIN: Pain++ on adduction of thumb; swelling over styloid

RX: 50% spontaneous cure over 18/12. In the rest, remove tendon sheath. Can use steroids and/or ultrasound

Tennis elbow

Supra-condylar region of outer side of humerus. Inflam of lat epicondylar muscle. Usually recover

RX: Best is rest but can use steroid, diathermy, ultrasound or procaine

Trigger Thumb & Finger

Nodules on flexor tendons in thumb around entrance to fibrous tunnel. Finger locks. Occ Cong. Ass c̄ Rh Arth

RX: Incise tunnel

SPINAL FRACTURES

Cervical Spine Fractures

Often fatal. Ass c̄ Whiplash inj, Head inj

a) Flexion inj → wedge compression #
b) Flexion ± rotation inj → subluxation, dislocation or #-dislocation
c) Hyperextension inj → # Atlas or Axis, extension subluxation or cord damage
d) Vertical compression inj → # Atlas or "burst" # of vert body

Distinguish between stable inj ie intact post ligs and unstable inj c̄ risk to spinal cord

CLIN: Local pain, tenderness & bruising. May cause root or cord damage eg Tetraplegia

RX: Stabilise. If paraplegia, open reduction & plating of #, prevent bed sores & rehabilitation

Thoracic and Lumbar Spine Fractures

Stable if interspinous lig intact

WEDGE COMPRESSION FRACTURE OF VERTEBRAL BODY

Common. 2° to fall on feet or buttocks. Local kyphosis

RX: Physio. Bed rest 1–4/52. Occ plaster jacket

FRACTURE–DISLOCATION

Uncommon. Unstable spine usually → cord inj

RIB FRACTURES

Usually 2° to direct inj. Severe pain

RX: Analgesia. Ribs unite spontaneously

COMPLICATIONS: (Esp if multiple rib #s). Haemothorax; Pneumothorax; Surgical emphysema; Pneumonia; Flail chest—paradoxical mvt

PELVIC FRACTURES

TYPES: 1. Avulsion
2. Pelvic ring # c̄ no displacement
3. Pelvic ring # c̄ displacement

Pelvic Ring # c̄ Displacement

Two or more fractures of ring. Ass c̄ complications. 3 types

HINGE TYPE

A-P crush injury → # pubic ramus c̄ # ilium or # dislocation SI jt

CLIN: Persistent SI pain

VERTICAL TYPE

Fall from height onto 1 leg → # pubic ramus & # ilium c̄ upward displacement → sciatic nerve damage

COMPRESSION TYPE

AP crush injury # pubic rami, central segment displaced backwards → bladder & membranous urethra damage

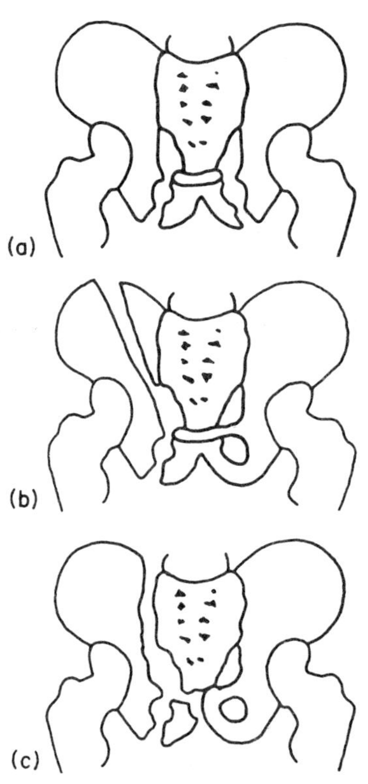

Figure 2 Fractures of pelvic ring. (a) Compression type (b) Hinge type (c) Vertical type

CLIN: 1. Due to #: Tenderness; Pain; Shock; Inability to stand
2. Due to sciatic nerve damage: Anaesthesia & weak leg
3. Due to GUS inj

Investigations

- X-R pelvis ± cysto–urethrograms

Management

1. CORRECT SHOCK

2. CATHETERISE

a) Catheter enters easily and only little urine obtained. Suspect bladder rupture. Op essential
b) Catheter will not pass. Suspect rupture of membranous urethra. Op essential

3. RX OF #

a) Hinge type: RUA. Nurse on hammock for 3/12
b) Vertical type: Leg traction on affected side for 3/12
c) Compression type: RUA ± int fixation. Bed rest for 3–4/52

4. RX OF BLADDER RUPTURE

a) Extraperitoneal Rupture: Suprapubic cystotomy. May need to open peritoneum & explore for any ass inj. Antibiotics
b) Intraperitoneal Rupture: Treat shock & haem. Close tear transperitoneally; Aspirate peritoneal fluid, catheterise; Antibiotics

5. RX OF MEMBRANOUS URETHRA RUPTURE

Try to pass catheter, if possible leave in place for 2wks. Repair urethra

FRACTURES & DISLOCATIONS (LOWER LIMB)

Femur Upper End

INTRACAPSULAR

ie Transcervical, Subcapital
Often in elderly c̄ little trauma

CLIN: Slow poor union; Lat rotation & shortening

RX: Internal fixation eg Smith Peterson nail. Occ remove head and replace c̄ metal prothesis (Thompson). Mobilise early to avoid pneumonia

EXTRACAPSULAR

ie Per-trochanteric, Sub-trochanteric & Basal
Commoner. Always union in 12/52, unless a pathological #

RX: Internal fixation c̄ blade plate & screw. If not fit then traction & "pin & plaster" for 14/52. Plaster prevents both sore heel and foot ending in equinus. Mobilise early

Complications of Arthroplasty (LIST 4 ORTH)

1. Infection
2. Dislocation
3. Hetertrophic bone formation
4. Femur
5. Loosening of cup in cement (if used)

Femur in Mid-shaft

Usually direct violence in young

RX: 1. Conservative: Fixed traction in Thomas Splint. Femur bent over a pad. Use 10–12lb traction. Union—12/52. Then active mvts in bed
2. Intramedullary nailing: For non-comminuted mid shaft # in young. Union—12/52

Around Knee Joint

Quite common. Tibial med & lat

condyles >femoral. Occ crush inj

RX: Thomas splint 4/52, then active mvts in bed. Wt bear in 12/52

Shaft of Tibia

UPPER 1/3

→ damage popliteal artery

MIDDLE 1/3

Common esp at junction c̄ lower 1/3

RX: Reduction in long leg plaster if possible. Otherwise fix c̄ plate & screws or use medullary nail
Any ass c̄ # fibula will unite spontaneously

LOWER 1/3

Poor union as few muscles & poor blood supply. At 8–10/52 can tell if bone graft needed
Two types of bone graft:
a) Cortical bone from other tibia
b) Ileal cancellous bone chips (Best)
If graft works it is firm in 10/52

Potts

#-dislocations of ankle. Several types: Ext rot >Abd & ext >Adduction >Dome of talus

RX: Manipulation, reduction and restoration of mortice. Below knee plaster for 6/52. No wt bearing for 6/52
N.B: #s of med malleolus running up and out from ankle are unstable & painful. This is usually an adduction injury

Rx: Open reduction. After 6/52 crepe bandage to control post-cast swelling

in the foot

OS CALCIS

Due to fall on heels. Always unites but may disable sub-talar jt interfering with walking on rough ground. Occ avascular necrosis

RX: If displaced, compression bandage. Early mobilisation. No wt bearing for 10/52

METATARSALS

A) WTS FALLING ON FOOT:

Rx: Reduction; Immobilisation 5/52

B) "MARCH" #: A stress fracture esp of 2nd metatarsal. Usually occurs when bone subjected to unusual or sudden stress eg long marches or walks or carrying backpack. Other stress #s include shaft of tibia, clavicle

Clin: Pain over dorsum of foot over 2nd metatarsal neck. Local tenderness and swelling. X-R +ve after 3/52. Always union

Dislocation of hip

Due to RTA. Femur out of jt backwards c̄ medial rotation

RX: MUA urgently. Delay → avascular necrosis of femoral head (femoral head is supplied by vessel running down ligamentum teres). Then immobilise for 6/52 to allow time for capsule to heal

COMPLICATIONS: 1. Avascular necrosis of femoral head
2. Occ damage to sciatic nerve

Causes of Avascular Necrosis (LIST 5 ORTH)

1. Fracture:
   Eg Femoral head; Scaphoid; Lunate; Talus
2. Drugs:
   a) Steroids
   b) Cytotoxic drugs
3. Cushing's Disease
4. Pancreatitis
5. Radiotherapy
6. Sickle cell Anaemia
7. Occlusive vascular disease
8. Fat embolism
9. Caisson Disease
10. Gaucher's Disease

Slipped Upper Femoral Epiphysis

Late childhood. ? cause. Ass c̄ obesity. Occ bilat

CLIN: Pain in hip or knee; Limp
X-R: Displaced epiphysis (Lat view needed)

RX: Fix femoral head c̄ pins. If severe MUA ± op

COMPLICATIONS: Occ OA; Avascular necrosis

Dislocation of Knee

Uncommon, unpleasant inj. Medial or lat lig is torn. Cruciate ligs often torn
Lat dislocation → lat popliteal nerve palsy c̄ foot drop

RX: Open op c̄ repair of ligaments. No wt bearing for 6–8/52
Exercises in bed

Dislocations of Mid-tarsal and Subtalar Joints

Uncommon. May be ass c̄ Potts #

RX: Reduction & fixation 6–8/52

RUPTURES

Rupture Supraspinatus

Fall on adducted arm stretching tendon

CLIN: Can't begin abduction of shoulder

RX: Open op if large tear → some disability

Knee Sprains

Cruciate and int lat lig sprains important. Int lat lig inj ass c̄ lat condylar #

INVESTIGATION: • Test jt stability

RX: Immobilise 6/52. Op if:
a) Ant cruciate lig damage c̄ a piece of bone pulled off tibia
b) Rupture of lateral or medial lig

Rupture of Achilles Tendon

Approx $2\frac{1}{2}$cm above insertion into os calcis. Usually due to indirect violence

CLIN: Difficulty c̄ walking; Can't stand on 1 leg on tip-toe; Palpable gap on tendon; Can't plantarflex v.R

RX: End to end suture. Above knee plaster c̄ knee flexed at 45° & foot in equinus for 4/52. No wt bearing. Then below knee plaster c̄ foot at 90° for 4/52. Some wt bearing. Then wt bear c̄ immobilisation. The equinus contracture corrects spontaneously

Rupture of Lateral Ligaments of Ankle

Rare. Adduction injury. More serious than Potts #

CLIN: Severe pain; Bruising++; Swelling

RX: Plaster cast no wt bearing 6–7/52. May need later tenodesis

INTERNAL DERANGEMENTS OF KNEE

Injury to Menisci (Semilunar cartilage)

TYPES: Ant horn tear; Post horn tear; complete longitudinal ie "bucket handle" tear (commonest)
Tear occurs due to rotational strain on tibia c̄ knee flexed & foot fixed
20 med: 1 lat semilunar cartilage inj because med cartilage attached to coronary ligament and tibia

CLIN: Sudden pain in knee, effusion in few hrs. No full extension ("Locking"). Will recover c̄ rest but will then recur on exercise. Wasting of quads

RX: Menisectomy

COMPLICATION: Risk of OA

Congenital Abnormalities of Menisci

Rare. Lat >med menisci. Presents at 10–12 yrs. Occ bilat

CLIN: Recurrent effusion; Loud noise on bending knee; Painful & wasted quads

RX: Often settle spontaneously. Occ Menisectomy

Loose bodies

OSTEOCHONDRITIS DISSECANS

Local articular surface necrosis → detached fragment → intra-articular loose body. Can occur elsewhere eg talus but 80% are in knee. Young M>F. ? cause

CLIN: Pain in knee after exercise; no history of trauma; Swollen & tender knee; quads wasted

INVESTIGATION: • X-R: Well circumscribed lesion of the bone at the articular surface

RX: If not detached, splint. No wt bearing for 6/52. Surgery if detached

OA

CLIN: Locking, painful, unstable knee jt

RX: Remove

OTHERS

1. Synovial Osteochondromatosis (See below)
2. Chip # of a jt surface

INFECTIONS OF BONES AND JOINTS

TB of bone

Esp small long bones, carpus, tarsus, & large jts

CLIN: Slow onset, mild malaise

RX: a) TB limb: Immobilise. Triple therapy for 12–18/12
b) TB spine: 6–8/12. Triple therapy then bone graft to arthrodese. Occ paraplegia results

DD: Septic bone infections which are distinguished by rapid onset, profound illness & predilection for metaphysis of long bones

TB METACARPUS

May be a 1° TB lesion

CLIN: Chr swelling of fingers c̄ sl pain & stiffness; Spindle shaped lesion. If jt involved more painful

TB KNEE

CLIN: Swollen knee. "Night Cries" as pain occurs when protective muscle spasm of day is lost; Swollen knee ± redness. May have pain referred to front of thigh, front of knee ± Trendelenberg's sign; Signs of primary TB

TB SPINE (POTTS DISEASE)

Thoracic, lumbar > Cervical

CLIN: Long history c̄ sl malaise; stiff back. Occ Abscess in loin c̄ swelling

TB HIP

Commonest bone TB. Child> Adult

CLIN: Hip mvts ↓; Gluteal & thigh muscles wasted. Occ Abscess

TB ARTHRITIS

Usually from TB bone when near a jt capsule

Acute Osteomyelitis

Child >Adult. Staph >Salmonella Usually metaphyseal. Medullary endarteries predispose to medullary cavity abscesses which go through bone into subperiosteum. Occ → destruction of diaphysis

CLIN: Sudden onset of pain & acute tenderness. Flushed, ill & feverish

INVESTIGATIONS: • X-R: Osteoporosis early; Later Periosteal reaction; Sequestrum (dead bone); Involucrum; Cloacae
• Blood culture

RX: Antibiotics. Drain pus, irrigate & splint

Chronic Osteomyelitis

Usually 2° to acute osteomyelitis. Staph > Strep. Long bones. Bone cavities ± sequestra. Often sinus to skin

CLIN: Purulent discharge. Flare-ups → pain, pyrexia & abscess

INVESTIGATION: • X-R: Thick bone c̄ patchy sclerosis ± sequestra

RX: Rest. Antibiotics. Drain abscess. Op to remove dead bone

Brodie's Abscess

Chr abscess near metaphysis. No preceding acute attack

CLIN: Deep boring pain

INVESTIGATION: • X-R: Oval cavity surrounded by sclerosis

RX: Op, drain abscess and obliterate dead space

Arthritis 2° to Burns

Always ass c̄ osteomyelitis. Deep seated infection

CLIN: Pain, distress. Occ Pathological dislocation

RX: Antibiotics ± arthrodesis. Immobilise until infection ↓

OSTEOARTHRITIS

Slow onset. Ass c̄ injury, articular surface damage
Commonly affects Knee, Hip, Lumbar spine (3–5), Cervical spine (C5–7). 1st CMC

INVESTIGATION: • X-R: Osteophytes; Loose bodies; Subluxations; Sclerosis; Pseudocysts

RX: Surgery:
Knee: Arthrodesis >Arthroplasty
Hips: Arthroplasty >Arthrodesis
Hand: Occ excise trapezium
Lumbar & Cervical spine: Occ laminectomy

EPIPHYSITIS

Esp childhood

CLIN: Pain, tenderness and swelling in epiphyses

Common types:

Femoral Head (Perthes Disease)

M>F. Esp 5–10 years. Occ FH. Cause unknown. Bilat in 30%

CLIN: Pain & stiffness in hip; Limp. Occ → OA as adult

INVESTIGATION: • X-R: Epiphysis is irregular & fragmented; Head of femur may deform and flatten

RX: Abduct & int rotate. Frame fixation for 2 yrs. Bed rest

Tibial Tubercle (Osgood Schlatter Disease)

At site of insertion of patellar tendon. Esp 8–14 yrs

INVESTIGATION: • X-R: Fragmented irregular epiphysis c̄ soft tissue swelling

RX: Reassure. 2–3 yrs to heal

Navicular (Kohler Disease)

Pain & swelling over dorsum of foot. No inversion & eversion of tarsus. Good prognosis. Occ OA as adult

Os Calcis (Severs Disease)

Harmless

RX: Rest

PAGET'S DISEASE

CLIN: Headache; Pain esp legs & back. Often no symptoms. Bowing of tibia and femur. ↑ head size. Kyphosis; Bones occ hot tender and painful. Occ Blindness; Deafness; 2° jt changes; ↑ BP; Cardiac failure. In long standing disease may → Osteosarcoma

INVESTIGATIONS: • X-R: Lytic & Sclerotic areas; Bony expansion; Cortical thickening; Coarse trabeculation; Kyphosis. Occ Path #; Incremental #; Osteosarcoma

• SXR: Lytic areas "Osteoporosis Circumscripta" → sclerosis; Frontal bossing; "Tam-o'-shanter" skull; Obliteration of foramina; Facial bone sclerosis (DD: Fibrous dysplasia)

DD of X-Ray Findings: 1. Sclerotic mets esp Ca Prostate
2. Reticuloses

CONGENITAL DEFORMITIES

Club Foot

2 Types:

1. CALCANEO–VALGUS

CLIN: Heel normal or large; Easy foot eversion; Exaggerated eversion and dorsiflexion; "Toes touch tibia"; ↓ inversion; ↓ plantar flexion. Occ 2° to abnormal tarsus

RX: Stretch strap foot into equinus and varus. Often normal by 5–6 yrs.

PROG: Good

2. EQUINO–VARUS

Bad prog if no early Rx. Tendency to recur. 2 Types:

a) **ALMOST PHYSIOLOGICAL:**

Clin: Newborn c̄ foot inverted & plantar flexed, inverted heel

Rx: Can be passively over corrected

b) **RIGID, ORGANIC EQUINO–VARUS:**

Clin: Inverted foot & heel, plantar flexed, metatarsal inturned. Passive correction to neutral impossible. R foot >L. Ass c̄ spina bifida & CDH

Rx: Manipulation not UA in first wk then plaster below knee c̄ foot everted & dorsiflexed, reapplying wkly. Often plaster will correct varus but not equinus. If uncorrected at 2 mths divide all tight bands. Relapses common

Rx of Relapses or Neglected Cases: Various ops: eg Tendon transfer; Calcaneal osteotomy; Arthrodesis of calconeo–cuboid jt. Above 12yrs, bony op needed

Pes Cavus

A hollow foot c̄ ass deformity of toes

CLIN: Effusion; Tenderness; Wasting of quads. Occ Pain under metatarsal head. Ass c̄ Spina bifida, Polio, Friedrich's Ataxia

RX: If mild: Chiropody & surgical shoe
If severe: Op on toes, soft tissues of sole or tarsal jt

Genu Valgum (Knock-knee)

80% children 0–2 yrs are knock-kneed. 1st child >others. F>M

CAUSES: 1. Benign idiopathic
2. # lower femur
3. Rh Arth
4. OA
5. Paget's
6. Dyschondroplasia
7. Osteomyelitis

RX: Most improve spontaneously. If severe, supracondylar osteotomy of femur is carried out

Genu Varum (Bow leg)

Common 1–3 yrs. Occ 2° to Vit D deficiency

RX: Observe. Rarely osteotomy

Congenital Dislocation of the Hip (CDH)

1 in 1000 GB children. F>M. Uni >Bilat
Cause malformed acetabulum or abnormal femoral head ± shallow socket

CLIN: Ortolani's Test is used to detect in perinatal period. If missed presents later c̄ delay in walking or abnormal gait

RX: To place femoral head in contact c̄ acetabulum & keep it there. Best treated young. Prog L>R
In neonate: Rx immediately by splint in abduction for 3 mths
In older children: Splint hips in abduction & medial rotation
N.B Occ get interposition of soft tissue between acetabulum and femur preventing reduction. Diagnose c̄ arthrogram. May need open reduction c̄ soft tissue removal

Torticollis

Contracture of sternomastoid

PATHOGENESIS: ? due to thrombosis of vessels to sternomastoid → degeneration of muscle

CLIN: Head rotated to one side

RX: Some respond to stretching & rotating head. If unsuccessful, Op at 3–5 years as prolonged torticollis → facial asymmetry.

Congenital Scoliosis

Uncommon. Abnormal vertebral bodies esp wedge shaped in dorsal spine

RX: Exercises

PROG: Good

Flat Feet See next section

ACQUIRED DEFORMITY

Cervical lordosis; Dorsal kyphosis; Lumbar lordosis are normal
Present by 7–8 yrs

Kyphosis

Causes of Kyphosis (LIST 6 ORTH)

1. Congenital:
   Cong spine anomaly
2. Infection:
   a) TB
   b) Polio
   c) Other eg Staph
3. Traumatic:
   Wedge compression fracture of vertebral body
4. Neoplastic:
   Eg Spinal Tumour
5. Metabolic & Endocrine:
   a) Osteomalacia
   b) Acromegaly
   c) Paget's Disease
6. Arthritides:
   a) Rheumatoid arthritis
   b) Ankylosing spondylitis
7. Osteoporosis
8. Scheuermann's Disease
9. Intervertebral Disc prolapse or degeneration
10. Neuromuscular diorders

May be local eg TB or general eg Polio
In Scheuermann's get pain in thoracic spine of teenager due to wedging of affected vertebra(e). Self limiting

Acquired Lordosis

Rare. Ass c̄ disc degeneration, prolapsed In.v disc

Scoliosis

Causes of Scoliosis (LIST 7 ORTH)

A. CONGENITAL
  1. Abnormal vertebral body
     Eg Butterfly vertebra, Hemivertebra
  2. Associated with congenital disorders:
     Eg Marfan's Syndrome; Friedrich's ataxia; Osteogenesis Imperfecta

B. ACQUIRED
  1. Structural—persists when bending over:
     a) Paralytic eg Polio; Syringomyelia; Muscular dystrophy
     b) Idiopathic
     c) TB
     d) Neurofibromatosis
     e) Bony tumour
  2. Postural—lost when bending over:
     Eg renal colic; muscular spasm
  3. Compensatory—due to unequal length of legs

Dorsal scoliosis is ass c̄ rib deformities

CLIN: "Humpback" due to angles of ribs forming peak of curve

IDIOPATHIC SCOLIOSIS

F>M

CLIN: Onset 4–14 yrs. Begins in dorsal region; Slow progressive scoliosis. Occ self limiting

RX: Observe—if progressing at 3–4/12 use Milwaukee brace or Risser cast (adjustable splints). Occ int splints (Harrington's rods)

PARALYTIC SCOLIOSIS

Unstable deformity. Esp marked if ass c̄ UMN lesion

RX: Correct c̄ spinal fusion

Flat Feet: Pes Planus

PATHOLOGICAL FLAT FEET

CLIN: Cong abnormality of tarsus. Feet flat & everted

RX: Remove "bony bar"; use insoles; tarsal arthrodesis

PARALYTIC FLAT FEET

Esp paralysis of tibialis ant. May be 2° to polio

RX: Tib post inserted into tarsus or peronei ± tarsal arthrodesis

Hallux Rigidus

OA of 1st MTP jt. Common in teens and >50 yrs. Rarely ass c̄ osteochondritis of 1st metatarsal head (Frieberg's Disease)

CLIN: Pain on "taking off" mvts. Thick swollen 1st MTP due to damage of epiphyseal cartilage

RX: In young, 5% need arthroplasty
In old, very painful stage → stiffness → painlessness. May need arthoplasty eg simple excision of base of proximal phalanx (Keller's op)

Hallux Valgus

2 types:

1. CONGENITAL

All toes in valgus. develop large exostoses

RX: Remove exostoses. Metatarsal osteotomy

2. ACQUIRED

Due to cramped feet, bad shoes. May dislocate 2nd toe due to P ↑.

CLIN: Very painful. May get infection of bursa on head of 1st metatarsal

RX: Exercise Exostosis, remove base prox phalanx, remove capsule on outer side, straighten toes. Leave bursa

Hammer toes

May be due to bad footwear

CLIN: Fixed flexion deformity. Esp 2nd toe

RX: Excise corn, excise IP jt, then arthrodesis. Occ amputate

POLIO

Spread by faecal–oral route. Invades the spinal cord, attacks ant horn cells

CLIN: 2 stages of disease:
a) Febrile stage: 10–14 days of Temp ↑; Limb pains; Backache; Headaches; Malaise; Mvts ↓; Sore throat ± Meningism. Most recover but some develop paralysis
b) Paralytic Stage: Temp normal; Tender painful muscles. Then feel better, muscle tenderness ↓ ± paralysis esp shoulder elevators, triceps, thenar gp; opponens (thumb)), tibialis ant, quads, calf muscles, abdominal muscles, diaphragm. Recovery starts 8–9/52, ends by 1yr

PREVENTION: Vaccination

RX: Prevent contractures by passive mvts c̄ splints
Surgery assess after 1yr:
i) Bony Ops: Arthrodesis—foot, ankle, hip, wrist
ii) Tendon & soft tissue Ops: Tendon transfer eg pectoralis major into biceps, esp if non-wt bearing jt affected
iii) Amputations: Rare eg painful blue ulcerated foot

COMPLICATIONS: 1. Circulation ↓ → blue cold limb
2. Respiratory failure
3. Short limb in child as epiphyseal growth ↓
4. Contractures

SKELETAL TUMOURS

Metastases

Commonest. Axial, proximal >distal. Most are osteolytic eg from breast, lung, thyroid, kidney. Others are sclerotic eg from prostate, breast, GIT
Path # ass c̄ hyperCa^{2+}

Tumour Like Lesions

DYSPLASIAS

Commonest fibrous dysplasia. Mono or poly-ostotic

CLIN: Present as #; Multiple #s → bony deformities. Ass c̄ Osteomalacia

INVESTIGATION: • X-R: lucent, ground glass & sclerotic areas. #s
Albright's syndrome is ass c̄ pigmentation, precocity

CARTILAGE CAPPED EXOSTOSES (OSTEOCHONDROMAS)

Bony outgrowths c̄ cartilage caps. Grow away from growth plate. Stop growth at maturity. Rarely → sarcoma. Usually asymptomatic

Diaphyseal Aclasis is multiple osteochondromata c̄ bone modelling abnormalities. Pre-malignant → chondrosarcomas

RETICULOENDOTHELIOSES

i) Eosinophil granuloma
ii) Schuller–Christian disease
iii) Histiocytosis X

MUCOPOLYSACCARIDOSES

i) Gaucher's
ii) Hurler's
iii) Niemann–Pick's
iv) Hunter's etc

BROWN TUMOURS OF HPT

Great mimic on X-R eg mimics Osteoclastoma
X-R: Lucent areas

SIMPLE BONE CYST

Children

CLIN: Asymptomatic. May present c̄ # or pain

INVESTIGATION: • X-R: Lytic, well defined areas esp humeral metaphysis. Occ #

RX: Spontaneous cure after #. If not, curettage c̄ bone chips. Also irrigation c̄ steroids

ANEURYSMAL BONE CYST

X-R: Lytic expansile area esp in immature bone inc axial skeleton

RX: Curettage, X-Rad

DD: Giant cell tumour

PREMALIGNANT CONDITIONS TO BONE TUMOURS

1. Diaphyseal Aclasis
2. X-Rad
3. Fibrous Dysplasia
4. Paget's Disease
5. Neurofibromatosis
6. Maffucci's Syndrome (See next Section)

Primary Tumour

A. Bone Forming—Benign

OSTEOID OSTEOMA

CLIN: Severe pain esp nocté, responds to Aspirin. Commonly cortex of long bones

INVESTIGATIONS:
- X-R: Lucent area c̄ central nidus. Sclerosis ++ if cortical
- Radioisotope bone scan: Very hot area

RX: Local excision

DD: Sclerosing osteomyelitis of Garré

OSTEOBLASTOMA

Children. Usually in spine

CLIN: Painful scoliosis

B. Bone Forming—Malignant

OSTEOSARCOMA

Occurs in 2nd decade and elderly when ass c̄ Pagets. Also ass c̄ X-Rad. Commonest primary. Long bone metaphysis. Parosteal type is a more benign form

CLIN: Swelling ± constant pain when periosteum elevated. Mets via blood to lung. Bone forming

INVESTIGATIONS:
- X-R: Periosteal reaction (Codman's △ & Sun ray spicules). Bony destruction, new bone formation & soft tissue mass
- Biopsy

RX: Amputate at 6/12 if no mets. Cytotoxic drugs (Kade method)

PROG: Parosteal > 1° > 2° to Paget's

C. Cartilage Forming—Benign

CHONDROMA

Mature cartilage affected. Short bones of hands & feet. Often spontaneous #. If widespread termed Ollier's disease (Hereditary chondrodystrophy) If ass c̄ angiomas (Maffuci's syndrome), pre-malignant

INVESTIGATION:
- X-R: Lucent areas c̄ specks of calcification

CHONDROBLASTOMA

M > F. Usually < 20yrs. Esp knee

INVESTIGATION:
- X-R: Lucent area, well defined c̄ reactive sclerosis. Both sides of epiphyseal plate

RX: Excise

D. Cartilage Forming—Malignant

CHONDROSARCOMA

Usually 30–60yrs. May be secondary to chondroma (10%). Usual sites proximal long bones, pelvis, shoulder girdle. Ass c̄ myxomatous change (rare)

INVESTIGATION:
- X-R: Lucent area, calcification, periosteal reaction, bone destruction, soft tissue mass

RX: Excise

PROG: Fair

E. Fibrous Forming—Benign

NON OSSIFYING FIBROMA (FIBROUS CORTICAL DEFECT)

Young adults. Metaphyseal circumscribed lesion. Path #

INVESTIGATION:
- X-R: Eccentric metaphyseal well defined lucent area

RX: Locally excise

F. Fibrous Forming—Malignant

FIBROSARCOMA

Usually 20–60 yrs. Spindle cell tumour producing collagen. Lysis, no reactive bone. Long bone metaphysis usually affected

INVESTIGATION: • X-R: Lytic area. Soft tissue mass, wispy calcification

RX: Excise widely

G. Vasoformative

ANGIOMA

Esp vertebral body. Occ multiple (Haemangiomatosis)

INVESTIGATION: • X-R:

←— Striated vert body. Occ #

DD: Paget's

H. Marrow Tumours

MULTIPLE MYELOMA

>50yrs. Paraproteinaemia

INVESTIGATIONS: • X-R: 3 presentations
a) Osteoporosis only
b) Well defined lytic punched out lesions (classical)
c) Sclerotic lesions (very rare)

RETICULUM CELL SARCOMA

Usually >20yrs. "Round cell tumour"

INVESTIGATIONS: • X-R: Medulla moth eaten. Periosteal reaction

RX: X-Rad

PROG: Fair

DD:
1. Osteomyelitis
2. Osteolytic mets
3. Fibrosarcoma
4. Lymphoma
5. Leukaemia
6. Malignant fibrous histiocytoma

EWING'S TUMOUR

Usually <20yrs. "Round cell tumour". Early mets
Usually affects pelvis, long bones (Metaphysis or diaphysis)

INVESTIGATION: • X-R: Moth eaten medulla. Periosteal reaction. Classical "Onion peel" appearance rare

RX: Local X-Rad

I. Osteoclastoma (Giant Cell Tumour)

Usually 20–40yrs. Usually affects tibia, 15% mets. Often recur

INVESTIGATION: • X-R: Subarticular lytic destruction. Expands bone ends. Rare in immature skeleton

RX: Excision. X-Rad

J. Chordoma

Usually >40yrs. 2M:1F. Malignant. Rare. Affects axial skeleton esp C1, C2 vert body & sacrum. Occ Cord compression

INVESTIGATION: • X-R: Destructive lesion

RX: Excision

K. Adamantinoma (Amelioblastoma)

Jaw or tibia

RX: Excision

SOFT TISSUE TUMOURS

Muscle

1. Myoma—rare
2. Fibrosarcoma—esp subsartorial canal. Mets. Poor prog
3. Rhabdomyosarcoma

Tendon & Tendon Sheaths

BENIGN FIBROMA

Rx: Occ excise

XANTHOMA

Fingers & toes. Yellowish

RX: Excise widely

PROG: Good

Fatty Tumours

LIPOMA

X-R: Lucent area of fat density. Occ Ca^{2+}. Rarely → liposarcoma

Peripheral Nerves

BENIGN NEURILEMMOMA (SCHWANNOMA)

Rx: Excise

NEUROFIBROMATOSIS

Familial. Cafe-au-lait spots. Scoliosis. Cord & nerve root irritation

RX: Excise neurofibromata

NEUROGENIC SARCOMA

Malignant

RX: Excise widely

Synovia (Jt capsule)

GANGLION

Benign, contains mucoid material

RX: Excise

SYNOVIAL OSTEOCHONDROMATOSIS

Multiple loose bodies in jt which calcify

PIGMENTED VILONODULAR SYNOVITIS (PVNS)

Chr proliferation of synovium pigmented c̄ haemosiderin. Swelling of jt esp knee initially painless but later pain & effusions

SYNOVIOMA

Highly malignant. Esp major jts eg knee. Spreads in soft tissue & rarely to bone. Early lung mets

CLIN: Indurated swelling of jt

INVESTIGATION: • X-R: destruction both sides of the jt. Soft tissue mass

DD of Destruction Both Sides of jt on X-R:

1. Infection
2. Synovioma
3. PVNS
4. Haemophilia

RX: Amputate or wide excision & X-Rad

Associations of Neurofibromatosis (LIST 8 ORTH)

1. Skin:
   a) Cafe-au-Lait spots
   b) Neurofibromata
2. Vascular:
   a) Aneurysms
   b) Renal artery stenosis
3. Tumours:
   a) Acoustic neuromas esp bilateral
   b) Dumbell neuromas
   c) Gliomas
   d) Meningiomas
   e) Fibrosarcomas
   e) Phaeochromocytomas
4. Orthopaedic:
   a) Pseudoarthroses
   b) Short segment scoliosis
5. Radiological:
   a) Ribbon ribs; Rib notching
   b) Hemihypertrophy; Hemiatrophy
   c) Pituitary fossa "J" shaped sella
   d) Posterior scalloping of vertebral bodies
   e) Lucent areas in lambdoidal suture
   f) Defective ossification of posterior, superior border of the orbit or sphenoid "The bare orbits"
   g) Asymmetric orbits
   h) Osteomalacia

BACKACHE & SCIATICA

Causes of Backache (LIST 9 ORTH)

A. INTRINSIC
1. Traumatic:
   a) Sprain
   b) Fracture esp compression
   c) Intravertebral disc prolapse
   d) Spondylolisthesis
2. Congenital:
   a) Spondylolisthesis
   b) Transitional vertebra eg Lumbar sacralisation
3. Neoplastic:
   Metastases commoner than primary tumours
4. Inflammatory:
   a) Rheumatoid Arthritis
   b) Ankylosing Spondylitis
   c) Osteomyelitis eg Staph >TB, Brucellosis
5. Idiopathic:
   "Lumbago". Occ psychosomatic
6. Degenerative:
   a) Kyphosis & Scoliosis
   b) Lumbar spondylosis
   c) Senile osteoporosis

B. EXTRINSIC
1. Gynaecological:
   Pelvic tumour invading sacral plexus
2. Abdominal:
   a) PU
   b) Pancreatitis
   c) Cholecystitis
   d) Biliary calculus
3. Hip Arthritis
4. Genito-urinary:
   Eg Renal calculus
5. Vascular:
   Eg Occlusion of aorta or iliac arteries
6. Malingering
7. Psychogenic:
   Eg Hysteria & Anxiety

General Features

GENERAL CLIN OF BACKACHE: a) Onset: If sudden—acute injury. If slow—inflam, tumours, congenital, idiopathic

b) Location: Over spine—Probably bone or disc. Over erector spinae—Probably muscular

c) Type: Constant dull—muscle. Knife like—disc

d) Sciatic radiation L45 S123: Worse on cough & sneeze. Due to In.v disc osteophyte or vert body collapse. Stabbing shooting pain from back to leg c̄ parasthesiae & numbness L4 dermatome—med calf. L5 dermatome—lat calf, big toe, med half foot. S1 dermatome—lat half of foot

e) Femoral radiation L234: Pain over front, med, lat, aspects of thigh

ASSOCIATED SYMPTOMS OF EXTRINSIC CAUSES: a) Pelvic Ca → Vaginal haem

b) UGS: Haematuria, frequency, bladder neck obst

c) GIT: Malaena

d) Vasc: Pulses ↓, intermittent claudication

e) Hip OA → fixed deformity, mvt ↓, limp

f) Psych: Headache, choking

GENERAL INVESTIGATIONS: • Spine X-R: A-P & Lat. Occ Obl
- FBC, ESR
- Acid phosphatase
- CXR
- Myelography
- CAT

SPECIAL INVESTIGATIONS: • Discography
- Plasma proteins
- Bone marrow
- LP
- Urinalysis—Bence Jones protein
- Vert body biopsy

GENERAL RX: Rest & physiotherapy helpful

Prolapsed Intravertebral Disc

CLIN: Sudden pain; Mvt ↓; Loss of lordosis. Lat tilt ("sciatic scoliosis") ± sciatica ± loss of Knee, ankle reflexes

RX: Traction. Analgesia, sedatives, tranquillisers, muscle relaxants. Laminectomy if symptoms persist. Urgent laminectomy if cauda equina symptoms

Muscular Ligamentous Sprain

CLIN: Dull ache; Tender over lat erector

spinae; Loss of lordosis

RX: Always conservative. Drugs: Anti-inflammatory eg Indomethacin; Sedatives & muscle relaxants eg Diazepam

Lumbar Spondylosis

CLIN: Pain. Loss of lordosis ± sciatica

RX: Analgesia, anti-inflammatory drugs. Occ op when ass c̄ sciatica

Spondylolisthesis

CLIN: Pain; Local tenderness; Step deformity on palpation; ± sciatica

RX: Analgesia, sedatives. Surgery if sciatica: Laminectomy ± fusion

Senile Osteoporosis

CLIN: Asymptomatic. Or sudden vertebral body collapse → pain, tenderness, undue prominence of spine on palpation

RX: Spinal support. Stilboesterol, Testosterone

Genito-urinary System

HAEMATURIA

Causes of Haematuria (LIST 1 GUS)

1. Tumours:
   a) Ca Bladder
   b) Ca Kidney
   c) Ca Prostate
   d) Mets
2. Infection:
   a) Pyelonephritis, Cystitis
   b) Urethritis
   c) Prostatitis
   d) Schistosomiasis
   e) TB
3. Glomerulonephritis
4. Stones in GUS
5. Vascular:
   Eg Renal infarct, Malignant BP ↑. Sickle cell trait, Arteritis
6. Renal cysts esp polycystic disease
7. SABE
8. Post X-Rad
9. Trauma
10. Renal papillary necrosis
11. Idiopathic
12. Bleeding diatheses:
    Eg Anticoag o/d, Blood dyscrasias
13. Drugs:
    Eg Cyclophosphamide
14. Exercise induced
15. Loin Pain & Haematuria syndrome
16. Primary Recurrent Haematuria

Primary Recurrent Haematuria

Aut Dom. Esp Young

CLIN: Haematuria soon after infection; Renal colic. Occ Malaise; Fever. No deafness

PROTEINURIA

Virtually all diseases of the kidney & the urinary tract cause proteinuria. Can be classified as Pre-renal eg CCF; Renal eg GN; Post-renal eg UTI. Degree of proteinuria is a guide to the cause. Mild proteinuria esp orthostatic proteinuria, tubular proteinuria; Moderate eg acute & chr infection; Heavy—causes of nephrotic syndrome

Orthostatic Proteinuria

A condition in which proteinuria is ass c̄ upright posture. Significance uncertain. Some later develop BP ↑

GLOMERULONEPHRITIS

GN describes a variety of lesions c̄ inflam in the glomeruli. Usually present c̄ acute nephritis or nephrotic syndrome. However 2–5% of "norm" people show presence of microscopic haematuria or proteinuria

Causes of GN (LIST 2 GUS)

1. Idiopathic
2. Infection:
   Eg Strep, Staph, Malaria, Schistosomiasis, Hep B, Sy, CMV, Leprosy
3. Drugs:
   Eg Penicillamine, Gold, Probenecid
4. Allergies:
   Eg Henoch–Schonlein
5. Autoimmune Disease:
   Eg SLE, Goodpasture's Syndrome, Wegener's

AETIOLOGY: The causes of most cases of GN is not known

PATH: Classification depends on histology

Classification of GN (LIST 3 GUS)

A. DIFFUSE LESIONS
1. Minor Glomerular lesions inc "minimal change" GN
2. Diffuse membranous GN
3. Diffuse endocapillary proliferative GN
4. Diffuse mesangial proliferative GN
5. Diffuse mesangiocapillary GN (Membranoproliferative)
6. Diffuse crescentic GN (Extracapillary)

B. FOCAL LESIONS
1. Focal & Segmental proliferative GN
2. Focal & segmental hyalinosis & sclerosis
3. Focal sclerosis

PATHOGENESIS: Some cases due to immune complex disease

GENERAL INVESTIGATIONS:
- Urinalysis
- U&E, creatinine clearance
- Blood & Urine Albumin
- Serum complement
- Measurement of selectivity of urine protein loss: In minimal change GN mainly low mol wt proteins
- Renal biopsy

N.B Lipids: Often LDL & VLDL ↑

Minimal Change GN (Lipoid Nephrosis)

M>F. Commonest cause of nephrotic syndrome in children esp 1–5yrs. Electron microscopy shows only minimal abnormalities in glomeruli inc foot process fusion

Factors against diagnosis of minimal change GN: Presence of BP ↑ or Haematuria; Girls; Unselective proteinuria; ↑ age; ↓ Complement

CLIN: Nephrotic syndrome. Rarely Haematuria; BP ↑

RX: High protein, low Na^+ diet. 90% respond to Prednisolone

PROG: Excellent. Rarely esp in non-steroid responders, histology alters & RF may occur

Diffuse Membranous GN

Commonest cause of nephrotic syndrome in adults. Sub-epithelial & granular deposits

CLIN: Nephrotic syndrome. Occ BP ↑; Haematuria

RX: Prednisolone or Cyclophosphamide, Dipyridamole & Warfarin

PROG: Mean survival 10yrs

Diffuse Endocapillary Proliferative GN

Usually post infective esp Strep. Esp children

CLIN: 10 days post infection. Often acute nephritic syndrome ie Oedema; BP ↑; Haematuria; Oliguria; Impaired renal function eg GFR ↓. Occ → ARF

RX: Supportive. Na^+ & fluid restriction ± diuretics

PROG: Excellent in children. May → ESRF esp in adults

Diffuse Mesangioproliferative GN

Common in S.Hemisphere esp Australia. An ↑ in mesangial cells. About 50% have mesangial IgA deposits (Mesangial IgA Nephropathy)

CLIN: Often Haematuria; BP ↑; Proteinuria. Occ Nephrotic syndrome. Rarely progress to RF

RX: Try steroids but usually no response

PROG: Excellent unless focal & segmental proliferative lesions develop

Diffuse Mesangiocapillary (Membranoproliferative) GN

Unusual. Double contours in capillary walls. In type I disease sub-endothelial deposits. In type II disease dense deposits in basement membrane & hypocomplementaemia

CLIN: Present c̄ proteinuria or nephrotic syndrome. Later BP ↑; RF

RX: Cyclophosphamide

PROG: Poor. May recur after transplantation

Diffuse Crescentic GN

Defined as patients c̄ crescents in >80% of glomeruli. Often underlying systemic disease eg SLE, PAN, Goodpasture's, Wegener's, Henoch-Schonlein purpura. Previously termed "rapidly progressive GN"

CLIN: ARF; BP ↑; Proteinuria; Haematuria

RX: Steroids & Azathioprine or Cyclophosphamide c̄ plasma exchange therapy

PROG: Much improved c̄ present Rx. Prog better if prompt Rx. Natural history is rapid progression to ESRF

Focal & Segmental Proliferative GN

Focal & segmental crescents. Often mesangial IgA deposits. Occ due to SLE, Goodpasture's syndrome, Wegener's, PAN. May progress to diffuse crescentic GN

CLIN: Haematuria. Occ Proteinuria; BP ↑. Variable progression to ESRF

RX: In SLE—Prednisolone. In PAN, Wegener's—Cyclophosphamide. In Idiopathic—Cyclophosphamide & plasma exchange

PROG: Best if GFR norm

Focal & Segmental Hyalinosis/Sclerosis

Usually deposition of IgM & C3

CLIN: Nephrotic syndrome or proteinuria; BP ↑. May progress to RF

RX: May respond to Steroids or Cyclophosphamide

Focal Sclerosis

Glomerular scarring. May be ass c̄ any form of GN

CLIN: Occ Nephrotic syndrome; Proteinuria; BP ↑; Microscopic haematuria

PROG: Quite good

Recurrence of GN in Transplants

Almost inevitable c̄ type II mesangiocapillary GN. Often occurs in mesangial IgA nephropathy & focal sclerosing GN

ACUTE NEPHRITIS

M>F. Esp young. Classically follows Gp A Strep throat infection. Similar picture in Henoch–Schonlein purpura; SLE; PAN; Goodpasture's; Wegener's

CLIN: Acute onset of Haematuria, Oliguria. Then Oedema; BP ↑, Renal function ↓. Occ ARF

INVESTIGATIONS:
- Urinalysis: Casts, Na^+ ↑, Osmolality ↑
- ASOT titre
- Throat swab
- ESR ↑
- U&E
- Occ Renal biopsy

RX: Antibiotics, Bed rest, Diuretics. Antihypertensives

PROG: Most recover fully esp Children

Alport's Syndrome

Commonest cause of hereditary nephritis. M>F

CLIN: M often more severely affected than F. Usually present in childhood. Haematuria; Proteinuria. Later BP ↑; CRF. Occ Nerve deafness; Eye defects. Rarely Nephrotic syndrome

INVESTIGATIONS:
- Renal biopsy: Splitting of basement membrane on electron microscopy
- Urine: "Foam" cells

RX: No specific Rx. Occ require transplant

SLE

Symptomless proteinuria common. Occ Nephrotic syndrome. Many forms of GN possible. Due to anti-DNA complex deposition

RX: Steroids, Azathioprine

NEPHROTIC SYNDROME

A syndrome characterised by Oedema, Albuminuria >0.05g/kg/day, Hypoalbuminaemia & Hyperlipidaemia

Causes of Nephrotic Syndrome (LIST 4 GUS)

1. GN:
   Esp Minimal change GN in children
2. Infections:
   Eg Malaria, Staph, HepB, Schistosomiasis, Sy, SABE, CMV
3. Metabolic:
   a) Diabetes
   b) Amyloidosis
   c) Hypothyroidism
4. Tumours:
   a) Ca
   b) Leukaemias
   c) Myeloma
   d) Sarcoma
5. Drugs:
   a) Gold
   b) Penicillamine
   c) Mercury
   d) Captopril
   e) Antiepileptics
   f) Probenecid
6. Vascular:
   a) Renal vein thromb
   b) Renal artery stenosis
   c) CCF
   d) IVC thromb
   e) Constrictive pericarditis
7. Collagen vascular disease:
   a) PAN
   b) SLE
   c) Henoch–Schonlein syndrome
8. Familial disorders:
   a) Cong nephrotic syndrome
   b) Alports syndrome
   c) Fabry's disease
9. Allergic reaction:
   Eg Serum sickness, Bee stings, Pollen, Vaccines
10. Chyluria
11. Cryoglobulinaemia

GN is the commonest cause

CLIN: Oedema; Ascites; Pallor. Occ Pleural effusions; Haematuria; BP ↑; SOB; Striae. May → RF

INVESTIGATIONS:
- Urinalysis
- FBC
- U&E
- Albumin
- BG
- PPE
- Serum Ca^{2+}
- Blood lipids
- Differential protein excretion index
- CXR
- IVU (After exclusion of myeloma)
- Renal biopsy
- Other tests for underlying disease

GENERAL RX: High protein, low Na^+ diet; Diuretics. Prompt Rx of infections. Steroids or immunosuppressives

COMPLICATIONS: 1. Protein malnutrition
2. Hypercoagulability → thromb
3. Infections ↑
4. Osteoporosis

Cong Nephrotic Syndrome

Rare. Esp Finland. Aut Rec

CLIN: Premature labour; Foetal distress; LBW. Develop oedema & ascites. Increased risk of infection

RX: Symptomatic treatment. Occ able to transplant

PROG: Most die in 1st yr of life

ACUTE RENAL FAILURE

Acute deterioration of renal function → disruption of int environment esp marked reduction in urine flow. Can complicate CRF (Acute on chronic renal failure)

Causes of Acute Renal Failure (LIST 5 GUS)

A. PRE-RENAL
1. Circulating vol ↓:
   a) Severe diarrhoea &/or Vom
   b) Haem
   c) Shock
   d) Severe burns
   e) Post-op esp if J
2. Cardiac Output ↓:
   Eg MI, Severe MSt, Cardiogenic Shock

B. RENAL
1. Vascular:
   a) Renal artery occlusion eg Trauma, Emboli, Aortic Dissection
   b) Renal vein thromb
   c) DIC
   d) Malignant BP ↑
   e) Thrombotic micro-angiopathy eg Haemolytic Uraemic syndrome, Post partum RF, Thrombotic Thrombocytopoenic Purpura
2. Acute GN:
   Eg Idiopathic, PAN, SLE, Goodpasture's Syndrome
3. Infections:
   a) Acute pyelonephritis
   b) Septicaemia
   c) Legionella
4. Drugs & chemicals:
   Eg Aminoglycosides, Amphotericin B, Sulphadiazine, CCl_4, Thiazides, Frusemide, Cis-platinum, Paracetamol, Paraquat, Ethylene glycol, Radiological contrast media
5. Collagen Vascular Disease:
   a) Systemic Sclerosis
   b) PAN
   c) SLE
6. Obstetric Accidents:
   Esp APH, PPH, Septic abortion, Eclampsia
7. Diabetes
8. Acute pancreatitis
9. Haemolysis/Haemoglobinuria:
   Eg Drugs in G6PD def, Sickle cell anaemia, Typhoid
10. Myoglobinuria:
   Eg Trauma, Alcohol, Coxsackie, Snake venom
11. Acute transplant rejection
12. ALF

C. POST-RENAL
1. Stone
2. Urethral Stricture
3. Neoplasm:
   Eg Prostate, Cervix, Bladder
4. Acute papillary necrosis
5. Schistosomiasis
6. Clot
7. Retroperitoneal fibrosis
8. Enlarged prostate
9. Cong urethral valves
10. Phimosis, Paraphimosis
11. Surgical tying of both ureters

Pre-renal RF

Renal Parenchymal damage occurs when renal plasma flow is 5% of normal

CLIN: Oliguria; Postural BP ↓; JVP ↓↓; Cool extremities. Occ Shock

INVESTIGATIONS:
- Urine Na <60mmol/l
- Urinary urea >2%
- Urea urine/plasma ratio >10
- Osmolality urine/plasma ratio >1.4
- U&E
- Creatinine clearance

RX: Rehydrate c̄ blood or saline IV c̄ CVP monitoring. Danger of LVF if overtransfused. When hypovolaemia corrected, diuretics used to promote diuresis. Occ Dopamine for unresponsive renal underperfusion

PROG: If hypovolaemia &/or ↓ CO corrected early, oliguria is reversible

Renal RF

The commonest cause of ARF is parenchymal kidney damage. There are a number of mechanisms of renal ARF: Acute tubular necrosis; Acute cortical necrosis; GN; Drug nephrotoxicity; Acute pyelonephritis ± papillary or medullary necrosis; Renal vascular disorders; Acute interstitial nephritis

ACUTE TUBULAR NECROSIS

Results from renal underperfusion or direct nephrotoxicity. Causes include acute haem, post-op, acute pancreatitis, burns, septic abortion, septicaemia, myoglobinuria

CLIN: Oliguria: Usually <400ml/24hrs; N&V; Anorexia; Uraemia. Occ Infection; Pulm oedema. Later Anaemia. Often oliguric phase lasts 2–3wks c̄ gradual increase in urine vol thereafter, less commonly a polyuric phase follows

INVESTIGATIONS:
- U&E: Urea ↑, K^+↑, Na^+ often ↓
- Creatinine ↑
- GFR ↓
- Urine Na^+: Low in incipient RF >40mmol/l established RF
- 5. Urea urine/plasma ratio: High in incipient RF, <4 in established RF
- Osmolality urine/plasma ratio: >1.5 in insipient RF, <1.5 in established
- Urine microscopy
- Blood, urine, sputum cultures
- FBC, reticulocytes
- CXR
- AXR
- Isotope studies
- PO_4, Ca^{2+}
- Urate
- Albumin

RX: Exclude obst. Prophylactic mannitol in complicated surgery. Restrict fluid intake to 500ml plus output in last 24hrs, monitor by weighing. Low protein, high calorie diet. Rx K^+ ↑↑ c̄ 50% glucose & insulin (1 unit insulin/4g glucose) or 10% Ca^{2+} gluconate or Ca^{2+} based resin. Prompt Rx of infection. Remove obst. Dialysis for resistant hyperK^+; Severe acidosis; Urea >50mmol/l; Poor clin condition esp LVF, severe D&V, pericarditis, fits; Fluid overload. In diuretic (polyuric) phase may need to give Na^+ & K^+ replacements

ACUTE CORTICAL NECROSIS

Usually 2° to severe rapid blood loss eg APH. Entire nephron is infarcted. If healing occurs calcification is seen on AXR. Poor prog. May need renal biopsy to distinguish from ATN

RX: Dialysis. Occ Transplantation

ACUTE GN

May be idiopathic or ass c̄ systemic disorder eg SLE. Previous h/o oedema, nephrotic syndrome or haematuria suggests diagnosis

ACUTE INTERSTITIAL NEPHRITIS

Usually due to drugs eg Sulphonamides, Frusemide

CLIN: Fever, Rash, Oliguria

Post-Renal RF

Common cause of anuria

INVESTIGATIONS:
- Ultrasound
- Ureteropyelography
- Cystoscopy

RX: Catheterise (often relieves obst). Occ require dialysis &/or percutaneous nephrostomy & drainage prior to surgery

DD OF TOTAL ANURIA: 1. Post-renal obst
2. Bilat renal infarcts
3. Acute GN

General Prognosis

ADVERSE FACTORS ARE: Septicaemia; Severe burns; Oliguria for >2wks; Serious co-existing disease; Rapidly rising urea; Post serious op RF; Acute cortical necrosis; Old age. Complications include: GI haem, 2° infections, Resp failure & CCF

CHRONIC RENAL FAILURE

Usually defined as creatinine clearance <12–15ml/min

Causes of Chronic Renal Failure (LIST 6 GUS)

1. GN
2. Chronic obstructive uropathy
3. Vascular:
   a) Ischaemia
   b) BP ↑
4. Infections:
   a) Chr pyelonephritis
   b) Renal TB
5. Collagen Vascular Disease:
   Eg SLE, Systemic Sclerosis, PAN
6. Metabolic:
   a) Diabetes
   b) Amyloidosis
   c) Gout
   d) Hypercalcaemia eg HPT, VitD excess, Sarcoidosis
7. Drugs:
   Esp Analgesic nephropathy
8. Primary tubular disease:
   a) Fanconi syndrome
   b) RTbA
9. Congenital/Hereditary:
   Eg Polycystic kidney, Renal hypoplasia, Alport's disease
10. Radiation

Course of ↓ renal function: Can be divided into 3 stages:
Diminished renal reserve: ↓ creatinine clearance, norm urea, asymptomatic
Renal insufficiency: Clearance 20–40% of norm, urea 6–8mmol/l, mild acidosis. Occ Nocturia
Renal failure: GFR ↓↓, Urea ↑↑. Rate of deterioration is variable

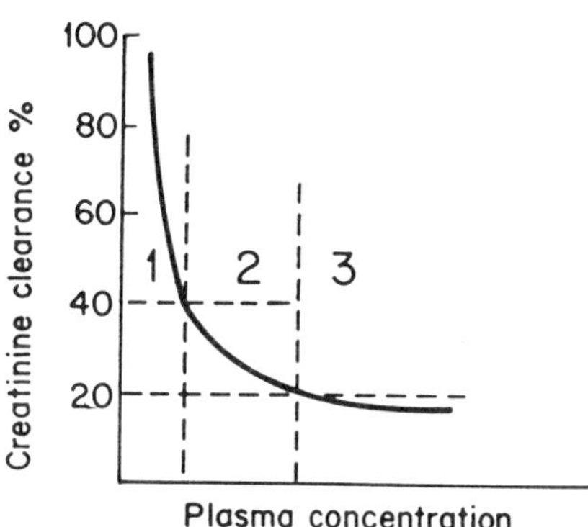

Figure 1 Stages of renal failure

PATHOPHYSIOLOGY: GFR ↓ → Urea ↑, PO_4 ↑, SO_4 ↑. Na^+ & water retained → ECF ↑, solute load per nephron ↑ (Can in rarer salt losing nephritis have Na^+ ↓). NH_4 production ↓, Urinary HCO_3 ↑ → Less H_2 secretion & metabolic acidosis. PO_4 ↑ → Ca^{2+} ↓ → PTH ↑ → HPT, also Vit D metabolism ↓ → ↓ Ca^{2+} absorption. Anaemia due to Erythropoetin ↓ & PO_4 ↑ → 2,3 DPG ↑. K^+ ↑↑ but may be balanced by loss due to anorexia, D&V. Mg^{2+} ↑; Urate ↑; Plasma creatinine ↑

Clin of CRF (LIST 7 GUS)

1. GIT:
   a) Nausea
   b) Vom
   c) Anorexia
   d) Hiccoughs
2. CVS:
   a) BP ↑
   b) CCF due to fluid overload
   c) Pericarditis
3. Skin:
   a) Pruritis
   b) Pallor

c) Purpura
d) Pigmentation
4. Neurological:
a) Ep
b) Confusion
c) Periph neuropathy
5. Haematological:
a) Anaemia
b) Bleeding tendency
6. Musculo-skeletal:
a) Growth failure
b) Osteomalacia
c) Osteoporosis
d) Proximal myopathy
e) 2° HPT
f) Bone pain
7. Respiratory:
a) Hyperventilation due to acidosis
b) SOB due to LVF
c) Foetor
8. Genitourinary:
a) Nocturia
b) Polyuria

Common causes of acute on chronic RF are: Fluid & electrolyte depletion; Infections; Obst; Drugs; Fluid overload; Uncontrolled BP ↑; Exacerbation of underlying disease eg diabetes, GI bleed

INVESTIGATIONS:
- FBC
- U&E
- Creatinine clearance
- Urine electrolytes
- Serum Ca^{2+}
- Alk phos ↑
- BG
- Urate
- X-R: Ultrasound, IVU, Isotope scanning, CXR, AXR, Skeletal survey
- Occ renal biopsy

GENERAL RX: Exclude Obst. Regular monitoring eg periodic creatinine clearance. Detect & treat reversible factors eg UTI, drugs, dehydration, obst. Low (high biological value) protein diet c̄ multidose amino acid & keto analogues supplements probably helpful. Adequate calorie intake. Restrict Na^+ & K^+ intake. Anti BP ↑ drugs. Phosphate binders eg Aludrox (Care to avoid hypophosphataemia). $CaCO_3$ unless moderate or severe PO_4 ↑ to help prevent osteodystrophy. Vit B, Folic acid & iron supplements. Treat pruritis c̄ Diphenhydramine

DIALYSIS RX: Aim to start dialysis when creatinine is approx 1000–1200 μmol/l, just before complications eg pericarditis, N&V usually occur. Usually access to dialysis is limited & therefore those c̄ better prog are selected eg the young. Types of dialysis are CAPD (SE: Peritonitis), Peritoneal dialysis (rarely used) & Haemodialysis. Haemodialysis is usually performed 3×/wk for 4–6hrs/session either at home, hospital or satellite unit. Dialysis obviates need for special diet but some fluid control is essential, it usually controls BP ↑, CCF, pericarditis, acidosis & CNS symptoms. Water purity is very important to prevent Aluminium toxicity → osteomalacia & dialysis dementia. Staff on units should be immunised against HepB

TRANSPLANT RX: Transplantation is the best long term solution both in terms of quality of life & cost effectiveness compared to dialysis. Dialyse prior to performing transplantation. Ensure ABO compatibility. HLA matching conveys small benefit. Prog best c̄ living related donor, in young & in non-diabetics. Use Azathioprine, Steroids & Cyclosporin A to ↓ risk of rejection

COMPLICATIONS OF TRANSPLANTATION:

1. **Acute Rejection:**
   Clin: Present early. Creatinine ↑. Occ Fever; Oliguria; Swollen tender graft. Can confirm diagnosis by biopsy, serial isotope scanning
   Rx: Methyl Prednisolone or Cyclosporin A
   Prog: Usually recover
2. **Urinary Leak**
3. **Lymphoceles:** Can diagnose & drain under ultrasound control. If recur, op
4. **Infections:** Eg CMV, Pneumocystis
5. **Chronic Rejection:** Much less common than acute rejection. Present late. Slow decrease in function usually ass c̄ BP ↑, Proteinuria
   Prog: Graft usually fails after variable periods of time
6. **Graft Artery Stenosis:** May → BP ↑; Bruit. Can diagnose & treat by arteriography & angioplasty
7. **Malignancy:** 2–3× ↑ risk of malignancy esp Ca cervix, Microglioma of brain, Skin cancer, Lymphoma
8. **Steroid SE:** Esp aseptic necrosis femoral head
9. **PU:** Can → post-op haem & perf. Prophylaxis by careful pre-op assessment & Cimetidine. Rx of any pre-existing PU

COMPLICATIONS OF CRF: 1. Metastatic Ca
2. Renal osteodystrophy
3. PU

PROG OF ESRF: Annual mort if on dialysis 5–15%. 10–30% of grafts are rejected. After 1st yr post transplant morbidity & mort are low. As anaemia is corrected by transplantation many are able to retun to work

Renal Osteodystrophy

Usually due to RF but occ due to renal tubular defect
Osteomalacia, Osteitis fibrosa, Osteosclerosis & Osteoporosis occur singly or in combination. Commonest abnormality is that of HPT

CLIN: Osteomalacia → bone pain, proximal myopathy, waddling gait, loss of height due to vertebral collapse. Osteoporosis may → bone pain & #. Pruritis (Esp 2° HPT); Red eyes, Corneal calcification

INVESTIGATIONS:
- Ca^{2+}
- PO_4
- Alk phos
- Albumin
- X-R Hands, Wrist, CXR, AXR, Spine, Lat Skull, Pelvis
- Bone biopsy
- PTH assay

In osteomalacia Ca^{2+} ↓, PO_4 norm or ↑, Alk phos ↑, Occ Looser's Zones. Osteoporosis & Sclerosis are radiological diagnoses eg "Rugger Jersey" spine

RX: Prevention by phosphate binders in early RF. Correct hypocalcaemia c̄ $CaCO_3$ or VitD analogues. Osteitis fibrosa can be treated by dialysis, VitD (risk of metastatic Ca^{2+}) or subtotal parathyroidectomy & VitD

ELECTROLYTE DISTURBANCES

Sodium Excess

Causes of Total Body Na Excess (LIST 8 GUS)

1. Ht failure
2. Iatrogenic—IV saline infusion
3. Hypoalbuminaemia:
   a) Nephrotic syndrome
   b) Peritoneal dialysis
   c) Cirrhosis
   d) Malabsorption
   e) Malnutrition
4. CRF
5. ARF
6. Conn's syndrome

CLIN: Periph oedema; Pulm oedema; Pleural effusions; Ascites. If cardiac function norm, hypervolaemia → BP ↑. In hypoalbuminaemia, oedema is ass c̄ signs of hypovolaemia due to leakage of fluid into interstitial space

INVESTIGATIONS:
- Na^+: Usually norm, ↑ in Conn's syndrome
- Albumin

RX: Low Na^+ diet; Diuretics c̄ care esp in hypoalbuminaemic. In RF dialysis

Sodium Def

Causes of Sodium Def (LIST 9 GUS)

1. GIT fluid loss:
   Eg D&V, Fistulae, PI
2. Addison's disease
3. Salt losing Nephritis:
   a) Chronic pyelonephritis
   b) Renal calculi
   c) Analgesic nephropathy
   d) Diabetes
4. Post relief of urinary obst
5. Excess diuretics
6. Excess dialysis
7. Polyuric phase of ARF
8. Excess sweating

CLIN: Sunken cheeks & eyes; Weakness; Cramps; Thirst; Cold extremities. Postural BP ↓ esp post exercise. Occ Periph cyanosis; PR ↑

INVESTIGATIONS:
- FBC
- Na^+: Norm or ↓
- Urinary Na^+

RX: IV isotonic NaCl usually required. Monitor c̄ CVP, serial weighing & serial K^+ estimations. In RF may give some Na^+ as $NaHCO_3$

Water Excess

Causes of Water Excess (LIST 10 GUS)

1. ARF
2. Inappropriate ADH secretion
3. Glucocorticoid def:
   a) Addison's disease
   b) Ant Pituitary failure
4. Excessive water intake in CRF
5. Post-op
6. Drugs:
   Eg Chlorpropamide, Carbamazepine
7. Iatrogenic:
   Esp IV therapy
8. Hypothalamic lesions

CLIN: N&V; Convulsions; Headache; Drowsiness; Oedema

INVESTIGATIONS: ● Plasma osmolality ↓
● Serum Na^+ ↓

RX: Restrict water. Rarely require hypertonic saline

Water Def

Causes of Water Def (LIST 11 GUS)

1. Drought
2. Inability to indicate thirst:
   Eg Coma
3. Nephrogenic DI:
   a) Hereditary
   b) Myeloma
   c) $HyperCa^{2+}$
   d) $HypoK^+$
4. Cranial DI
5. Osmotic diuresis:
   Eg Diabetic ketotic coma

CLIN: Dry tongue; Thirst. Later Confusion; Coma

INVESTIGATIONS: ● Plasma osmolality ↑
● Serum Na^+ ↑

RX: Water orally if tolerated or slow infusion of 5% Glucose

Hyperkalaemia

Causes of Hyperkalaemia (LIST 12 GUS)

1. ARF
2. CRF
3. Iatrogenic:
   Eg Excess K^+ supplements, Drugs given as K^+ salts
4. Addison's disease
5. Spurious:
   Eg Partially haemolysed blood analysed in lab
6. Relative $HyperK^+$ (ie K^+ shift into ECF from cells):
   Eg Acidosis, Glycogen breakdown, Catabolism

CLIN: Usually asymptomatic until sudden cardiac arrest

INVESTIGATIONS: ● K^+
● HCO_3
● ECG: Peaked ˆTˆ wave, loss of ˆPˆ wave, ˆQRSˆ splaying

RX: 5% Ca^{2+} gluconate. IV Insulin & glucose c̄ $NaHCO_3$ if no Na^+ ↑. In RF may require Ion exchange resin or dialysis. Remove drugs & may need to restrict dietary K^+

Hypokalaemia

Causes of Hypokalaemia (LIST 13 GUS)

1. Renal loss:
   a) Thiazide or loop diuretics
   b) Uncontrolled diabetes
   c) Iatrogenic—IV or dialysis fluids c inadequate K^+
   d) Systemic alkalosis
   e) Renal tubular acidosis
   f) Conn's syndrome
   g) 2° hyperaldosteronism eg Accelerated BP ↑, Renal artery stenosis, Renin secreting tumour
   h) Cortisol excess eg Cushing's syndrome, ACTH producing Ca
   i) Polyuric phase of ARF
2. GIT loss:
   a) Prolonged vomiting
   b) Severe diarrhoea
   c) Fistulae
   d) Laxative abuse

e) Diuretic abuse
f) Aspiration
g) PI
h) Uretero-sigmoid anastomosis
i) Mucus secreting Ca
3. Decreased intake:
a) Poor diet
b) Malabsorption
4. Relative HypoK (ie K^+ shift from ECF into cells):
a) Familial periodic paralysis
b) Alkalosis
c) Glycogen deposition

CLIN: Muscle weakness; Thirst; Polyuria; Constipation; Fatigue. Occ Ileus; Sudden death from arrhythmias. Rarely Nephrogenic DI

INVESTIGATIONS: • K^+
- HCO_3
- Cl^- : Usually ↓ but ↑ in RTbA & uretero-sigmoid anastomosis
- Urinary K^+
- Urinalysis: Mild proteinuria
- ECG: Arrhythmias, ^U^ wave, ^ST^ depression

RX: Treat underlying cause. Replace c̄ KCL
N.B: ↑ digoxin sensitivity

RENAL TUBULAR DISORDERS

Renal Tubular Acidosis

H_2 is actively secreted, Proximal >Distal tubule. RTbA can be due to lack of functioning nephrons eg in CRF or due to 1° distal or proximal renal tubular disease

RTbA TYPE 1 (DISTAL)

Commoner form of RTbA. 1° form usually presents in infancy. Aut Dom. 2° causes inc Hypercalciuria, HPT, CAH, Vit D toxicity

PATHOPHYSIOLOGY: Failure of distal H_2 secretion → urine pH ↑ → ↑ Urinary HCO_3 → ↑ serum Cl^- → hyperchloraemic acidosis

CLIN: Failure to thrive in infancy; Dehydration; Polyuria; Constipation. Usually Renal stones; Rickets & Osteomalacia. Occ HypoK$^+$ symptoms

RX: Small amounts of alkali

PROG: Good if nephrocalcinosis not advanced

RTbA TYPE 2 (PROXIMAL)

Very rare. Children >Adults. May be 1°, Aut Dom, or 2° to Cystinosis, Fanconi syndrome, Nephronophthisis, Medullary cystic disease, HPT

PATHOPHYSIOLOGY: A HCO_3 leak → ↑↑ HCO_3 in urine → Hyperchloraemic acidosis. Can form acid urine in presence of severe acidosis

CLIN: Growth failure; Vom

RX: Large amounts of alkali. Thiazide diuretics & K^+

PROG: Good

Fanconi Syndrome

A syndrome of glycosuria, phosphaturia, aminoaciduria & tubular acidosis due to a tubular disorder. 3 main types: Cystinosis (Lignac–Fanconi syndrome); Idiopathic adult Fanconi syndrome; 2° Fanconi Syndrome

CYSTINOSIS

Rare. Aut Rec. Due to transport mechanism abnormality. Proximal tubule abnormality. Cystine crystals deposited in soft tissues

CLIN: Failure to thrive in infancy; Rickets; Polyuria; Thirst; Vom; Weakness. Later Photophobia; Gritty eyes

INVESTIGATION: • Cystine crystals in cornea

RX: No specific Rx. Transplant may help

ADULT FANCONI SYNDROME

Presents in young adults. May be FH

CLIN: Weakness; Osteomalacia → bone pain

RX: Replace Vit D, Alkali & K^+

PROG: Good

SECONDARY FANCONI SYNDROME

Occurs in Glycogenoses; Wilson's disease; Tyrosinosis; Myeloma; Heavy metal poisoning; Galactosaemia; Outdated Tetracyclines

RX: Treat underlying condition

Hypophosphataemic Vit D Resistant Rickets

Rare X-linked Dom. Due to defective tubular PO_4 resorption
Presents in childhood

CLIN: Rickets

RX: Large doses of Vit D analogues c̄ PO_4

1° Nephrogenic DI

Rare. X-linked Rec. Presents in infancy

CLIN: Polyuria; Dehydration

RX: Thiazides may help

Aminoacidurias

May be 1° due to specific transport defects eg Cystinuria, Hartnup disease or 2° to general tubular damage esp Fanconi syndrome; or an overflow due to hyperaminoacidaemias eg PKU

URINARY TRACT INFECTION

Very common. 4F:1M esp F 15–65yrs, however in infants M>F due to cong abnormalities of GUS in M. About 5% adult F have bacteriuria. Esp common in pregnancy, catheterised, neurogenic bladder. Usually due to *E.coli*
N.B Also see section on Cystitis

PATHOGENESIS: Commoner in F due to short urethra. Ass c̄ residual urine; Intercourse. Acute pyelonephritis predisposed to by: Obst; Pregnancy; Calculi; HypoK^+; Analgesic nephropathy; X-R procedures; Hydronephrosis. Pyelonephritis often ass c̄ vesico–ureteric reflux

PATHOLOGY: In childhood, pyelonephritis may → "U" shaped scar c̄ later contraction of adult kidney which may → CRF ± BP ↑

CLIN: Bacteriuria may be asymptomatic. Dysuria; Frequency. Occ Suprapubic pain; Haematuria; Foul smelling urine; Fever; Rigors; Loin pain. Difficult to identify site of infection from symptoms

INVESTIGATIONS:
- MSU: If no bacteriuria termed urethral syndrome. Sterile pyuria seen in TB, Analgesic nephropathy, Partially treated infection
- IVU: Indicated in M, & in F if failure of single dose Rx, h/o acute pyelonephritis or symptoms of underlying disease
- Rarely: Suprapubic aspiration, Urethral catheterisation

RX: In acute uncomplicated UTI adequate fluids & single dose or 5–7 days antibiotic Rx. In recurrent UTI advise prophylactic p/u after intercourse. Give prophylactic antibiotic eg Amoxycillin to F c̄ covert bacteriuria of pregnancy. If underlying urinary tract abnormality treat even covert bacteriuria

COMPLICATIONS: 1. Scarring due to reflux nephropathy ± asc infection
2. Renal Abscess via blood

PROG: Upper tract infections generally more serious

Reflux Nephropathy

Strongly ass c̄ vesico–ureteric reflux. Often FH. Reflux is generally worse in the young. Approx 20% of bacteriuric schoolchildren have reflux. Predisposing factors for reflux inc Cong defects of vesico–ureteric junction; Obst; Ureteric surgery; Neurogenic bladder. Often → CRF in adults

CLIN: Often UTI; Nocturnal enuresis in childhood. In adults often h/o acute pyelonephritis; BP ↑; Proteinuria. May present in pregnancy. Later CRF

INVESTIGATIONS:
- Micturating Cysto–urethrography
- IVU

N.B In adults frequently reflux not demonstrated but classical reflux kidney scarring seen

RX: In children anti-reflux op may help.

Relieve any outflow obst. Prompt Rx of UTI & BP ↑. Very close supervision if pregnant

DD: 1. Obst uropathy
2. Analgesic nephropathy

Renal Abscess

Often Staph via blood eg from carbuncle

CLIN: Fever; Malaise. Gradually increasing pain & tenderness. Occ Rigors

INVESTIGATIONS: • WCC ↑
• Blood cultures
• Ultrasound

RX: Drain abscess, Antibiotics

Renal TB

Always due to 2° spread of TB. Although both kidneys infected, often one kidney worse affected

CLIN: Frequency then urgency, dysuria. Later Haematuria; Lumbar pain

INVESTIGATIONS: • Urinalysis (EMUs): Sterile pyuria; Protein ↑; Stain & culture for TB
• AXR: Occ Ca^{2+}
• IVU
• Cystoscopy

RX: Triple TB therapy for 6/12 continuing c̄ Isoniazid & PAS acid for further 12mths. If one kidney grossly affected nephroureterectomy

COMPLICATIONS: 1. Spread to ureter & bladder → TB hydronephrosis
2. TB cystitis may heal → contracted bladder
3. Spread to epididymis
4. CRF in bilat cases

RENAL CALCULI

Very common. M>F. Esp higher social class. Occ FH. Approx 80% of renal stones are Ca^{2+} Oxalate, 10% triple PO_4 (esp alkaline urine), 5–10% uric acid (esp acid urine), 1% cystine stones

PATHOGENESIS: 1. ↑ Excretion of relatively insoluble crystalloid
2. Variation of urine pH → ↓ crystalloid solubility
3. ↓ urine vol
4. Def of substances which aid crystalloid solubility eg GAGS

Causes of Renal Stones (LIST 14 GUS)

A. CALCIUM STONES
1. With normocalcaemia:
a) 1° Distal RTbA
b) Idiopathic hypercalciuria
c) Immobilisation
d) Recurrent UTI
e) Hyperoxaluria
f) Medullary sponge kidney
2. With hypercalcaemia:
a) 1° HPT
b) Sarcoidosis
c) Vit D excess
d) Idiopathic hypercalcaemia
e) Milk–alkali syndrome
f) Malignancy, Myeloma

B. URIC ACID STONES
1. With normouricaemia:
a) Idiopathic
b) Low water intake eg desert climate
2. With hyperuricaemia:
a) Gout
b) Increased cell turnover eg PRV, Leukaemia
c) Chr metabolic acidosis eg Glycogen storage diseases
d) Lesch–Nyhan syndrome
e) Uricosuric drugs

C. CYSTINE STONES
1. Cystiniuria
2. Cystinosis

D. TRIPLE PHOSPHATE STONES
UTI

CLIN: Many stones asymptomatic. Occ Obst → Ureteric colic (sometimes recurrent; haematuria) &/or acute pyelonephritis. Chr obst may → pyonephrosis. Sometimes calculus grows → "staghorn" calculus filling renal pelvis & parts of calyces which may → pyonephrosis, perinephric abscess, CRF

GENERAL INVESTIGATIONS:
- AXR
- IVU: Radio-opaque stones are Ca^{2+}, Oxalate & cystine
- Urine: C&S, pH
- Stone analysis
- Fasting blood Ca^{2+}, PO_4, Albumin (×3)
- Fasting blood HCO_3, Uric acid, Creatinine, PTH
- 24hr urine for Ca^{2+}, Oxalate, Mg^{2+}, PO_4, Uric acid, Cystine
- Cyanide nitroprusside test for cystinuria (if no stones available)
- Tests for underlying disorders

RX: Analgesia. Many stones passed spontaneously. Op if—symptomatic stone not passed spontaneously; Progressive renal function ↓; Staghorn calculus. Occ can use less invasive percutaneous or perureteric stone removal methods. ESWL is being evaluated

Calcium Oxalate Stones: Prevention by high fluid intake >2l/day. Diet: High fibre; ↓ intake of Ca^{2+} &/or oxalate only if high dietary intake identified. Rx c̄ Thiazides ± Allopurinol. Alternatives are inorganic phosphates (orthophosphates) (SE: Diarrhoea; c/i Triple PO_4 stones); Mg^{2+} supplements

Triple Phosphate Stones: Careful surgical removal & prompt Rx of UTI. If op c/i Antibiotics & Thiazides

Uric Acid Stones: High fluid intake >3l/day. Alkalinisation of the urine eg c̄ $NaHCO_3$. If disturbed uric acid metabolism add Allopurinol

Cystine Stones: High fluid intake & alkalinisation of urine. If this fails add Penicillamine & Pyridoxine

Nephrocalcinosis

A ppt of Ca^{2+} in the kidney esp tubules & parenchyma. Often coexists c̄ calculi

Causes of Nephrocalcinosis (LIST 15 GUS)

1. All causes of hypercalcaemia Eg HPT, Sarcoidosis, Vit D intoxication
2. Idiopathic hypercalciuria
3. Rarely:
   a) Renal TB
   b) RTbA
   c) Medullary sponge kidney
   d) Cyst, Tumour, Haematoma calcification
   e) Oxalosis
   f) Old cortical necrosis
   g) Chr GN

CLIN: No specific symptoms. Complaints of 1° disease

INVESTIGATIONS:
- FBC
- Urine C&S, pH
- U&E
- Creatinine clearance
- AXR
- Ca^{2+}, PO_4, Alk phos
- 24hr urine
- IVU

RX: Treat underlying condition

COMPLICATIONS:
1. Infection
2. Calculi
3. ↓ renal function

Medullary Sponge Kidney

Occ FH. Ass c̄ cystic disease of liver. Rare developmental abnormality. Esp 20–40 yrs. Ass c̄ hemihypertrophy

CLIN: May present c̄ haematuria, calculi or UTI

INVESTIGATION:
- IVU

RX: Prompt attention to UTI or calculi

Oxalosis

Rare. Aut Rec. Enzyme def → ↑ oxalic acid synthesis

CLIN: Present in 1st decade c̄ calculi, nephrocalcinosis. Crystal deposists in retina, Ht, bone & brain. Later RF

RX: High Pyridoxine diet c̄ phosphate supplements

POLYCYSTIC KIDNEY

Infantile Polycystic Disease

Aut Rec. Often presents at birth. Also Aut Dom form, M=F

CLIN: Usually Oligohydramnios; "Potter" facies (Low set ears; Micrognathia); Large kidneys. Often die early. May present later c̄ Liver ↑; Kidney ↑; BP ↑

INVESTIGATION: • Ultrasound

RX: Treat RF & portal BP ↑

Adult Polycystic Disease

Aut Dom. Esp 40yrs. Ass c̄ polycystic disease of liver & pancreas, Haemangioma of pancreas, "Berry" aneurysms

CLIN: Asymmetric renal enlargement. Often Renal pain; Calculi; Haematuria; UTI; BP ↑. Later CRF

INVESTIGATIONS: • Ultrasound
• IVU

RX: Treat CRF. Control BP ↑

DIURETICS

Act at sites of water resorption ie Proximal tubule eg Mannitol, Acetazolamide; Asc loop of Henle eg Frusemide, Bumetanide, Ethacrynic acid; Cortical diluting segment (Asc loop of Henle) eg Thiazides; Distal tubule (Na^+/K^+, H_2 exchange mechanism) eg Amiloride, Spironolactone, Triamterine. Aminophylline acts by ↑ GFR. Spironolactone is also an Aldosterone antagonist

CAUSES OF INADEQUATE RESPONSE:

1. Insufficient dosage
2. Acidosis → Thiazide action ↓ Acetazolamide ↓↓
3. Progression of 1° disease
4. GFR ↓ → Thiazide action ↓

METABOLIC COMPLICATIONS:

1. Hypovolaemia
2. Uric acid ↑
3. BG ↑ (except Ethacrynic acid)
4. K^+ depletion unless distal tubular action
5. ↓ Ca^{2+} excretion c̄ Thiazides
6. Alkalosis due to loss of K^+, Cl^-, H_2 & retention of HCO_3

Other SE: Thiazides: Rashes, Thrombocytopenia, Pancreatitis
Frusemide: Ototoxicity
Ethacrynic acid: Ototoxicity (M), Dysmenorrhoea (F)

Causes of Drug Induced Renal Disease (LIST 16 GUS)

1. Acute Tubular Necrosis:
   Esp Aminoglycosides
2. Acute Interstitial Nephritis:
   a) Sulphonamides
   b) Penicillins
   c) Thiazides
   d) Phenylbutazone
   e) PAS acid
3. Nephrotic syndrome:
   Eg Gold, Penicillamine
4. SLE-like state:
   a) Hydrallazine (esp slow acetylators)
   b) Procainamide
   c) Isoniazid
   d) Oral contraceptives
   e) Sulphonamides
5. Retroperitoneal fibrosis:
   Methysergide; ?Hydrallazine; ??β blockers
6. Analgesic Nephropathy:
   a) Phenacetin
   b) NSAID
7. Hypokalaemic Nephropathy:
   a) Diuretics
   b) Steroids
   c) Laxatives
   d) Carbenoxolone
   e) Tetracycline
   f) Amphotericin B
8. Renal calculi:
   a) Vit D excess
   b) Thiazides
   c) Milk–alkali syndrome
   d) Cyt.T
   e) Sulphonamides
9. ISADH:
   a) Chlorpropamide
   b) Thiazides
   c) Carbamazepine
   d) Vincristine
   e) Cyclophosphamide
   f) Clofibrate
10. Nephrogenic DI:
    a) Prolonged hypoK^+
    b) HyperCa^{2+}
    c) Li^+ salts
    d) Analgesic nephropathy
    e) Old Tetracycline
    f) Amphotericin B
    g) Methoxyfluorane
11. Acute obst:
    a) Causes of renal calculi
    b) X-Ray contrast
12. Hypovolaemia:
    a) Excess use of loop diuretics
    b) Drugs → D&V
13. Hypernatraemia & BP ↑:
    a) Carbenicillin
    b) Fusidic acid

Tetracyclines, c̄ the exception of Vibramycin should not be used in RF as they ↓ GFR & tend to ↑ blood urea due to catabolic action on protein metabolism. They have a direct nephrotoxic effect which may → exacerbation of RF

Analgesic Nephropathy

Major cause of CRF. Esp countries c̄ high per capita consumption of analgesics. F>M. Esp 30–70 yrs

PATHOGENESIS: Chr analgesic ingestion eg Phenacetin & Aspirin → interstitial nephritis & papillary necrosis

CLIN: Headache; Haematuria; Recurrent UTI. Occ Depression; Polyuria; Obst; Dyspepsia; Anaemia. Occ → Transitional Cell Ca

INVESTIGATION: • Urinary Salicylate & Paracetamol estimation

RX: Discontinue analgesics

RENAL ARTERY STENOSIS

Usually due to atheroma or occ fibromuscular hyperplasia, tumours, aortic aneurysm, trauma, SABE, MI. May be uni- or bilat

CLIN: Occ BP ↑. Occ h/o loin pain c̄ haematuria

INVESTIGATIONS:
- IVU: In unilat sten, small kidney c̄ delay in opacification of pelvicalyceal system on affected side
- Arteriogram
- Isotope renogram
- Renal vein renin
- Ureteric catheterisation studies

RX: Anti-BP ↑ drugs. If medical Rx unsuccessful, angioplasty esp for fibromuscular hyperplasia. Occ Nephrectomy

RENAL VEIN THROMBOSIS

Causes of Renal Vein Thrombosis (LIST 17 GUS)

1. Amyloidosis
2. 2° to Nephrotic syndrome
3. 2° to maternal diabetes & dehydration in infants
4. Hypernephroma
5. Thrombophlebitis
6. Trauma to renal vein

About 50% of cases occur in infancy & are ass c̄ ARF. May be uni- or bilat. Uncommon

CLIN: Acute loin pain & swelling; Haematuria; Fever; D&V; Kidney ↑. Occ Cyanosis; Purpura. Often → ARF. In adults more insidious onset often → nephrotic syndrome, PE or CRF

INVESTIGATIONS:
- IVU
- FBC
- Angiography
- Biopsy

RX: Nephrectomy in children

RENAL INFARCT

Major causes are SABE, Atheroma, PAN, Trauma & Thrombi

CLIN: Partial renal infarction usually asymptomatic. Complete infarction → loin pain, haematuria. Occ BP ↑

INVESTIGATIONS: • IVU
• Angiography

RX: Prompt embolectomy occ indicated. Occ anticoags

Causes of Small Kidneys (LIST 18 GUS)

A. UNILATERAL
1. Reflux uropathy
2. Post obst atrophy
3. Post inflam atrophy
4. Post traumatic atrophy
5. Post renal vein thromb
6. Renal infarct
7. Congenital hypoplasia
8. Radiation nephritis
9. Surgery

B. BILATERAL
1. CRF
2. Chr GN
3. Papillary necrosis
4. Bilat ischaemia
5. Amyloidosis (late)
6. Urate nephropathy
7. Medullary cystic disease

RENAL TUMOURS

Benign Tumours

HAMARTOMA

Rare. Ass c̄ Tuberous sclerosis. Often multiple & bilat

CLIN: Haematuria

INVESTIGATION: • Angiography

RX: Conservative

ADENOMA

Commonest benign tumour. Usually asymptomatic

Malignant Tumours

RENAL CELL Ca (HYPERNEPHROMA)

2M:1F. Esp late middle age. In UK causes 2% of deaths from malignancy

PATH: Ca arises in tubules usually at pole of kidney. Spread is direct to perinephric tissue, via lymph to Para-aortic LN & via renal vein to the IVC. Mets esp lung, bone & brain

CLIN: Painless haematuria; Unilat palpable expansile mass; Loin pain; Anaemia; Wt ↓. Occ PUO; "clot colic"; HyperCa^{2+}; Liver ↑; Bone pain; Polycythaemia. Rarely Amyloidosis; IVC thrombosis

INVESTIGATIONS: • FBC: Occ Erythrocytosis
• Ca^{2+}
• Alk Phos.
• Urinalysis
• AXR, IVU
• Ultrasound
• Angiography
• Rarely CAT scan

RX: Nephrectomy ± pre-op embolectomy. Post-op X-Rad may help

PROG: 5yr survival 50%. Some mets regress after nephrectomy

RENAL PELVIS TUMOURS

SQUAMOUS CELL Ca: Rare. Often ass c̄ calculi
Clin: Recurrent UTI. Symptoms of mets
Rx: Nephro–ureterectomy

TRANSITIONAL CELL Ca: Uncommon. Arise in pelvis or ureter. May be 2° to Analgesic Nephropathy. Often multifocal
Clin: Haematuria; Ureteric colic. Occ Hydronephrosis
Investigations: • Urinalysis
• IVU
• Ultrasound
Rx: Nephro–ureterectomy. Occ local excision. Follow-up as occ recurrence

KIDNEY INJURIES

Usually due to direct trauma. Potentialy serious. Often ass inj

CLIN: Haematuria. Retroperitoneal bleeding → N&V, Ileus. Occ Shock; Kidney ↑

INVESTIGATIONS:
- FBC
- AXR
- IVU
- Ultrasound
- Isotope scan
- Occ angiography

RX: Bed rest, careful monitoring. Treat shock & Haem. May need antibiotics. Occ nephrectomy required esp if severe haem

PROG: Contusions: Excellent. Rupture: Occ complications

HYDRONEPHROSIS

May be uni- or bilat. Esp middle aged men

CAUSES: 1. Cong—Urethral stricture, bladder neck obst c̄ reflux eg pinhole meatus, urethral valves, phimosis
2. Acquired—Urethral stricture; Phimosis; Prostatic tumours; Retroperitoneal fibrosis & Other obsts. Rarely in Pregnancy. Unilat causes include Ureteric stricture, Calculi, Tumours

CLIN: May be asymptomatic. Occ Backache; Loin pain; Renal swelling; Haematuria; UTIs; Pyelonephritis. May → IVC obst, RTbA or renal DI. Later CRF if bilat

INVESTIGATIONS:
- Ultrasound
- IVU

RX: Remove obst. Occ Nephrectomy

Causes of Enlarged Kidneys (LIST 19 GUS)

A. UNILATERAL
1. Compensatory hypertrophy
2. Acute pyelonephritis
3. Obst uropathy
4. Haematoma
5. Renal cysts
6. Renal vein thromb
7. Renal tumours
8. Congenital
9. Xanthogranulomatous Pyelonephritis

B. BILATERAL
1. Acute GN
2. PAN
3. SLE
4. Diabetes
5. Malignancy: Esp Leukaemia, Lymphoma
6. Amyloidosis
7. Polycystic kidneys
8. Acromegaly
9. Wegener's granulomatosis
10. Bilat obst (Usually asymmetrical)

URINARY TRACT OBSTRUCTION

Due to obst to urinary flow at any point from renal calyx to exterior. In children, cong anomalies are commonest cause. Between 20–60yrs F>M. In >60yrs, M>F as commonest cause is prostate ↑. Bilat obst usually due to prostate ↑, calculi or bladder tumour. Commonest cause of unilat obst are calculi & neuromuscular dysfunction at PUJ

Causes of Urinary Tract Obst (LIST 20 GUS)

A. WITHIN LUMEN
1. Calculus
2. Clot
3. Ca
4. Sloughed papilla

B. WITHIN WALL
1. Neuromuscular PUJ dysfunction
2. Vesico-ureteric stricture: Eg Congenital, Calculus, Ureterocoele, Schistosomiasis
3. Ureteric stricture: Eg Calculus, TB
4. Cong Megaureter
5. Cong bladder neck obst
6. Urethral stricture: Eg Calculus, Trauma, Gonococcal
7. Neurogenic bladder
8. Cong urethral valve
9. Pinhole meatus

C. OUTSIDE PRESSURE
1. Prostatic obst
2. Tumours: Eg Ca Colon, Diverticulitis, Aortic aneurysm, Ca Cervix
3. Retroperitoneal fibrosis
4. Aberrant vessels, Bands
5. Phimosis
6. Accidental ureteric ligation

Commonest cause of acute urinary retention are Benign prostatic hypertrophy, Ca prostate & post-op

GENERAL CLIN OF UPPER TRACT OBST: May be symptomless or mild Backache or Malaise; Fever; Loin pain; Recurrent UTIs. Loin pain may be ppt by high fluid intake

GENERAL CLIN OF BLADDER OUTFLOW OBST: Hesitancy; Dribbling; Incomplete voiding; Frequency. Occ Acute retention; Recurrent UTIs; ARF; Polyuria

INVESTIGATIONS:
- AXR
- Ultrasound
- IVU
- Isotope scan
- Percutaneous antegrade pyelography & nephrostograms
- Retrograde pyelography
- Cystoscopy
- Urethrography

RX: Remove obst

PUJ Obst

Common cong condition due to abnormal muscle function interfering c̄ peristalsis. Acquired obst may be due to kinks, bands, adhesions, aberrant vessels

CLIN: May present in infancy c̄ Vom; Failure to thrive; Abdo mass (hydronephrosis). In older children may present c̄ Colicky abdo or loin pain occ ppt by large fluid intake or minimal trauma; Haematuria

INVESTIGATIONS:
- IVU ± Frusemide load: Often hydronephrosis
- Serial DTPA scans ± Frusemide load

RX: Surgical widening of narrow segment by pyeloplasty eg Anderson–Hynes

Retrocaval Ureter

Rare cong abnormality due to persistent embryonic postcardinal veins. The ureter passes medially behind & around vena cava

CLIN: Often asymptomatic. May → upper tract obst ± infection

INVESTIGATION: • IVU

RX: Divide ureter & reanastomose ant to vena cava

URETERIC STONE

Originate in kidney. Usually cause partial obst if not passed spontaneously

CLIN: Ureteric colic; N&V; PI. Occ Haematuria; UTI; Fever. May → hydronephrosis

INVESTIGATIONS:
- AXR
- IVU

RX: Analgesia. If stone not passed spontaneously then perureteric removal or surgery

Causes of Ureteric Stricture (LIST 21 GUS)

1. Congenital
2. Trauma
3. Ca
4. Chr infection
5. TB
6. Schistosomiasis
7. Retroperitoneal fibrosis
8. Stone
9. Endometriosis
10. Ext compression: Eg Ca, LN ↑, Aortic aneurysm, Severe constipation

RETROPERITONEAL FIBROSIS

An inflam fibrosis of retroperitoneal tissues causing symptoms by strangulation of retroperitoneal structures esp ureters. May be idiopathic, 2° to Methysergide or rarely due to Hodgkins disease, Mediastinal fibrosis, Sclerosing Cholangitis, Ca, LSD

CLIN: Occ Backache; Loin pain; IVC obst. Rarely IC; CRF

INVESTIGATIONS:
- FBC: Hb ↓
- ESR ↑
- IVU: Medial deviation of dilated ureters
- CAT scan

RX: Steroids. Ureterolysis ie freeing & transplanting of ureters

BLADDER CALCULI

M>>F. Common in India, Middle East, China. Ass c̄ dehydration. Most stones occur 2° to infection of residual urine which is ass c̄ neurogenic bladder, prostate or bladder neck obst, cystocoele & bladder diverticula. A kidney stone or foreign body lodging in bladder can act as a nidus for ppt of further stones

CLIN: Frequency; Subphrenic, perineal, pubic pain esp end of p/u; Terminal haematuria; Flow of p/u dependent on posture

INVESTIGATIONS:
- Urinalysis: Bacteriuria, Haematuria
- AXR
- Ultrasound
- IVU
- Cystoscopy

RX: Cystoscopy & surgical removal. Occ chemical dissolution used

COMPLICATIONS:
1. UTI ± Squamous metaplasia
2. Vesico–ureteric reflux
3. Obst → Hydronephrosis

BLADDER DIVERTICULA

M>>F. Usually 2° to obst but occ cong

CLIN: Usually asymptomatic. Rarely "pis en deux"

INVESTIGATIONS:
- IVU
- Cystoscopy

RX: Relieve obst. Occ large diverticula requires excision

COMPLICATIONS:
1. Infection
2. Calculus
3. Malignancy
4. Contralat hydronephrosis

CYSTITIS

Acute Cystitis

F>>M. Ass c̄ coitus. In M always 2° to other path eg prostatits

CLIN: Frequency; Dysuria; Urgency. Occ Incontinence; Haematuria; Fever; Nocturia

INVESTIGATIONS: • WCC ↑
• Urinalysis

RX: Increase fluid intake. Antibiotics

COMPLICATION: Acute pyelonephritis

Chronic Cystitis

Usually 2° to chr infection of upper tract but occ 2° to conditions causing residual urine

CLIN: May be symptoms of acute cystitis & renal infection. Occ asymptomatic

INVESTIGATIONS: • FBC
• U&E
• Cystoscopy
• AXR

RX: Antibiotics. Treat underlying condition

Interstitial Cystitis (Hunner's Ulcer)

Esp middle-aged. F>M. ?Auto-immune disease

PATH: Bladder fibrosis, thin mucosa. Small contracted bladder

CLIN: h/o severe progressive frequency & nocturia. Suprapubic pain relieved by voiding. Occ Haematuria

INVESTIGATIONS: • Urinalysis: Usually abacteriuric
• Cystoscopy

RX: Enlarge bladder volume to relieve pain. Try Steroids, Antihistamines or instil hypochlorous acid

COMPLICATION: Ureteric sten → hydronephrosis

PROG: Poor

DD: TB cystitis

Radiation Cystitis

Commonly seen some mths after X-Rad for Ca Cervix

Non-infectious Haemorrhagic Cystitis

Occurs c̄ Cyclophosphamide or following X-Rad. Haem is intermittent but often serious

RX: Stop drug. Instil formalin into bladder

Abacterial Cystitis

A condition of dysuria & frequency in absence of bacteriuria or obvious bladder abnormality

Malakoplakia

A chr granulomatous process c̄ yellow–brown plaques

NEUROPATHIC BLADDER

Due to interruption of either sensory or motor nerves of bladder. Commonest cause is spinal cord trauma. Other causes include Spina bifida; MS; Tabes

Spastic (Automatic) Neuropathic Bladder

An UMN lesion usually due to trauma & MS

PATH: ↓ capacity; Involuntary muscle contractions; Bladder wall hypertrophy; Sphincter spasm

CLIN: Incomplete involuntary p/u; Recurrent UTIs; Impotence. Often renal complications eg hydronephrosis, calculi. Later may develop 2° amyloidosis

INVESTIGATIONS: • Cystometry
• Urinalysis
• IVU
• Cystoscopy

RX: Train to initiate voiding by manual stimulation. May require permanent catheter or ureterostomy

Uninhibited Neuropathic Bladder

A mild form of spastic bladder. May be due to a CVA, MS, Brain tumour, Prolapsed In.v disc or Parkinson's disease

CLIN: Frequency; Nocturia; Urgency. No residual urine

INVESTIGATION: • Cystometry

Flaccid (Autonomous) Neuropathic Bladder

Due to injury of sacral cord or cauda equina roots impairing reflex arc of bladder. Common causes are Trauma; Tabes; Tumours; Cong anomalies eg meningomyelocoele

PATH: Large bladder, low P

CLIN: No sensation of fullness. Overflow incontinence; Sensation ↓; Overdistended bladder. Residual urine

INVESTIGATIONS: • FBC
• Urinalysis
• U&E
• AXR
• IVU
• Cystoscopy
• Cystometry

RX: Manual voiding of bladder 2hrly. Intermittent catheterisation to remove residual urine. Occ TUR of bladder neck. Parasympathetic drugs

COMPLICATIONS: 1. UTI
2. Bladder & renal calculi
3. Hydronephrosis
4. Impotence

INCONTINENCE

Stress Incontinence

Incontinence due to high intraperitoneal P eg cough. F>M. Common. Esp multiparous. Bladder neck weakness

CLIN: Incontinent when straining in upright position

INVESTIGATION: • Videocystourethrogram

RX: Exclude DD. If cystocoele use a vaginal repair to support bladder neck. Otherwise a retropubic urethrovesical suspension (Marshall–Marchetti) op is preferred

DD:
1. Neurogenic bladder
2. Senile urethritis
3. Urethral diverticulum
4. Ectopic ureter
5. Cystitis/Urethritis

Urge Incontinence

An inability to reach the WC in time following strong urge to p/u. Many causes inc local bladder or urethral irritation eg cystitis, calculus & UMN lesions eg MS. Occ no cause found esp in anxious F

INVESTIGATIONS: • Urinalysis
• Videocystourethrogram

Incontinence due to Sphincter Damage

May develop after prostatectomy esp after TUR. Damage to sphincteric smooth muscle

CLIN: Able to stop PU temporarily but permanent control not possible (due to fatigue of striated muscle of voluntary sphincter)

RX: Insert prosthesis or reconstructive surgery

Incontinence due to Neuropathic Bladder

RX: Condom catheter or indwelling catheter is usually needed

Overflow Incontinence

A paradoxical feature of chr urinary retention or 2° to flaccid bladder

Incontinence due to Fistula

RX: Treat underlying cause

BLADDER FISTULAE

Rare. Usually due to diverticulitis, Ca colon, Crohn's disease, Ca cervix, Trauma inc surgery or X-Rad

RX: Proximal colostomy & when inflam settles closure of bladder opening. Then close colostomy

Vesico–Colic Fistula

CLIN: Passing of faeces through urethra; Pneumaturia; Change in bowel habit

INVESTIGATIONS: • Ba Enema
• Sigmoidoscopy
• Cystoscopy
• Cystogram

Vesico–Vaginal Fistula

CLIN: Constant leakage of urine

INVESTIGATIONS: • Cystoscopy
• IVU

RX: Surgical repair

SCHISTOSOMIASIS

S.haematobium endemic in Africa, Middle East
Principally affects urogenital system esp bladder, ureters & seminal vesicles

CLIN: Pruritis; Malaise; Fever; Sweating; Backache; Terminal haematuria. Later Frequency; Suprapubic & back pain; Haematuria; Pyuria. Occ Fever; Rigors; Uraemia

INVESTIGATIONS: • Urinalysis: Often find ova
• FBC: Occ Hb ↓, Eosinophilia
• U&E
• AXR: Bladdder &/or ureteric Ca^{2+}
• IVU: Occ hydronephrosis, hydroureter, ureteric stricture, contracted bladder
• Cystoscopy

RX: Antimony potassium tartrate. Antibiotics for 2° infection

COMPLICATIONS: 1. Bladder contraction
2. Calculi
3. Hydronephrosis
4. Fistula
5. Squamous cell Ca Bladder
6. Vesico–ureteric reflux
7. Recurrent UTIs

BLADDER TUMOUR

Common. M>F. Esp Elderly; Smokers; Aniline dye industry workers

PREDISPOSITIONS: 1. Ectopica vesicae, Urachus
2. Cystitis glandularis (to AdenoCa)
3. Cystitis cystica (to TCCa)
4. Leukoplakia (to Squamous cell Ca)
5. Schistosomiasis (to Squamous cell Ca)
6. Diverticulae (to Squamous cell Ca)
7. Chemicals eg Aniline, β-naphthaline, Trytophan

TYPES: Transitional cell tumours commonest; Squamous cell Ca 5%; AdenoCa, Sarcoma rare. Papillary growths are common & typically are of low malignancy. Tumours are graded by degree of cell differentiation & depth of penetration of tumour into bladder wall or beyond. Commonest site is the bladder base

SPREAD: Direct → Hydronephrosis; Lymph to Iliac, Para-aortic LN; Blood (late) to Liver, Lung, Bones

CLIN: Painless haematuria. Occ UTI; Urgency; Frequency; Nocturia; Hesitancy. Later Pain; Uraemia; Hydronephrosis; Wt ↓

INVESTIGATIONS: • FBC
- WCC
- Urinalysis
- U&E
- IVU
- Cystoscopy & biopsy
- Serial CEA studies

RX: Screen Aniline dye & rubber workers periodically. Low grade & stage are excised by TUR or diathermied & reviewed by periodic repeat cystoscopies. Adjuvent intravesical chemotherapy is indicated if recurrent multiple supf tumours. If infiltration of muscle then pre-op X-Rad & Total cystectomy c̄ urinary diversion ileal conduit. Occ radical X-Rad. Cyt.T is being evaluated

COMPLICATIONS: 1. UTI & Pyelonephritis
2. Obst, Hydronephrosis & uraemia
3. Severe haem
4. Retention
5. Rarely Fistula, ARF

PROG: Prog of early stage Ca is very good if patient well reviewed so that recurrences are quickly treated. Prog correlated to stage & grade. If mets approx 5–10% 5yr survival

BLADDER RUPTURE

GENERAL INVESTIGATIONS: • FBC
- WCC ↑
- Urinalysis if possible
- X-R for #
- Cystogram

Intraperitoneal Rupture

Usually due to abdo trauma when patient has full bladder or surgery

CLIN: h/o injury. Slowly developing peritonitis; Anuria or Haematuria

RX: Treat shock & haem. Close tear transperitoneally; Aspirate peritoneal fluid, catheterise; Antibiotics

Extraperitoneal Rupture

Ass c̄ injury to bony pelvis eg # of pelvis & surgery. May be ass urethral inj

CLIN: h/o injury; Lower abdo pain; Shock; Anuria or Haematuria; ↑ suprapubic tenderness; Pelvic swelling

RX: Suprapubic cystostomy. May need to open peritoneum & explore for ass injury. Antibiotics

COMPLICATION: Infections

DD OF EXTRAPERITONEAL RUPTURE: Urethral (Membranous) rupture

PROSTATITIS

May be acute or chronic. Causes inc TB, Staph, Strep, *E.coli*, GC. Occ bacteria not isolated

Acute Prostatitis

CLIN: Dysuria; Frequency; Urgency; Nocturia. Occ Haematuria; Purulent discharge; Fever; Perineal pain; Myalgia. Tender hot prostate. Often ass c̄ acute cystitis

INVESTIGATIONS: • WCC ↑
- Urinalysis
- Prostatic massage c/i due to risk of bacteraemia
- Stamey Test

RX: Cotrimoxazole. Bed rest

COMPLICATIONS: 1. Abscess
2. Acute retention
3. Acute pyelonephritis
4. Acute epididymitis

Chronic Prostatitis

Usually 2° to infection spread from urethra

CLIN: May be asymptomatic or perineal or low back pain; Mild dysuria; Mild fever. Occ → acute retention, acute epididymitis. Hard fibrotic prostate

INVESTIGATIONS: • WCC: Often norm
• Urinalysis: Occ sterile pyuria
• Stamey test

RX: Difficult. Try 2wks of Cotrimoxazole Rx. If fail try Vibramycin, Erythromycin, or Metronidazole. TUR may be needed if palpable abnormality of prostate

BENIGN PROSTATIC HYPERTROPHY

Very common esp >50yrs

EFFECTS: Prostate ↑ → bladder neck obst → bladder hypertrophy, trabeculation of wall, diverticulae. Then ureters & calyces dilate. Later acute retention. Often UTIs; Stones; Prostatitis. Occ RF

CLIN: Hesitancy; Poor stream; Dribbling; Frequency; Nocturia; Prostate ↑. Often UTIs. Occ Terminal haematuria. May → retention. Later may be uraemic

INVESTIGATIONS: • Urinalysis
• U&E
• Acid phos
• IVU
• Ultrasound

RX: Prostatectomy if renal function ↓ or marked symptoms. If acute retention catheterise & then prostatectomy. 4 types of op

1. **TUR:** Popular. Mort 1–2%. No Scar. Potency maintained
   Common Indications: Small benign prostate; Prostatic Ca
2. **Retropubic Extravesical (Millin op):** Bladder not opened. Mort 1–2%. Potency maintained
   Common Indication: Large benign prostate
3. **Transvesical:** Open op. Mort 1–3%. Excellent result & potency maintained
   Common Indications: Benign prostate with other bladder path eg stone, diverticulum (but not bladder Ca)
4. **Perineal:** Low risk but often → impotence & occ → incontinence, recto–urethral fistula

COMPLICATIONS OF PROSTATECTOMY:
1. Haem
2. Infection
3. Obst
4. Suprapubic fistula esp c̄ transvesical
5. Incontinence due to sphincter damage esp perineal
6. Inguinal hernia
7. Retrograde ejaculation

DD: Ca prostate

Ca PROSTATE

Incidence ↑ c̄ age. Common in very elderly. Often found in autopsies of elderly M. Occ FH. Usually AdenoCa. Often arises from post lobe

SPREAD: Local, via Lymph & blood esp to bone (Osteosclerosis) & liver

CLIN: Frequency; Nocturia; Hesitancy; Dribbling; Hard prostate usually enlarged, loss of sulcus if advanced. Often acute retention. Occ Uraemia; Symptoms of mets eg Bone pain

INVESTIGATIONS: • FBC
• Acid Phos: Often ↑
• CXR
• Prostatic Biopsy
• Bone scan
• Ultrasound

RX: In fit c̄ no obvious mets: X-Rad or radical prostatectomy. If mets: Approx 85% are androgen dependent &

respond to bilat orchidectomy or Oestrogens (SE: Gynaecomastia; CVS complications; Impotence). Testosterone & radioisotope Rx can be tried if tumour is androgen independent. X-Rad may help cure & certainly palliates esp bone pain. TUR for symptomatic relief. Monitor c̄ serial acid phos & X-rays

PROG: Approx 25% 5yr survival

URETHERAL INJURIES

Bulbous Urethral Injuries

Usually due to falling astride an object

CLIN: Local pain; Bleeding; Tenderness; Bruising. Occ 2° infection

INVESTIGATION: • Urethrogram

RX: If perineal haematoma not extensive manage conservatively. Drain any infected haematoma. If urinary extravasation, catheterise if possible. In extensive injuries partial repair, secure haemostasis & catheterise; Later urethroplasty

Membranous Urethral Injury

May be due to # pelvis → extravasation of blood & urine into perivesical & periprostatic tissues

CLIN: Perineal pain; Urethral bleeding or haematuria. Often unable to p/u; Suprapubic mass; Displaced prostate. Occ Shock; 2° infection. Later, often Stricture; Impotence

INVESTIGATIONS: • FBC: Occ Hb ↓
• WCC ↑
• Urethrogram
• IVU

RX: Try to pass catheter, if possible leave in place for 2wks. Repair urethra

URETHERAL STRICTURE

M>F. Rare. May be due to GC urethritis; Post urethral trauma or Ca

CLIN: Poor stream, improved by straining. Occ Acute retention; UTIs

INVESTIGATION: • Urethrogram

RX:
1. Dilatation
2. Urethrotomy
3. Occ surgical reconstruction

PHIMOSIS

An inability to retract the penile foreskin over the glans. Maybe cong; 2° to infection; or 2° to trauma

CLIN: On p/u, prepuce seen to balloon, stream ↓. Often local infection

RX: Antibiotics. Later circumcision

PARAPHIMOSIS

Foreskin cannot be retracted from behind glans penis → contracture & obst of venous return

CLIN: Pain; Swelling of glans. If unrelieved may → gangrene

RX: Attempt manual reduction. If fails try ice packs. Occ require dorsal slit & later circumcision

BALANITIS

An acute inflam of foreskin & glans. Usually due to *E.coli*, Staph, Strep. Ass c̄ diabetes. May cause phimosis

RX: Antibiotics

PRIAPISM

Rare. Prolonged painful erection. Cause often unknown, occ due to leukaemia, mets, sickle cell disease

RX: Difficult. Ice water enemas. Occ embolisation or op (Corporo–sapheno bypass)

PEYRONIE'S DISEASE

Rare. A fibrosis of the covering sheath of the corpora cavernosa. Esp >45yrs

CLIN: Penis bends due to fibrosis. Painful erections

RX: Low dose X-Rad or op. May try steroid injection

Ca PENIS

Esp China, Africa & S.E.Asia

AETIOLOGY: Follows chr inflam. Leukoplakia, Erythroplasia of Queyrat & Bowen's disease (Ca in situ) are premalignant. Circumcision is protective

SPREAD: Mainly local & via lymph

CLIN: Usually growth on glans or foreskin. Ulcer c̄ bloody, purulent discharge

INVESTIGATION: • Biopsy

RX: In local tumour excision & or X-Rad. If necessary amputate penis. If local LN spread try X-Rad

PROG: Very good if no spread

EPIDIDYMAL CYST

Painless cystic mass containing sperm. Seprate from testis. Often multiple & bilat. Old name—spermatocoele

CLIN: Small mobile transilluminating cystic mass

HYDROCOELE

A collection of fluids within the tunica or processus vaginalis usually surrounding the testicle. Cause unknown but occ 2° to orchitis, Ca, TB, epididymitis, trauma. In young boys may be due to connection between peritoneal cavity & tunica vaginalis

CLIN: A rounded non-tender transilluminating cystic mass enclosing the testis

INVESTIGATION: • Occ ultrasound

RX: May require aspiration. Occ surgery

COMPLICATIONS: 1. Haematocoele
2. Testicular atrophy (rare)

VARICOCOELE

Varicosities of pampiniform venous plexus. L>R side. Esp young M. Rarely due to renal Ca

CLIN: A mass of dilated tortuous veins ("Bag of worms") above & post to testis. Often tender. Relieved by recumbence. Occ ass c̄ subfertility

RX: Occ require scrotal support or ligation of int spermatic vein

EPIDIDYMITIS

Acute Epididymitis

May occur 2° to prostatitis or following prostatectomy

CLIN: Sudden severe scrotal pain & swelling; Fever; Thickened spermatic cord. Occ Urethral discharge; Cystitis. May → hydrocoele. Often concurrent prostatitis

INVESTIGATIONS: • Urinalysis
• WCC ↑

RX: Infiltrate spermatic cord c̄ LA; Antibiotics; Bedrest; Analgesia

DD: TB epididymitis

Chronic Epididymitis

A rare irreversible complication of acute epididymitis

ACUTE ORCHITIS

Many causes including Mumps, Coxsackie

CLIN: Sudden onset of Testicular pain & swelling; Red swollen scrotum; Fever. No urinary symptoms. Occ Bilat

RX: Bed rest, testicular support. No specific Rx for mumps orchitis. Antibiotics

COMPLICATION: Rarely → sterility

TORSION OF TESTIS

Torsion of spermatic cord. Esp pre-pubertal M. May be 2° to cong abnormality of tunica vaginalis or spermatic cord

CLIN: Sudden severe pain in testicle followed by swelling & redness of scrotum, lower abdo pain; N&V; Fever

RX: If within few hrs of onset, try manual detorsion—if successful, surgically fix both testes later. If fails immediate surgical decompression & fixing. If detorsion delayed for >48hrs often require orchidectomy

DD:
1. Ac Epididymitis
2. Strangulated ing hernia
3. Traumatic orchitis
4. Mumps orchitis

TESTICULAR TUMOURS

Account for approx 0.5% of all M malignancies. Whites >Blacks. Cause unknown. Testicular tumours 30× more frequent in undescended testes. About 40% of testicular tumours are seminomas, 30% teratomas & 15% combined tumours ie seminomas & teratomas

GENERAL INVESTIGATIONS:
- Histology of testis removed at op
- CAT scan
- CXR
- αFP
- β HCG
- Occ lymphangiography
- FBC
- LFT
- U&E

Seminoma

Esp 30–40yrs. Arise from seminiferous tubules. Malignant

SPREAD: Slow growing. Lymph spread to para-aortic LN

CLIN: Firm smooth enlargement of testes, usually painless. Occ 2° hydrocoele. Later signs of mets

RX: Orchidectomy & X-Rad (Extent dependent on stage). In diffuse disease use Cyt.T eg Cyclophosphamide

PROG: Very good if no mets or mets confined to abdo nodes. Tumour often radiosensitive

Teratoma

TERATOMA & TERATOCARCINOMA

Moderately well differentiated tissue. Esp 20–30yrs. Arise from germ cells. Malignant

SPREAD: Early via blood & lymph esp to lungs & liver

CLIN: Often enlargement of testes, usually painless. Occ 2° hydrocoele. Cell contents variable eg bone, cartilage. Later signs of mets

RX: Orchidectomy & X-Rad. In more advanced disease add Cyt.T & excise residual bulk disease at laparotomy

PROG: If no LN spread, 80% 5yr survival. If LN spread or mets Cyt.T offers improving 5yr survival

UNDIFFERENTIATED MALIGNANT TERATOMA (EMBRYONAL CARCINOMA)

Tend to secrete chorionic gonadotrophin

SPREAD: Early mets via blood

INVESTIGATIONS:
- Urinary HCG
- αFP ↑

RX: Orchidectomy. Later Cyt.T

PROG: Poor

CHORIOCARCINOMA (MALIGNANT TROPHOBLASTIC TERATOMA)

Rare. Contains true trophoblastic elements

Interstitial (Leydig) Cell Tumours

Esp 30–40yrs. Usually benign. Secrete oestrogens

CLIN: In young, sexual precocity. In adults, gynaecomastia, impotence & sterility

INVESTIGATION: • Urinary 17-ketosteroids ↓

RX: Orchidectomy. Chemotherapy

Sertoli Cell Tumour

Rare. Benign. Usually feminising

MALE INFERTILITY

Causes of Male Infertility (LIST 22 GUS)

1. Endocrine:
   a) Hypopituitarism
   b) Hypothyroidism
   c) Hyperadrenalism
   d) Klinefelter's Syndrome
   e) Isolated gonadotrophin def
2. Infections:
   Eg Mumps orchitis, TB, Epididymitis, Gonococcus
3. Irradiation
4. Congenital:
   Eg Germinal cell aplasia, Absent vas, Anorchia
5. Sperm abnormalities
6. Sperm antibodies
7. Varicocoele
8. Maldescent of testes
9. High body temperature inc wearing of tight underwear
10. Drugs:
    Eg Oestrogens
11. Testicular Tumours
12. Trauma
13. Surgery:
    Esp Orchidectomy, Prostatectomy
14. Cirrhosis
15. Haemochromatosis
16. Impotence

GENERAL INVESTIGATIONS:
- Sperm: Count, motility (usually >60% motile), morphology (usually >70% norm) & vol (usually 2.5–6mls)
- TFT
- Testicular biopsy (if Azoospermia)
- Chromosomes
- FSH
- Testosterone
- HCG test
- Urinary 17-ketosteroids
- Sperm antibodies
- Vasography

RX: Remove any varicocoele. Treat underlying cause if possible. Idiopathic oligospermia may respond to Cortisone or Clomiphene. If normal spermatogenesis but azoospermia, op may help eg epididymovasostomy. In 1° androgen def give testosterone. In 2° hypogonadism give HCG ± FSH to stimulate spermatogenesis

Impotence

Most cases are due to psychogenic causes. Esp elderly

Causes of Impotence (LIST 23 GUS)

1. Psychogenic:
   Eg 2° to guilt, anxiety, jealousy
2. Surgery:
   Eg Prostatectomy, Abdo–perineal resection
3. Autonomic neuropathy:
   Esp Diabetes, Tabes
4. RF
5. Leriche Syndrome
6. X-Rad
7. Trauma:
   Eg To membranous urethra
8. Neurological:
   Eg MS, Spina bifida, Spinal cord transection
9. Drugs:
   Eg Oestrogen, Methysergide, Heroin, TCAD
10. Genital abnormalities:
    Eg Epispadias, Hypospadias
11. Endocrine:
    Eg Cushing's, Addison's, Testicular failure, Acromegaly, Hypopituitarism
12. Leriche syndrome

CLIN: Complaints can inc inability to gain or maintain an erection, lack of emission c̄ orgasm, loss of libido, premature ejaculation. In psychogenic cases impotence may be related to situation. Rarely Hypogonadism, Gynaecomastia

RX: Discontinue drugs. In Psychogenic gp, re-education concerning technique & attitude

Community Medicine

Community medicine is the branch of medical practice that is concerned to promote, to maintain, & when necessary to restore the health of human communities. The function of the community physician is analagous to that of other physicians in the need to give timely, relevant & soundly based advice to the solution of problems related to health & sickness. Whilst the clinician mainly deals c̄ the individual, the community physician mainly deals c̄ problems at a pop/community level. The basic science of community medicine is epidemiology. Epidemiology is that branch of medical science concerned c̄ the study of health in communities Many health phenomena become apparent only when analysed at the pop level eg the link between smoking & lung cancer. Studying the characteristics of pops in respect to health & illness has often → the formulation of hypotheses regarding the aetiology of illness

Community medicine is also concerned c̄ the study of the effectiveness & efficiency of health services. Thus Planning; Factors affecting service uptake eg service organisation, the doctor–patient relationship; Priorities in resource allocation, are also the province of the community physician. The areas of Community Medicine interest have also been summarised as: Need & Demand; Provision; Process; & Outcome

THE EPIDEMIOLOGICAL APPROACH

Epidemiological methods can be divided into various stages: Hypothesis formulation & design of investigation; Data collection; Data analysis; Data interpretation. Broadly, epidemiological studies can be divided into descriptive, analytic & intervention studies

Descriptive studies eg cross-sectional surveys, identify the patterns in which diseases are distributed in pops. Comparisons may be drawn between the incidence & prevalence in respect to time, place & other variables. Usually routinely collected data are used. Such studies alone rarely demonstrate causality but may allow hypothesis generation

Analytic studies are planned investigations designed to test specific hypotheses. The two principal types are termed case-control & cohort studies. Data are collected in a systematic manner

Intervention studies eg randomised control trials are experiments designed to determine the efficacy of particular health care interventions. They may be used to assess the comparative effectiveness & efficiency of different treatments/services

Efficiency is chiefly applicable to the conversion of money, manpower, premises & equipment into items of service. Effectiveness is a measure of the success c̄ which items of service are converted into improved health. Efficacy is a term used to describe the effectiveness of a procedure carried out at the individual level

Epidemiological comparisons aim to show whether some aspect of health status & some other defined characteristic tend to coincide in individuals eg lung cancer is commoner amongst smokers compared to non-smokers. Such comparisons may be of: Diseased & non-diseased; Exposed & unexposed; Correlation studies

Epidemiological studies may also be classified as: Cross-sectional ie data on health & other characteristic collected at same point in time; Retrospective ie data on health at present & of characteristic in the past; Prospective ie data on characteristic at start of study c̄ health monitored in future

Routine Sources of Data

In general, routine sources of data are more extensive & more reliable in the "developed" world than elsewhere. It is convenient to consider routine data under 3 headings: Mortality & other denominator data (N.B mortality can be both a numerator & denominator); Morbidity data; Data related to characteristics ass c̄ health

As mortality is an easily defined concept & data concerning death are relatively easy to collect, such data are generally more accurate & more available than morbidity data. Occ mortality is used as a rough proxy for morbidity. Much routine morbidity data are measures of the administrative health process rather than health outcome

In UK the following routine sources of data are available: Mort & other denominator data inc: Records of births & marriages from General Register office; 10yrly census data on pop size & demographic characteristics; Mort from death certificates. Cause of deaths are routinely analysed by age, sex etc

Morbidity data inc: HAA; HIPE (a 10% sample of death & discharges from hospital excluding mental illness); SH3s (a hospital return relating to hospital & outpatient usage eg number of beds, bed occupancy); Mental health enquiry; Confidential enquiry into maternal deaths; Cancer registries; Disabled person's register; Notification of statutory infectious diseases; Cong malformation notification; Abortion notification; % of working pop drawing sickness & injury benefit

Data related to characteristics ass c̄ health inc: Information on social trends eg The OPCS General Household Survey, HMSO publication "Social Trends"; EMAS & HSE reports; Drug misuse notifications to Home Office

The Korner reports, soon to be implemented in the UK, will establish a series of basic data sets for component services of the NHS

Many ad-hoc studies have been carried out eg surveys of morbidity in general practice

Sources of error in routine data are that: Not all cases are correctly diagnosed; Not all diagnosed cases are included ie def in certification, registration, notification, coding, processing &/or interpretation; Not all cases experience the type of service contact being monitored eg not all diabetics receive hospital inpatient care. Changes in diagnostic fashion can occur eg in the decade 1969–78 cases of SIDS in UK rose, but this rise was counterbalanced by a fall in infant deaths ascribed to resp infection, inhalation & mechanical obst. Coding changes can account for variations in disease prevalence over time eg the ICD is in its ninth revision

Descriptive Studies

Descriptive studies are usually based on the frequency of disease related to time, place &/or person

VARIATIONS IN TIME

3 major patterns of disease incidence

c̄ respect to time can be recognised. These are long term (secular trends), periodic (cyclic) trends inc seasonal trends, & epidemics

LONG TERM TRENDS: Changes in the incidence of a disease over a number of yrs. The change does not necessarily indicate changes in underlying causality, but a change of large magnitude is more likely to warrant the testing of a specific hypothesis. An example of a secular trend is the ↑ in M deaths from lung Ca in UK in the 20th century, this later trend being highly correlated c̄ the national consumption of cigs during the same period
A period effect occurs when a causal event affects all age gps at the same time eg prevalence at birth of NTD ↑ in 1955–59 in UK for each age gp of mothers. A cohort effect occurs when a pop experiences an effect at a particular time & thereafter show a different disease incidence than other cohorts eg F born in 1920s & 1930s have higher rates of cervical Ca than cohorts born at different time when compared at similar ages

PERIODIC CHANGES: Cyclic changes in the incidence of disease eg the irregular epidemics of whooping cough in UK every 3–4yrs. Many illnesses show a seasonal periodicity eg resp infections are commoner in winter compared to summer

EPIDEMICS: Epidemics are temporary significant increases in the incidence of disease in a pop. The term is usually applied to infectious diseases

VARIATIONS IN PLACE

Variations in place can be analysed at different levels eg international, national, regional, district, small areas. Often analysis may involve aggregation of similar places eg urban/rural, places c̄ soft water. Geographical differences in disease incidence often generate hypotheses about factors such as race, climate, diet & vectors. Racial hypotheses are often studied by observing the disease incidence of migrant gps. In broad terms, if a migrant gp has a similar disease incidence to that of the country of birth a genetic cause is suggested, whereas a change in incidence towards that of the host country suggests an environmental cause

At national & lower levels, variations of health experience c̄ place are common. In UK, mort rate varies geographically c̄ large regional variations in mort & morbidity. Differences between urban & rural health risks inc ↑ risk of chr bronchitis in town dwellers. Illness can often be ass c̄ very specific geographic location eg a dirty water supply → cholera, a restaurant → food poisoning
Diseases c̄ low frequency require special analytic techniques often involving large study numbers, long-term aggregation of data & space–time interaction analysis

VARIATIONS IN PERSON

Commonly analysed variables inc age, sex, ethnic gp, marital state & occupation

AGE: Most diseases vary both in frequency & severity c̄ age eg children are generally more susceptible to infectious diseases than adults
The fact that most diseases vary considerably in incidence in relation to age means that to allow true comparisons of pops c̄ different age structures requires an adjustment procedure termed standardisation.
The variation of disease incidence c̄ age may represent a cohort effect eg the number of people c̄ lung cancer aged 60–70yrs is dependent on their smoking habit over the past 40–50yrs, thus the incidence of lung Ca reflects the amount of smoking present in that cohort

SEX: Many diseases show a sex difference in frequency & severity. In most countries, M have a lesser life expectancy than F. In most studies, it is sensible to standardise pops for sex as well as age

ETHNIC GROUP: It is often difficult to define an ethnic gp accurately. Nonetheless studies based on skin colour or religious grouping have demonstrated disease associations eg Tay–Sachs disease is commoner & cervical Ca less common amongst Jews; Sickle cell disease is commoner in Blacks

MARITAL STATUS: Marital status is a significant marker of lifestyle. Certain gps eg physically & mentally handicapped people, are less likely to marry. Marital status is ass c̄ contact c̄ children & sexual behaviour. Many diseases are significantly related to marital status eg cervical Ca incidence is highest in divorcees & lowest in single F esp nuns

OCCUPATION: There is a social class gradient for most diseases. Usually disease prevalence is highest in the lower social classes. Occ a specific occupational hazard can be linked c̄ a disease eg CS_2 exposure & coronary Ht disease, or particular occupations are linked c̄ a disease eg wives of deep sea fishermen c̄ cervical Ca, but usually the effect of social class seems to be multifactorial ie occupation itself is linked c̄ lifestyle, education, housing, diet & wealth

A possible bias in studies of occupation & health is the "well worker" effect. In some industries, people may change their jobs because of their worsening health & an investigation of the health of people performing that job may give a spurious impression eg coal face workers moving to lighter duties if their health deteriorates, unless workers leaving the industry are also followed up

TWIN STUDIES: Twin studies are a particularly useful way of discriminating between genetic & environmental aetiological factors. Types of study inc Twins reared apart; Monozygous versus dizygous twin's health experience

Descriptive & Hypothesis Testing Studies of Specially Collected Data

Often routine data are inadequate to answer an hypothesis. In these cases, original data must be collected eg a descriptive cross-sectional survey which relies on data collected in a systematic way from a defined pop in order to compare individuals exposed & unexposed to a suspected causal agent

The requirements for a successful study include an appropriate choice of: Hypothesis & aim; Study gp eg a sample or total pop?; Type of sample; Size of study; Categories of data needed; Methods of data collection (eg questionnaire, personal interview) to achieve accurate results c̄ an acceptable pop coverage; Methods of analysis & interpretation

It is usually impossible & often undesirable to study the whole of a pop. Techniques are available to draw a sample which is representative of the pop under investigation. The method of sample selection depends on the nature of the investigation. Common types of sample are: Simple random sample ie each individual in the parent pop has an equal probability of being selected; Stratified sample (where the pop is first divided into sub-gps according to one or more characteristics eg sex, & random sampling is then performed independently in each sub-gp) ie ensuring the representativeness in the sample of certain variables within the parent pop; Cluster sampling involves the use of groups rather than individuals as the sampling unit; Systematic multistage sampling involves a combination of the above techniques

Attempts to minimise bias are crucial if the investigation is to be worthwhile. Potential sources of selection bias are: Replacement of previously selected individuals by other persons; Using volunteers (this is self-selection); Omission of hard to identify people from study (non-responders are generally different eg often are iller); Low response ratio. A response ratio of >90% should usually avoid bias

All surveys contain errors, but good surveys manage to minimise errors so that sensible conclusions may be drawn from their outcome. Sources of error include: Intra–observer variation ie failure of same observer to record same result on repeated examination of same material; Inter–observer variation ie failure of different observers to record the same result; Subject variation ie different responses by same individual on different occasions to same test eg BP variability; Test of poor sensitivity & specificity; Faulty equipment; Inappropriate test

Errors can be minimised by the use of: Clear definitions; Relevant, reliable & validated tests; Standardised methods; Training of observers; Standardised equipment; Unambiguous questions

Where possible test should be validated. Validity is partly assessed by how well it detects those c̄ disease (sensitivity) & how well it rejects those without disease (specificity)

An example was screening by the Haemoccult test of 4000 people aged >40yrs for large bowel tumours when the test was 98% specific & 52% sensitive

	With Disease	Without Disease	Total
+ve Test	a	b	a + b
−ve Test	c	d	c + d
Total	a + c	b + d	

$$\text{Sensitivity} = \frac{\text{True +ves}}{\text{All } \bar{c} \text{ disease}} = \frac{a}{a + c}$$

$$\text{Specificity} = \frac{\text{True −ves}}{\text{All } \bar{c} \text{ no disease}} = \frac{d}{b + d}$$

Fig 1: Screening Test Sensitivity & Specificity

An example of a hypothesis testing, cross-sectional study was one that considered possible links between bronchitis, smoking & urbanisation. It was found that there was a dose-response relationship between the prevalence of bronchitis & the number of cigs smoked ie the relative risk of bronchitis in smokers compared to non-smokers increased c̄ amount smoked. The power of a study to be certain that it has uncovered a true difference between variables is dependent on the sample size

Retrospective Studies

Generally are case-control studies. Individuals who are known to have the disease have their history analysed eg by reference to clin records, for suspected causal agents & the same data are collected in the same way from a control gp of disease-free individuals. Controls are often matched for some characteristics c̄ the cases eg age & sex Particular risks of bias in these studies inc: Differential recall rate eg if malformations are investigated, parents are more likely to recall events during the pregnancy than a gp of parent controls; Differential response rate; Different approach by interviewers to cases & controls; Inability to check reliability of records; Inability to select random sample of cases &/or controls eg it is easy to identify cases of a disease who happen to be in contact c̄ hospital, however these cases are probably at the more severe end of the spectrum of the disease
An example of a case control study was an investigation of lung Ca & smoking carried out by Doll & Hill. Previous smoking habit, assessed by questionnaire, of lung Ca patients & controls who were drawn from British hospitals (individually matched by place & date of hospitalisation & by age gp) revealed a dose-response relationship between number of cigs smoked before illness onset & likelihood of developing lung Ca

Prospective Studies

Prospective studies are often used to test hypotheses generated from retrospective, case controlled or cross-sectional studies. The study should define its objectives & outcome measures at the start. The study pop is a gp of people (who often are healthy) usually chosen either because they have been particularly exposed to some agent that is under investigation or they have characteristics which makes their follow-up easy eg professions c̄ a register of members. These cohort studies can investigate the prevalence, incidence & risk of disease in relation to suspected causal agents. If the study pop is a group selected because of exposure to a presumed noxious agent, a control gp is required. It is important not to lose people at follow-up. Methods of analysis inc: "Person–years" at risk; Life table analysis
Examples of prospective studies are: The British National Child Development Study which has followed a cohort of all children born during 1wk in March 1958 to investigate the effects of obstetric care & socioeconomic factors on subsequent morbidity; A study of a gp of F who took analgesics in the first 16wks of pregnancy & a control gp of F who took no drugs in early pregnancy, showed that on follow-up the children from the 2 gps had no significant difference in their cong malformation rates
Prospective studies usually require large numbers & are slow & expensive to carry out compared to retrospective studies, but prospective studies are more free from outcome bias, can determine pop disease incidence & offer stronger evidence of causal links

Intervention Studies

These are prospective studies in

which an intervention procedure which it is hoped will protect against some undesirable outcome is tested. For ethical reasons it is usually unacceptable to deliberately expose a gp to a suspected causal agent, although this is sometimes done in animal experiments. In these experimental studies randomly selected intervention & control gps are compared in terms of a defined outcome. The commonest intervention studies are clinical trials

The study pop should be: Readily accessible; Of sufficient size to meet the power (ie the degree of certainty that there is a real difference of a specified magnitude at a chosen significance level between the two gps) & significance (ie the level of probability chosen to represent a real difference between the gps eg $p < 0.05$) requirements of the study; Of sufficient stability to avoid significant loss to follow-up; Representative of the pop in which it is intended to apply the procedure being tested

In principle, individuals should be allocated to intervention & control gps at random so that differences in outcome are not merely the result of sampling method. To avoid bias in reporting illnesses & other factors, subject should, if possible, not know to which gp they have been allocated. It is also often valuable to avoid bias, if the observers of the study do not know if the individual is in the control or intervention gp. If the subjects do not know to which gp they have been randomised it is termed a single blind trial, whilst if both subjects & observers do not know it is termed a double blind trial

In UK, intervention studies usually require agreement by an ethical committee

An example of a double blind RCT was the MRC trial of whooping cough vaccine. Children were randomised into 2gps, one receiving 3 inoculations of whooping cough vaccine, the other gp three inoculations of anti-catarrh vaccine. The incidence of pertussis per 1000 person–mths follow-up was calculated. The protection given by the whooping cough vaccine was then calculated & found to be 78%. (% efficacy of whooping cough vaccine = incidence of pertussis in control gp minus incidence of pertussis in intervention gp × 100 divided by incidence in control gp)

Data Interpretation

INCIDENCE & PREVALENCE

Many studies are carried out to determine the incidence &/or prevalence of disease. The incidence rate is the proportion of a defined gp developing a condition within a stated period of time. Point prevalence is the proportion of a defined gp having a condition at one point in time. Prevalence = incidence × average duration of disease. Although prevalence is usually measured at a point in time (point prevalence), it is sometimes necessary to measure the period prevalence ie the proportion of a defined gp having a condition at any time within a stated period

Incidence rates & prevalence ratios form the basis of comparison between pop gps. The numerator is usually the frequency of an observed state or event, & the denominator the total number in whom this state or event might occur. To allow comparison between different rates, standardisation procedures are usually required eg because of different age/sex structures in the pops, these include the methods of direct standardisation, indirect standardisation & regression techniques

INFERENCE OF CAUSALITY

Many studies are valuable even if their result is the disproving of a hypothesis. Studies which show support for a hypothesis do not necessarily prove causality. There are many examples of associations between agents & disease which are non-causal. Associations between exposure to a risk factor & occurence of disease are esp likely to be causal if the association is: Strong eg relative risk of 30 (relative risk = the risk ratio between the exposed & unexposed, the unexposed by definition having a risk of 1); Repeatedly found; Unidirectionally related in time ie postulated cause precedes effect; Specific; Graded ie a dose-response relationship; Biologically plausible; Between variables about which there is independent evidence to support a link; Analagous to associations already known to be causal. Evidence of causality is also present if disease incidence in those who have been exposed to risk factor declines when they remove themselves from it

MAJOR CAUSES OF & TRENDS IN MORTALITY & MORBIDITY

In most countries in the Western world age-specific death rates have fallen markedly since records were first routinely collected (in UK, since about 150yrs ago). The reduction has been almost entirely due to the elimination of the major endemic infectious diseases

In the UK overall mort fell at age 3–45yrs throughout 19th century. In 20th century fall has extended into infancy & later middle-age. Most of the fall for most diseases occured before 1930. In the last 50yrs mort rates have been more stable, but further improvement in lowering PNMR & increased life expectancy has occured.

In recent yrs hospital admission rates have ↑, sickness absence has sl ↑ but indices of general health eg Hgh, nutritional status have improved.

The position of the UK in relation to other Western countries has generally declined in respect of major mort rates eg PNMR

Factors accounting for the decline in mort, point to the conclusion that general environmental changes eg proper sanitation, clean water, good diet, safer working conditions, better housing have been the most significant determinants of health. Advances in therapeutic medicine & its wider availability have been a minor factor in the decline, as the falling mort had largely been completed before these advances began. Some advances in preventive (community) medicine have had a significant effect on mort eg some vaccinations

The major causes of morbidity & mort in the UK can be summarised by reference to a number of markers eg deaths, operations, handicaps, ave duration of in-patient stay

Major Causes of Death in UK (LIST 1 CM)

1. IHD
2. Cancer:
   Esp Resp, Bowel, GU, Lymph & Blood
3. Cerebrovascular disease
4. Pneumonia
5. Bronchitis & emphysema
6. BP ↑ disease

Commonest Symptoms in UK Adults (LIST 2 CM)

1. Headache
2. Cough, catarrh or phlegm
3. Aching limbs or jts
4. Backache
5. "Nerves"
6. Trouble c feet
7. Indigestion
8. Colds
9. Sleeplessness
10. Tiredness
11. SOB
12. Eyestrain

(Source: General Household Survey)

Commonest Presentations to GP in UK (LIST 3 CM)

1. Acute pharyngitis & tonsillitis
2. Acute nasopharyngitis
3. Bronchitis
4. Anxiety neurosis
5. Depressive neurosis
6. Acute D&/orV
7. Cough
8. Acute OM
9. Wax in ear

Commonest Causes of M Sickness Absence Spells in UK (LIST 4 CM)

1. Influenza
2. Bronchitis
3. D&V
4. LRTI & URTI
5. Gastritis
6. Rheumatism

The commonest cause of M sickness absence in respect of days lost are Bronchitis, Influenza, IHD, Neuroses, Arthritis, Surgical Rx

Commonest Causes of Long Hospital Stay (LIST 5 CM)

1. Senility
2. Cerebrovascular disease
3. MS
4. Ep
5. # of femur
6. Arthritis
7. Mental handicap
8. Chr mental illness

In the developed world the major problems for the health services are the chr disorders. This is partly due to the success of eliminating infectious diseases & the change in pop structure (there are relatively more elderly who have a higher risk of chr disease eg arthritis, senility, CVAs). These generally require caring rather than curative services. To an extent all Western health services are still geared to the curative treatment of acute disease which was appropriate for the management of infectious diseases

The major causes of mort in the UK in different age gps are:

0–1yrs: Cong malformations; Birth trauma
2–15yrs: Accidents & violence
16–40yrs: Accidents & violence
41–60yrs: IHD (esp M)
>61yrs: Ca; IHD; CVA; Chr bronchitis

In the developing world, the causes of death follow a similar pattern to that seen in the 19th century in the West. It is therefore inherently plausible that environmental changes eg clean water, better housing, improved diet & preventive medicine eg immunisation programmes should be the route to major falls in mort in these countries

Examination of the prevalence of specific diseases in different parts of the world can generate hypotheses about causation. Migrant studies help to evaluate whether a cause is environmentally determined

The UK has particularly high prevalence of Ca lung, Ca breast & IHD. Ca uterus & colon are common in Latin America. Japan has high rates for Ca stomach & CVAs but low rates of Ca breast

SOCIAL DETERMINANTS OF HEALTH

There is much evidence that social factors have been important in determining the health of pops. Sometimes the causal link between health & a social factor has been unifactorial eg that between unclean water supply & cholera, but more often social factors seem to exert an influence on health in a more complicated fashion. As social factors eg trends in fertility & marital status, housing are early elements in the causal chain → many diseases, changes in social factors & hence lifestyle often exert a considerable influence on the pop's experience of many diseases

Social Class & Health

In the UK, a measure of social class is based on the Registrar General's classification of occupation. In the case of married couples the man's occupation is used for classification purposes. This classification divides the pop into 6 gps:

Social Class I: Professional workers eg doctors (Approx 5%)
Social Class II: Managerial workers eg teachers (Approx 17%)
Social Class IIINM: Skilled non-manual workers eg draughtsman (Approx 12%)

Social Class IIIM: Skilled manual workers eg butchers (Approx 36%)
Social Class IV: Semi-skilled manual workers eg postmen (Approx 17%)
Social Class V: Unskilled manual workers eg labourers (Approx 8%)
Not Classified: eg Unemployed (Approx 5%), armed forces

An alternative classification used in the UK is that of socioeconomic gp. This classification has many more groupings which allows each class to contain occupations of much greater similarity than is the case c̄ Social Class. Social Class is often used in studies rather than SEGs due to its greater simplicity (although neither classification allows rapid coding of occupations)

Social Class gradients are very common in relation to disease incidence & prevalence. A worse experience of disease by the lower social classes is seen in a large majority of diseases eg infections, IHD

The worse health experience of the lower social classes in the UK relative to the higher social classes has not diminished since the inception of the NHS. Although social class gradients have not diminished, disease frequency in both gps has fallen

Examples of social class gradients in E&W for major causes of death are shown by the disease-specific Standardised Mortality Ratios (SMRs) for M aged 15–64yrs (N.B By definition SMR for E&W = 100):

IHD: SCI 88, SCIIIM 107, SCV 111
Cerebrovascular Disease: SCI 80, SCIIIM 106, SCV 136
COAD & Asthma: SCI 36, SCIIIM 113, SCV 188
Ca lung: SCI 53, SCIIIM 118, SCV 143
Ca stomach: SCI 50, SCIIIM 118, SCV 147

The SMR for all causes in M aged 15–64, is almost double in SCV as compared to SCI

Morbidity rates are also strongly ass c̄ social class eg the attack-rate of depression in the inner city areas is 3× higher in F from SCIV & SCV compared to SCI & SCII; Home & playground accidents are commoner in lower social classes

The reason for the often strong ass between social class & health usually seems to be multifactorial & not simply due to the occupation which is used to determine the social class. There is a very strong correlation between the health experience of husbands & wives, which obviously cannot be explained by occupation as wives rarely have the same jobs as the husband. Social class is itself highly correlated c̄ education, dietary habit, housing conditions, wealth & other determinants of lifestyle eg family size, leisure activities, smoking. It is presumed that these complex interrelated factors are important in determining health experience

Social class is not only implicated in the causation of many diseases, but also as a determinant of the type of health care received. In the UK, the lower social classes find access to PHC more difficult for a number of reasons eg employers unwilling to allow time off work, cost of travelling to surgery, larger list size of their GPs, ↑ number of single handed GP practices c̄ inadequate deputising service esp inner cities. On reaching the GP the service is generally less acceptable eg poorer surgery equipment, less time spent in consultation, GP less likely to hold post-graduate degrees, referral to hospital less likely for similar condition. Higher use of GP surgeries is made by the lower social classes but not as much as would be expected given their greater burden of disease. Some of this usage is simply a result of administrative need eg requirement to obtain a sick note

Partly as a result of these service defs the lower social classes are more prone to use the A&E depts for minor health problems. Fortunately many of the major hospitals in the UK are located in the inner city areas

These trends were summed up by the inverse care law of Hart "that the availability of good medical care tends to vary inversely c̄ the needs of the pop served". In general those regions of the UK c̄ the highest proportion of lower social class people have a lower per capita expenditure & worse capital stock ie buildings

The lower social classes are less likely to carry out the advice of the health agencies for a number of reasons eg failure to understand the doctor's instruction (the doctor is likely to use different language & have less understanding of the patient's lifestyle), competition c̄ health beliefs of the patient (eg the patient may equate surgery c̄ early death & therefore not comply c̄ advice), expense of Rx or

advice
The lower social classes are less likely to utilise preventive health measures eg cervical screening, regular brushing of teeth, attendance at ANC, V&I programmes. Smoking & drinking are more prevalent in the lower social classes
In the NHS, the principle that it is free at the point of access (apart from prescription charges) is an advantage over the systems of many countries where wealth is an obvious determinant of the access to & quality of care.
For emergency conditions, there is little social class difference in access to health care in the UK. However for non-acute conditions, wealth can improve the access &/or quality of health care eg earlier op for hip replacement in private hospital, ability to afford care in a private nursing home
As the lower social classes represent a high risk gp for disease, many health programmes have been specifically targeted on this gp. In addition, attempts to change the organisation of health services have taken place eg general practice is regulated to encourage GPs into underdoctored areas & the RAWP introduced a system to equalise the regional differences in revenue & capital

Occupation & Health

Can be divided into the effects of health on work & the effects of work on health
The effects of health on work can be divided into specific factors eg a HGV driver may have to give up work following an epileptic fit, & non-specific factors eg the greater difficulty of the physically & mentally handicapped, & mentally ill in finding & keeping work compared to the general pop.
The effect of physical illness can have psychological consequences affecting work eg the man who has an MI & becomes a "cardiac cripple" despite good physiological recovery
In the UK, certain occupations have been reserved for the disabled eg lift & car park attendants, & larger firms are expected to have at least 2% of their workforce composed of disabled persons
The effects of work on health can be considered as non-specific, indirect & direct. Occupation is used to classify people into social class & although social class is strongly correlated c̄ many health experiences, this often does not appear to be a direct effect of occupation. The occupation may be indirectly ass c̄ ill health when the job gives a greater than usual opportunity of exposure to a health hazard eg both the deep sea fisherman & his wife are more likely to have extra-marital sex & thus the F is at more risk of developing Ca cervix, brewery workers are more likely to drink alcohol & thus have a greater risk of developing cirrhosis. In a number of occupations the job itself can directly cause disease either in the long term eg Pb poisoning in battery factory workers, pneumoconiosis in miners, bladder Ca in aniline dye industry or in the short term eg accidents, contact dermatitis
Lung cancer is ass c̄ a range of occupational hazards inc: Asbestos; Radon; Chloromethyl ethers; Polycyclic aromatic hydrocarbons eg from coke ovens, coal gas & tar; & probably Ni, Cr & As
Occupational health legislation has been introduced in most countries to prevent disease & compensate for injury & illness. In the UK, the Factories Acts prevented young children from working. The 1974 Health & Safety at Work Act set up a Health & Safety Commission. Other legal provisions are Factory Inspectors, Safety Officers & committees & the Employment Medical Advisory Service. In the UK there are about 50 Prescribed Industrial Diseases & 15 Notifiable Industrial Diseases, in which the factory inspectorate has a role in prevention & for which compensation in the form of industrial benefit can be paid
Some countries have a comprehensive OHS. In the UK, about 33% of the work force have a full service, about 33% have a partial service & the rest have no service. The functions of an OHS inc: Immediate Rx at the workplace; Biological monitoring eg of Pb levels; Health education; Accident prevention; Control of industrial hazards; Employment rehabilitation; Advice on diagnosis of occupational diseases
Methods of reducing risk inc: Substitution of materials eg carbon fibre for asbestos; Protective clothing;

Machine guards; Machine design; Monitoring of known hazards eg r-a; Health & Safety committees
Problems c̄ monitoring occupation & health can occur as the views of management & staff may conflict. There have been examples of industries not wishing to have the health experience of their workers analysed

Unemployment & Health

Many countries have significant levels of long-term unemployment, but some Western nations have recently experienced ↑ levels of unemployment due to structural changes in their economy. In the UK the unemployed are common amongst the disabled, unskilled, young, elderly, ex-prisoners & some minority ethnic gps eg New Commonwealth immigrants. Unemployment also varies c̄ place, being highest in Scotland, Wales, N.Ireland & N.England esp in the inner cities. The health experience of the unemployed is often similar to those in Social Class IV & V
There is increasing evidence that unemployment has a direct – ve effect on both physical & mental health. Work apart from the direct benefit of earning money also provides the individual c̄ a gp of fellow workers who share similar experiences & therefore often provide friendship, interests outside the family, a daily routine & social status
It is intuitively plausible that the threat of losing one's job & actual redundancy are important factors in diminishing the psychological well being of individuals. There is a strong statistical association between unemployment & poor psychological health in respect of the following variables: Suicide; Neuroses; Psychotic disorder; Unhappiness; – ve self esteem; Anxiety; Depression
The effects of unemployment on physical health are less easy to determine. Some authorities have estimated that unemployment in the UK results in excess deaths, perhaps 3000/yr. Unemployment is strongly related to poverty & poor diet. There is some evidence that the young unemployed are more likely than the employed to take illicit drugs

Diet & Health

Worldwide the major influence on health is undernutrition. This esp effects the developing world eg Ethiopia & is a major factor in mort in the <5yr age gp. The Brandt report summarised factors in Third World undernutrition as: Inadequate food production; Individual poverty; Misconceptions about infant feeding; High prevalence of infections & infestations. Protein calorie malnutrition c̄ <1500 cals/day → ↓ perinatal birth wt
Nutrition is presumed to be a very important factor in the determination of many diseases. It is difficult to study the effect of diet on long term health because of the complexity & variability of diet & the long follow-up that would be necessary in any intervention trial. The general advice on diet in Western countries is to eat more fibre & less sugar, salt & fat

SPECIFIC DEFICIENCIES

1. **DIETARY FIBRE:** Burkitt hypothesised that the high fibre diet of the "underdeveloped world" protected them against a range of diseases eg Diverticulitis, Bowel Ca. Evidence supporting Burkitt's theory has accumulated in respect of bowel disease eg IBS, Diverticulitis, Large bowel Ca. It is now generally believed that fibre protects the body: By modifying the bowel flora; Diluting carcinogens in the bowel; Speeding transit time so that carcinogens have less time in contact c̄ the bowel wall; Giving the bowel musculature less work to do in propelling the faeces; & ↓ faecal bile acids (which may promote Ca). In addition, the high fat content of Western diets promotes the formation of bile acids. The use of high fibre diets is now part of the standard Rx of many conditions eg IBS, Diverticulitis, Haemorrhoids
There is some evidence from retrospective studies that Crohn's disease is ass c̄ a low fibre, high refined sugar diet
2. **VITAMIN DEFS:** The clin effects of vit defs are well known eg Vit C → scurvy, Vit D → rickets. There is some evidence of an ass between low Vit A levels & squamous Ca eg lung

Ca. NTD have been linked c̄ poor maternal diet in the periconceptual period & intervention studies in which higher risk mothers have been given a multivitamin preparation led to a ↓ incidence of NTD. Further studies of the possible link between NTD & diet are in progress

SPECIFIC EXCESSES

1. **FAT:** It is hypothesised that dietary fat esp animal → high sat fatty acids → high cholesterol → IHD. It is known that high serum fatty acid & cholesterol levels are ass c̄ IHD, but is less certain that diet is directly related to ↑ serum levels. Some intervention studies have found that decreasing serum levels by dietary means led to ↓ IHD
Obesity is ass c̄ IHD & this appears to be mediated via ↑ serum lipids & BP ↑. Obesity is also ass c̄ endometrial Ca, non-insulin dependent diabetes, CVAs & digestive disease
2. **SUGAR:** ↑ sugar consumption is strongly ass c̄ the development of dental caries
3. **SALT:** In communities c̄ low salt intakes there is an ass c̄ low levels of BP ↑ & BP does not increase c̄ age. Analytical studies have generally not supported the hypothesis that low salt intake → ↓ BP
4. **NITROSAMINES:** It is well established that nitrosamines are ass c̄ Ca stomach & oesophagus. Various factors have been proposed to explain the mechanics of the ↑ nitrosamine levels. Nitrosamines are derived from nitrates, nitrites & 2° amines. These compounds are esp derived from preserved food, fertiliser, drinking water in infected areas (esp Columbia), foods in high risk areas. The bacteria & fungi involved in nitrosamine synthesis are inhibited by gastric activity; thus the ↓ gastric activity in PA, atrophic gastritis & post gastrectomy is explained as a risk factor for Ca. Vit C inhibits nitrosamine synthesis & explains the risk factor of a low intake of fruit & vegetables esp seen in Iran. Nitrosamines themselves are particularly found in diet in high risk areas. Some studies do not support the hypothesis that nitrosamines cause upper GIT Ca
5. **AFLATOXIN:** Aflatoxin in foodstuffs is well correlated geographically c̄ chr hepatitis & Ca liver. Aflatoxin is formed when food is stored c̄ the mould Aspergillus flavus in warm damp conditions
6. **ALCOHOL:** Alcohol is ass c̄ ↑ risk of accidents, Ca oesophagus, cirrhosis, psychiatric & social morbidity. Alcohol in small dosage → ↑ HDL levels which are cardioprotective & there is some evidence that a regular small alcohol intake → ↓ rates of IHD. There is certainly no cardioprotective effect if large amounts of alcohol are imbibed. Alcohol may be ass c̄ Ca rectum: Brewery workers have high incidence & international correlations between alcohol intake & incidence of Ca are supportive
7. **CRUCIFERA FAMILY VEGETABLES (eg cabbage, sprouts, broccoli):** Case control studies support an ass between low crucifera family vegetable intake & Ca large bowel. Indoles in cruciferous vegetables appear to induce aryl hydrocarbon OHlase activity which may inhibit tumour (as it does in rats)

FOOD POISONING

A notifiable illness in the UK (about 12000 cases/yr). In the UK, ↑ incidence. Roughly 50% are sporadic cases. About 25% of outbreaks occur in hospital.
In hospitals esp young, old, immune deficient. Main bacterial causes are Salmonella >*Cl.perfringens* >Staph, *V.parahaemolyticus*, *B.cereus*. Main foodstuffs implicated are beef, turkey, chicken, pork & ham
General control of infection inc: General investigations of an outbreak; General preventative advice; Investigation of kitchens inc food, environment & staff; Screening of patients & staff (esp if F–O spread). Occ Isolation; Early discharge from institution; Restrict staff transfer

Major Contributing Factors to Food poisoning outbreaks in UK (LIST 6 CM)

1. Preparation of food too far in advance
2. Storage of food at ambient temperature
3. Inadequate cooling
4. Inadequate reheating
5. Contaminated processed food
6. Undercooking
7. Inadequate thawing
8. Cross-contamination

SALMONELLA: Commonest cause in UK. Often sporadic cases. About 10,000 incidents/yr. Two types of outbreak: Enteric fever due to host-specific salmonella eg *S.typhi* & GE due to host-adapted salmonella (food poisoning). Incub Pd 12–24hrs

Pathogenesis: Salmonella is endemic in poultry & not uncommon in other domestic animals. There are >1500 serotypes, the commonest isolated from man being *S.typhimurium* & *S.hadar*. Initial infection occurs from eating contaminated food but outbreaks can be enhanced by F–O spread. Source of infected foodstuff is usually meat esp poultry but occ milk. Inadequate heat processing of meat inc inadequate thawing is usually responsible

Clin: D&V; Abdo pain; Fever

Investigation: • Stool culture: Large numbers of organisms

Prevention: Heat processing of animal feeds & protein (US advise temperature of 70°C). Proper thawing of meat & sufficient cooking time (approx 20mins/lb cooking time required for poultry). Health education of catering staff, advise good general hygiene. Isolate patients admitted c̄ diarrhoea

Rx: Supportive treatment eg may require fluid replacement. Advice to help prevent F–O spread

Prog: Usually excellent. Dangerous in very young & very old

CLOSTRIDIUM PERFRINGENS: Due to an anaerobic organism which produces heat resistant spores. Foodstuffs involved are esp Beef, pork, mutton & poultry. Common. Usually → large outbreaks involving >30people. Incub Pd 12–18hrs

Pathogenesis: Conditions for spore generation occur if food is inadequately cooled or reheated. Endotoxin released in GIT causes symptoms. Commonest cause of outbreaks are preparation too far in advance combined c̄ storage at ambient temperature, inadequate cooling & inadequate reheating

Clin: Diarrhoea; Abdo pain

Investigation: • Stool culture: Large numbers of organisms

Prevention: Health education re food preparation

Rx: Supportive treatment

Prog: Usually excellent

STAPH AUREUS: Common commensal of skin (approx 40% of pop are carriers). ↓ in incidence in UK. Incub Pd 2–4hrs. Usual cause of infection from contaminated canned food

Pathogenesis: Relatively heat resistant toxin formed in food eg cooked meats, dairy products. Often spread by infected food handlers

Clin: Vom. Occ Diarrhoea

Investigation: • Stool culture: Toxin present, small numbers of organisms

Prevention: Health education re food preparation. Screen for food handlers in catering industry

Rx: Supportive treatment

BACILLUS CEREUS: Uncommon cause. Esp Chinese restaurants. Foodstuffs involved esp rice & other cereals. Incub Pd 2–15hrs

Pathogenesis: *B.cereus* produces heat-resistant spores which produce toxin in food left at room temperature. Toxin is relatively heat-resistant. Typical history is 3 days supply of rice boiled together & left at room temperature, & then only quickly fried before serving

Clin: Vom. Occ Diarrhoea

Investigation: • Stool culture

Prevention: Health education re food preparation. Advise refrigeration of rice

Rx: Supportive

VIBRIO PARAHAEMOLYTICUS: Uncommon cause. Tropics, Asia >UK. Foodstuffs involved esp raw fish, shellfish. ?may be toxin. Incub Pd usually 10–15hrs

Clin: D&V; Abdo pain; Mild fever

Investigation: • Stool culture: Large number of organisms in acute phase

Prevention: Health education re food preparation

Rx: Supportive

CAMPYLOBACTER JEJUNI: Common. Causes about 8% of cases of diarrhoea in UK. Summer >Winter. Usual source is raw milk >raw water. Rural >urban. spread by F–O route. No toxin

Clin: Often prodromal phase c̄ Malaise; Headache; Pyrexia. Then Diarrhoea, occ chr. ± blood; Abdo pain. Occ Vom; Myalgia. Rarely Arthritis

Investigations: • Stool culture
• CFT

Prevention: Treatment of raw milk & water. Health education re food preparation

Rx: Supportive. Erythromycin may be beneficial

BOTULISM: Due to *Cl.botulinum*. Very rare. Usually ass c̄ consumption of preserved or canned foods eg meat, fish, fruit which have been inadequately heat treated. Incub Pd 12–36hrs

Pathogenesis: Organism multiplies in anaerobic conditions producing a potent neurotoxin

Clin: Present c̄ Tiredness; Vom; Paralysis of ocular & swallowing musculature; Thirst; No pyrexia. Within a day, flaccid paralysis of limb & trunk muscles which may → death from resp failure. Recovery (if it occurs) is slow but complete

Investigation: • Demonstration in guinea pigs of toxin in blood or vomit

Prevention: Efficient canning techniques. (Some recent outbreaks have been due to inadequate home preservation)

Rx: Supportive Rx eg Tracheostomy, Respirator. Botulinus anti-toxin is of doubtful value

Prog: High case fatality

FOOD HYGIENE & THE LAW

Enforcement of the law is carried out by environmental health officers & the community physician (environmental health). In UK, current regulations on food labelling require information on food composition eg preservatives used

FOOD & DRUG ACT 1955: Main food legislation in E&W. Two main objectives are:

1. To prevent fraud & deception ie food offered for sale must be of the nature, substance & quality demanded
2. To safeguard public health eg it is a criminal offence to sell food unfit for human consumption

Registration of some food premises is required eg where ice cream & sausages are sold. Registration can be refused if hygiene standards are not met

FOOD HYGIENE (GENERAL) REGULATIONS 1970: Applies to all premises where food is manufactured, stored or sold (excludes abattoirs). Requirements inc Adequate lighting, ventilation, washing facilities etc; Appropriate protective clothing; Reporting of certain illnesses; Minimum temperature for many hot foods; Maximum temperature for some cold foods; Measures against vermin & insects; Health education. Fines can be imposed on any insanitory premises or other failure to comply c̄ regulations

FOOD & DRUGS (CONTROL OF FOOD PREMISES) ACT 1976: If a local authority thinks there is a risk to public health from a food premises they can apply for a closure order

Housing & Health

Can be considered in two gps, the effects of ill health on housing & the effects of housing on health

Housing is strongly correlated c̄ social class & there are strong gradients in health experience between owner–occupiers, private renters of accomodation & council tenants. Indeed even amongst the same social class, owner–occupiers have signf lower SMRs

The scientific evidence demonstrating causal links between ill health & housing is sparse. There is good evidence that poor sanitation, overcrowding & high housing density are linked c̄ communicable diseases & that improvements in sanitation → ↓ in enteric infections. Households c̄ poor amenities have higher than expected mort from resp disease, circulatory disease & accidents. Many aspects of home safety could be introduced at minimal cost. Poor housing esp the lack of play facilities &/or high rise deck access flats are ass c̄ ↑ minor morbidity eg dissatisfaction, diminished social life, ↑ psychiatric illness. Many reports link overcrowding & lack of amenities c̄ delinquency. The importance of housing conditions eg dampness in the causation of resp illness esp in children is disputed. Badly heated houses may → hypothermia esp in the elderly. Infestation c̄ rats & mice may → *S.typhimurium* infections

Rehousing has achieved variable results. In general, the moving gp are satisfied but high rates of mental ill-health have been noted in some studies perhaps due to the higher cost of living eg ↑ rents, ↑ cost of travel to work, &/or the breakdown of supportive family &/or community networks

The special housing needs of particular gps eg physically disabled, elderly, mentally handicapped are increasingly recognised. The elderly often require ground floor accommodation, minor aids & adaptions eg handrails, some community support. Community support may be supplied by a warden, meals on wheels, relative eg daughter. Often it is possible to adapt ordinary houses to meet the functional abilities

of the individual
Slum areas can be cleared by compulsory purchase orders. Various grants are available to improve the fitness of housing. Most L.Auths in determining the allocation of housing, take into account health factors. Recommendation for rehousing on medical grounds is usually assessed by the community physician. The building materials themselves may cause ill-health eg asbestos, Pb from pipes

PHYSICAL ENVIRONMENT & HEALTH

Environmental health activities are those which seek to maintain & improve the human ecosystem by maximising the benign environmental components & minimising or eliminating the malignant ones. The factors which may place health in jeopardy can be classified as: Physical or chemical; Biological; & Socio–cultural. Physical factors inc climate, soil, water, radiation & noise. Chemical factors inc asbestos, SO_2, I_2, flouridation, Pb & pesticides. Biological factors inc zoonoses. Socio–cultural factors inc industrialisation, diet

Many environmental health issues are supervised by central & local government eg

DHSS: Communicable diseases, Food hygiene, Toxicology
DoE: Pollution, Transport
MAFF: Animal welfare, Food additives
Dept of Employment: Factory inspectorate
Dept of Energy: Fuels
Home Office: Register of drug misusers
Regional Water Authorities: Water
Local government: Waste disposal, Housing

Air Pollution

Air pollution may be natural eg eruption of Mount St.Helens or man-made eg domestic or industrial pollution. Air pollution is worse in industrial areas esp due to combustion of hydrocarbon fuels ie coal & oil.

Air pollution can be compounded by topographical or climatic factors eg Smog in Los Angeles valley; Wind; Temperature inversion ie a warm air blanket covering a layer of cold air & trapping pollutants near ground level. The major pollutants are SO_2, Nitrogen oxides, CO & Pb

Air pollution can cause short & long term health effects. The acute effects eg malaise, headache, N, sore eyes, throat & chest complaints are most serious in the elderly, & those c̄ pre-existing chr cardiac or resp disease. The 1952 London smog caused 4000 excess deaths

The long term effects on health are an ↑ in acute & chr chest illnesses in urban areas. Chr bronchitis is ass c̄ low social class, smoking & urban residence, & exacerbations may be due to changes in SO_2 levels. LRTIs in infancy are ass c̄ level of atmospheric pollution & have been implicated in the aetiology of COAD. It is postulated that polluted air → ↑ resp irritants → ↑ mucus production & damage to cilia → ↑ AWR → COAD. Lung Ca is commoner in urban areas, but this effect is mainly explained by smoking.

Pollution from the exhaust of motor cars can also be a hazard

Some authorities believe that the ↑ ozone layers in industrial countries will → a "greenhouse effect" adversely affecting the climate

Air pollution control has been the subject of legislation in many countries. In the UK, Clean Air Acts were passed in 1956 & 1968, enpowering L.Auths to establish smoke control areas. The HSE advise factories on pollution control eg use of "scrubbers", higher chimneys. The Clean Air Acts have proved successful eg ↑ visibility, ↑ hours of sunshine, ↑ cleanliness, ↑ flora, ↓ smell & ↓ erosion to buildings in the smoke controlled areas

Water Pollution

Adequate safe water supplies are extremely important to health. Water

is an important carrier of many pathogenic organisms & potentially harmful chemicals
The main water-borne infections are typhoid, cholera & dysentery. They are caused by the contamination of water supplies by human excreta. Animals are also important in the transmission of pathogenic organisms esp in stored or still water eg Salmonella from sea-birds. Water is also involved in the life cycle of organisms causing many diseases eg malaria, schistosomiasis
Man-made chemical pollution may arise from effluent discharge from factories into rivers or the use of pesticides & fertilisers reaching water. The chemical composition of water depends on the composition of the river bed & banks esp rocks; Soft water occurs when water runs over relatively non-porous rocks & contains few ions. Soft water areas are ass c̄ an ↑ incidence of IHD but some evidence that this is not a causal relationship
The prevention of water-borne disease depends on the purification, monitoring & protection of water supplies. In the UK, a series of Acts have been introduced to ensure chemical, bacteriological & radiochemical standards. Water should be colourless, tasteless, odourless, non-pathogenic, without sediment & relatively non-corrosive. Water purification is achieved by the combination of a number of processes: Defence of catchment water supply; Storage in reservoir (→ sedimentation of suspended matter); Biological filtration eg sand or chemical filters; Adjustment of pH eg acid water leaches out Mn; Chemical coagulation; Chemical disinfection eg Cl_2; Monitoring by regular sampling at various points in distribution system. The water is distributed through a closed system of pipes & service reservoirs. Storage plants are used to meet the fluctuating demand
In many countries, some piping is made of Pb which may → ill-health
The prevalence of dental caries is signf lower in areas c̄ a high Fluoride content (which can be obtained by artificial flouridation). A level of 1ppm is protective & is esp beneficial during childhood. There is no good evidence that flouridation is harmful to health but nonetheless some Water Authorities have not flouridated their supplies

Sewage & Waste Disposal

An efficient sewage & waste disposal system is one of the most signf public health measures & contributed greatly to the fall in mort rates that occured in Western industrial countries in the late 19th & early 20th centuries. The Rx of sewage includes: Separation of solids by filtration & sedimentation; Biological oxidation of liquid sewage
Special methods are required for the disposal of many chemicals & r-a materials

Radiation

There are 3 types of r-a decay ie α (the nucleus of He atom) which has no effect on skin but is a problem if ingested; β (the electron); & γ (non particulate based electromagnetic energy). Different r-a sources may produce one or more types of decay eg C14 decay → β emission. The source of radiation may be natural eg Uranium ores or man-made eg diagnostic imaging
The effect on man depends on the absorbed dose & the type of r-a decay. For X-Rays & α rays, the unshielded dose rate varies inversely as the square of the distance from the source. The rate of decay of a r-a source is variable & depends on the r-a half-life ie the time taken to reduce the radioactivity by half eg Iridium 192 T1/2 = 74 days
The biological effects depend on tissue responsiveness eg sperms are very radiosensitive. The effects depend on the stage of cell differentiation, metabolic activity & division rate.
The effects may be stochastic ie no threshold or non-stochastic ie a threshold effect. Once the threshold, if any, is reached severity depends on radiation dose
Stochastic effects inc Ca eg ↑ rates in Hiroshima survivors, watchmakers; Genetic abnormalities inc SBs
Non-stochastic effects inc the acute radiation syndrome, cataracts, growth retardation & ↓ fertility
The atomic bomb is capable of enormous death & destruction. The Hiroshima bomb, which was only about 2% of the size of present day bombs, killed all those fully exposed within 0.5 miles of ground zero & most within

0.75 miles. Acute radiation syndrome was present in those 2 miles from ground zero. Signf mort & morbidity has continued to the present day Radiation has a number of potentially beneficial usages eg medical diagnostic imaging, nuclear energy. Stringent monitoring of industries & occupations involved c̄ radiation have been introduced, advisory bodies inc the Atomic Energy Commission, NRPB & the ICRP. The disposal of r-a waste is strictly controlled but is difficult due to the long T1/2 of some waste products

ACUTE RADIATION SYNDROME

A non-stochastic effect. Whole body threshold is approx 1Gy

CLIN: Depends on immediate whole body dosage. 1–2Gy → N; Diarrhoea; Hair loss; Fever; Mort rate of approx 25% at 9mths. Dosages of 2–6Gy → earlier & more severe symptoms c̄ a mort rate of 25–75% at 9mths. Dosages of 6–8Gy → CNS symptoms eg coma, Ep & a mort rate >75% within a few days. Dosages >8Gy → death
Different parts of the body have very different sensitivities to radiation eg breast & eyes >skin, extremities

INVESTIGATION: • WCC: Changes occur at low dosage

RX: Prevention eg rigorous safety checks on equipment. Supportive therapy

Temperature/Latitude

↑ sunshine → ↑ Vit D synthesis but is ass c̄ ↓ incidence of Skin Ca & Melanoma. In E&W, the regional incidence of melanoma is +vely correlated c̄ the mean daily hrs of sunshine. "Rheumatism" sufferers have a subjective improvement in warm climates. Rates of many diseases increase in the winter eg many infectious diseases, IHD. MS appears to be much commoner in individuals who have spent their childhood in temperate climes

Lead & Health

Lead poisoning is a prescribed industrial disease. Esp Children (show effects at lower blood levels & absorb Pb quicker than adults); May occur 2° to Pica. The major sources of environmental Pb are petrol, food, tap water & air. In the UK it is estimated that 45–95% of blood Pb is derived from food, 0–45% from water, & 3–20% from air
Pb from food can occur from: Soil & crop contamination; Weathering of Pb ores; Tap water used in cooking; Pb solder in canning
Pb from tap water depends on: Concentration of Pb in tap water; Amount consumed; Transfer between water & food during cooking. The amount of Pb in water depends on Length of piping; Length of time water stored in pipe or tank; Temperature; Chemical constituents of water ie acid, soft water → ↑ levels
Pb in air is mainly derived from petrol. Pb conc depends on Traffic density & speed; Weather conditions; Local topography.
Industrial sources of Pb inc Paints; Solders; Glazes; Eye cosmetics & medicines; Mining; Coal combustion

CLIN: Anorexia; Malaise; Headache. Occ Abdo pain; Anaemia; Nephritis; Periph neuropathy; Blue lines on gums. Rarely Encephalopathy → Coma; Ep; Spasticity; Blindness. In children may → Failure to thrive; Sl IQ ↓

INVESTIGATIONS:
- FBC & film: Occ Hb ↓, Sideroblastic anaemia, Punctate basophilia
- Serum Pb: Satisfactory level is <0.35ppm
- Enzyme assay eg ALA
- X-R bones

PREVENTION: Food regulations in UK allow level <0.2mg/Kg in baby foods. Tin solder. Washing crops, discarding outer layer of foodstuffs eg peeling fruit. Replace Pb pipes. Chemical Rx of water to ↓ plumbosolvency. Reduce Pb emissions from cars. Regulations re use of Pb paints

RX: EDTA

INFECTIOUS DISEASE CONTROL

Infectious diseases are now much more prevalent in the underdeveloped world compared to the West. Nonetheless infection remains important in the West, as: New infections become recognised eg Legionnaire's disease, AIDS; ↑ foreign travel → ↑ imported disease; Infection remains a signf cause of morbidity & mort. In E&W there are 29 statutory notifiable diseases where it is the legal responsibility of the clinician to notify the community physician

Statutory Notifiable Infectious Diseases in E&W (LIST 7 CM)

1. Acute encephalitis
2. Acute meningitis
3. Acute poliomyelitis
4. Anthrax
5. Cholera
6. Diphtheria
7. Dysentery
8. Food poisoning
9. Infective J
10. Lassa fever
11. Leprosy
12. Leptospirosis
13. Malaria
14. Marburg disease
15. Measles
16. Ophthalmia neonatorum
17. Paratyphoid fever
18. Plague
19. Rabies
20. Relapsing fever
21. Scarlet fever
22. Smallpox
23. Tetanus
24. TB
25. Typhoid fever
26. Typhus fever
27. Viral haemorrhagic fever
28. Whooping cough
29. Yellow fever

In the UK, infections can be monitored by routine mort data, statutory notifications, RCGP reporting, laboratory reports, sickness absence, & hospital & OPD records. The OPCS has also carried out national morbidity studies in general practice. Responsibility for the investigation & control of notifiable disease lies c̄ the Community Physician & within hospital, the Control of Infection Officer. Many areas have a control of infection team. Specialist advice is available from the PHLS & CDSC
The most common imported diseases in the UK are Malaria & Enteric fever. The most important vector is the aeroplane. Serious but rare imported diseases inc Lassa fever & Marburg disease. Certain diseases can occur in pandemic form affecting both industrialised & non-industrialised countries eg Influenza. Health monitoring at ports & airports, & the use of quarantine before animals are imported into the country is a useful means of preventing disease spread eg Rabies
In the developing world, infectious diseases are a major cause of morbidity & mort. The inadequacy of public health measures eg clean water, proper sanitation, good diet, good housing is often a major cause of the prevalence & severity of infection. Many communicable diseases are endemic eg typhoid, hepatitis, kala–azar. Zoonoses ie infections naturally transmitted between vertebrates & man are also commoner

Investigation & Control of an Outbreak

An outbreak is two or more related cases or infections. Investigation requires swift & methodical action to allow early & effective control measures. The approach can be considered as the following activities: Preliminary inquiry inc confirmation of diagnosis; Identification of cases; Data collection; Data analysis; Control; Further epidemiological & laboratory studies
Preliminary inquiry inc Diagnosis verification; Formulation of working hypothesis. In some cases eg suspected Lassa fever, immediate control measures must be instituted
Identification of cases inc Definition of a "case"; Attempt to identify additional cases eg laboratory screening, review of notifications, contact tracing. To calculate attack-rate & gain more representative information about

outbreak, a denominator of persons at risk is required
Data collection inc data both from cases & those apparently exposed to risk but unaffected. Information collected eg by questionnaire, usually inc: Name; Age; Sex; Address; Occupation; Travel history; Immunisations; Dates & description of any illness; Food history
Data should be analysed by the three major parameters of time, place & person. Analysis of time may show: Point source; Relationship to exposure to suspected source; Seasonal pattern. Analysis by place may provide evidence of the source & mode of disease spread. Analysis by person may suggest vehicle of infection. In foodborne outbreaks, food-specific attack rates are calculated
Control measures may involve: Removal of infection source eg remove infected animal; Rx of infected; Preventive measures for those at risk eg immunisation, chemotherapy of close contacts; Health education eg advice re food preparation; & Control of the mode of transmission eg isolation of patient, barrier nursing. Surveillance follows control measures. A written report of the outbreak should be made & information may be required for other professionals & the media
Further epidemiological & laboratory studies may be indicated eg longitudinal studies, microbiological serotyping

IMMUNISATION

Immunisation is the means by which specific immunity to micro-organisms is acquired. Immunity can be natural or artificial ie achieved by deliberate exposure to an Ag stimulus before natural exposure to a similar or related Ag occurs. Both natural & artificial immunity may be passive or active. Immunisation has been a signf factor in the control of certain infectious diseases. Infections which are specific to man can potentially be eradicated by effective immunisation programmes. Smallpox has probably been so eradicated
Passive immunity is the transference to a non-immune individual, of Ab preformed in another person or animal. Natural passive immunity occurs in the transfer of IgG from mother to fetus. Examples of artificial passive immunity are Hep-specific human Ig & human anti-tetanus serum. Passive immunity has a rapid onset but immunity is short lived
Active immunity is acquired by the formation of an active immune host response to a foreign Ag. The immunity may be naturally acquired after infection or induced by vaccination. Vaccines may consist of killed or live attenuated organisms or toxins. Vaccines must be safe ie no longer produce disease but remain immunogenic. Toxoids eg Tetanus & Diphtheria toxoids, are non-pathogenic forms of toxins whose immunogenicity is usually enhanced c̄ adjuvants ie substances which ↑ immune response. Live attenuated vaccines are preferred to killed vaccines as they stimulate antigenic response in a manner to the natural pathogen, require smaller doses & may obviate need for multiple doses. Some live vaccines can be given by a natural route eg Polio. Live attenuated vaccines inc Measles, Rubella, Yellow fever, TB & Rabies. Killed vaccines inc Cholera, Pertussis & Typhoid, require at least 2 doses & are less effective than live vaccines. Full immunity c̄ killed vaccines is not achieved until all the doses have been given
An ideal vaccine should be safe, reliable, necessary, protective, free of side effects, cheap, easy to store & transport, acceptable to the pop & easy to administer
Although immunisation primarily protects the immunised individual, contagious infections depend on there being sufficient susceptible individuals in the pop to allow spread. The effect of immunisation can therefore potentially extend protection to greater numbers than have actually been immunised, an effect termed herd immunity. The "threshold" level of pop uptake of a vaccine required to achieve herd immunity varies according to the infection, but is generally between 70–95%

Routine Immunisations

Most countries have a routine immunisation schedule in early childhood. In the UK, parental consent is mandatory before immunisation can be given. In the USA, many immunisations have to be administered before the child is allowed to attend school unless there are specific medical c/i

Routine Immunisation Schedule in UK Children (LIST 8 CM)

3–12mths	3 doses of Dip/Tet/Pert & oral Polio c interval of 6–8wks between 1st & 2nd dose & 4–6mths between 2nd & 3rd dose
12–15mths	Measles
5–6yrs	Dip/Tet & oral Polio
10–13yrs	BCG & Rubella (in F). Interval of >3wks between BCG & Rubella vaccination
15–19yrs	Oral polio & Tetanus toxoid

DIPHTHERIA

Active immunisation by diphtheria toxoid. Immunisation introduced in UK in 1940s was followed by dramatic drop in notifications. Cases are now rare in countries c̄ immunisation programmes. Herd immunity occurs at about 75% immunisation rate. 3 doses of the vaccine are given in the 1st yr of life c̄ a booster at school entry. Inject vaccine IM or deep sc

c/i are: h/o allergy or convulsions; Defer if child unwell. Reactions to vaccine are generally mild eg Local swelling; Malaise; Sl temperature ↑. Rarely allergic reaction

TETANUS

Active immunisation by tetanus toxoid. Passive immunisation by human anti-tetanus serum. Tetanus cases are uncommon in developed countries, but still occur esp 2° to dirty wounds. Immunisation has no effect on the natural history of the disease & hence confers no herd immunity. 3 doses of the vaccine are given in the 1st yr of life c̄ a booster at school entry. Boosters are also given at time of injury, & to high risk gps eg farmworkers. Usually boosters should not be required at intervals of <5yrs. Inject vaccine IM Reactions to vaccine are commoner in adults & inc Local swelling, pain & redness; Urticaria ± angioneurotic oedema; & Rarely serum sickness

PERTUSSIS

Active immunisation by killed vaccine. Introduced officially in UK in 1957. Major reason for the fall in disease prevalence has been social factors, no dramatic drop in mort or incidence was noted c̄ introduction of vaccine. However the public dissatisfaction c̄ the vaccine in the 1970s led to ↓ uptake rates & subsequently notifications increased. The vaccine is now 90–95% efficacious, but earlier vaccines were less efficacious due to less resistance to some pertussis serotypes. To achieve herd immunity uptake rates of about 80% are required. At present UK uptake rates are approx 50%. Morbidity & mort rates from the disease are highest in the 1st yr of life & thus it is important that older siblings should have been immunised to prevent spread to those most at-risk

3 doses of the vaccine should be given between 3–12mths. Usually vaccine given in 1° course is the triple vaccine (Dip/Tet/Pert), a monovalent pertussis vaccine is available. Inject deep sc or IM

c/i are: Neonatal cerebral disorder; Ep; Convulsions. Caution should be used in children c̄ a FH of Ep or other neurological disease. Eczema is not a c/i. Children c̄ acute illnesses should have their vaccination delayed. If severe general reactions or convulsions occur following vaccination, do not continue c̄ further doses. Reactions are less common c̄ modern vaccines. Mild transient reactions eg irritability, mild fever are common. Rarely major reactions occur inc Convulsions; Collapse; Encephalopathy. Very rarely chr encephalopathy ensues (National Childhood Encephalopathy Study estimated freq of 1 in 310,000 doses). Most authorities agree that the risks of the disease far outweigh the dangers of the vaccine & strongly advise vaccination. Compensation is available for vaccine damaged children

POLIOMYELITIS

A live attenuated oral vaccine (Semple) is used in UK. Previously an inactivated virus vaccine (Salk) was used. Immunisation was introduced in UK in 1958 & was followed by a

dramatic drop in cases & fatalities. The oral vaccine contains strains of the 3 polio virus types. Three doses are needed as only one strain colonises the GIT after each administration. The oral route has the advantage of mimicking natural infection. They are given between 3–12mths usually along c̄ the triple vaccine. Further doses are given at school entry & school leaving. Vaccine should also be offered to unimmunised parents as there is a very slight risk of spread of a virulent strain following immunisation of the child. Herd immunity occurs at high acceptance rates
c/i inc agammaglobulinaemia, patients on steroids or immunosuppresives, pregnant F earlier than the 4th mth. Delay vaccine if acute or intercurrent illness. Reactions are rare inc vaccine-associated polio

MEASLES

A live attenuated vaccine. Introduced in UK in 1968. Acceptance rates in UK have not been high (approx 50%), but USA experience shows that vaccine can be extremely effective. Herd immunity occurs at very high pop acceptance rates. Maternal Ab persists for about 12mths & therefore immunisation is usually carried out at about 15mths. Morbidity & mort of the disease are greatest in infancy & thus it is important to protect older siblings thereby reducing spread to the at-risk. Protection rate is 85–90%. Inject vaccine IM
c/i are diseases or conditions → deficient immune mechanisms. Careful consideration should be given if there is a personal or FH of convulsions or allergic disease, these children may be offered vaccine c̄ the concurrent use of specific Ig. Pregnant at risk F are passively immunised c̄ specific Ig. Mild reactions are quite common eg transient rash, fever lasting <2 days. Severe reactions rarely occur eg convulsions, SSPE, encephalitis. Measles vaccine → signf ↓ chance of developing SSPE. The immune response to vaccination may be impaired by blood transfusion or human Ig given within previous 3mths. Measles vaccine may depress response to tuberculin test for up to a month

RUBELLA

A live attenuated vaccine. Importance of disease is its teratogenic potential esp if disease acquired in early pregnancy. In the UK, immunisation policy is to offer vaccine to: F aged 10–13yrs; F found to be sero – ve during pregnancy (vaccine given in puerperium); Sero – ve F c̄ an occupational risk of acquiring disease eg health staff. Other countries have differing policies eg in the USA immunisation of children of both sexes is undertaken. Rubella vaccination protection probably lasts throughout the childbearing period. Seroconversion following the single dose is approx 98%
c/i inc: Pregnancy; Diseases or conditions → deficient immune mechanisms. Occ reactions which resemble mild rubella eg Fever; Rash; LN ↑. Rarely esp in adult F, Arthralgia; Arthritis; Myeloradiculitis. It is most important that F take effective precautions against becoming pregnant for at least 3mths after vaccination

BCG

A live attenuated strain of bovine TB. Major decline of TB cases due to improvements in social conditions. Definite benefit from anti-TB Rx & probable benefit from immunisation. Vaccine introduced in UK in 1951. In the UK, BCG is usually offered to: Children aged 10–13yrs; Close contacts of TB cases; Neonates born into household where there is active TB; Health workers. A Mantoux or other tuberculin test is first done to identify +ve reactors in whom vaccine is c/i. In some areas the vaccine is routinely offered in the neonatal period
The most commonly used tuberculin tests are the intradermal (Mantoux) or multiple puncture (Heaf). The test requires careful standardisation & dosage. Test results are graded. A Mantoux → a reaction of >5mm diameter is evidence of previous Mycobacterial infection. A reaction c̄ >15mm induration is strongly +ve & requires further investigation. Absence of reaction usually indicates absence of TB but occ is due to immunological defs or other illness eg active leprosy, sarcoidosis. Mantoux reactions can also be suppressed by recent measles, mumps or rubella vaccination
Injection is given intracutaneously or percutaneously. Faulty technique may → ulceration, local abscesses
c/i inc +ve tuberculin test reactors;

Immunodepressed; Those suffering from other infectious disease. BCG should not be given within 3wks of the administration of another live vaccine. Reactions inc Local ulcers or abscesses; LN ↑ (mild adenitis is common)
The efficacy of BCG is disputed. BCG appears to modify disease experience & probably prevents CNS disease. Some studies of effectiveness eg the Madras study have shown that BCG offers little protection whilst other studies have shown up to 80% protection. The WHO suggest that in areas of high TB prevalence, BCG should be given as early in life as possible. In the UK the withdrawal of routine vaccination to low risk gps is being actively considered

Other Active Immunisations

MUMPS

A live attenuated vaccine. A routine vaccination in the USA. Has been considered for use in susceptible post-pubertal M in UK

INFLUENZA

Inactivated vaccine. There are 3 influenza viruses & many antigenic strains. The tendency of the virus esp influenza A, to produce new strains ie antigenic shifts & drifts means that vaccines against previous infections may subsequently be ineffective. Vaccines often require to be raised against the most recent circulating strain & as this process is time consuming an epidemic may spread through many countries before an effective vaccine is available in sufficient quantities. Vaccine offered to high risk gps inc: Elderly esp in institutions; Children in institutions; People c̄ chr Ht, Pulm or renal disease; Diabetics; Health workers. Injection by deep sc or IM
c/i if egg allergy. Use c̄ caution in young children. Reactions are common esp in children eg Local soreness & redness; Malaise; Headache; Fever. Rarely Guillain–Barré syndrome

HEPATITIS B

Vaccine prepared from blood of carriers. Expensive. Recently developed. At present offered to: Health care personnel working c̄ high risk patients; Renal dialysis patients; Sexual partners of infective carriers. Highly effective. Reactions rare. Potentially the vaccine is of enormous worldwide importance

PNEUMOCOCCAL INFECTIONS

The pneumococcal vaccine contains Ag of various serotypes, inc Ags of the most prevalent strains. It is offered to persons at particular risk of pneumococcal infection eg those without properly functioning spleens

ANTHRAX

Vaccine is offered to workers c̄ occupational disease risk eg Woolsorters, Workers c̄ animal hides or bone meal

YELLOW FEVER

A live attenuated vaccine. Required for travel to Central & W. Afr; Central & S.Am. Only one dose usually necessary. International Certificate following vaccination is valid 10yrs
c/i in infants & egg allergy. Reactions are uncommon

RABIES

A killed vaccine prepared from human diploid cell cultures. Vaccine is offered pre-exposure to workers at occupational risk & is given by 2 sc injections 4wks apart followed by yrly boosters. Post-exposure vaccination is offered to any person in contact c̄ a known or suspected rabid animal. 6 injections are given over a pd of 90 days c̄ anti-rabies Ig. Reactions are uncommon

MENINGOCOCCAL INFECTIONS

Vaccines are available against GpA & GpC serotypes but not GpB which is the commonest cause in the developed world. Vaccine indicated for travel to endemic infection areas eg Central Afr, S.Am

CHOLERA

A killed vaccine. Vaccine indicated for travel to endemic infection areas eg Middle & Far.E. Vaccine is of limited efficacy & of short lasting effect. 2 sc injections about 4wks apart. Control of disease should be primarily based on public health measures. International Certificate is valid for 6mths

TYPHOID

A killed vaccine. Vaccine indicated for: Travel to endemic areas; Control of institutional outbreaks; Family or close contacts of known carrier. 2 sc injections about 4–6wks apart. Offers about 40–80% protection. Control of disease should be primarily based on public health measures
Reactions are common eg Fever; N; Malaise; Headache, usually starting within a few hrs & lasting for a few days
N.B There is no evidence for the efficacy of the Paratyphoid A & B vaccine

ENDEMIC TYPHUS

An inactivated vaccine given by 2 sc injections 4wks apart followed by yrly boosters. Indicated for travellers to rural parts of endemic countries

Passive Immunisations

IMMUNOGLOBULINS

Norm human Ig can be used for Measles & HepA prophylaxis. Disease specific Ig can be used for prophylaxis in HepB, Chickenpox, Shingles, Tetanus, Mumps & Rabies

ANTITOXINS

Animal derived & therefore more likely to cause allergic response & more rapidly eliminated than human Igs. Must be used c̄ caution as risk of anaphylaxis esp if h/o allergy or previous serum Rx. One or more test doses required before use. Can be used for prophylaxis & Rx of Diphtheria, Gas gangrene & Botulism

PRIORITIES IN RESOURCE ALLOCATION

Expectations re health are almost infinite & probably no amount of money spent on health could satisfy all demands. The Health Service & other health related agencies often have to function as rationing devices. There is an increasing realisation by both the public & health professionals of the gap between what is done & what could be done eg relative underprovision of renal dialysis in UK. Societies need to formulate objectives, appraise problems, review potential for intervention & thus devise health policy. A series of basic choices can be considered inc: Health versus other social objectives eg Defence, Education; Health services versus indirect health measures eg better housing, improved social services & safer roads; Prevention versus Cure versus Rehab & Care; Resources given to acute versus chr illness Rx; Hospital versus non-hospital services eg PHC, Preventive care; Doctors versus other health personnel; Capital ie buildings versus Revenue monies. The geographical spread of resources is also subject to social choice. It may also be policy to try to minimise inequality between gps eg social class differences
Basic questions are: How much money should be spent?, Who decides how much?, Which areas should money be spent on?, & Who decides those areas? Esp in Western societies there are large P to ↑ health spending for 3 major reasons: The ageing pop structure → ↑ numbers of elderly persons who generally require ↑ health resources; The development of new technologies; ↑ in public & professional expectations. The first 2 factors require a real growth of the health service of about 1% p.a

Health Policy

Health policy can be considered as a series of rational steps → the implementation of the most cost-effective measures. Inevitably "non-rational" factors eg personality of individuals, lack of scientific knowledge about intervention, & politics interfere c̄ the determination of policy. The steps in policy formulation inc: Problem definition eg importance of condition; Potential for intervention eg are any procedures of proven value?; Review in light of national, regional or local objectives; Level of intervention eg national, regional &/or local; Financial & other costs of possible interventions; Formulation of options; Option appraisal; Organisational factors in possible intervention; Monitoring & evaluation methods

Health policy in the UK is decided at distinctive levels eg Minister of Health, DHSS, RHAs, Health Districts. In general terms, the Central Govt's role is to: Impose a national standard; Ensure value for money; Set national health objectives & priorities; Issue guidelines on good practice; Ensure collation of national statistics; Represent country in international health matters; Liaise c̄ other govt depts; Uphold some statutory duties; Negotiate Terms & Conditions of Service of Employees; Coordinate activities relying on large economies of scale. The local health services have a role in adapting to local circumstances the health services offered eg particular needs of local pop, policies & practices of other agencies, state of capital stock. Decision making in the NHS is increasingly a multidisciplinary activity eg most Authorities have a specialised planning team of a community physician, administrator, nurse & treasurer. Decentralised decision making is strong in the NHS mainly due to historical factors eg the influence of the medical profession

Many gps are involved in the monitoring of health policy. They inc the: DHSS; RHAs; HAS; Health Districts; Medical Committees; CHCs; P gps eg Trade Unions, NSPCC, Media; Other statutory bodies. The RHAs & Health Districts both have a gp of members to decide on health policy which has usually been formulated by the authority's officers eg RGM, DMO or local health workers. The authority membership includes Local Councillors, GP, Consultant, Nursing, Trade Union & often University nominees. The CHCs have observer status on Health Authorities & have been recently introduced in the NHS to represent the views of the consumer

The techniques used in decision making are varied, rational methods inc: Double blind RCT; Cost benefit analysis; Cost effectiveness studies; Operational research. There are of course many constraints on reallocation & rationality eg The presence of buildings designed & staff trained to deal c̄ a problem in a particular way can impose great inertia on change; The power of certain gps eg hospital consultants, to retain their traditional role in the health service; The difficulty in attaching quantified values to suffering & mort; The fact that not all costs involved fall upon the NHS ie a new procedure may overall be more expensive but may cost less to the NHS

Cost Effectiveness Studies

Four broad requirements: Objective must be stated in terms of final & not intermediate output eg lives saved & not number of treatments; Alternative methods identified; Effect of each option quantified; Total cost of each option measured. The analysis will show which is the best alternative. However the analysis will not determine whether the best option is worth pursuing as benefits are not completely assessed

N.B It is often useful to distinguish between effectiveness of procedures at the individual & pop level. Effectiveness at the individual level may be termed efficacy. A procedure may be efficacious at the individual level eg Rx of abnormal cervical cytology & yet relatively ineffective at the pop level

Cost Benefit Analysis

A comparison of all costs & benefits to society of a policy, inc intangible psychological costs & benefits. The analysis is expressed in monetary terms for the convenience of a common measure & is related to a particular point in time. As it is widely accepted that consumption now is prefered to consumption in the future, future costs & benefits are "discounted" at a rate which reflects the society's preference for immediate consumption

Marginal Analysis

When a health programme is already in operation, it is often valuable to analyse the marginal costs & benefits of increasing the programme. It is often found that once a certain level of operation is reached, that increasing the programme will involve an increased cost per +ve result eg a single screening test may detect 90% of cases & cost £X/case detected, adding a 2nd screening test may raise detection to 95% but ↑ costs to £X+Y/case detected. Marginal analysis allows planners to consider "how much of a service" is justified ie whether the extra £Y/case detected is worth the ↑ number of detected cases. All money spent in the NHS imposes an "opportunity cost" ie if money is spent on one activity out of a finite budget the opportunity is lost to spend it on an alternative activity

Finance of Health Care Systems

The NHS spends about 6% of the GNP compared to about 10% spent on the health care system in the US, W.Germany, Holland & Sweden. This major difference may be partly due to different relative priorities re health vis a vis other national objectives eg defence but are generally agreed to be mainly due to the efficiency of the NHS system

The following factors have been put forward as the cause of the relative cheapness of the NHS: NHS is subject to budget limits; Finance is primarily from tax revenue; NHS is in competition for finance c̄ other public services; Quotas for medical school entry ie restriction of number of expensive doctors; No fee for service payment for curative measures; Strongly developed PHC system; Low administration costs (large numbers of people are required to manage insurance based systems). The NHS being centrally organised can set priorities between different care gps, insurance based systems have little incentive to provide preventive & community based services

The NHS is financed mainly from taxation & is free at the point of access apart from prescription charges. About 72% of the money is spent on hospital services, 18% on family practitioner services (excluding GPs salaries), 5% on community services & 4% on admin. By client gp, about 40% is spent on acute services, 19% on PHC & community services, 15% on the elderly & physically handicapped, 8% on chr mental illness & 5% on mental handicap. Tagged NHS "Joint Finance" monies are available for schemes related to personal health to be carried out by social services & other agencies

There has been little change in recent yrs in the relative amounts of money spent on different sections of the NHS, despite evidence that health priorities demand a change in the balance of care in favour of PHC rather than 2° & 3° care, community rather than hospital care, & preventive services. One exception has been some redress in the regional imbalance of health resources achieved since the introduction of the RAWP formula eg more to N.England & less to London

Most of W.Europe & Canada have insurance based health system. It is generally based on occupation eg in France premium is 16% & employee pays 2%. Most countries have a compulsory part to the system eg in W.Germany 90% pop coverage, top 5% income earners are excluded. The cost of Rx may not be fully reimbursed eg in Belgium only 80% of cost is reimbursed, & many people take out a separate insurance to cover the shortfall. In Holland, the state will pay after a person has been >1yr in a hospital or nursing home. The insurance based systems have developed massive bureaucracies & premiums have steadily risen

A potential problem of the NHS is that it provides little impetus for the economic use of resources by the major spenders ie doctors. For this & other reasons eg to ↑ resources for the health service without raising tax levels, people have considered the virtues of private health care systems. Potential problems c̄ the expansion of private health insurance in Britain would be: Fragmentation of unified social policy & planning; Development of a two-class system eg better health care for the rich who already have the best health experience; Diversion of staff from the public sector (this might involve increased training requirements on the NHS as well as the loss of experienced staff); Rise in the total cost of care; Discouragement of non-technological aspects of patient care ie care of the elderly, mentally handicapped, mentally ill, PHC & prevention. Health is a desirable commodity & a market could exist for it, however willingness to pay depends on ability to pay & therefore discriminates against the poor. Also there is understandable consumer ignorance about the worth of a service

RAWP

RAWP was set up "To review the arrangements for distributing NHS capital & revenue to RHA, AHA & Districts, c̄ a view to establish as soon as practical a method of distribution responsive objectively, equitably & efficiently to relative need & to make recommendations. The RAWP reported in 1976 & their Formula was introduced on the basis that pops c̄ the same level of need should have equal access to health facilities but accepted that time was required to equalise geographical inequalities & thus recommended a realistic pace of change. The RAWP formula was mainly concerned c̄ the setting of revenue targets & it was decided to base this target mainly on age/sex structure of the pop, condition-specific SMRs, & cross boundary flows. The RAWP formula assumed that SMR was a reasonable proxy for morbidity
Since the introduction of RAWP geographical inequalities have lessened but the London area still has signf more resources. The RAWP formula has been critisised as: FPC & L.Auth expenditure is not taken into account; Social class inequalities are insufficiently accounted for; SMR may not be a good proxy for morbidity eg disabling diseases c̄ low fatality; There is no reward for efficiency; Formula is insensitive esp at sub-regional level; Pace of change to equity is too slow; Cross-boundary flow adjustments are insensitive

SCREENING OF POPULATIONS

For most health service interactions it is the patient who initiates the doctor/patient relationship. Screening involves the detection of a disease or condition at a pre-symptomatic stage & requires the doctor to initiate contact c̄ the screened community. Appropriate criteria for the justification of screening procedures are thus particularly pertinent

Criteria for the Evaluation of a Screening Test (LIST 9 CM)

1. Is the disease important?
2. Is there a safe reliable screening test?
3. Does the test discriminate well between +ves & −ves?
4. Can −ves be reassured?
5. Are false +ves harmed?
6. Is the natural h/o the disease known?
7. Is successful intervention possible?
8. Can the target pop be reached?
9. Is the cost reasonable?

An example of the evaluation of a screening test can be made c̄ reference to cervical Ca screening:

1. Is the disease important?:
   Cervical Ca is a major cause of morbidity & mort, causing approx 2,500 deaths/yr in UK
2. Is there a safe reliable screening test?:
   Cervical cytology is a safe procedure c̄ relatively few hazards
3. Does the test discriminate well between +ves & −ves?:
   Cervical screening for Ca-in-situ has a sensitivity of approx 85% & a specificity of approx 98%. Smears often require repeating
4. Can −ves be reassured?:
   Test merely indicates present freedom from pre-malignant cervical epithelial changes. Further tests are periodically required
5. Are false +ves harmed?:
   False +ves undergo unnecessary psychological & occ surgical trauma. The confirmatory & curative biopsy

is reasonably safe. Some F c̄ true pre-malignant cervical changes would have reverted to normality spontaneously

6. Is the natural h/o the disease known?:
   The natural h/o is reasonably well known but it is thought that a more aggressive form of the disease occurs in the young & is increasing in incidence. This lack of knowledge of the future course has led to some uncertainty re age of onset of screening & screening interval
7. Is successful intervention possible?:
   Rx is efficacious at an individual level but in the UK, trends in the incidence of cervical Ca have not obviously been altered by the screening programme (in some countries the screening programme has been ass c̄ ↓ Ca incidence)
8. Can the target pop be reached?:
   The UK screening programme has been bedevilled by poor attendance of high risk gps eg low social class middle-aged F & overuse by low risk F. The programme appears to be relatively inaccessible & unacceptable to high risk F. Improvements in call/recall systems may benefit the situation
9. Is the cost reasonable?:
   The cost per life saved is high compared to other screening procedures

Some screening tests appear well justified eg αFP screening for NTDs in N.Ireland. It is important to recognise that just because a screening test & Rx are effective at an individual level, the screening programme will not work if the high risk gps are not attracted to use the service. Service organisation is often critical if a service is to be efficient & effective. The service should be acceptable, available & accessible to the public; this may involve recognition of social or cultural factors eg many F from Indian sub-continent prefer to be examined by a F doctor

Some authorities distinguish between screening & case finding. Case finding is the opportunistic use of a health service/patient interaction to carry out a screening procedure eg the identification of BP ↑ by screening of people of defined ages presenting to GPs. If, as is the case c̄ BP ↑ screening by GPs, a large proportion of the at-risk pop present to the doctor, case finding can be a cheap & efficient practice

REGISTERS

The characteristics of registers are that data: Relates to a total defined pop; Relates to individuals rather than events; Collection is standardised & systematic; Records are prospective & cumulative. Registers can provide information about the natural h/o a condition, trends, & the effect of Service practices on the condition (N.B The lack of a control gp differentiates registers from prospective studies). There are many registers eg UK National Cancer Registry

Data collected inc Personal data eg demographic characteristics; Service contact data eg contact c̄ hospitals, GPs, Social services. The register method is to: Collect contact data from relevant agencies (data must relate to a defined pop); Identify appropriate individuals; Collect descriptive data for new individuals; Collect new or changed data on all previously recorded individuals eg change of housing or marital state; Collate & link all data relating to one individual on a cumulative case file; Process & store data; Allow information retrieval in a standardised form

The register output generates: Standardised information based on a defined pop; Routine operational information for service planning & evaluation; Centralised record of the accumulated individual's experience; Facilities for monitoring trends; Sampling frame for research

Problems which registers have to overcome are: Confidentiality; Data collection & recording practices must be correct from the start (otherwise problems c̄ for example, cohort comparisons); Divising standardised classifications; Ensuring system works administratively eg training of clerks; Ensuring proper data storage

& processing availability eg some registers depend on record linkage which requires a complex computer programme to analyse

PREVENTATIVE HEALTH & DISEASE CONTROL

Prevention, cure & amelioration are embraced by the single notion of control. In most communities, a dynamic quasi steady state has been reached in which important diseases are present but not readily eradicable. The health service has the broad objectives of minimising disease incidence, treating such cases as occur & modifying their disabling effect. All diseases are amenable to some control. Control of disease can be considered at a number of levels

Levels of Control

For convenience, levels of control can be divided into discrete areas but often control is required at many if not all of the levels. The systematic approach does allow health planners to consider which methods of control are likely to be the most efficient & effective for the pop

Levels of Control (LIST 10 CM)

1. General health promotion
2. Specific protection
3. Early diagnosis
4. Active treatment
5. Rehabilitation
6. Continuing & terminal care

The control of Ca can be used as an illustration:

1. General health promotion:
   To encourage a healthy life style eg anti-smoking publicity, good dietary advice, ie health education & promotion measures; Research
2. Specific protection:
   Inc: Protection against occupational hazards eg asbestos; Monitoring of environmental hazards eg radiation; Control of new compounds eg testing drugs for carcinogenicity. Research eg will HepB vaccine protect against Ca liver ?
3. Early diagnosis:
   Inc: ↑ public awareness of signf symptoms eg by health education; ↑ acceptability & accessibility of diagnostic facilities eg ↓ public fear of Ca which may have delayed presentation; Screening of at-risk gps or more general screening eg cervical cytology; Identification of at-risk gps; Development of screening tests; Training of doctors & other staff in diagnosis & referral; Research
4. Active treatment:
   Inc: Provision of personnel, buildings & equipment; Avoidance of delay in Rx; Development & evaluation of therapy; Use of properly trained experienced staff (many cancers have better Rx outcomes if treated in centres of special expertise eg childhood Ca); Research
5. Rehabilitation:
   Inc: Minimisation of mutilation eg lumpectomy rather than mastectomy; Advice & support eg re colostomy; Retraining; Help to adjust to any new lifestyle
6. Continuing & terminal care:
   Inc: Advice & support inc family; Education of health staff; Procedures to allow death c̄ dignity eg Hospices; Control of troublesome symptoms esp pain relief; Evaluation of care procedures; Research

Health Education & Promotion

There are many definitions of health education. It is sometimes simply regarded as information & advice about factors which promote health. Usually it is more useful to define health education more widely as a formalised activity aimed at either reinforcing or changing behaviour & initiating actions related to the prevention of disease & maintenance of health. Health education is principally an applied behavioural science c̄ a theoretical basis in the social & behavioural sciences. Good health education often requires an understanding of the medical rationale of what is proposed. In particular it is the study of processes such as: Decision-making; Communications; Learning; Socialisation; Introduction of change; Community organisation; Gp dynamics; & Personal interaction. The term health promotion is sometimes preferred as it suggests a subject of wider scope

To an extent everybody is a health educator as health at its basic level is about how we learn to survive. Health education can be divided into formal & informal aspects ie mothers are informal educators & doctors formal

THEORY OF HEALTH EDUCATION

Various models have been put forward to explain why people act in certain ways & how their behaviour might be influenced

The simplest model is that of Knowledge → Attitude → Practice (KAP) & that ↑ knowledge will → a rational change or reinforcement of practice. Unfortunately the KAP model is rarely of value in practice as so many factors can influence this common sense approach eg cultural norms, psychological factors, memory, situation, language

Individual & social factors influencing action inc: Personal readiness eg perceived seriousness, predisposition & ability to act, motivation, knowledge; Social control eg social pressure, acceptability of action; Situation. In many cases it is possible to identify a process by which a person adopts a new health influenced role eg symptom experience → assumption of sick role → medical care contact → dependent patient stage → recovery or rehab. Some models attempt to take into account both social & medical factors, partly by reference to the processes & norms of health related behaviour. Some health educators use a social intervention model & believe that health can be influenced through changing social norms & roles

Norms impose a definitive ordering & regulation to society & have a coercive power → conformity. Norms vary in their specificity & permanence. In general, norms introduced during 1° socialisation are difficult to alter. Health educators may seek to introduce new norms eg it is wrong to smoke in pregnancy. Although norms are usually adhered to, variant or deviant reactions may occur eg gangs of young adults who contravene norms by vandalising property. The recognition of differing norms may be important for health educators eg advice about diet would need to be tailored to the religious & cultural norms of some minority gps

Evidence from psychological research gives some insight into how attitudes change. Factors important if a communication is to be persuasive inc:

Communicator credibility: It has been found that a highly credible source is advantageous as long as the recipient later remembers the nature of the source

Message factors: It has been found that Fear arousing messages may not be effective; Giving both sides of the argument is more effective than a one sided presentation; Recommendation is more persuasive if seen as painless & effective. It was found that the recommendation is more effective if the probability of development of disease was felt to be high

Receiver factors: Inc personality, intelligence & the descrepancy between the person's present role & the message. If subject's position & message are not perceived as discrepant (latitude of acceptance) or if message is perceived as highly discrepant & threatening (latitude of rejection) little change is likely, whereas change is most likely in latitude of indifference between these extremes

COGNITIVE DISSONANCE: Attitudes are organised in a systematic way. People are disturbed by inconsistencies between attitudes & behaviour & will attempt to reduce or abolish them. 2 cognitions are said to be dissonant if one implies the opposite of the other. According to cognitive dissonance theory, cognative dissonance is assumed to be an uncomfortable tension-like state incorporating a motivation to reduce dissonance. It has been observed that it is often easier to manipulate cognitions to reduce cognitive dissonance rather than change belief. The amount of dissonance experienced depends on the importance of the two cognitions involved &

their resistance to change. Methods of maintaining a belief inc: Repression; Selective attention; Maximising consonant factors; Minimising dissonant factors. Smokers, for example, have been divided into dissonant (agree c̄ health hazards, wish to give up) & consonant gps. Evidence that dissonant smokers may have resolved cognitive dissonance by lowering self esteem or resigning themselves to an addiction ie they explain their inability to give up cigs, despite knowledge of the hazards, as the result of an addiction

Cognitive dissonance can be aroused in various ways eg in an experiment one gp were offered a small reward & another a large reward in what they were told would be a painful experiment, & it was subsequently found that the poorly rewarded gp experienced less pain as measured by a galvanometer than the well rewarded gp. It is postulated that cognitive dissonance resulted from the insufficient justification of the reward → pain experience being reduced. It has been argued that the placebo effect may be partially explained by cognitive dissonance

Health Education Practice

Health education is carried out by many people. It is part of the job content of all health workers esp HEOs, HVs & Community Physicians. It is a component of many doctor–patient interactions as well as being involved at a pop level eg through use of the media

The broad aims of health education can be gained by analysing the WHO sponsored document "Health for All by the Year 2000"

"HEALTH FOR ALL BY THE YEAR 2000": This 1978 document was based on the following premises: Health is a human right; Pop health has not ↑ at the same rate as knowledge & services; Behaviour related illnesses are increasing; Inequality of distribution of health care availability & utilisation; Too little money spent on PHC & prevention compared to hospital; A change of priorities towards prevention, PHC & self-care is required; Economic factors are important & demand greater awareness of health economics; Social & cultural factors are of great importance to health

The strategy was for health to be seen as part of the socioeconomic development of societies, that health should be seen as a priority for societies & that underprivileged areas should be initially treated. The 4 basic principles underlying the strategy are equity, participation, prevention & cost effectiveness

The achievement of HFA2000 is via 3 main routes: Promotion of lifestyles conducive to health; Reduction in the number of preventable conditions; Provision of adequate & accessible health care for all

Actions to promote lifestyle inc: Improvements in conditions that promote health eg housing, employment; Reduction of exposure to self-imposed risks eg smoking cessation gps; Research into lifestyle; Imaginative health education starting early eg in homes & schools

Actions to ↓ preventable conditions inc: V&I; Family planning; Safety at work, home & on the roads eg seatbelts; Legislation eg re food composition

Actions to provide adequate health care inc: Improved PHC; Improved quality of service ie more relevant to community needs; ↑ co-operation between different agencies inc both statutory & non-statutory; Special care for high risk gps esp physically & mentally handicapped, elderly & young; Greater community participation & self-care; Improved indicators of the cost effectiveness of health care; Better indicators of morbidity & mort to allow evaluation of health care

SMOKING & HEALTH

Cig smoking has become prevalent in many countries this century. Smoking is the major known preventable cause of ill health. M>F. Esp lower social class. Cig smoking can → to the development of many diseases. There is good evidence for a causal ass between smoking & various cancers, COAD,

IHD, PU & the birth of LBW babies to F smokers. Other relationships may be due to the general lifestyle of the smoker eg ↑ likelihood of being a heavy drinker. Total mort is much higher for smokers than non-smokers, it has been estimated that the ave life expectancy from age 25 for cig smoking M is 4–8yrs less than for non-smokers. Total mort is not simply due to the excess risks of known causally related diseases. Risks are higher for cigs compared to cigars & pipes

Smoking Related Disease (LIST 11 CM)

1. Lung Ca
2. Chr bronchitis & emphysema
3. IHD
4. PU
5. LBW babies
6. Ca bladder, pancreas, oesophagus, larynx, mouth
7. PVD
8. Resp TB
9. Cirrhosis & alcoholism
10. Suicide & poisoning

Trends in most industrialised countries are for falling rates of cig smoking in M & ↑ rates in F, whilst in many developing countries smoking is ↑ in both sexes. As some cohorts of heavy smokers have not yet fully experienced the expected high rates of smoking related disease, it will be some yrs before the effects of the present lower smoking rates in some pops are reflected in the mort figures

Smoking & Lung Ca

Lung Ca is a maj cause of death in many countries. In UK it accounts for 9% of all M deaths. Numerous studies both case-control & cohort show that lung Ca risk is: Higher for smokers than non-smokers; ↑ c̄ amount smoked; Higher c̄ cigs than c̄ other tobacco products; Highest for those who started smoking youngest; Lower for ex-smokers than current smokers. There is also evidence that there is a ↑ risk for inhalers. In a classic study, it was shown that in British doctors, relative risk compared to lifelong non-smokers was 2 for those who had stopped smoking >15yrs before enquiry, 16 for all smoking cigs at that time & 30 for those smoking >25/day at time of enquiry. The time relationship between smoking habit & lung Ca also provides strong evidence of causality ie the large ↑ in smoking popularity in the early 20th century was followed by a large ↑ in lung Ca incidence, & the ↓ in the number of British doctors smoking was followed by a drop in Ca incidence

It has been hypothesised that smoking → bronchial tree sq metaplasia & formation of polycyclic aromatic hydrocarbons → Ca. The risk of lung Ca starts to fall as soon as smoking is stopped. Although low tar cigs are sometimes felt to be safer than high tar, there is little reliable evidence

Smoking & exposure to asbestos seem to act in a multiplicative manner re the risk of developing lung Ca. Exposure to both factors → very high risks which are greater than simply the addition of the risks of the individual factors

Smoking & Chr Bronchitis & Emphysema

A maj cause of morbidity & mort esp UK. The prevalence & morbidity of COAD rises c̄ the quantity smoked & the degree of inhalation. The prevalence & mort of COAD in non-smokers is low. COAD may be worsened by high tar cigs. Smoking → mucus hypersecretion ("smoker's cough") & airflow limitation. An important study showed that the decline in FEV c̄ advance in age is particularly accelerated in about 15% of light & 30% of heavy smokers

It has been hypothesised that smoking → ↑ macrophages & polymorphs → ↑ elastase release → emphysema. In British doctors, smokers of >25cigs/day have about a 40× ↑ mort from COAD compared c̄ non-smokers

Smoking & IHD

The relationship between smoking & IHD is complex. The relative risk for IHD is greatest below the age of 45yrs eg risk to British doctors smoking >25cigs/day relative to non-smokers was 15 at <45yrs, 3 at 45–54yrs & 2 at 55–64yrs. The lower relative risk at high ages suggests that any ass at these ages is indirect. Ex-smokers show a decline in IHD esp those who give up below the age of 45yrs. As the death rate from IHD is higher at older ages the absolute number by which death rate in smokers exceeds that in non-smokers is highest after age 55yrs

Prevention

Health education is usually introduced at the asymptomatic or early disease stage. At the personal level, health education methods inc: Teaching children not to start smoking; Advice of health professionals; Example of health professionals ie not smoking or, if a smoker, not smoking in professional situations. At the pop level, health education methods inc: Anti-smoking information in the media eg TV adverts; Anti-smoking health warnings on tobacco products; Smoking cessation gps eg stop smoking clinics. Other +ve influences on cig consumption inc: ↑ Level of cig taxation; Prohibition of cig advertising; Prohibition of smoking in specified places eg hospitals, trains. There is some evidence that banning of sponsorship of health related events by cig manufacturers eg sport would → ↓ consumption

A problem for health educators is that the money available for anti-smoking propaganda is far outweighed by that used by the cig manufacturers in promoting their products. A rapid decline in cig consumption would also → loss of jobs & signf loss of tax revenue in many countries

Nonetheless there is no doubt that health education can be effective. A doctor simply advising patients to give up smoking during consultations will result in about 5–10% giving up & remaining non-smokers for >1yr. A trial of health education designed to persuade M to give up smoking post MI showed that intensive health education led to ↑ rates of smoking cessation. Smoking cessation gps can offer a supportive climate assisting smokers to stop (it is relatively easy to stop smoking but it is initially difficult to remain an ex-smoker, hence the Rx results are usually assessed at 1yr). Aversion therapy, hypnosis & acupuncture are occ of benefit.

A nicotine containing gum used in gradually decreasing dose over 6mths may be of benefit

ASPECTS OF CHILD HEALTH

In the developed world there have been large falls in mort & morbidity in the paediatric age gp. This beneficial change has been mainly due to socio-environmental factors. Preventive measures esp immunisation have proved beneficial & there is evidence that improvements in medical care are partly responsible for the ↓ in PNMR.

In the developing world, childhood mort & morbidity remains high esp due to infectious diseases & malnutrition.

Morbidity & mort are highest in the lower social classes

In the UK the major causes of deaths are:

- In the post-neonatal period: Cong malformations; SIDS; Infections esp Resp
- In those aged 1–4yrs: Accidents, Poisoning & Violence; Resp disease
- In those aged 5–14yrs: Accidents; Cancer

Deaths are commoner in M

Many countries have a policy of concentrating their preventive activities on this age gp. This appears sensible on a number of criteria eg disease prevention can potentially → many productive extra yrs of life. Older parents are generally better than young in bringing up children, this appears to be partly due to likelihood of already having raised children, being wealthier & having greater maturity ie experience of life

In the UK, for historical reasons 2 parallel services have evolved concerned c̄ 1° preventive care ie the Community Health services & General Practice.

Developmental assessment starts in the hospital c̄ a paediatric examination. The community health services monitor the development of a child by a series of periodic examinations carried out, principally by doctors & HVs, at clinics, home & schools. Routine screening tests are performed for the detection of certain diseases & conditions eg PKU & other metabolic disease (by blood test at 10 days); Cong hypothyroidism (by blood test at about 10 days); CDH; Maldescent of testes; Hearing disorders; Disorders of vision. The sequential monitoring of child development should allow rapid detection of developmental delay esp if examination evidence is taken in conjunction c̄ the mother's observations. Community health doctors carry out the V&I schedule but do not prescribe medicines. GPs have the potential advantages of knowing all the family & being able to prescribe, they may however be untrained in developmental assessment or ascribe more importance & hence more time to their Rx rather than prevention role Hearing is usually tested at 7mths & vision at 3yrs c̄ a further examination at school entry or nursery. A UK National cohort study found the following disabilities in 7yr olds: 3% squint; 8% mod or severe defect in at least 1 eye; 6% speech impediment; 9% discharging ear; 1% hearing loss in both ears. An Isle of Wight study found the age–specific rates/1000 children aged 10–12yrs for physical disorders were highest for: Asthma; Eczema; Ep; Cerebral Palsy; Orthopaedic conditions; Heart disease

Sudden Infant Death Syndrome (Cot Deaths)

Large ↑ in diagnosis in 1970s, but probably due to change in classification preference rather than true increase. In UK, incidence 2–3/1000 live births. M>F. Esp 3–6mths. Esp Low social class; Young parents; Poor maternal obstetric history. Winter>Summer. Bottle fed >breast. Unknown cause, ?viral infection of bronchi & bronchioles. ↑ risk to siblings. May be >1 disease. A few cases may be due to child abuse

CLIN: Sudden infant death esp nocte. Occ short h/o mild LRTI, URTI, Diarrhoea, Drowsiness or Poor feeding

PREVENTION: Good antenatal & obstetric care. Advise breast feeding. Observe closely siblings of infants who have died. Apnoea alarms

RX: Family support

Non-Accidental Injury

True incidence unknown. Serious injuries or death inflicted non-accidentally by parents are not rare. Esp low social class

Factors Ass c̄ NAI (LIST 12 CM)

A. PARENTAL FACTORS
1. Lack of support from extended family
2. Unreasonable expectations of baby
3. h/o abuse during their childhood
4. Rigid authoritarian personalities
5. Impulsiveness
6. Aggressive personality
7. h/o psychiatric illness

B. FACTORS RELATED TO CHILD
1. Unwanted child
2. Child separated from mother at birth:
   Eg Required prolonged Rx in SCBU
3. Hyperactive child
4. Poor sleeper
5. Illness
6. Stepchild

C. SOCIAL FACTORS
1. Life crises:
   Eg Loss of job, Poor housing
2. Poverty
3. One parent working away from home
4. Marital discord

CLIN: Often pattern of injuries which do not appear accidentally caused or fit explanation of parent. Wide range in severity & type of inj eg head inj, #s, bruises, abrasions, burns. Usually detected by agency involved in child care eg Dr, HV, Soc W, NSPCC. Occ Failure to thrive eg poor wt gain

INVESTIGATIONS:
- Skeletal survey ± isotope bone scan
- Coagulation studies

RX: Formal procedures to notify other child care agencies. Appropriate investigations often in hospital. Assessment of case at multi-agency case conference, & if NAI suspected, child put on register & a recommended surveillance programme agreed eg Soc W to be key worker, HV to visit monthly & appointments to Paediatric OPD. Closely monitor growth & development eg hgh & wt charting. Occ child is placed in care. Child is removed from register if satisfactory reports from involved agencies. Parents may require psychiatric assessment N.B Child sexual abuse is also increasingly recognised occ in ass c̄ NAI

FAMILY PLANNING

Although the desire to plan family size is common in human societies, the demand for safe, harmless contraceptives has markedly increased recently due to social factors inc Less need to have many children to support parents in old age; ↓ risk of death in early childhood; Desire to have "risk-free" intercourse inc outside marriage. Rarely countries eg China, India have been worried about pop growth & offered incentives to those who restricted their family size Wide choice of contraceptives. A good contraceptive should be: Effective; Safe; Compatible with enjoyable coitus for both partners; Cheap. Important for success at community level that contraceptives are easily available to public. In UK, Family Planning advice can be obtained at community clinics as well as from GP

Methods of Birth Control Used by F Partner

HORMONAL CONTRACEPTION

COMBINED PILLS: Combination of synthetic progestogen (to suppress ovulation) & oestrogen (to control breakthrough bleeding). Widely used. Introduced in 1960's. Very efficient & safe. Single daily dose from Day 5 to Day 25–27 of cycle. Regular checks of BP, Wt, Breast & pelvic examination, Cv cytology. SE: N&V; Breast tenderness; Wt ↑; Amenorrhoea (may persist after stopping pill); Depression; Thrombophlebitis esp if >35yrs, smoker. May benefit F suffering c̄ dysmenorrhoea or menorrhagia. c/i: H/o Thrombophlebitis; Severe Ht disease; Recent infective Hep; Sickle cell disease. Low dose Oestrogen ie <0.05mg Ethinyl Oestradiol/day, → ↓ risk of thrombophlebitis & is also recommended following conflicting reports on the risk of breast & cervical Ca c̄ higher dose pills

PROGESTOGEN ONLY PILLS: Not as effective as the combined pill. Taken every day. Occ used if medical c/i to combined pill. SE: Irregular bleeding; Amenorrhoea

INJECTABLE PROGESTOGENS: Used only when other methods unsuitable. Effective & easy to administer. Depot IM preparations are effective for about 2–3mths. No inhibition of lactation. Disliked, as once given none of its actions can be reversed including SE of irregular bleeding, wt ↑, & amenorrhoea

INTRA-UTERINE DEVICE

Now usually made of plastic ± copper. Many types eg Lippes loop. Probably act by preventing implantation. IUCDs are cheap, effective & do not impair enjoyment of coitus. After the first few mths the F can almost forget about them as the follow-up is undemanding. Must be fitted by trained Dr towards end of menstruation to avoid insertion during pregnancy. SE: Uterine perf; Expulsion; Bleeding & Abdo pain esp soon after insertion; Infection. c/i to insertion: Genital tract infection; Large fibroid; Genital tract Ca; Abnormal genital tract bleeding

DIAPHRAGM

An occlusive pessary. Safe & effective esp if used c̄ a spermicide. Advantage over the condom is that they do not have to be inserted at height of sexual activity. Important that correct size of diaphragm is selected & F instructed in its use. User should reattend to check fitting after 1 week & then 6mthly.

Diaphragm should not be removed for at least 8hrs post-coitus

SPERMICIDES

Variety of preparations eg creams, jellies, pessaries, sponges. Prescribed in conjunction c̄ barrier method

F STERILISATION

Sterilisation is the deprivation by surgical means of the capacity to reproduce. Indications may inc conditions which could constitute a risk to the future physical or mental health of the F eg h/o 3 LSCS. Various ops designed to interrupt continuity of Fallopian tubes

RHYTHM METHOD

Method based on calculating infertile phase of F cycle when unprotected coitus carries least risk. In a 28 day cycle, "safe period" is during the 7 days before menstruation & the first 7 days of cycle. Disadvantages inc unreliability if cycle is irregular (thus unsuitable after childbirth or abortion, or in F near menopause) & need for self-control to restrict coitus to "safe" period. May be advised if religious practice of partners prevents use of more effective measures

Methods of Birth Control Used by M Partner

CONDOMS

A thin rubber sheath inserted over penis & disposed of following coitus. Popular. Reasonably safe esp c̄ spermicide, but rarely leak or burst. May affect enjoyment of coitus. Use of condom → ↓ risk of spread of infection

VASECTOMY

Relatively minor op of bilat division of vas deferens. After op, other forms of contraception should be used until 2 consecutive seminal specimens at an interval of at least 2 weeks show aspermia. This may take >3mths

COITUS INTERRUPTUS

M withdraws from F before reaching orgasm. Widely used. Relatively ineffective but better than no contraception at all. Reduces pleasure of coitus

Post-coital Contraception

Recently introduced emergency technique for use soon after unprotected intercourse. 2 methods, insertion of IUCD or hormones eg Eugynon 50. Offers limited protection

ASPECTS OF CARE OF THE MENTALLY HANDICAPPED

Mental retardation is a syndrome where the individual has signf reduced intellectual functioning & a marked impairment in the ability to cope c̄ society's demands

Many cases of unknown cause. In UK, about 20% of severe cases due to genetic/chromosomal disorder esp Down's Syndrome

2 major groups: Severe & Mild

Severe Mental Retardation: In developed countries, about 3–4/1,000 school-aged children. IQ <50. Often Single causative factor; CNS signs. No social class gradient

Mild Mental Retardation: In developed countries, about 25/1,000 school-aged children. IQ 50–70. Esp lower social class. Minority have CNS signs. Many are independent in adulthood

Age-specific prevalence rates appear to be falling in developed world

Causes of Mental Handicap (LIST 13 CM)

1. Chromosomal Aberrations:
   a) Down's Syndrome
   b) "Cri du Chat" Syndrome
   c) Patau's Syndrome
   d) Edward's Syndrome
   e) Klinefelter's Syndrome

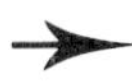

2. De Lange Syndrome
3. Tuberous Sclerosis
4. Metabolic Disorders:
   a) PKU
   b) Galactosaemia
   c) Hurler's Syndrome
   d) Hypothyroidism
   e) Hypercalcaemia
   f) Tay–Sachs Disease
   g) Batten's Disease
5. Ante-natal causes:
   a) Severe Rhesus incompatibility
   b) Infections eg Rubella, Toxoplasmosis
   c) Foetal Alcohol Syndrome
   d) Chemicals eg Hg
   e) X-Rad
6. Peri-natal Factors:
   a) Trauma
   b) Hypoxia
   c) Cerebral Haem
7. Post-natal Factors:
   a) Trauma eg RTA
   b) Meningo–encephalitis esp TB
   c) Encephalopathy eg Whooping Cough
   d) Pb
   e) Poor nutrition eg High solute feeds
8. Idiopathic

CLIN: ↓ intellectual ability inc slowness in learning, problems c̄ basic ADL. Occ, esp in severe cases, supplementary handicaps eg Ep, Cerebral Palsy, Sensory handicap. Occ Behaviour problems eg Hyperactivity, Destructiveness, Non-communication; Sleep disturbance; Dental problems

INVESTIGATIONS: • Tests for Metabolic & infectious causes

PREVENTION: General measures eg Family Planning advice to older F; Good antenatal & paediatric care. Rubella vaccination. Genetic counselling eg for Tay–Sachs in high-risk gp. Screening for Cong Hypothyroidism, PKU & other metabolic causes. Monitoring of environmental Pb. Early specific Rx eg special diet for PKU, Thyroxine for Hypothyroidism

RX: Many people still wrongly regard mentally handicapped people negatively eg menace, object of pity, dread or ridicule, burden of charity, eternal child. Carers have to counteract these misconceptions. Traditionally early in the 20th century, mentally handicapped persons were institutionalised. Now problems of institutionalisation are increasingly recognised & care is based on multi-agency teamwork & community care wherever possible. Individual programmes with short & long term goals are agreed c̄ client & family, & usually seek to increase independence

Once detected, child is placed on handicap register & family receives support & assessment from Soc W & Health workers. Often care provided by a Community Mental Handicap Team inc Soc W, Dr, Psychologist, Community Drug Misuse Nurse. Psychosocial amelioration inc Building up of social competence of family unit; Involving parents as carers. Occ Behaviour modification techniques; Fostering; Adoption. Severe cases require Special schooling. Detection, Rx & care of ass conditions eg Dental problems, Ep, Sensory defects

As adult will require variable amount of formal help. Often Reside in minimum support home; Use Adult Training Centre; Crisis intervention team c̄ alternative accommodation if required. Occ work in "sheltered" job

Individuals who have resided in large mental handicap hospitals require "deinstitutionalisation" before returning to community

Institutionalisation

Many large institutions caring for the chronically sick and/or handicapped esp mentally handicapped have a poor record. A "total institution" has been defined as "a place of residence and work where a large number of like-situated individuals, cut off from wider society for an appreciable time, together lead an enclosed, formally administered round of life". People within such institutions often become "institutionalised" ie lacking in initiative & detatched from events in the outside world

Processes likely to → Institutionalisation inc Batch management eg meals at same time & place; Highly structured day; Discouragement of individuality eg lack of choice of clothing & furnishings; Paucity of links c̄ outside society; Poor staff attitudes. Large,

geographically isolated residences c̄ severely handicapped clients and poor staff:resident ratios are esp likely to → institutionalisation
Staff may value chr carer role negatively; most health staff have been trained to deal c̄ cure & short-term care. Often the desire for administrative efficiency → routinisation of tasks.

Staff may ↓ resident's personal choice & ↑ individual's dependence on staff
Rarely large institutions can be resident-orientated & geared to ↑ personal freedom & ↑ personal skills. In such places there can be a risk of distressing the handicapped person by asking him to achieve a task beyond his capabilities

DISABILITY & HANDICAP

Often the terms, disability & handicap are used in an ill-defined manner. Determinants which ascribe people into able & not able gps are complex & sometimes contradictory, they inc: Person's perception & personality; Sub-cultural milieu esp the family; Socio–cultural norms; Medical legitimization partly based on clin details
Health Impairment can be defined as any loss or abnormality of psychological, physiological or anatomical structure or function. A **Disability** is any restriction or lack of ability to perform an activity in the manner or within the range considered normal for a human being consequent upon an impairment. A **Handicap** is an impairment or disability, that constitutes a disadvantage for an individual in that it limits or prevents the fulfilment of a normal role for that individual. Thus impairment is a problem at the organic level, disability at the functional level, & handicap at the social level. For example, myopia is an impairment & disability but not a handicap, whilst a facial deformity is an impairment & handicap but not a disability
Disability & handicap are commonest in low social class, poor, elderly, & socially isolated. Often → premature retirement
Often handicap does not merely effect the disabled person, but secondarily affects others esp family eg elderly person has CVA → residual problems → daughter giving up work to look after mother → less money, ↓ freedom of action for daughter
Impairments are reasonably age-specific. In the UK:
In infancy about 1% of cases occur esp due to Cong malformations; CP;
In youth about 1% of cases occur esp due to Ep; Muscular dystrophy
In early maturity about 15% of cases occur esp due to Sensory organ problems; Amputations; Injuries esp RTA; MS
In late maturity & old age about 70% of cases occur esp due to Arthritis; Ht disease; Chest disease; CVA; Senility; Infections
About 15% of cases are generally not age specific eg Allergic & metabolic disease, GU disease, Skin disease
In UK about 3–4% of adult pop are severely disabled.

PREVENTION: Important 1° control measures inc Compulsory seat belts; Screening for cong malformations; Stopping smoking; Monitoring & Rx of BP ↑; Screening for sensory organ impairments

RX: Drugs are useful in the control of some conditions eg Ep; Arthritis; Infections; Mental illness
Community action is needed to prevent disability → handicap. Community attitudes are an important determinant of the priority given to disabling conditions by the Govt, social services, Drs & voluntary agencies
The Govt can provide state benefits which should be adequate & easy to claim. Legislation can improve lifestyle eg the UK Chronic Sick & Disabled Act instructed the L.Auths to find out the number & needs of its disabled, to inform the disabled of the availability of services & to improve housing, parking, access & toilet facilities. In UK, large firms are expected to employ at least 3% of their workforce from the Disabled Register
Medical intervention inc the use of remedial professions eg physiotherapy, OT, speech therapy, chiropody. Specialist rehab may be given by

Consultants in Rehab, Limb fitting centres. GPs & Community Physicians are important in liaison. Rx must be a dialogue c̄ the patient as the therapy is such an important & longlasting determinant of lifestyle
Social services are often involved in care, often providing support staff eg Home helps & equipment eg aids & adaptations
To improve employment prospects often requires retraining. In UK, this is partly the task of the DRO

The family & voluntary agencies have traditionally played a large role in the care of the disabled

PROG: The disabled have traditionally received relatively poor services. Training of Drs has generally undervalued caring & rehab roles. Legal sanctions are often not fully enforced. Claiming of benefits is often complex & inequitable ("no fault compensation" obviates some of the difficulties)

ACCIDENTS

Important cause of morbidity & mort esp in children & young adults

Road Traffic Accidents

Major cause of death & morbidity. Many of deaths are in young adults esp 15–19yrs. Predominant cause of death in children & young adults in many countries. Esp lower social classes. Death & inj rates are improving in many countries, but the pop at-risk is rising
Of the UK RTA deaths:
About 10% are children & 20% young adults
About 33% are pedestrians, 40% are in cars, 17% are on motorcycles, 5% are on bicycles & 5% on some other motorised vehicle
About 60% occur in towns, 35% in country & 5% on motorways
In UK, ave length of stay in hospital after RTA is about 14 days & about 1.5% of all hospital beds are used by these patients. About 1% of hospital admissions have severe chr disabilities. Death & severe inj are esp common in pedestrians, motorcyclists & bicyclists. Pedestrian & motorcyclist accidents often → leg injs. Head injs are commonest in bicyclists & vehicle occupants. Motorcyclists & pedal cyclists have the highest casualty rate/km

Major Factors Contributing to RTAs (LIST 14 CM)

A. HUMAN ERROR IN DRIVERS
1. Lack of care
2. Driving too fast
3. Poor observation
4. Distraction
5. Inexperience
6. Wrong path
7. Improper overtaking

B. HUMAN ERROR IN PEDESTRIANS
1. Lack of care
2. Fail to look
3. In dangerous position
4. Distracted
5. Misjudged speed & distance

C. VEHICLE DEFECTS
1. Tyre defect
2. Brake defect
3. Mechanical failure
4. Light defects
5. Steering defects

D. ROAD ENVIRONMENT FACTORS
1. Adverse road design: Eg Inadequate signs, markings, lighting
2. Adverse road weather or traffic conditions
3. Obstructions

The cause of accidents is often multifactorial. Pedestrian & driver factors are commonest, adverse environmental factors are not infrequent & vehicle defects are uncommon. Amongst drivers common contributory factors are alcohol, tiredness, drugs & illness

Alcohol intake is strongly dose related to risk of having an accident. In UK, about 35% of drivers killed in RTAs had a blood alcohol concentration above 80mg/100ml (the UK legal limit). Alcohol tends to impair the judgement of drivers, they may overrate their capacity to drive & have a euphoric sense of security

Speeding is dangerous esp if carried out on the wrong type of road. Motorways have low accident rates per passenger miles travelled (alternative denominator of hours travelled is less favourable to motorways). Some evidence that it is drivers going much faster or much slower than the ave on a particular road who are the major causes of accidents

Road design is important eg many accidents occur close to junctions. Poor lighting & inadequate road signs are occ contributory factors

Some weather conditions esp fog & black ice are ass c̄ ↑ risk of accidents. Accidents are commoner in the dark

PREVENTION: Legal constraints inc Speed limits; Breathalyser; Driving tests; Wearing of seat belts. Health education campaigns eg "Green Cross Code", "Don't drink & drive". Environmental improvements inc Improvement in road layout; Better street lighting; Better road surfaces; Improved road signs. Improved vehicle design eg better impact resistance

Most countries have a driving test to ensure the competence of potential road users. Some countries eg New Zealand have a periodic driving test. Stringent tests of competence & instruction by qualified tutors is probably beneficial

In UK, the 1967 Road Safety Act made it illegal to drive c̄ a blood alcohol [>80mg/100ml] & led to a ↓ in alcohol-related RTAs which unfortunately was later not maintained. In some countries eg Sweden, drink/driving legislation has led to a persistent improvement in accident rates. The Act also required special licences for HGV drivers which led to a decline in HGV accident rates. Most country's law allows for the fining or disqualification of drivers for motoring offences

Illness & disability are uncommon causes of road accidents. The elderly can be medically assessed periodically for fitness to drive (the elderly are more likely to be involved in accidents but often these are minor). Most forms of Ep are a bar to driving. MIs are probably the commonest cause of illness → serious RTAs & in the UK, IHD may disbar a person from holding a HGV licence. Vision testing is part of the statutory driving test used in many countries. Tiredness is a recognised factor in some RTAs & many countries control the hours of work of commercial vehicle drivers eg by use of tachograph

Most evidence shows that realistic speed limits improve road safety. A realistic limit being a speed that most experienced drivers consider safe for a particular road. Speed checks by police have a powerful temporary deterrent effect. Other methods of speed control inc speed governors, "sleeping policemen", "rumble areas", bar pattern on roads to give illusion of ↑ speed

Road signs should be conspicuous & unambiguous. Prominent signs near accident blackspots are helpful. Often investigation of a "blackspot" → alteration in local road design. Well lit roads → a fall in accident rates

In bad weather conditions, journeys should be avoided if possible. Systems that can quickly respond to changes in road conditions, such as bad weather or road works, by altering information to motorists eg changing speed limits, are useful

Seat belts, esp for front seat occupants, are an important preventer of death & inj. Legislation increases wearing rates & hence → ↓ inj rates. It is estimated that seat belts reduce serious inj by 45–70% & deaths by about 40%. Serious inj from seat belts are extremely rare

Crash helmets are compulsory for motorcyclists in many countries. They signf ↓ the risk of fatal & non-fatal head inj

Bicycle inj are reduced if cyclists have reduced exposure to traffic eg not allowing children to cycle in road, providing designated cycle tracks

Health education campaigns usually have a beneficial but short lasting effect. Some training schemes in road safety for young persons appear to have a longer lasting effect. Road safety officers, Police, teachers & parents can all provide useful information to children re road safety. Systematic advice for child pedestrians eg the

Green Cross Code is probably useful. Accident rates are lowest in cul-de-sacs, segregated housing estates & in areas c̄ plentiful protected play areas. Whenever possible, children & the elderly should be accompanied by an adult
If the public believes that the police are vigilant & the penalties for offences are high, they are generally likely to behave better on the roads

RX: Depends on type of inj. Often requires prompt action & may inc use of all emergency services ie Police, Fire, Ambulance. Usually require first-aid & use of A&E Depts. Occ expensive medical techniques eg intensive care, surgery
N.B Accidents from rail and air transport are much less common than RTAs. Rail & air travel both carry ↓ risk compared to road travel

Accidents in the Home

Common cause of mortality & morbidity. Many injs not officially reported. Esp Young children, Elderly. In elderly, major cause of deaths is from falls. In children, major causes of mortality & morbidity are burns, scalds, suffocation & poisoning. Esp low social class, handicapped eg mentally handicapped child. In young, M>F
Many possible causes of accidents eg deep stairwells, poor lighting, insecure flooring, lack of fireguards, faulty electrical wiring, unprotected blades, accessible tablets, dangerous toys

PREVENTION: Govt action can inc laws: To ensure safe design & construction of dwellings; To oblige manufacturers & vendors to provide goods of merchandisable quality. Govt may also recommend products to public as being of a safe standard eg in UK by meeting requirements of British Standards Institute. Good construction & design
Advice to family esp by HV & District Nurse. Fireguards. Inflammable clothing. Keep sharp objects, tablets & noxious materials out of reach of children. Handrails. "Non-slip" surfacing materials
Parents should be advised to teach good practices re home safety to their children, starting at an early age
Advice on good practice via media (probably only of minor value)

Playground Accidents

Not uncommon. Many injs not officially reported. Esp occur if equipment poorly designed or badly maintained, & playground surface is hard

PREVENTION: Make playground surfaces softer. Don't allow steep slides. Place slides on sloping ground. Provide swing seats of soft material. Regular inspection of equipment. Encourage supervision of children by parents. Provide trained playground attendants

Accidents ass c̄ Water

Common. Esp children; Non-swimmers. Common sites inc Unguarded static water eg ponds, wells, tanks; Hazardous areas of sea eg strong currents, rocks. Immersion in cold water may rapidly → hypothermia & death. Sailing accidents often due to lack of seamanship esp in poor weather
Drowning is usually due to aspiration of copious amounts of fluid ("wet drowning"), but may be due to asphyxia 2° to intense glottic spasm, the immersion syndrome (ie cardiac arrest 2° to intense parasympathetic stimulus), or development of ARDS following extraction from water

CLIN OF DROWNING: Drowning is ass c̄ Severe metabolic acidosis; O_2 ↓; Arrhythmias; Cerebral oedema; Wet heavy lungs
Near-drowning has variable signs. Often Cyanosis; Coughing; Frothy sputum; Coma or agitation. Occ Hypothermia; Arrhythmias; ARDS; Cerebral oedema. Rarely DIC; ARF

INVESTIGATIONS:
- FBC
- U&Es
- WCC: Usually ↑
- Astrup
- ECG: Often tachycardia, non-specific ˆSTˆ & ˆTˆ wave changes
- CXR: May be norm but usually pulm infiltrates

RX OF NEAR DROWNING: Establish airway. May require cardio–pulm resus. High concentrations of O_2. Steroids for cerebral oedema & possibly for pulm lesions. Standard Rx of hypothermia. Monitor closely

PREVENTION: Fencing in of static water. Don't leave young child during bath.

Teach children to swim early. Training in seamanship. Wear lifejackets. Easy availability of lifebelts. Lifeguards. Clear signs to indicate hazardous stretch of water. Teach resus techniques

Electrical Accidents

Deaths usually due to high voltage electricity esp a.c, or lightning. Danger esp if Voltage >1000; a.c >60 cycles/sec; Current passes through Ht or resp centre; Long duration of current passage; Skin is moist

CLIN: High voltage injs often → Arrhythmias, Cardiac arrest. Burnt skin. Occ ARF; K^+ ↑↑; GI perf; CNS damage eg polyneuritis; Haem; Long bone #. Occ late organ damage eg cataracts, GI dysfunction

RX: If arrest, cardio–pulm resus. Continuous ECG monitoring for at least 2 days. Monitor urine output. Standard Rx of K^+ ↑↑. Once haemodynamically stable, assess tissue damage. May require debridement ± amputation

PROG: Prompt resus is often lifesaving esp in lightning inj

ASPECTS OF CARE OF THE ELDERLY

The age of 65yrs is commonly taken to define the onset of old age. In most countries, changes in the pop structure & size this century have → an increase in the proportion & absolute numbers of elderly persons in the pop. In the UK, for example, between 1900–1940, the total pop increased by 15% & those aged >65yrs by 94%, whilst between 1940–1970, the total pop rose by 15% & those aged >65yrs by 54%. At present about 14% of the UK pop is aged >65yrs. For the rest of the century, only a small rise in the numbers of elderly is forecast, but those aged >85yrs will increase significantly

The demand for health & health related services increases markedly in old age. It has been estimated that those aged >85yrs receive about 8× the ave in health services. Death & morbidity rates are much higher in the older age gps esp due to Ca, IHD & CVAs. Compared to other age gps, the elderly are much more likely to concurrently suffer from more than one disease process. As M tend to die earlier, about 60% of all aged >65yrs are FAs most

As most people retire in their 60's, old age also → change in lifestyle. For many, old age is ass c̄ poverty. In the UK, of elderly people living at home, about 33% live alone. As social trends have led to smaller family size & ↑ geographic mobility, many of the elderly have become isolated from family support

The special requirements of the elderly for health care were late in recognition, the speciality of geriatrics starting in the 1940s or later in many countries. As the elderly are more likely to suffer from chr disease & often take longer to recover from acute disease, their Rx conflicted c̄ the prevailing model of medical Rx propounded at medical schools ie curing of young persons c̄ acute disease was the fundamental role of drs. Hospital beds for the elderly still tend to be in old buildings distant from the DGH & without good investigative or rehabilitative services (the elderly under the care of non-geriatricians are more likely to be admitted to the DGH)

The combination of physical & psychiatric conditions is commonest in the elderly age gp. Dementia prevalence is strongly age related. Depression & suicide are common. Rx requires close co-operation between geriatrician & psychiatrist

Day hospitals offer a range of services usually to people who have been previous inpatients. Patients can be medically reviewed as well as receive nursing & rehabilitative care eg physio, OT, speech therapy. Relatives can also be educated in the care of old people

Facilities for care of the dying should allow a pain-free dignified death. Drs often require better training in the care of the dying (see Psych chapter). For those who prefer to die at home, health & social service input eg district nurse, provision of commode, is usually helpful. Hospices can provide an atmosphere geared to the demands of the dying person & a focus for expertise in pain relief

Social services provide many facilities for the elderly eg Old people's homes, meals on wheels. The degree of L.Auth provision in the UK is variable geographically & unrelated to the degree of hospital provision. In most areas there is a lack of facilities & services for the elderly

Hypothermia

Esp poor low social class elderly in cold climates. Factors inc: Poverty & high fuel costs; Unawareness of dangers of cold; ↓ physiological ability to withstand cold in the elderly. Rarely 2° to drugs eg Phenothiazines, hypothyroidism. Not uncommon

CLIN: At temperatures below 32° C: Clouding of consciousness; Ataxia; Tremulous speech; Sluggishness. Occ Rigidity; Oliguria; BP ↓; PR ↓; Reflexes ↓; Stupor; Coma; Dysarthria; Vom; BG ↓; Arrhythmias

INVESTIGATIONS:
- Low reading thermometer p.r
- ECG: Widening of ˆQRSˆ complex, ˆJˆ waves, bradycardia. Occ Arrhythmias eg VEs, VF
- BG
- U&Es
- T4

PREVENTION: Advice to at-risk gps re dangers of cold eg use many layers of clothing, cover head & if unable to heat all of house ensure that one well heated room is available. Special financial allowances for heating available to at-risk gps in some countries

RX: Medical emergency. If comatose, ensure patent airway & aspirate gastric contents. Minimise stimulation to avoid ppt of VF. Close monitoring of BP, PR, Temperature, ECG, Urine output & neuro signs
Rewarm at rate of about 0.5° C/hr.
If moderate hypothermia, passive rewarming c̄ metallised reflective blankets. If severe hypothermia or haemodynamic disturbance, active rewarming eg warm IV fluids & heated O_2. Risk of "rewarming shock" → severe lactic acidosis, BP ↓↓
Occ HCO_3 for metabolic acidosis; Ventilation for severe hypercapnoea; Hydrocortisone. Glucose if BG ↓. Prophylactic antibiotic may benefit

COMMUNITY CARE

The concept of "Community Care" has been emphasised by many health care policy makers since the 1960's. The stimulus to this perspective included the inadequacy of care provided in institutional settings & the perceived cheapness of community care
The concept is ill-defined, for example, it can mean care in the community or care by the community. Care in the community predominantly refers to plans for residential homes for people c̄ chr handicapping conditions within towns rather than in geographically isolated large institutions eg in UK the 1959 MHAct advocated caring for psychiatric patients in the community. Care by the community envisages care by voluntary & informal networks as well as by the formal services
Community care is mainly carried out by the family esp F, spouses & close relatives. Often large economic, social & psychological "costs" to family eg a household c̄ a disabled member is usually poorer than ave esp if disability is severe. In chr conditions, help from distant relatives, friends & neighbours tends to diminish over time. Families may be less able to offer help compared to former times due to social trends inc:↑ geographic & social mobility; ↓ family size; ↑ fragility of family life eg ↑ divorce rate, ↑ numbers of single parent families. Little evidence that people are nowadays more likely not to want to look after their parents
Community care for most client gps has been shown to be more expensive than institutional care designed to meet approx similar levels of client need. The paucity of growth monies in the UK Health & Social Services in recent yrs & the P not to redistribute funds from the hospital sector has → the formal community services being sometimes unable to provide little more than a crisis intervention service. Often the better funded services are in areas of lower need, an example of the "inverse

care law". Targets set for provision of service for the elderly, mentally handicapped & mentally ill have rarely been reached eg in the UK targets for day care places for the mentally ill are far less than those proposed by DHSS. However complaints re the formal agencies may be muted, for whilst large institutions were relatively easy to monitor, community care is difficult to assess both by the formal agencies (it is much more time consuming) & the client and his family who may lack comparative information or feel less able to comment when not part of a gp

Even when services are available, many eligible people may not be aware of their existence. In addition, some services may not be acceptable to the client &/or family eg many feel that the sort of care provided in a short-stay accommodation is deleterious to their dependent relatives' well-being

Nonetheless, community care offers large potential social benefits eg the client remains c̄ family & friends & avoids institutionalisation

THE DOCTOR–PATIENT RELATIONSHIP

Most societies have accepted the value of division of labour including the setting up of a gp of specially trained persons to advise about the general pop's health. These gps have usually become parts of formal institutions. The study of the interaction between the public & these specialised gps esp Drs can elicit how the system works in particular settings & suggest action to improve the value of the relationship

A basic discrimination can be drawn between the community level, where it can be the doctors esp Community Physician's or Govt that initiates contact c̄ the public, and the individual level, where it is usually the public which generates the initial consultation c̄ the clinician

In a perfect system, the public would only consult the health professional for significant health problems, the patient would consult at an early stage & the transaction c̄ the Dr would allow compliance c̄ the Rx and an early cure. Most health complaints never reach the doctor's consulting room, this may be appropriate if the complaint is self-limiting, trivial or amenable to successful Rx based on local cultural knowledge eg plaster for a cut, Aspirin for a headache, but other problems which could benefit from professional advice present late or not at all, & are occ compounded by inappropriate lay therapy

The process by which people become socially recognised as sick contains culturally-specific patterns. Attainment of the sick role generally grants certain rights & obligations to the sick person. Deviations from the normal pattern of illness behaviour (ie the usual roles in the stages from being well to being sick) can disrupt the success of the Dr–Patient relationship eg late presentation c̄ a disease making cure more difficult

The Dr–Patient relationship is rarely simply the objective application of medical science. The human interaction between Dr & patient is crucial for a successful relationship, & is dependent not only on the knowledge & personality of the Dr & patient but on the general sociocultural matrix & those of the specific relevant sub-culture eg the views of the medical profession & those of the patient's family. Problems at any of these levels can disrupt a successful relationship. However an understanding of the possible reasons for the failure of the relationship can allow the Dr to take corrective action

The Sick Role

In Medical Sociology: Disease is defined as a pathological state; Illness as an individual's subjective perception; & Sickness as a socially recognised status

Parsons, a Sociologist, proposed an idealised typification of the role of the sick person. The sick role accorded 2 rights ie exemption from blame for the condition & from certain obligations & responsibilities esp work, & 2 obligations ie the desire to get better & the acceptance of technically competent Rx of the health service esp Drs

The model assumes that the Dr is an instrument of social control who can officially legitimate & define sickness. It further assumes that technically competent Rx is the exclusive province of the health professions
Although the model is useful, there are many significant variations from the role:
Exemption from blame: Not true of many health conditions eg o/d, alcoholism, STD
Exemption from obligations esp work: Occ not true esp for housewives
Duty to accept state as undesirable: May be inappropriate eg if condition becomes chronic
Duty to accept Rx from health profession: May be inappropriate for a variety of reasons eg absence of useful medical Rx (esp if non-medical Rx of value) or conflict of medical advice c̄ important norms of the patient. Compliance is usually low if the Dr fails to appreciate the social context of an illness

Illness Behaviour

A series of stages in illness behaviour can usually be identified: Well → Experience symptoms → Explore Social environment eg may seek views of family & friends → Medical care contact → Legitimization & adoption of Sick Role (Dependent patient stage) → Relinquishment of Sick Role, eg → Recovery, Rehab Stage, Chr Sick Role, or Death
Factors involved in the patient making contact c̄ the Dr inc: Whether symptom considered abnormal; Whether symptom considered medical; Whether symptom considered medical & serious (depends on factors such as: Degree of disability, degree of pain, freq & duration of symptoms, familiarity of symptoms); Whether symptom considered medical & serious but disregarded; Whether competing service used eg Osteopath for backache
An individual may disregard perceived serious medical symptoms for 3 major reasons: Competing interests eg obligations to work; Denial eg the commonly observed delay when Ca suspected; Poor availability or acceptability of service eg cost, previous poor relationship c̄ Dr
The individual's perception of symptoms are partly socially determined eg backache & bronchitis may not be considered noteworthy by middle-aged lower social class UK M, Headache more likely to be defined as migraine by a middle class person. Evidence that dissatisfaction c̄ family life or work → ↑ illness & ↑ medical consultation rate
When the patient & doctor meet, there are many potential barriers to a successful relationship. 3 models of satisfactory interaction have been proposed: "Dr active, patient passive" is appropriate in some medical emergencies eg unconscious patient; "Guidance—Co-operation" where patient seeks help & follows advice ie paternalistic model, is appropriate for some acute illness; "Mutual participation" where both Dr & patient have approx equal power & mutual interdependence, is often appropriate in chr illness. Successful Drs from the client's viewpoint are generally those perceived to be interested in the client, honest (esp important as the information passed between Dr & patient should be confidential), approachable, good at listening & explanation, & technically competent
The Dr's common expectation that a person should make an active assessment of trivial illness (& not bother him) & yet be a passive responder to his advice about more serious illness, is a dichotomy which may result in relationship problems
The power differential between individuals in negotiations can be an important factor in a relationship. The Dr is a powerful figure due to: Expert knowledge; High social status; The mystique of health inc perceived control over life & death, & understanding of the mind; Organisational factors eg setting of interview. Compared to the Dr, the client has a greater knowledge of community, social gp & family norms, less knowledge about disease & increased scepticism of medical practices. Research has shown that Drs find successful relationships easier to forge c̄ patients from similar backgrounds eg GP consultation times exhibit a social class gradient c̄ longer ave times spent c̄ higher social class patients. Thus as might be expected, the gp of patients closest in power to the Dr c̄ the greatest similarity in

lifestyle, language & norms are most likely to enter into a mutually satisfying relationship
Compliance c̄ Drs advice & Rx at the 1° care level has been shown to be between 50–70% for a wide range of different illness eg BP ↑ Rx, diet regimes, drugs for Psychiatric conditions, Anti-TB drug Rx. Factors ass c̄ compliance can be divided into 5 categories:

1. Situational: Inc Culture; Economics; Family Support; Physical Environment
2. Nature of Illness: Compliance increased in acute & serious illness
3. Treatment Regime: Compliance increased if regime simple
4. Demographic Characteristics: Usually ↑ compliance in higher social class & well educated persons
5. Doctor–Patient Interaction: Usually ↑ compliance if clear directions, Dr perceived as friendly & approachable, Dr is good at non-verbal communication

Drs can be trained to minimise their problems in the Dr–Patient relationship. Such training can inc: Greater awareness of potential problems in Dr–Patient relationship; ↑ instruction about the lifestyle, language & norms of the public esp lower social class & chr ill persons; Practice of listening & explanation skills eg by use of video analysis of Dr–Patient interviews; Advice on organisational setting eg communication is improved if a desk is not interposed between Dr & patient; Training in Non-Verbal Communication skills eg importance of direct eye contact, body posture & tone of voice. Rx regimes should be as simple to follow as possible. Some evidence that supplying supportive simple written advice for the patient may further improve compliance
In chr illness, successful Rx relies heavily on medical advice being compatible c̄ the patient's lifestyle preferences. Thus mutual participation is usually the model of choice for this client gp

Placebo Effect

A placebo is an inactive substance or preparation formerly given to please a patient but now often used in controlled studies to determine the efficacy of medicines, the patient being unaware that the substance is inactive. It has been found in many circumstances that giving a substance known to be physiologically inactive in a particular condition to a patient ignorant of this fact, leads to an improvement in health in a substantial number of people c̄ the condition (the "placebo effect"). The explanation for the effect is not fully understood, factors may inc Inherent variability in symptomatology & course of many diseases; Subjective feeling of improvement by the patient because of belief in expert. Some evidence that placebos may indirectly cause physiological change eg "dummy" analgesics may → ↓ response to pain
Due to the existence of this effect, it is essential in the testing of new medicines to include a control gp who receive a placebo (if possible morphologically indistinguishable from the "true" medicine). It is desirable if both doctor & patient are unaware of which preparation is the placebo (ie a double-blind trial)

THE PROFESSION OF MEDICINE

The existence of professions rests on the development of specialisation & the division of labour. The divisions between professions eg law & medicine & occupations, in terms of work content is fairly arbitrary. Nonetheless there are general criteria whereby professions can be distinguished from occupations

General Characteristics of Professions (LIST 15 CM)

1. Prolonged specialised training
2. Service orientation
3. Monopoly of a particular kind of knowledge
4. Non-substitutable skills
5. High social status

6. Legitimate, organised Autonomy: Eg Control of entry into profession, Self-regulation re conduct & standards
7. Exercise authority over others

Medicine clearly meets the criteria for being a profession. The practice of medicine is dependent on a vast theoretical knowledge passed on by a prolonged period of training. Admissions, curriculum, exams & training posts are all regulated almost exclusively by the profession. In the UK, the GMC (an almost exclusively medical body) regulates standards of professional conduct. In many areas, medical monopoly on knowledge has → public dependency on non-substitutable skills. Prestige for drs is high eg surveys of the public have repeatedly ranked medicine as one of the most valuable jobs, & has been recognised in most countries by comparatively high wages. Other occupations in the health field derive their activities from the medical profession & are ultimately under its control eg Nursing

Within the medical profession, there are differences in the extent of autonomy & status of gps eg acute specialities such as Surgery are perceived to have a higher status than specialities concerned c̄ care of chr conditions such as Mental Handicap. There is a concentration of F & immigrant drs in the "low status" specialities

Acceptance that the profession should be largely autonomous is based on the trust of society regarding its service ethic. There are some trends that the public believes doctors to be abusing their power eg the campaigns to demedicalise pregnancy & to allow death c̄ dignity

As professional status usually accords c̄ better working conditions & increased rates of pay, it is possible to interpret the actions of other health occupations as increasing their attempts to become a profession. In the UK, for example, in recent years, there has been a large increase in the number of university trained nurses & a phasing out of the lesser trained SEN grade

The process by which the non-professional medical student becomes a professional dr is an example of anticipatory socialisation. The attitudes & behaviours of role models in the profession & other influences of the environment of the medical school & teaching hospitals, gradually equip the medical student for his or her forthcoming role, thereby anticipating the requirements for success in the job of doctoring

NON-MEDICAL HEALTH AGENCIES

Health has been defined in many ways ranging from the utopian WHO definition of "complete physical, mental & social well-being" to the narrower concept of absence of illness. Common to the operationalisation of any of these definitions is the recognition that health can not simply be the province of the formal medical services. Thus, for example, the promotion of positive health involves the sport & leisure industry. Indeed, many non-medical agencies eg Social Services have an important role in the promotion of health. Inter-agency co-operation is required to help in the management of individuals & gps whose health needs cross agency boundaries eg mentally handicapped persons

Social Services

In the UK, L.Auth Social Services Depts were set up concerned largely c̄ children, the elderly & the disabled. Their duties are broadly based & often underpinned by legislation. Their objective has been stated as "To assist members of society who are handicapped or deprived to lead &/or establish as full & satisfactory lives as possible within the community"

Duties concerned c̄ children inc: Protection, control & supervision of children deemed by courts to require care (may inc assumption of parental rights); Provision & regulation of nurseries & child minders; Fostering & Adoption; Provision for children deprived of normal home life eg

"Children's Homes" for orphans; Supervision of voluntary child care agencies; General child welfare promotion eg Soc W support to families under stress; Involvement in NAI procedures

Duties concerned c̄ the elderly inc: Provision & Supervision of EPHs; Provision of domestic & home help facilities; Assessment of needs eg for Aids & Appliances, Laundry, Telephone; Soc W support to at-risk elderly inc Casework & Crisis intervention; Supervision of voluntary agencies; Day care provision; Social Clubs

Duties concerned c̄ the disabled inc: Provision of sheltered work; Ascertainment of chr sick & disabled in community; Residential provision & supervision; Supervision of voluntary agencies; Provision of aids & appliances; Role in compulsory admission of mentally disordered to hospital; Registration & welfare of sensory handicapped persons; Adult Training Centres eg for mentally handicapped persons; Alterations to homes; Social Clubs

Techniques employed by Soc W inc Regulation enforcement; Inspection of facilities; Casework inc problem solving facilitation; Crisis intervention; Community Development; Advocacy of client eg to DHSS, Housing Dept; Screening eg re Bus passes; Long-term surveillance; General information & advice

Social Services play an important role in informing people about the benefits for which they may qualify. In the UK, the benefit system is complex & often requires the explanation of experts (a role principally undertaken by Social Services & the Citizen's Advice Bureau). Possible benefits inc Supplementary Benefit, Rent & Rates rebates, Family Income Supplement, Mobility Allowance & Attendance Allowance

Some Soc Ws have developed specialisation eg in care of mentally handicapped persons. Others (Community Soc Ws) have specific geographic base & try to identify needs & resources of local community, & +vely develop the community by promoting community self-help (which may inc community action such as a sit-in to complain about housing conditions) & advocacy to the formal agencies

Drs & Soc Ws regularly meet at a number of forums inc: Hospital via Hospital Soc W; PHC via Soc W attachment to GP's team; JCPTs; NAI case conferences; Medical inspections of Social Service establishments; Mental Health Tribunals; Joint Working Parties esp re Elderly, Children, Mentally Ill & Mentally Handicapped. The Community Physician has a specific role in liaison c̄ the Social Services

Relationships between Drs & Soc Ws are sometimes not good. Reasons put forward for this finding inc: Differences in training, knowledge & expertise esp emphasis on biological sciences in medicine compared to Soc W's social science orientation; Misperceptions of respective roles eg some GPs are unaware of therapeutic role of Soc W & may not see the relevance of the individual's functioning in the total social setting; Differences in work tempo & method inc the Dr's tendency to act decisively eg rapid examination, diagnosis & Rx formulation, whilst social work often depends on the slow process of building a relationship & the field worker's proposed action may require acceptance by senior Soc Ws; The Dr's power to direct many gps of staff eg Nurses, Paramedical occupations is not present in respect of Soc Ws which may → frustration; Soc Workers do not have a formal code of ethics; Differences in social status inc related factors eg use of language, may → poor communication; Drs are often unaware of the legal responsibilities of Soc Ws; GP is likely to be middle-aged & highly experienced whilst the Soc W is often young & relatively inexperienced (In the UK, many Soc Ws have not been formally trained)

Areas of large overlap between roles of GP, HV & Soc W inc Personal counselling; Mild Neuroses; & Bereavement counselling

Education

Schooling is an important determinant of the personality & practices of the future adult. Increasingly schools are appreciating the need for teaching about personal development & life

skills. Teachers are important health educators & there are good grounds for believing that good lifestyle practices learnt during schooling are likely to persist in adult life. Thus children should be presented c̄ the information necessary to make informed choices about their lifestyle eg Cig smoking, drugs, alcohol, diet, sexual practice
School meals are an important dietary influence, both in determining long-term dietary habits & occ in providing the most nutritious meal of the day. Many countries provide a school meal service which may be subsidised thereby benefiting children from poor families. There have been some campaigns to improve the dietary composition of school meals, but the child's preference for chips & sweets is often difficult to overcome
In many countries, all school children receive medical examinations & some vaccinations. There is a debate about the best way to school handicapped children. In the UK, the trend is to educate the handicapped where possible in "normal" schools. The 1981 Education Act imposed a duty on the health & education services to identify & assess handicapped children, & make recommendations about the type of schooling appropriate for children in consultation c̄ the parents. Placing handicapped children in a norm school setting has potential benefits in their socialisation & it may make their non-handicapped contempories more accepting of handicapped persons. Special schools have the advantage of concentrating expert resources & facilities in one centre, but may stigmatise the child & are often relatively inaccessible to the parents
Whether the place of schooling is a special, normal or hospital school, there is a need for collaboration between the education & health services esp in respect of handicapped children. The community physician has a specific role in liaison c̄ the education dept
School phobia, delinquency, truancy & emotional upsets are all relatively common. The health workers may need to liaise c̄ the Ed Psych, Educational Welfare Officer, Youth Worker or Child Guidance Service in the management of these & other conditions
The Education Dept is also concerned c̄ careers advice & further education. Finding employment for the handicapped is often difficult & requires the advice of various agencies eg Health, Education, & Employment officers such as the DRO

Voluntary Agencies

Non-statutory organisations can play an important role in the management of health-related conditions. Their roles may inc: Fund raising; Campaigning eg for changes in Rx or improvement in facilities; Independent monitoring; Innovation in care or Rx; Setting up support gps for clients &/or their families; Providing information & advice often via individuals who have experienced a particular health condition; Promoting community self-reliance
Fund raising is a common undertaking of voluntary gps. Funds may be raised for a variety of purposes eg research, equipment
Some voluntary gps have played an important role in commenting on the type of care received by particular client gps. In the UK, for example, MIND was an important influence in the framing of the 1983 MH Act which strengthened the rights of mentally ill patients. Voluntary agencies concerned c̄ maternal & child health have been important in improving conditions in antenatal clinics & labour wards, & helping to stop the medical profession treating pregnancy as a disease
The independent monitoring role of voluntary gps can be esp valuable in respect of chr conditions eg the exposure of poor conditions at mental illness, mental handicap or elderly institutions
As voluntary agencies are not hampered by the constraints of formal agencies, they may be in a position to innovate eg the development of therapeutic self-help gps
Many workers in voluntary agencies have themselves had direct or indirect experience of the specific health condition covered by their agency. This experience is often the basis of an advisory & information service eg those c̄ stomas advising potential stoma patients. Some voluntary agencies eg NSPCC, Citizen's Advice Bureau have

an extensive information service
Self-help gps eg Alcoholics Anonymous have grown in popularity in many countries. Their perceived advantages inc Easy availability of other gp members throughout day; Equality of participants; Social contact; Being less impersonal than contact c̄ formal agencies. Some gp members find they lose autonomy in the gp &/or may find it difficult to function outside the gp
Where possible it is useful to seek the community's view in planning & evaluation of services. It is often appropriate to use representatives of voluntary organisations to represent a community viewpoint eg some teams planning services for mentally handicapped people inc representatives of voluntary agencies usually including a parent of a mentally handicapped child. In the UK, CHCs have been specifically created to monitor the health services & have observer status on health authorities

ALTERNATIVE MEDICINE

There are many alternative health strategies outside of the formally recognised health agencies which nonetheless have the confidence of significant numbers of the pop. They are a disparate gp of strategies, but are usually linked by the lack of scientific evidence for their efficacy & a long h/o usage. Some of these techniques are likely to become part of the formally recognised armoury of the health service
Alternative health strategies inc Holistic medicine; Acupuncture; Herbalism; Meditation; Chiropraxy; Homeopathy; Faith healing; Osteopathy; Optometry
Some alternative medicine is highly culturally specific eg Witch doctoring in Africa, use of Hakkims in India & amongst immigrants from India in the UK. Much non-Western medicine has a strong non-scientific strand. It also often places great emphasis on the Rx of the whole person & the mind/body relationship (these concepts gradually becoming more appreciated in the West). In general, alternative medicine is more used by the less well educated. It has been found that the introduction of Western medicine into developing countries is often best achieved by working c̄ the traditional healers & explaining the action of treatments in terms relevant to the local culture
Reasons for the apparent effectiveness/attractiveness of some alternative medicine may inc: Large amount of time devoted to patient by practitioner ie attraction of "personalised" service; Cost of therapy ie feeling that what one pays for must be of more value than a "free" service; Inherent variability of symptomatology in many diseases; Pride ie not wishing to admit to oneself &/or others that time & money has been wasted; Placebo-like effect; Desperation eg if traditional medicine holds out little hope of symptom relief or cure; Strength of cultural belief in therapy. Of course, the Rx may in time be recognised as effective even on "scientific" criteria

Acupuncture

Traditional Chinese Rx. Based on a theory that the functioning of int organs can be influenced by the stimulation, usually by sc needles, of the skin at particular points (NB These points seem to bear no relation to Western knowledge of anatomy & physiology). The technique is used for a very wide range of conditions
There is some evidence that acupuncture stimulates the production of pain relieving opiate-like substances. Certainly acupuncture can be used for pain relief in surgery. For many conditions there are anecdotal reports of successful Rx but there have been few controlled trials
The technique appears very safe as long as the needles are properly sterilised. Paradoxically the absence of reports that acupuncture can cause problems suggests that the technique may not usually have a direct effect
Some UK Drs are already using acupuncture in their practice

Herbalism & Other Diet-Related Theories

Therapies related to diet are common in many cultures. In Western countries, there has been a movement to see "natural products" as advantageous. This movement, which is subscribed to in many adverts, is based on some truths eg that the removal of fibre from food was not beneficial to health, & some mainly unsubstantiated speculation eg food additives are harmful

In the therapeutic field, there have been many examples of herbs providing the basis for pharmacologically active drugs (& there are likely to be more in the future). However, some herbal remedies, despite their "naturalness" have been found to be harmful either intrinsically or due to impurities

The "food allergy" theory remains a subject of great debate, but is accepted by a minority of Drs

Meditation

Various meditation techniques are used esp in non-Western medicine. It is well demonstrated that meditation techniques can induce profound physiological changes eg reduction in PR. Such techniques eg transcendental meditation may be of benefit in the management of mild psychiatric & emotional illness. Biofeedback techniques were initially based on traditional meditation techniques & are of some benefit in the control of BP ↑

Chiropraxy

A system of therapeutics based upon the claim that disease is caused by abnormal function of the nervous system. It attempts to restore normal function of the nervous system by manipulation & Rx of the structures of the human body esp the spinal column. Little scientific evidence for its benefits

Homeopathy

A system of therapeutics based on Rx c̄ minute doses of drugs which in larger doses produce symptoms akin to those of the disease being treated. Although practiced by some Drs (in the UK there is even a homeopathic hospital), in the vast majority of diseases there is no evidence to justify its use

Faith Healing

Usually based on a belief that a divine being can act through a human (who is usually a devout believer) to heal an ill person. There are many anecdotal examples to support claims for faith healing

Osteopathy

A system of therapeutics based on the theory that the body can make its own remedies against disease & other toxic conditions, if it is placed in a normal structural relationship & has favourable environmental conditions & adequate nutrition. It stresses the importance of manipulative methods of detecting & correcting faulty structure. It is mainly used in the diagnosis & Rx of musculo–skeletal conditions. Scientific support for its effects is generally lacking, but there are many anecdotal reports of its benefits & many orthopaedic specialists are willing to sanction its use

Bibliography

Whenever possible the latest edition is noted except when the edition is a first one, where the date of publication is given.

General:

British Medical Journal.

The Lancet.

New England Journal of Medicine.

British Journal of Hospital Medicine.

Hospital Update.

Medicine International. The Medicine Group.

The "Lecture Note" series of books published by Blackwell.

The "Short Textbook" series of books published by Unibooks.

The "Recent Advances" series of books published by Churchill Livingstone.

Medical Lists for Examinations. Gabriel, R., Gabriel, C. M. Butterworths, 1983.

Aids to Undergraduate Medicine. Burton, J. L. 3rd Ed, Churchill Livingstone.

Aids to Postgraduate Medicine. Burton, J. L. 3rd Ed, Churchill Livingstone.

Cecil Textbook of Medicine. Ed Wyngaarden, J. H., Smith, L. H. W. B. Saunders & Co, 1985.

Davidson's Principles & Practice of Medicine. Ed Macleod, J. 14th Ed, Churchill Livingstone.

Price's Textbook of the Practice of Medicine. Bodley Scott, Sir Ronald. 12th Ed, Oxford University Press.

Dorland's Illustrated Medical Dictionary. 26th Ed, W. B. Saunders & Co.

Obstetrics & Gynaecology

Principles of Gynaecology. Jeffcoate, Sir Norman. 4th Ed, Butterworths.

Practical Obstetric Problems. Donald, I. 5th Ed, Lloyd–Luke (Medical Books) Ltd.

Obstetrics Illustrated. Garrey, M. M. *et al.* 3rd Ed, Churchill Livingstone.

Gynaecology Illustrated. Garrey, M. M. *et al.* 2nd Ed, Churchill Livingstone.

Fundamentals of Obstetrics & Gynaecology, Vol I Obstetrics. Llewellyn–Jones, D. 3rd Ed, Faber & Faber.

Fundamentals of Obstetrics & Gynaecology, Vol II Gynaecology. Llewellyn–Jones, D. 3rd Ed, Faber & Faber.

"Cancer of the Female Reproductive System". Ed Williams, C. J., Whitehouse, J. M. A. Vol 3 in series *Cancer Investigation & Management.* John Wiley & Sons, 1985.

A Practical Guide for The Obstetric Team. Read, M. D., Welby, D. John Wiley & Sons, 1985.

Essential Management of Obstetric Emergencies. Baskett, T. John Wiley & Sons, 1985.

Principles & Practice of Obstetrics & Perinatology. Ed Iffy, L., Kaminetzky, H. A. John Wiley & Sons, 1981.

Neonatology & Paediatrics

Textbook of Paediatrics. Forfar, J. O & Arneil, G. C. 3rd Ed, Churchill Livingstone.

Nelson Textbook of Pediatrics. Ed Behrman, R. E., Vaughan III, V.C. 12th Ed, W. B. Saunders & Co.

Common Symptoms of Disease in Children. Illingworth, R. S. 8th Ed, Blackwell Scientific Publications.

The Normal Child. Illingwoth, R. S. 8th Ed, Churchill Livingstone.

Practical Paediatric Problems. Hutchinson, J. 5th Ed, Lloyd–Luke (Medical Books) Ltd.

Neonatal Medicine. Chiswick, M. L. Update Publications, 1978.

The ABC of 1–7. Valman, H. B. British Medical Journal Publications. 1982.

First Year of Life. Valman, H. B. British Medical Journal Publications, 1980.

Ellis & Mitchell, Disease in Infancy & Childhood. Mitchell, R. G. 7th Ed, Churchill Livingstone.

Psychiatry

Oxford Textbook of Psychiatry. Gelder, M., Gath, D., Mayou, R. Oxford University Press, 1983.

An Outline of Modern Psychiatry. Hughes, J. John Wiley & Sons Ltd, 1981.

Psychiatry. Trethowen, W. H. 4th Ed, Ballière–Tindell.

Neurology

Brain's Diseases of the Nervous System. Ed Walton, S. N. 8th Ed, Oxford University Press.

Diseases of the Nervous System. Matthews, W. B., Miller, H. 2nd Ed, Blackwell Scientific Publications.

Ophthalmology

Basic Clinical Ophthalmology. Phillips, C. I. Pitman, 1984.

Ear, Nose & Throat

Diseases of the Nose, Throat & Ear. Hall, I. S., Colman, B. H. Churchill Livingstone, 1983.

Respiratory System

Respiratory Diseases. Croften, J., Douglas, A. 3rd Ed, Blackwell Scientific Publications.

Cardiovascular System

Clinical Heart Disease. Oram, S. 2nd Ed, William Heinemann Medical Books.

Gastroenterology

Scott, An Aid to Clinical Surgery. Ed Dudley, H. A. F. 3rd Ed, Churchill Livingstone.

Diseases of the Liver & Biliary System. Sherlock, Dame Sheila. 6th Ed, Blackwell Scientific Publications.

Practical Management of the Acute Abdomen. Keddie, N. C. Lloyd–Luke (Medical Books) Ltd, 1967.

A Concise Textbook of Gastroenterology. Langman, M. J. C. S. Ed, Livingstone Medical Texts, 1973.

Haematology

De Grouchy Clinical Haematology in Medical Practice. Ed Pennigton, D., Rush, B., Castaldi, P. 4th Ed, Blackwell Scientific Publications.

Essential Haematology. Hoffbrand, A. V., Pettit, J. E. 2nd Ed, Blackwell Scientific Publications.

Endocrinology, Metabolic Disorders & the Breast

Fundamentals of Clinical Endocrinology. Hill, R., Anderson, J., Smart, G. A., Besser, M. 3rd Ed, Pitman Medical Publications.

Infectious Diseases

Infectious Diseases, Epidemiology & Clinical Practice. Christie, A. B. 3rd Ed, Churchill Livingstone.

AIDS, A Basic Guide for Clinicians. Ed Ebbesen, P., Biggar, R. J., Melbye, M. Munksgaard 1984.

Dermatology

Dermatology an Illustrated Guide. Fry, L. 3rd Ed, Butterworth/Update.

Textbook of Dermatology. Ed Rook, A., Wilkinson, D. S., Ebling, F. J. G. 2nd Ed, Blackwell Scientific Publications.

Rheumatology

Copeman's Textbook of Rheumatic Diseases. Ed Scott, J. T. 5th Ed, Churchill Livingstone.

Rheumatology in General Practice. Rogers, M., Williams, N. Churchill Livingstone 1981.

Orthopaedics

Outline of Fractures. Crawford Adams, J. 8th Ed, Churchill Livingstone.

Outline of Orthopaedics. Crawford Adams, J. 8th Ed, Churchill Livingstone.

Genito–urinary System

Renal Disease. Ed Black, Sir Douglas. 3rd Ed, Blackwell Scientific Publications.

A Course in Renal Diseases. Berlyne, G. M. Blackwell Scientific Publications.

General Urology. Smith, D. R. 9th Ed, Lange Medical Publications.

Community Medicine

Survey Methods in Community Medicine. Abramson, J. H. 2nd Ed, Churchill Livingstone.

An Introduction to Community Medicine. Florey, C. du V. Churchill Livingstone, 1983.

Immunisation. Dick, G. Update Books, 1978.

Preventive Medicine. Leavell, H. R., Clark, E. G. McGraw Hill.

Sociology as Applied to Medicine. Ed Patrick, D. L, Scambler, G. Ballière–Tindell, 1982.

A Study Guide to Epidemiology & Biostatistics. Morton, R. F., Hebel, J. R. University Park Press, Baltimore 1980.

Epidemiology & Policies for Health Planning. McCarthy, M. King Edward's Hospital Fund for London 1982.

Health Crisis 2000. O'Neill, P. Published for WHO by William Heinemann Ltd.

Alphabetical List of Lists

Index

I